VENTILATOR MANAGEMENT
STRATEGIES FOR CRITICAL CARE

LUNG BIOLOGY IN HEALTH AND DISEASE

Executive Editor

Claude Lenfant

Director, National Heart, Lung and Blood Institute
National Institutes of Health
Bethesda, Maryland

ADDITIONAL VOLUMES IN PREPARATION

The opinions expressed in these volumes do not necessarily represent the views of the National Institutes of Health.

VENTILATOR MANAGEMENT STRATEGIES FOR CRITICAL CARE

Edited by

Nicholas S. Hill
Mitchell M. Levy

Rhode Island Hospital
Brown University School of Medicine
Providence, Rhode Island

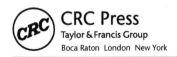

CRC Press
Taylor & Francis Group
Boca Raton London New York

CRC Press is an imprint of the
Taylor & Francis Group, an **informa** business

CRC Press
Taylor & Francis Group
6000 Broken Sound Parkway NW, Suite 300
Boca Raton, FL 33487-2742

First issued in paperback 2019

© 2001 by Taylor & Francis Group, LLC
CRC Press is an imprint of Taylor & Francis Group, an Informa business

No claim to original U.S. Government works

ISBN-13: 978-0-8247-0522-0 (hbk)
ISBN-13: 978-0-367-39726-5 (pbk)

A CIP record for this book is available from the Library of Congress.

Visit the Taylor & Francis Web site at
http://www.taylorandfrancis.com

and the CRC Press Web site at
http://www.crcpress.com

SERIES INTRODUCTION

> Because a three-fold division of function may exist in science, between the instrument-maker, the laboratory worker, and the theorist, it has always been possible, and still is, for the strategic thinking in science to take place outside the laboratory. . . .
> The progress of science demands originality at all three levels. . . . .
>
> *A. R. Hall* (1)

This statement is applicable in many ways to ventilator management in critical care. Ventilatory assist has had a long history—one has only to read Chapter 2 in this volume to know it. Since the mid-nineteenth century, there have been two turning points; interestingly, they were not driven by the instrument-maker, but by the theorist. The first was a shift in concept from *inflation of the lungs* to *ventilation*. Initially, the goal was to keep the lungs inflated, but then, particularly with the advent of anesthesia, clinicians resurrected the practice of rhythmic assisted ventilation that had been recognized in the sixteenth century by Andreas Vesalius. The second turning point was the description by Ashbaugh et al. in 1967 of "adult respiratory distress syndrome" (2). Although it appears that ventilatory failure may have initially been thought to be the cause of ARDS rather than its consequence, work on that condition has truly established and revolutionized the concept of critical care in patients with ARDS as well as in patients with many other conditions.

The exact prevalence of critically sick patients in need of ventilatory management is really unknown, but one can safely say that it is a very large number with tremendous public health impact. Over many decades, the "theorist" (or the physiologist) and the "laboratory worker" (or the clinician), joining with the instrument-maker, have advanced the field remarkably.

Today, in the era of genomics and genetics research, the hope has emerged that these disciplines will resolve many pathogenetic problems, especially those we do not understand. While the pathogenetic process of critically ill patients may indeed become better understood, this understanding will not eliminate respiratory failure and the need for ventilatory management, and, for this management to be effective, we will still require a triad made up of engineers, physiologists, and clinicians.

This volume, *Ventilator Management Strategies for Critical Care,* edited by Drs. Nicholas S. Hill and Mitchell M. Levy, brings to the readers theories and applications. In some ways, it demonstrates that "progress of [medical] science demands originality at all three levels. . . ." The editors assembled a cadre of experts who are well recognized for their experience and successes in critical care medicine. From my viewpoint as Executive Editor of the Lung Biology in Health and Disease series, this volume symbolizes what I want the series to be about: the merging of basic research, clinical investigation, and excellent medicine. I am grateful to the editors and authors for illustrating so well my goal, and I am proud to present this volume to our readership.

Claude Lenfant, M.D.
Bethesda, Maryland

References

1. Hall AR. The Scientific Revolution, 1500–1800. The Formation of the Modern Scientific Attitude. London: Longmans Green, 1954.
2. Ashbaugh DG, Bigelow DBB, Petty TL, Levine BE. Acute respiratory distress in adults. *Lancet* 1967; 2:319–323.

PREFACE

Ventilator management of patients with respiratory failure has undergone revolutionary changes during the past century. The polio epidemics of the 1920s through the 1950s led to the widespread use of negative pressure ventilation. Positive pressure ventilation, which had been the province of the anesthesia suite, saw increasing use during the late 1950s and 1960s, which paralleled the creation of intensive care units. The difficulty in managing pressure-limited positive pressure ventilation during the 1960s presaged the virtual rejection of such modes during the 1970s and early 1980s, as well as the predominance of volume-limited ventilation. During this time, assist/control and intermittent mandatory ventilation modes were commonly used to give patients more control over their breathing patterns.

Progress made through the late 1980s was remarkable and undoubtedly saved many lives. However, the advances made over the past dozen years have outpaced previous developments. The development of microprocessor controllers has given ventilator manufacturers great flexibility in the creation of new ventilator modes. Advances in ventilator monitoring technology have made it possible to administer pressure-limited modes safely, which has led to a resurgence of their use. Hybrid modes are now available that combine features of pressure-limited and volume-limited ventilation. These new modes are directed by algorithms that incorporate breath-by-breath measurements of respiratory mechanics.

Efforts have been directed at ventilating patients more safely and comfortably, leading to the increasing proliferation of noninvasive ventilation as well as the use of settings to protect against injury induced by the ventilator. Efforts are also underway to understand how patients with different pathophysiological mechanisms for their respiratory failure are best managed. With advances in microprocessor technology, it has become possible to apply both disease- and patient-specific ventilator therapy. In addition, the increasing use of evidence-based medicine is expanding the scientific foundation for ventilator management. More recently, protocolized therapy has become an important tool in liberation from mechanical ventilation.

The purpose of the present volume is to serve as a thorough and current treatise on ventilator management practices in critical care that brings recent developments into perspective. Our intention is to provide the reader with practical strategies for achieving identifiable goals based on the patient's pathophysiological defects. Carefully prepared and thoroughly referenced chapters, which highlight new and evolving concepts, have been included from leading authorities in their fields. The contributors were also encouraged to be provocative.

Part One consists of four chapters. Chapters 1 and 2 lay the epidemiological and historical foundation for the chapters that follow. Chapter 3 presents a number of international surveys, with observations on how mechanical ventilation is administered in different parts of the world. Chapter 4 examines economic aspects of ventilator use.

With the economic perspective as a backdrop, Part Two examines ways in which mechanical ventilation can be administered more efficiently in the critical care setting. In Chapter 5, the application of protocol-driven strategies that shorten the duration of mechanical ventilation is described. Chapter 6 discusses the application of noninvasive ventilation to improve outcomes and resource utilization. Chapter 7 explains how advances in microprocessor technology have enabled enhancements in patient–ventilator synchrony. As an extension of this approach, Chapter 8 elaborates how microprocessor algorithms can be incorporated into feedback loops to permit the development of "smart" ventilators—devices that can adjust automatically, based on frequent measurement of respiratory mechanics, to achieve desired targets.

Although sedation and analgesia are widely regarded as essential for successful ventilator management, overuse can retard the weaning process. In Chapter 9, methods for the optimal use of sedation and analgesia during mechanical ventilation are described. Critical care specialists are well aware that proper airway management during mechanical ventilation is essential to favorable outcomes. Accordingly, Chapter 10 provides a comprehensive review of proper airway management, including recent advances regarding intubation.

Part Four focuses on specific pathophysiological causes of respiratory failure that necessitate the application of different strategies for optimal management.

In Chapter 11, optimal management of the patient with severe acute asthma is discussed. Chapter 12 proposes an approach to mechanical ventilation in COPD patients that includes noninvasive ventilation as a first step, and applies basic pathophysiological concepts to the management of invasive mechanical ventilation. Chapter 13 thoroughly reviews the various approaches to optimizing mechanical ventilation in patients with ARDS with an eye toward lung protection strategies. Chapter 14 discusses the use of noninvasive ventilation in patients with non-COPD causes of respiratory failure, in whom indications are not as clear as in COPD patients.

Part Four examines new approaches to weaning from invasive mechanical ventilation. Chapter 15 offers a perspective on which predictors of weaning should be used. Chapter 16 describes an approach to weaning that includes daily screening and spontaneous breathing trials, a method that may shorten the weaning process by days. Finally, Chapter 17 discusses the application of noninvasive ventilation for facilitation of weaning, another approach that can be used to improve weaning efficiency.

Part Five focuses on the avoidance of complications during mechanical ventilation. Chapter 18 describes the problem of ventilator-induced lung injury and avoidance strategies. Ventilator-associated pneumonia (VAP) is another serious and all-too-common complication of invasive mechanical ventilation, and Chapter 19 describes ways to diagnose, treat, and avoid VAP. Finally, Chapter 20 lays the foundation for a pathophysiologically based strategy to optimize hemodynamics during mechanical ventilation.

Part Six is concerned with outcomes of mechanical ventilation. Chapter 21 examines the mechanisms and outcomes of extubation failure, and proposes methods that might enable clinicians to predict and avoid this morbidity. And finally, Chapter 22 offers thoughts on the ethical implications of different strategies for mechanical ventilation.

We are certain that readers will find this volume a thoroughly researched and referenced source of current information on the management of mechanical ventilation in the critical care setting. We believe we have achieved our two goals for the volume: first, to present balanced, but sometimes provocative, views of conceptual as well as technical developments in mechanical ventilation; and second, to provide the critical care clinician with practical strategies to guide the use of mechanical ventilation in critically ill patients. We are very grateful to the contributors for their outstanding chapters, which reflect their knowledge and expertise. We can all share pride in the fruit of their labors. We would also like to thank our wives and children for indulging us the many hours necessary to bring this volume to fruition.

Nicholas S. Hill
Mitchell M. Levy

CONTRIBUTORS

Massimo Antonelli, M.D. Università "La Sapienza" Policlinico Umberto I, Rome, Italy

Arunabh, M.D. Division of Pulmonary and Critical Care Medicine, North Shore University Hospital, Manhasset, New York

Antonio Anzueto, M.D. Associate Professor, Department of Pulmonology/ Critical Care, University of Texas Health Science Center, San Antonio, Texas

David L. Bowton, M.D. Wake Forest University School of Medicine, Winston-Salem, North Carolina

Richard D. Branson Associate Professor of Surgery, University of Cincinnati, Cincinnati, Ohio

George B. Buczko, M.D., F.R.C.P.(C) Clinical Assistant Professor, Department of Surgery/Anesthesiology, Brown University School of Medicine, Providence, Rhode Island

G. R. Scott Budinger   Loyola University of Chicago Stritch School of Medicine, Maywood, and Hines Veterans Administration Hospital, Hines, Illinois

Dean R. Chittock, M.D., F.R.C.P.C.   Associate Director, Department of Critical Care Medicine, Vancouver Hospital and Health Sciences Centre, Vancouver, British Columbia, Canada

Giorgio Conti, M.D.   Università ''La Sapienza'' Policlinico Umberto I, Rome, Italy

Thomas Corbridge, M.D.   Director, Medical Intensive Care Unit, and Associate Professor, Department of Medicine, Northwestern University Medical School, Chicago, Illinois

David Crippen, M.D., F.C.C.M.   Associate Director, Department of Emergency and Critical Care Medicine, St. Francis Medical Center, Pittsburgh, Pennsylvania

Didier Dreyfuss, M.D.   Professor, Medical Intensive Care Unit, Hôpital Louis Mourier, Colombes, and IFROZ, Faculté de Médecine Xavier Bichat, Paris, France

E. Wesley Ely, M.D., M.P.H., F.A.C.P., F.C.C.P.   Center for Health Services Research, Vanderbilt University Medical Center, Nashville, Tennessee

Scott K. Epstein, M.D.   Associate Professor, Tufts University School of Medicine, and Associate Director, Medical Intensive Care Unit, Department of Pulmonary and Critical Care, New England Medical Center, Boston, Massachusetts

Andres Esteban, M.D.   Director, Intensive Care Unit, Hospital Universitario Getafe, Getafe, Spain

Alan M. Fein, M.D.   Director, The Center for Pulmonary and Critical Care Medicine, Department of Pulmonary Medicine, North Shore University Hospital, Manhasset, New York

Jesse B. Hall, M.D.   Chief, Section of Pulmonary and Critical Care Medicine, Department of Medicine, University of Chicago, Chicago, Illinois

Edward F. Haponik, M.D.   The Johns Hopkins Medical Center, Baltimore, Maryland

Dean Hess, Ph.D.   Assistant Professor of Anesthesia, Harvard Medical School, and Assistant Director of Respiratory Care, Massachusetts General Hospital, Boston, Massachusetts

Nicholas S. Hill, M.D.   Director, Pulmonary and Critical Care Medicine, Miriam Hospital; Director, Critical Care Services, Rhode Island Hospital; and Professor, Department of Medicine, Brown University School of Medicine, Providence, Rhode Island

Sean P. Keenan, M.D., F.R.C.P.(C)   Associate Director, Intensive Care Unit, Royal Columbian Hospital, New Westminster, British Columbia, Canada

Brian A. Kimble   Brown University School of Medicine, Providence, Rhode Island

James R. Klinger, M.D.   Assistant Professor, Department of Medicine, Brown University School of Medicine and Rhode Island Hospital, Providence, Rhode Island

Marin H. Kollef, M.D.   Associate Professor, Department of Pulmonary and Critical Care, Washington University School of Medicine, St. Louis, Missouri

Mitchell M. Levy, M.D.   Director, Medical Intensive Care Unit, and Associate Professor, Department of Medicine, Brown University School of Medicine, Providence, Rhode Island

Denis Lin, M.D.   Brown University School of Medicine, Providence, Rhode Island

John M. Luce, M.D.   Professor, Department of Medicine and Anesthesia, University of California, San Francisco, California

Dana Lustbader, M.D.   Division of Critical Care Medicine, North Shore University Hospital, Manhasset, New York

Neil MacIntyre, M.D.   Professor of Medicine, Department of Pulmonary and Critical Care, Duke University, Durham, North Carolina

William T. McGee, M.D., M.H.A.   Director, ICU Quality Improvement, Critical Care Division, Baystate Medical Center, Springfield, and Assistant Professor of Medicine and Surgery, Tufts University, Boston, Massachusetts

G. Umberto Meduri, M.D.   Professor, Department of Medicine, University of Tennessee, Memphis, Tennessee

Joseph V. Meharg, M.D.   Assistant Professor, Division of Pulmonary Medicine, Roger Williams Hospital, Providence, Rhode Island

Stefano Nava, M.D.   Head, Respiratory Intensive Care Unit, Department of Pneumology, S. Maugeri Foundation, Istituto di Pavia, Pavia, Italy

Michael R. Pinsky   University of Pittsburgh Medical Center, Pittsburgh, Pennsylvania

Jean-Damien Ricard, M.D.   Medical Intensive Care Unit, Hôpital Louis Mourier, Colombes, and IFROZ, Faculté de Médecine Xavier Bichat, Paris, France

Fiorenzo Rubini, M.D.   Department of Pneumology, S. Maugeri Foundation, Istituto di Montescano, Montescano, Italy

Georges Saumon, M.D.   IFROZ, Faculté de Médecine Xavier Bichat, Paris, France

Martin J. Tobin, M.D.   Professor, Department of Pulmonary and Critical Care Medicine, Loyola University of Chicago Stritch School of Medicine, Maywood, and Hines Veterans Administration Hospital, Hines, Illinois

CONTENTS

Part Two **STRATEGIES FOR OPTIMAL UTILIZATION OF MECHANICAL VENTILATION IN CRITICAL CARE**

5. Mechanical Ventilation: Protocol-Driven Strategies   **111**

Marin H. Kollef

6. Noninvasive Ventilation: A Strategy to Improve Outcomes and Resource Utilization in Critical Care   **137**

Nicholas S. Hill and Denis Lin

1

Epidemiology of Acute Respiratory Failure

SEAN P. KEENAN

Royal Columbian Hospital
New Westminster, British Columbia,
    Canada

DEAN R. CHITTOCK

Vancouver Hospital and Health Sciences
    Centre
Vancouver, British Columbia, Canada

I. Introduction

Understanding the specific cause and appropriate treatment for acute respiratory failure (ARF) is the backbone upon which critical care medicine has been built. Epidemiology has been defined as the study of the incidence, prevalence, and spread of a disease or disorder (1). Loosely applying this definition to the clinical entity of acute respiratory failure, we will provide an overview of the evolution of this disorder over the past two to three decades. To do this, we will begin by defining acute respiratory failure, including a description of its varied pathophysiology. Patients with acute respiratory failure often require some form of assisted ventilation, the most common of which involves placement of an endotracheal tube. Following a review of acute respiratory failure, we will outline other indications for intubation and ventilation.

Acute respiratory failure is caused by a number of different disorders that result in similar physiological abnormalities. We will describe this spectrum of underlying disease processes and try to determine whether their relative contributions appear to be changing over time. While space prohibits our covering all etiologies of acute respiratory failure in depth, we will focus on two processes whose underlying pathophysiologies closely approximate the hypothetically pure

1

hypoxemic respiratory failure and hypercapnic failure. The acute respiratory distress syndrome (ARDS), while relatively uncommon, continues to be the most challenging form of respiratory failure for the intensivist to manage. Chronic obstructive pulmonary disease, in contrast, presents primarily as hypercapnic respiratory failure. We will describe the etiologies and prognoses for both types of patient, including short-term and long-term survival as well as impact upon quality of life.

While the ability to recognize acute respiratory failure dates back to early times, our ability to effectively treat this entity is still evolving. The large number of patients developing ventilatory failure during the polio epidemics of the 1950s far exceeded the number of available iron lungs. This led a group of Danish anesthesiologists to adopt the use of positive pressure ventilation with endotracheal tubes for prolonged ventilatory support because many of these patients required manual ventilation (2). The adoption of pressure-cycled ventilators and the organization of the first respiratory units, led by the group in Denver, resulted in the birth of critical care medicine in the 1960s (2). In this chapter, we will not discuss treatment of acute respiratory failure in any depth because that is the focus of the remaining chapters of this book.

II. What Is Acute Respiratory Failure?

In order to understand the pathophysiology of acute respiratory failure, a review of the normal function of the respiratory system is necessary. The primary role of the respiratory system is to provide a means of removing carbon dioxide from the body in exchange for oxygen. Oxygen is vital to the functioning of all body systems, and the delivery of oxygen to cells is directly proportional to three variables: oxygen saturation of hemoglobin, hemoglobin concentration, and cardiac output. In order to provide effective gas exchange, the following are required: sufficient surface area for gas exchange to occur, adequate airways to conduct air to and from the gas-exchanging surface, and the ability to move gas in and out of the lungs. The latter function relies upon a functional neuromuscular system comprised of a sufficiently intact sensorium, normal brain stem respiratory center, spinal cord, peripheral nerves, neuromuscular junction, and respiratory muscles. Finally, optimum movement of gas requires normal anatomy of the thorax, including rib cage, alignment of the spine, and pleural space.

Acute respiratory failure occurs when abnormalities in at least one of the above factors leads to a rapid and significant compromise in the system's ability to adequately exchange carbon dioxide and/or oxygen. Arbitrary values have been used to define respiratory failure, most commonly a partial pressure of oxygen of less than 55 or 60 mmHg or a partial pressure of carbon dioxide of greater

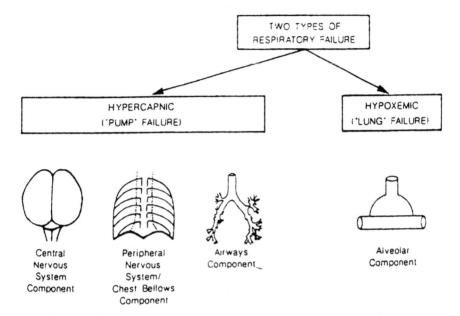

Figure 1 The two classic types of respiratory failure: Hypercapnic failure can arise from one of three major components of the respiratory system (CNS, peripheral nerves/ chest bellows, or conducting airways), while hypoxemic failure generally arises from the fourth component, the alveoli. (From Lanken PN. Respiratory failure: an overview. In: Carlson RW, Gebb MA, eds. Principles and Practices of Medical Intensive Care. Philadelphia: W. B. Saunders Company, 1993:754–763, with permission.)

than 45–50 mmHg. While acute respiratory failure has many etiologies, a simplified approach is to consider that all these can be grouped under one of two pathophysiological processes (Fig. 1). The first is a failure to oxygenate and the second a failure to ventilate (remove carbon dioxide). These are commonly referred to as Type 1 and Type 2 acute respiratory failure, respectively.

III. Type 1 Acute Respiratory Failure

The primary problem with patients presenting with Type 1 failure is impaired gas exchange. This can arise from an absolute reduction in the surface area for gas exchange due to either loss of blood flow (e.g., pulmonary embolus) or ventilation (e.g., alveolar filling due to pulmonary edema) or an inefficient matching of ventilation and perfusion (e.g., obstructive lung disease). The primary gas exchange abnormality seen in this setting is hypoxemia, the partial pressure of

Table 1 Causes of Acute Respiratory Failure

Type 1 respiratory failure	Type 2 respiratory failure
Parenchymal process	Increased load
Pneumonia	Upper aiway obstruction
Pulmonary edema	Asthma
cardiogenic	COPD
noncardiogenic	
Pulmonary hemorrhage	Neurological etiology
Progressive interstitial process	Central respiratory depression
	Spinal cord injury
Pulmonary vascular	Peripheral nerve
Pulmonary embolism	Neuromuscular junction
Pulmonary hypertension	

carbon dioxide being preserved by its ability to diffuse across capillary membranes 20 times more rapidly than oxygen. Patients present acutely short of breath with rapid respiratory and heart rates and use of their accessory muscles of respiration. Common examples of Type 1 acute respiratory failure are listed in Table 1. Patients may initially compensate for impaired gas exchange by increasing their minute ventilation, which leads to an improvement in oxygen levels but a fall in carbon dioxide levels. In more severe settings even a marked increase in minute ventilation does not adequately correct gas exchange abnormalities. In some cases, the large increase in work of breathing eventually leads to muscle fatigue and a gradual reduction in minute ventilation with associated hypercarbia in addition to hypoxemia (Fig. 2). If support of ventilation is not initiated, respiratory arrest may ensue.

IV. Type 2 Acute Respiratory Failure

In contrast to Type 1 acute respiratory failure, the abnormality of concern in Type 2 acute respiratory failure is impaired ventilation. The patient is unable to generate sufficient minute ventilation to clear carbon dioxide, and hypercarbia results. Associated with hypercarbia is a reduction in arterial partial pressure of oxygen that is not usually clinically relevant, requiring minimal if any supplemental oxygen to correct. Indeed, patients requiring supplemental oxygen in this setting generally have underlying impaired gas exchange due to chronic lung disease, not the acute event. Impaired minute ventilation can occur in patients with either normal respiratory mechanics or those with increased work of breathing due to increased airways resistance (either upper airway or lower airways) or

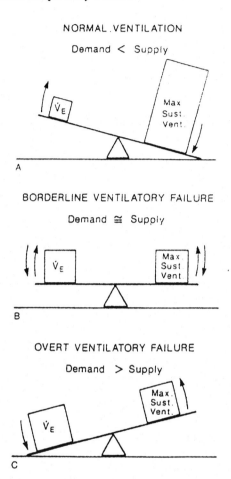

NORMAL VENTILATION

Demand < Supply

BORDERLINE VENTILATORY FAILURE

Demand ≅ Supply

OVERT VENTILATORY FAILURE

Demand > Supply

Figure 2 The evolution toward respiratory failure due to increasing imbalance between demand, represented by V_E or minute ventilation, and supply, Max. Sust. Vent. (maximal sustainable ventilation). (From Lanken PN. Respiratory failure: an overview. In: Carlson RW, Gebb MA, eds. Principles and practices of medical intensive care. Philadelphia: W. B. Saunders Company, 1993:754–763, with permission.)

decreased lung or chest wall compliance (abdominal, chest wall, or pleural space abnormalities). In the setting of normal respiratory mechanics, a decrease in minute ventilation may occur as a result of a decrease in respiratory drive (cerebrum or brain stem), spinal cord injury, abnormality of peripheral nerves (e.g., Guillain-Barré syndrome), neuromuscular junction (e.g., myasthenia gravis), or respiratory muscles (e.g., steroid-induced myopathy). In Table 1 we have presented selected causes of Type 2 acute respiratory failure. As noted previously, patients with an initial "pure" picture of Type 1 respiratory failure who develop respiratory muscle fatigue secondary to high minute ventilation also present with hypercarbia and are described as having a mixed picture.

V. Indications for Intubation with or Without Assisted Ventilation

While acute respiratory failure is the most intuitively obvious reason for intubation and ventilation, intubation is also required in a number of other important settings (Table 2). Airway protection, the "A" in the ABCs of resuscitation, is of vital importance. Impending upper airway obstruction is an absolute indication for securing an airway, either by inserting an endotracheal tube or, if necessary, establishing a surgical airway. Once the airway has been established, the need for additional assisted ventilation is variable and may depend more upon the requirements for adequate patient sedation than underlying cardiopulmonary status.

Airway protection is also important in at least three other settings. In patients with a decreased level of consciousness resulting from anesthesia, drug ingestion, or a variety of metabolic aberrations, intubation is required to avoid aspiration of pharyngeal secretions and gastric contents. The degree of assistance with ventilation required depends on the degree of impaired ventilatory drive. A second setting in which airway protection is required is to prevent aspiration in patients with impaired bulbar function but a normal level of consciousness, such as those with myasthenia gravis or amyotrophic lateral sclerosis. Finally, patients with massive hemoptysis may require intubation followed by direct visualization of their airways to determine the source of bleeding. At times it is prudent to consider providing independent routes of ventilation for each lung to prevent aspiration of blood into the nonbleeding lung. Patients in this setting require assisted ventilation to compensate for the heavy sedation—and occasionally paralysis—used to avoid coughing or gagging that may provoke further bleeding.

Table 2 Indications for Intubation and/or Ventilation

1. Upper airway obstruction
2. Inability to protect airway
3. Inability to oxygenate
4. Inability to ventilate
5. Hemodynamic collapse

VI. Etiology of Acute Respiratory Failure

In the 1950s the primary cause of respiratory failure receiving ventilatory support was polio (2). With the gradual introduction of intensive care units in the 1960s, exacerbation of chronic obstructive pulmonary disease (COPD) was one of the more common reasons for mechanical ventilation (2,3). The list of etiologies of acute respiratory failure requiring mechanical ventilation grew quickly, as did the resources dedicated to care of the critically ill patient (4). Attempting to determine the relative contribution of the varied etiologies of acute respiratory failure to the total population of ventilated patients is problematic. While the literature provides a wealth of studies that describe various reasons for needing assisted ventilation in their respective populations, generalizing these findings outside of the specific center or centers is difficult. Few studies exist that include a thorough description of the etiology of respiratory failure and associated outcomes of all patients ventilated in a specific intensive care unit (ICU). One recent multicenter study did identify specific etiologies for acute respiratory failure demonstrating 52% of pulmonary origin and 47.9% of nonpulmonary origin (5). Some studies deal with all ICU patients (6–9), including nonventilated patients, while others, assessing the effectiveness of therapies aimed at preventing ventilator-associated pneumonia (and hopefully improving survival), only included patients ventilated longer than 24–72 hours (10–14). Still other studies, evaluating the effectiveness of different weaning strategies, only included patients who had progressed to the stage where weaning is possible (15–18). Finally, most studies have been conducted in academic centers, and generalizing these findings to community hospitals may misrepresent true practice. Keeping these limitations in mind, we will explore the various etiologies of respiratory failure and see whether there appear to be any trends over time.

The most common reason for intubation and mechanical ventilation is elective surgery. In general or nonspecialized ICUs, postoperative surgical patients made up the majority of ventilated patients in North America during the 1970s and 1980s (3,6–9,19–21) (Table 3). A study by Zimmerman and colleagues (9) suggested that this relative proportion might have decreased in the 1990s. This study included 285 ICUs at 161 hospitals, but the hospitals were not sampled randomly and generalizations must be made with caution. However, if the decreasing proportion of postoperative patients is representative of North American practice, it may reflect a move toward caring for a larger proportion of postoperative patients in intermediate care units or regular floors rather than intensive care units. Such a move may have been prompted by a number of early studies reporting that a significant proportion of patients who were admitted to ICUs required only intensive monitoring, which could be provided at a lower level of care (22–25).

Table 3 Relative Proportion of Patients Receiving Mechanical Ventilation in the ICU for Postoperative Versus Nonoperative Conditions

Study	Years	n	No. centers	Postoperative (%)	Nonoperative (%)
Pontoppidan et al., 1972 (20)	1961–70	923	1	59.7	40.3
Petty et al., 1975 (3)	1964–74	1,877	1	53.8	46.2
Knaus et al., 1985[a] (6) (all patients)	1979–82	5,030	13	52.5	47.5
Knaus, 1989 (19) (ventilated patients)	1982	1,886	12	70	30
Knaus et al., 1991[a] (7) (all patients)	1988–89	17,440	40	42	58
Seneff et al., 1996 (21) (ventilated patients)	1988–89	5,915	40	50.6	49.4
Le Gall et al., 1993[a,b] (8)	1991–92	3,732	28	46.5	53.5
Zimmerman et al., 1998[a] (9)	1993–96	37,668	161	28.5	72.5
Esteban et al., 1999 (26)	March 1998	3,250	18 countries	21.4	78.6

[a] Includes all patients admitted (ventilated and not ventilated).
[b] North American centers only.

The focus of this chapter is acute respiratory failure. To understand the relative proportion of conditions causing patients to present with this disorder requires a closer look at the nonoperative ventilated ICU population. While published data are somewhat limited, we identified and selected four North American studies that cover different periods over the last three decades to explore the relative importance of nonoperative conditions requiring mechanical ventilation (3,19,21,28). In addition, we have included a large international study by Estaban and colleagues, as it is unique in its scope (26,27) (Table 4). All these studies had few, if any, exclusion criteria relevant to nonoperative patients. Two studies were conducted at single centers (3,28), two were derived from the large databases of APACHE II (19) and APACHE III (7), and the fifth was a one-month prospective study of mechanical ventilation in selected ICUs of 18 countries (26,27). Overall, by grouping patients into general categories, the primary reasons for mechanical ventilation were found to be as follows: respiratory conditions accounted for 20–25% of patients; cardiac conditions comprised a further 20%; infection or sepsis another 20%; and trauma and neurological disorders approximately 10–15% each. The relative proportion will obviously vary depending on the type of ICU and the patient population it serves.

Data available from our own institution spanning the 10 years from March 1988 to March 1998 may provide some insight into changes that have occurred in various patient populations who require mechanical ventilation. The database collects information on all patients admitted to the ICU at the Vancouver Hospital and Health Sciences Centre (VHHSC), Vancouver, British Columbia (BC), Canada, and follows them for the duration of hospital stay. The VHHSC is the largest teaching, research, and referral hospital in western Canada. VHHSC is a university-affiliated, tertiary care hospital for the province of BC and acts as the provincial center for trauma, solid organ transplantation, and neurosciences as well as the only center in western Canada providing bone marrow transplantation.

The ICU at VHHSC is a 21-bed multidisciplinary medical/surgical/trauma unit that cares for all critically ill patients for the hospital except for uncomplicated cardiac, cardiac surgery, and spinal cord patients. The total number of patients admitted to the ICU over this 10-year period was 6935, with no significant changes in the number of patients admitted each year. Patients who received mechanical ventilation accounted for 83% ($n = 5768$) of this population and had a mean APACHE II score of 26.9. For purposes of comparison we divided the ventilated population into two groups. Group I represented the first 5 years (1988–1993) and Group II the last 5 years (1993–1998). The relative proportion of patients receiving mechanical ventilation in Group II was significantly greater than Group I, 88% vs. 77%, respectively. Table 5 summarizes the results according to primary admitting diagnosis. Some proportional changes have occurred in each diagnostic group over the 10 years. The largest relative increase in a single diagnostic category is that of septic shock at 50%. Gastrointestinal

Table 4 Reason for Mechanical Ventilation Among Nonoperative ICU Patients

	Petty et al., 1972 (3)	Knaus et al., 1989[a] (19)	Cohen et al., 1991 (28)	Seneff et al., 1996[a] (21)	Esteban et al., 1999 (26)
Respiratory	28.5%				
COPD	15.3%	2.1%	4.1%	5.8%	14%
ARDS		3.5%	4.8%	2.7%	7%
Respiratory arrest			3.4%		3%
Other	13.2%	13.0%	11.5%		
Cardiac					
CHF		2.6%	17.4%	8.6%	11%
Cardiac arrest		11.9%	15.0%		2%
Infection					
Pneumonia		9.4%	14.8%	11.0%	16%
Sepsis		11.7%		6.5%	9%
"Shock"			16.1%		
Neurological	13.1%				
Intracranial		6.0%			23% (coma)
Peripheral			1.1%		3% (NMD)
Overdose	16.5%		5.9%		
Trauma	19.1%		5.9%	7.9%	7%
GI bleed		4.6%			
Other	22.8%		16.1%		5%

[a] Not all categories were available; therefore, those presented do not add up to 100%.
NMD = Neuromuscular disease.

Table 5 Relative Proportion of Mechanically Ventilated Patients by Diagnostic Category Over a 10-Year Period

Admitting diagnostic category	Group I, 1988–1993 (N = 2639)	Group II, 1993–1998 (N = 3129)
Respiratory	31.3	30.1
Cardiovascular	21.2	20.2
Neurological	12.4	16.3*
Trauma/burns	16.8	16.6
Gastrointestinal	7.6	9.9*
Metabolic/renal	10.8	7.1*
Septic shock	3.7	7.5*
APACHE II score (mean)	27.5	26.2
Predicted hospital mortality (%)	59.8	59.1
Actual hospital mortality (%)	37.7	32.2*

* $p < 0.05$.

diagnoses have had a relative increase of 23%, while metabolic/renal (mostly renal failure) have had a relative decrease of 34%. Neurological cases increased in the last 5 years, most likely due to the transfer of the university's neurosurgical program to VHHSC in 1994. According to the APACHE II scoring system, no changes in severity of illness were observed, but hospital mortality decreased significantly from 37.7 to 32.3%. This represents a relative risk of mortality in Group II of 0.89 (95% CI 0.84, 0.94).

A closer look at four specific respiratory diagnoses from the VHHSC database reveals some interesting trends over time. Specifically, we looked at mechanically ventilated patients with admitting diagnoses of asthma, COPD, ARDS, and pneumonia. The outcomes of these diagnostic groups and their changes over time are presented in Table 6. Significant increases in the proportion of patients with pneumonia and ARDS have occurred with a decrease in COPD. The decrease in COPD patients is temporally related to the introduction of noninvasive forms of ventilation on the wards at VHHSC. Again, striking decreases in mortality in the latter 5 years appear without changes in APACHE II scores among COPD, pneumonia, and ARDS patients. The most significant change is found in the ARDS population, with a decrease in mortality from 62.8% to 37.3%.

The data suggest that, compared to the 1960s and 1970s, infection and sepsis account for a larger proportion of patients with acute respiratory failure, while COPD accounts for a smaller portion. As more research networks are established that collect large amounts of descriptive data on patients requiring mechanical ventilation, trends in patient populations will be easier to appreciate (26,27,29–31).

Table 6 Comparison of Outcomes of Patients with Acute Respiratory Failure Over a 10-Year Period

	1988–1993 (N = 292)				1993–1998 (N = 360)			
	Asthma	COPD	ARDS	Pneumonia	Asthma	COPD	ARDS	Pneumonia
Age (years)	51.8	66.9	47.5	54.4	45.2	67.8	49.6	56.8
% total ICU admissions	1.7	2.3*	1.2*	3.6	1.4	1.3*	3.2*	5.3
ICU length of stay (mean, days)	7.3	14.7*	12.7	10.5	9.1	10.4*	10.9	11.3
Hospital length of stay (mean, days)	17.2	27.7*	35.4	29.1	16.3	18.3*	38.4	26.5
APACHE II score (mean)	22.0	27.2	32.3	29.5	21.4	25.2	31.1	28.6
Predicted mortality (%)	38.5	57.1	71.2	65.1	48.5	50.0	66.8	62.3
Hospital mortality (%)	4.3	31.8	62.8*	54.6*	4.9	22.7	37.3*	39.4*

*$p < 0.05$ for Group I versus Group II comparison.

The short-term and long-term prognosis for patients with acute respiratory failure requiring mechanical ventilation is very dependent on the underlying disorder that caused respiratory failure. Data are available describing mortality over 90 days for patients with ARF while controlling for severity of illness and age (Figs. 3,4) (5). While data can be presented for pooled outcomes for all patients with acute respiratory failure, they are not useful for clinicians treating specific patients. Clinicians are generally more interested in knowing the outcomes of the individual etiologies of acute respiratory failure. While space precludes discussion of all disorders resulting in acute respiratory failure in depth, we have summarized the recent findings by Estaban and colleagues for ICU and hospital mortality (26,27) (Table 7). In addition we will review the available literature on two examples in greater depth.

The remainder of this chapter will present the epidemiology of two specific causes of acute respiratory failure: ARDS, representing a classic example of hypoxemic respiratory failure, COPD, a good example of hypercarbic respiratory failure.

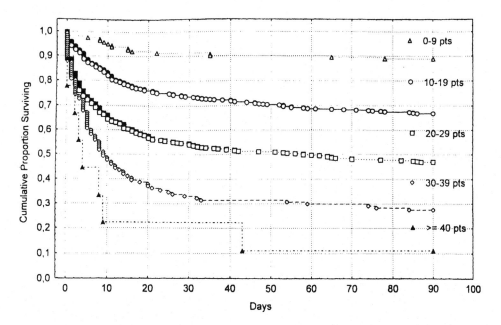

Figure 3 Cumulative proportion of surviving acute respiratory failure patients by APACHE II score intervals. (From Luhr O, Antonsen K, Karlsson M, et al. Incidence and mortality after acute respiratory failure and acute respiratory distress syndrome in Sweden, Denmark, and Iceland. AJRCCM 1999; 159:1849, with permission.)

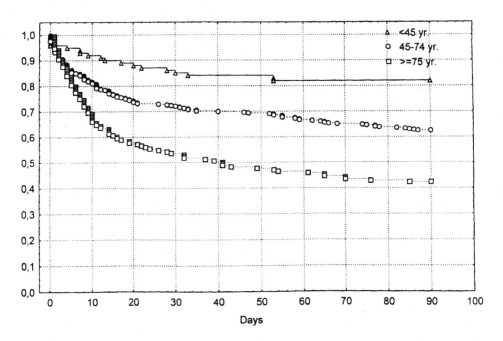

Figure 4 Cumulative proportion of surviving acute respiratory failure patients by increasing age intervals. (From Luhr O, Antonsen K, Karlsson M, et al. Incidence and mortality after acute respiratory failure and acute respiratory distress syndrome in Sweden, Denmark, and Iceland. AJRCCM 1999; 159:1849, with permission.)

VII. Acute Respiratory Distress Syndrome

While acute lung injury (ALI) encompasses a broad range of severities for acute lung damage, ARDS represents the more severe end of the spectrum. ARDS generally presents in the setting of the systemic inflammatory response syndrome (SIRS) and may be associated with dysfunction of other organ systems (32). The diagnostic criteria for ARDS have evolved over the last 30 years. In 1967 Ashbaugh and coworkers first described ARDS, identifying a group of patients presenting with specific clinical signs, physiological aberrations, and radiographic findings (33). Over the years variable aspects were added to the definition, including objectively defined abnormalities in lung compliance and gas exchange as well as identification of the underlying cause or risk factor for the disorder. In 1988, Murray and associates created the Lung Injury Score (LIS), which incorporated the various pathophysiological features of ARDS (34). Despite the popularity of the LIS, concerns continued regarding a general lack of consensus on the definition of ARDS (35). Having a universally accepted definition was considered extremely important, not simply for diagnostic purposes but to allow studies of

Table 7　Factors Associated with In-Hospital Mortality for Patients with COPD Exacerbations

Study	Nutrition	General health status/comorbid illness	Severity of underlying lung function	Severity of respiratory failure	Cause of exacerbation
Menzies et al., 1989 (113)	Albumin	Lifestyle score	Lower FEV_1	Hypoxemia/ Dyspnea severity	
Portier et al., 1992 (103)	Cachexia	Low sodium	Lower FEV_1		Non-COPD cause
Rieves et al., 1993 (114)					Infiltrates present Atrial fibrillation
Fuso et al., 1995 (111)		Age		Higher PA-a gradient	Ventricular dysrhyth- mias
Seneff et al., 1995 (115)		Nonrespiratory physi- ology abnormality		Longer pre-ICU hos- pital stay	
Vitacca et al., 1996 (116)	Nutrition index			Higher APACHE II score	

risk factors, prognosis, and therapy to be interpreted on an international level. To address this concern, a consensus conference including investigators from North America and Europe was convened (36). After much deliberation, this group defined 4 criteria for ARDS: (1) acute onset, (2) bilateral pulmonary infiltrates on chest x-ray (CXR), (3) an arterial oxygen tension to inspired oxygen concentration ratio of less than 200, and (4) a pulmonary artery occlusion pressure of ≤18 mmHg or the absence of left heart failure (if a pulmonary artery catheter was not available).

Despite general acceptance of this definition, reflected in its adoption for clinical trials, it is readily apparent to those treating patients with ARDS that ARDS represents a syndrome comprised of a heterogeneous group of patients. In the past, "lumping" has been partly justified by the assumption that these various types of lung injury lead to a uniform pulmonary pathophysiological response (37). Recent data, however, suggest that even this assumption may not be correct. Due largely to the work of Gattinoni and colleagues, there is an increasing belief that ARDS arising from a direct pulmonary insult should be considered as a separate entity from that arising from extrapulmonary disease. In a recent publication, this group demonstrated a different response in respiratory mechanics to the application of increasing amounts of PEEP between pulmonary and extrapulmonary ARDS patients, consistent with the predominance of consolidation in the former group compared to edema and alveolar collapse seen in the latter (38). Recognition of differences in pulmonary mechanics between these two disorders may lead to therapeutic strategies that are type-specific that will lead, hopefully, to an improvement in outcome.

A. Incidence

There exists a large discrepancy in the reported incidence of ARDS in the literature largely attributable to the type and quality of the studies as well as to the variability in the definition of ARDS (39). It has been widely quoted that about 150,000 cases of ARDS occur per year in the United States. This would translate into approximately 65–75 cases per 100,000 individuals and is consistent with the NIH estimate of 60 cases per 100,000 persons per year (40). However, this may be an overestimate of the true incidence of ARDS. Prospective cohort studies in the Canary Islands, Utah, and Berlin, as well as a retrospective survey conducted in Britain, all reported appreciably lower incidence estimates (41–44). Villar and Slutsky reported an incidence of 1.5–3.5 per 100,000 people, depending upon how ARDS was defined, in the Canary Islands (41), while estimates from Utah and Berlin were very similar at 5.3 and 3.0 per 100,000 respectively (43,44). Although they adopted a weaker study design, Webster and coworkers reported a similar incidence of 4.5 per 100,000 people, as did Valta et al., at 4.9 cases per 100,000 inhabitants per year (42,45). A recent article looking at the incidence and mortality of ARDS in Sweden, Denmark, and Iceland found the incidence of acute respiratory failure, acute lung injury, and ARDS to be 77.6, 17.9, and 13.5 per 100,000 persons per year, respectively (5). The 90-day mortality for the three separate patient groups was surprisingly similar at about 41%. A primary pulmonary cause for ARDS was noted in 77.9% of cases. This body of work deserves particular attention because it is a large prospective population-based study that utilized the American-European Consensus Conference definition of ALI and ARDS.

B. Demographics

ARDS is most commonly seen in previously healthy patients suffering from an acute illness. The development of lung injury after the onset of the triggering event is usually rapid, often occurring within 24–48 hours. According to a multicenter registry of patients with ARDS, the average patient is 49 years of age, more frequently male, and less likely to be a smoker (35). In general, the mean length of stay for these patients is longer than most other ICU patients, lasting about 12 days. The associated hospital stay for a survivor is also prolonged, being approximately 1 month (35). This agrees closely with the demographics from the VHHSC database (Table 6).

C. Risk Factors for ARDS

In a recent systematic review, Garber and colleagues rigorously assessed the evidence supporting a causative role for the various risk factors reported in the literature to be associated with the development of ARDS (39). These authors developed a "causation score" and reported the strongest evidence for the risk factors of sepsis, aspiration of gastric contents, pulmonary contusion, pneumonia, near drowning, and smoke inhalation/burns, all scoring 11 out of 18. Trauma, pancreatitis, and multiple transfusions scored 10 out of 18; the presence of shock or fractures scored 9 out of 18; and fat embolism, disseminated intravascular coagulation, and cardiopulmonary bypass all scored an 8. In reviewing this study it is important to realize that the strength of causation was influenced by the quality of the primary studies. The most common risk factors for ARDS have generally been reported to be sepsis, aspiration, and multiple trauma (46). The risk of developing ARDS increases with the number of risk factors. One study demonstrated a fourfold increase in risk for patients who had two or more risk factors compared to patients with a single risk factor (47).

While a great deal of research has been conducted to identify early predictors of acute lung injury among patients who present with one or more of the various risk factors for developing ARDS, no variables have been found to be useful from a clinical perspective. Despite plausible rationales, studies of levels of different mediators of inflammation have not been found to have the level of sensitivity and specificity necessary to predict the development of ARDS (48).

D. Outcome from ARDS

Short-Term Mortality

ARDS has a high in-hospital mortality, reported to be 40–60% for all comers (46,47,49). There is a general feeling that survival has improved over the past 20 years, although a recent review of 101 ARDS studies could not detect a significant trend in mortality reduction, averaging 53% before 1990 to 51% in 1994 (50). However, the great heterogeneity among studies of both severity of disease and the underlying etiology of ARDS may have obscured a change in prognosis over time. In a single-center study of ARDS using a consistent definition and adjusting for age, gender, and risk factors for ARDS, Milberg and coworkers reported a reduction in hospital mortality from 54% to 40% from 1983 to 1993 (49). The ARDS registry has also reported an overall decline in ARDS mortality (35). A recent European study has also indicated an improvement in mortality rates over the past decade (51). Data collected over 10 years at VHHSC also suggests an improvement in ARDS mortality (Table 6). These improvements in mortality have occurred with no change in case mix severity. Finally, Suchyta and associates noted that patients fulfilling the eligibility criteria for extracorporeal membrane oxygenation that were recruited to the extracorporeal CO_2 removal trial had a mortality of 55% compared to 89% in the original ECMO trial (52). In balance, there is an optimistic belief that patients with ARDS have a higher short-term survival now than 15–20 years ago.

The prognosis for patients with ARDS has been shown to vary in relation to premorbid factors as well as the etiology of ARDS. Increasing age has been demonstrated to be associated with poorer outcome (35,53,54), and in the study by Milberg and coworkers the relative risk of age appeared to be increasing over the past 10 years (49). Suchyta and colleagues found a greater mortality in patients with underlying liver disease or malignancy (mortality rates reaching up to 90%). Other investigators have found a similar increased risk associated with significant chronic co-morbid illness including cirrhosis, HIV, organ transplantation, malignancy, and increasingly abnormal MCABE score (measure of severity of underlying medical disease) (53,55). The severity of acute nonpulmonary organ dysfunction has also been demonstrated to be associated with survival (56). Monchi and colleagues found a higher SAPS 2 score and right ventricular dysfunction to be associated with increased mortality (55). Others have also found the development of nonpulmonary organ dysfunction to be a poor prognostic sign (5,32,57), and it has been demonstrated that ARDS patients generally die from multiple organ dysfunction rather than progressive respiratory failure (58,59). The effect that gas-exchange severity on either presentation or later during ICU stay has on survival is less clear, with some investigators observing positive associations with mortality (55) and others detecting no such association (53). Finally, the etiology of ARDS influences outcome with a poorer prognosis for patients presenting with ARDS secondary to pneumonia or sepsis and a better prognosis for multiple trauma (35,53,46,47,60–62).

Long-Term Survival

Does recovery from ARDS have an impact on long-term survival? Data to answer this question are sparse. There has been increased interest in survival beyond hospitalization for patients admitted to the ICU over the last decade, but most studies report on general, not specific, ICU populations (63–75). Studies indicate that mortality is increased for ICU patients over the first few years after hospital discharge compared to an age- and gender-matched general population (63,64,71,73). It appears that younger patients and patients with trauma have little increased long-term mortality (63). Patients with underlying malignancies or other significant comorbidity do not fare as well (63). Most studies of ARDS report a mortality rate at 30 days or hospital discharge as most deaths are felt to occur within this time frame (47). A recent study of 90-day mortality reported a rate of 41.2%, almost identical to the 30-day rate in the same study (5). One study, however, did report 16.3% mortality during an 18-month period following discharge from the ICU after an episode of ARDS (76).

The only data on long-term survival comes from a recent Seattle study group (77). This was a cohort study of survivors of ARDS secondary to trauma or sepsis matched to a group of critically ill patients with trauma or sepsis who did not have ARDS. The median follow-up time for the cohort was 753 days. Total mortality of the ARDS cohort over this observation period was 38%. Hospital mortality constituted 80% of all deaths and varied in rate from 14% for trauma-related ARDS patients to 43% for sepsis-related ARDS patients. The median time to death after the onset of ARDS was 10 days. Survival plots for the cohort are depicted in Figure 5. There was a 10% late mortality rate, with no difference in mortality between subjects and controls. A multivariate analysis demonstrated no independent effect of ARDS on survival after hospital discharge. It appears that long-term survival in ARDS patients is related to associated comorbid disease or risk factor for ARDS, as age and comorbid illness were found to be independent risk factors, while sepsis patients had a sixfold increase in mortality over trauma patients (77).

Long-Term Morbidity

At the time of extubation, abnormal pulmonary function is the rule among ARDS patients, including a reduction in lung volumes, a more pronounced reduction in diffusing capacity, and, in some patients, an increase in airway resistance (78,79).

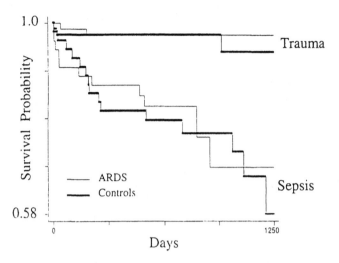

Figure 5 Survival plot of ARDS patients and controls after hospital discharge. (From Davidson T, Rubenfeld G, Caldwell E, Hudson L, Steinberg K. The effect of acute respiratory distress syndrome on long-term survival. AJRCCM 1999; 160:1838, with permission.)

Follow-up over the first year has demonstrated an improvement in all of these measures of lung function, often to within normal limits (80,81). Significant respiratory impairment in the long term has been identified in only 4% of patients (80). It appears that prolonged positive pressure ventilation, high FiO_2 levels, increasing age, and severity of hypoxemia during the acute illness strongly correlate with pulmonary impairment after recovery (78,80). Interestingly, the degree of abnormality on open lung biopsy does not correlate with lung function one year later (82). It is possible that the current practice of ventilating ARDS patients with smaller tidal volumes and low pressures may lead to even less long-term respiratory impairment and disability.

E. Quality of Life After ARDS

Concern with not just quantity of life but its associated quality has led to an emphasis on understanding patient quality of life beyond the ICU. This area of study is still in its infancy, and most investigators have reported on heterogeneous groups of ICU patients (63,65–75,83–85). McHugh and coworkers used the Sickness Impact Profile (SIP), a tool designed to assess a subject's self-perceived physical and psychological status, to measure quality of life in ARDS patients over time (86). They found that patients improved significantly by 3 months after extubation and that younger patients continued to improve up to one year. In another study, 24 patients with ALI completed the SF-36, a well-validated generic health-related quality of life (HRQL) survey, 6–43 months after extubation (87).

Forty-three percent of these patients met criteria for depression, and 43% had self-reported significant functional limitations. These authors concluded that ARDS patients have significantly poorer quality of life than the general population. Schelling and associates reported a similar reduction in all domains of the SF-36 in a study of 80 ARDS survivors, most notably in physical functioning (76). Interestingly, they found a large number of these patients also fulfilled criteria for the posttraumatic stress syndrome.

All of these studies are open to selection bias and do not control for prior level of quality of life, which may lead to an overly pessimistic conclusion regarding long-term outcome for these patients. Davidson and coworkers performed a prospective, matched cohort study composed of 73 pairs of ARDS survivors and controls matched for clinical risk factors for ARDS and severity of illness (88). Compared to controls, a clinically meaningful and statistically significant reduction in the quality of life scores for ARDS were seen in most domains of the SF-36 as well as the St. George's Respiratory Questionnaire, a respiratory disease–specific HRQL tool. The largest decrements in the quality of life were seen in physical functioning and pulmonary symptoms and limitations. These differences in HRQL were found to be consistent within the two subgroups of trauma and sepsis risk factors. These authors concluded that survivors of ARDS had a clinically significant reduction in quality of life, most notably in physical functioning and respiratory symptoms that appeared to be caused exclusively by ARDS and its sequelae. It is important to emphasize that this study only looked at trauma and sepsis patients with ARDS (65% of the total). Of these patients, approximately 75% of those eligible, or 50% of the total number of patients with ARDS secondary to trauma or sepsis, were contacted. While selection bias may be a problem for all these studies the evidence available in the literature to date suggests that ARDS has a negative impact on future HRQL. Further careful study, especially of patients treated with low tidal volume, low pressure ventilation should be undertaken and for a more prolonged follow-up period (beyond the one year maximum in most studies) because many of these patients require extensive rehabilitation for underlying polyneuropathy of critical illness.

In summary, there appears to be a trend to lower in-hospital mortality for acute respiratory failure in ARDS patients in recent years, the reasons for which remain unclear. A similar improvement in long-term survival has not been as clearly demonstrated. Survivors appear to have a reduction in their QOL for at least the first year, largely in the domains of physical functioning and pulmonary symptoms.

VIII.   Chronic Obstructive Pulmonary Disease

COPD describes an abnormality of pulmonary function testing consisting of irreversible or incompletely reversible obstruction of the airways. The obstruction arises as a result of loss of lung tissue elasticity, narrowing of airways, or, more commonly, a combination of the two. The most important risk factor for the development of COPD is smoking (89), though it is important to recognize that up to 80% of smokers do not develop COPD. Other factors that are believed to lead to an increased risk of COPD include exposure to certain organic dusts (cotton, grain, or wood), air pollution, hereditary (α_1-antitrypsin deficiency), and prior viral infections (89).

COPD is common, affecting approximately 16 million adults in the United States according to the 1994 National Health Interview Survey (90). It is the fourth leading cause of death in the United States, with an age-adjusted death rate of 21 per 100,000, leading to 106,146 deaths in 1996 (91). While the death rate for men reached a plateau in the mid-1980s, it continues to rise in women. The economic impact within the United States is huge, estimated at $14.7 billion dollars in direct health care costs in 1993 (92).

From the studies in Table 4, it appears that COPD accounts for approximately 5% of nonoperative patients requiring mechanical ventilation in North American ICUs (3,19,21,28). While early studies would suggest that the relative proportion of patients requiring ventilation because of an exacerbation of COPD has decreased since the 1960s and 1970s, the absolute number continues to increase with the increasing prevalence of the disease and growing number of total ICU beds. Of more importance, when one looks at patients ventilated for longer than a few days, the relative proportion of patients with COPD increases further (10–14), while studies of weaning from mechanical ventilation in U.S. centers have reported that COPD and asthma comprise 10–15% of nonoperative patients (15–18).

A. Outcome for COPD Patients Presenting with Acute Respiratory Failure

Short-Term Mortality

The traditional outcome of most concern to clinicians caring for patients with COPD has been hospital survival. In North America, an aggressive approach to acute respiratory failure in the setting of COPD has historically led to routine institution of mechanical ventilation when patients deteriorate to the extent that intervention was deemed necessary for patient survival. In contrast, other nations, such as the United Kingdom, have been more conservative in offering mechanical ventilation to patients with COPD in acute respiratory failure (93,94).

A large body of literature has been published on hospital mortality of patients admitted with COPD exacerbations. Weiss and Hudson conducted a thorough review of the literature up to 1992 and noted that there appeared to be a trend toward an improved survival if one compared studies published prior to 1975 to those published afterward, with hospital mortality averaging approximately 26% and 10%, respectively (95). These mortality figures included all patients presenting with acute respiratory failure due to an exacerbation of COPD whether mechanical ventilation was required or not. Mortality was appreciably higher among those requiring ventilation, ranging from 30 to 80%. These authors acknowledge the potentially large problem that selection bias may play in interpreting study results and drawing comparisons over time.

Figure 6 plots hospital mortality versus the year of publication of the studies included in Weiss and Hudson's review (96–106) plus several further studies published since that review (93,107–117). These studies suggest that mortality in patients with COPD treated conventionally has not improved over time to the extent previously suggested, though selection bias remains a possibility. It still appears that mortality was higher in the studies published prior to 1975, averaging 26%. However, the studies since 1975 now appear to have a higher average mortality than previously thought, in the range of 15–20%. It is possible that patients admitted to ICUs in more recent studies were more severely ill than those in earlier studies, reflecting more strict admissions policies, thus obscuring a greater improvement in outcome. Alternatively, as a result of changes in practice, mechanical ventilation may have been offered less frequently in later studies leading to higher short-term mortality. Once again, mortality appears appreciably higher among patients requiring mechanical ventilation.

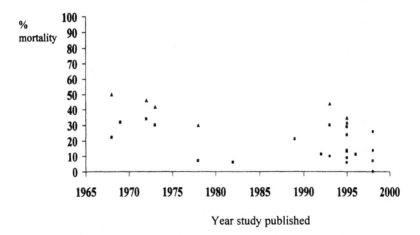

Figure 6 Summary of the literature on hospital mortality for COPD patients. Each marker represents an individual study plotted against the year of publication. The squares represent studies including all COPD patients admitted to hospital with respiratory distress regardless of the need for mechanical ventilation. The triangles represent studies that include only patients who required mechanical ventilation. The circles represent studies that included patients ventilated with noninvasive positive pressure ventilation.

One encouraging finding from Figure 6 is the decreased mortality in trials evaluating the effectiveness of noninvasive ventilation in COPD. Mortality rates in these trials are consistently 10% or less (93,107–109,112). While concerns may be raised that these trials selected patients who were less ill as a group than those in other studies, the control groups of these trials have mortality rates in keeping with other studies of conventionally treated patients. In conclusion, it appears that hospital mortality may have improved over the past 30 years for patients presenting with acute exacerbations of COPD leading to acute respiratory failure. Furthermore, a major contributor to the increase in survival is the introduction of noninvasive ventilation.

Investigators have tried to determine which variables are predictive of hospital mortality in COPD patients admitted with acute respiratory failure. Despite variability in study size, patient severity, and variables included, consistent themes emerge from reviewing the literature. As nicely summarized by Weiss and Hudson (95), the major predictors of in-hospital mortality are: (1) prior comorbid illness and underlying nutritional status, (2) baseline degree of obstructive lung disease, (3) severity of acute respiratory failure upon presentation, and (4) the etiology of the acute exacerbation.

In a summary of studies published over the last 10 years (Table 7), these risk factors are well illustrated. Patients with more advanced COPD represented by a lower FEV_1 on pulmonary function testing had a worse prognosis (113,114). Other indicators of advanced COPD or significant comorbid illness including poor nutritional status, measured by specific indices or serum albumin, advanced age, and higher lifestyle scores (representing greater disability), also portended a poor prognosis (111,113,114,117). Not surprisingly, patients presenting with more severe respiratory failure are more likely to require mechanical ventilation and have a higher mortality (111,113,117). It is notable that the etiology of the exacerbation was also found to be of importance prognostically (103,111,114). Patients with infiltrates on chest x-ray (most commonly pneumonia, but occasionally due to congestive heart failure) had a higher mortality (114). The development of dysrhythmias is also a poor prognostic sign (111), representing either a more severe episode of acute respiratory failure or significant underlying cardiac disease.

Long-Term Survival

COPD, in contrast to ARDS, is a chronic condition, and patients presenting with an acute exacerbation requiring mechanical ventilation are generally entering into the more severe stages of the underlying progressive disease process. Survival is not guaranteed by the provision of mechanical ventilation, and some patients may have a prolonged and uncomfortable ICU stay prior to their death. For these reasons, greater emphasis has been placed on understanding the long-term prognosis for these patients. To do this requires an assessment of both the quantity of life remaining and, perhaps even more important, the quality of that life. Eight studies including long-term follow-up of COPD patients beyond an index admission for acute respiratory failure are summarized in Table 8 (101,110,114,115, 117–119).

A true inception cohort study of a chronic process such as COPD would ideally identify all patients at a similar stage of their disease and follow them forward from there until death. The resultant survival curve would include data gathered at regular intervals to describe the average stage of disease represented by pulmonary function, symptoms, and, perhaps, quality of life. Such a study would allow more accurate prognostication by providing data for physicians that they could then apply to any patient by matching the patient's stage of disease with the survival curve. Unfortunately, this ideal cohort study would be very difficult to orchestrate and would require early identification of a large number of COPD patients for prolonged follow-up. In its stead we have studies that include patients with a relatively broad spectrum of severity of underlying COPD, a spectrum that varies from study to study. For example, the study by Martin and associates had no patients with clinical cor pulmonale (101), while in other studies 37% (118) and 60% (119) of patients presented with this feature. These differences in severity of illness likely account, in part, for the respective differences in long-term survival. The relative proportion of patients requiring mechanical ventilation also impacts on the average long-term survival, explaining in part the apparently lower survival in the study by Menzies and colleagues (113).

Overall it appears that prior to noninvasive ventilation, the average one-year survival after an acute exacerbation with associated acute respiratory failure was in the neighborhood of 50%. Two more recent studies suggest an improvement in long-term survival to 70% with use of noninvasive ventilation (117,120). However, both these studies are small, and larger prospective studies are required to determine whether these results can be generalized outside of a selected population.

While average values for long-term survival are useful, more prognostic precision can be accomplished by identifying specific factors associated with long-term survival. For patients who survive their index hospitalization, the factors that are associated with survival reflect both the severity of the underlying COPD and comorbid illness. Lower baseline FEV_1, dyspnea severity, and functional status were all demonstrated by Menzies and coworkers to be associated with 1-year survival (113). This group also reported that hypercarbia at the time of presentation portended a poorer long-term prognosis (113).

Seneff and colleagues noted that, while respiratory physiological variables did not predict hospital survival well, patients with abnormal values were more likely to die in the long term (115). In a very interesting study, Costello and associates noted that the response of arterial blood gas during the index hospital-

Table 8 Long-Term Survival of COPD Patients Presenting with an Acute Exacerbation

Study	Total N	Available for follow-up	2 months	3 months	6 months	1 year	2 years
Gottlieb et al., 1973 (119)	30	30				30%	
Martin et al., 1982 (101)	36	36					72%
Menzies et al., 1989[a] (1984–1987) (113)	95	95				38%	
Seneff et al., 1995 (1988–1990) (115)	362	167		58%	52%	48%	
Connors et al., 1996 (1989–1994) (110)	1,106	1,106	80%		67%	58%	51%
Confalonieri et al., 1996 (120)							
(1991–1992;	24	24			54%	50%	
1993–1994 [NPPV])	24	24			71%	71%	
Vitacca et al., 1996 (117)							
NPPV group	30	30		77%		70%	
MV group (2 years prior)	29	29		52%		37%	
Costello et al., 1997[b] (5-year follow-up) (118)	85	85				61%	46%

[a] All received conventional mechanical ventilation.
[b] Estimated values from original graphical data.

ization predicted long-term outcome—patients with persistent hypercarbia at discharge faring the worst over 5 years of follow-up compared to patients who either did not present with hypercarbia or whose initial hypercarbia reversed to the normal range prior to discharge (118). Another marker of respiratory status, the need for mechanical ventilation, was felt to be associated with higher long-term mortality, but recent data suggest otherwise (115). Finally, factors indicative of poor nutritional status such as albumin level and patient age correlate with survival.

B. Quality of Life After COPD Exacerbations

Relatively little work has been conducted assessing the quality of life of COPD patients who survive a bout of acute respiratory failure. The SUPPORT group followed up a group of patients at 6 months after discharge and found that 21% considered their quality of life to be excellent or very good, 30% good, and 49% fair or poor (110). Just over half of these patients, 54%, required assistance with at least one activity of daily living. Cydulka and coworkers reviewed all elderly (>65 years) patients admitted with the diagnosis of COPD or asthma in the Health Care Financing Administration computerized database of hospital discharge for patients receiving Medicare from 1984 to 1991 (121). They found that an increasing proportion of patients were being transferred to other care facilities rather than home over this 7-year period, rising from 5% to 15%. Those patients returning home were more likely to be receiving home health care, an increase from 2.5% to 10%. While the latter observation may reflect more appropriate home planning with time, the two observations together support a population requiring significant assistance with activities of daily living. Finally, Seemungal and colleagues followed a total of 73 patients with COPD over a 1-year period (122). They found that quality of life, as measured by the St. George's Respiratory Questionnaire at the end of one year, was significantly worse in patients experiencing more frequent acute exacerbation of their disease (122).

Over the past decade in North America, an increasing emphasis on quality of life and a better understanding of prognoses for disorders treated in ICUs has been associated with an increased proportion of patients dying following the withdrawal of life support rather than after failed resuscitation (123–125). Recognizing that intubation and mechanical ventilation does not cure COPD patients, and may, in some settings, lead to unnecessary suffering, has resulted in ventilation no longer being routinely offered to all COPD patients. While physicians in some countries makes decisions on end-of-life care without consulting with the patient, in North America these decisions are more often made in conjunction with the patient and family. In a Canadian survey of 279 respirologists, most acknowledged that these discussions were not conducted until advanced stages of the disease (126). The majority of respirologists completing the survey favored a shared approach to decision making, but most admitted to framing the discussion in order to influence the decision (127). These authors' findings suggest that more work is needed to assure that patient decisions regarding the institution of mechanical ventilation are truly informed.

In summary, there appears to be a trend toward a higher in-hospital survival for acute respiratory failure in COPD patients in recent years, in part due to the adoption of noninvasive ventilation. A similar improvement in long-term survival has not been as clearly demonstrated, although recent case-control studies of patients receiving noninvasive ventilation are intriguing. Finally, a large proportion of patients' quality of life after discharge is fair to poor, and dependence on others is high. All these factors strongly support the promotion of an organized approach to end-of-life decision making for COPD patients, the primary objective of this approach being to facilitate informed decisions regarding life support interventions well in advance of crises.

IX. Summary

In this chapter we have summarized information from different types of studies to give an overview of acute respiratory failure over the past 3 decades. While it appears that there have been changes over time in the types of patients being ventilated in our ICUs, the process we have been forced to use to reach these conclusions—extracting data available from the literature, reported for other purposes—is of unclear validity. With the current adoption of increasingly comprehensive databases and the increasing ease with which they can be used, we look forward to the availability of data that will better describe the epidemiology of acute respiratory failure in the future. The data provided by Estaban and his international colleagues is a good example of this (26,27). We have also explored the epidemiology of two causes of respiratory failure—ARDS and COPD—in greater depth, including a look forward at both the quality and quantity of life for those that survive the ICU.

References

1. Stedman's Medical Dictionary. 23rd ed. Baltimore: The Williams & Wilkins Company, 1973.
2. Petty T, Cherniak R. The origins and evolution of critical care. In: Hall JB, Schmidt GA, Wood LDH, eds. Principles of Critical Care. New York: McGraw-Hill, 1992: xxxi–xxxviii.
3. Petty TL, Lakshminarayan S, Sahn SA, Zwillich CW, Nett LM. Intensive respiratory care unit: review of ten years experience. JAMA 1975; 233:34–37.
4. Jacobs P, Noseworthy TW. National estimates of intensive care utilization and costs: Canada and the United States. Crit Care Med 1990; 18:1282–1286.

5. Luhr OR, Antonsen K, Karlsson M, et al. Incidence and mortality after acute respiratory failure and acute respiratory distress syndrome in Sweden, Denmark, and Iceland. AJRCCM 1999; 159:1849.
6. Knaus WA, Draper EA, Wagner DP, Zimmerman JE. APACHE II: a severity of disease classification. Crit Care Med 1985; 13:818–829.
7. Knaus WA, Wagner DP, Draper EA, et al. The APACHE III prognostic system: risk prediction of hospital mortality for critically ill hospitalized adults. Chest 1991; 100:1619–1636.
8. Le Gall JR, Lemeshow S, Saulnier F. A new simplified acute physiology score (SAPS II) based on European/North American multicenter study. JAMA 1993; 270:2957.
9. Zimmerman JE, Wagner DP, Draper EA, et al. Evaluation of acute physiology and chronic health evaluation III predictions of hospital mortality in an independent database. Crit Care Med 1998; 26:1317–1326.
10. Cook D, Guyatt G, Marshall J, Leasa D, Fuller H, Hall R, et al. A comparison of sucralfate and ranitidine for the prevention of upper gastrointestinal bleeding in patients requiring mechanical ventilation. N Engl J Med 1998; 338:791–797.
11. Dreyfuss D, Djedaini K, Gros I, et al. Mechanical ventilation with heated humidifiers or heat and moisture exchangers: effects on patient colonization and incidence of nosocomial pneumonia. AJRCCM 1995; 151:986.
12. Gastinne H, Wolff M, Delatour F, et al. A controlled trial in intensive care units of selective decontamination of the digestive tract with nonabsorbable antibiotics. NEJM 1992; 326:594.
13. Kollef MH, Shapiro SD, Fraser VJ, Silver P, Murphy DM, Trovillion E, et al. Mechanical ventilation with or without 7-day circuit changes: a randomized controlled trial. Ann Intern Med 1995; 1995:168–174.
14. Valles J, Artigas A, Rello J, et al. Continuous aspiration of subglotic secretions in preventing ventilator-associated pneumonia. Ann Intern Med 1995; 122:179.
15. Ely EW, Baker AM, Dunagan DP, et al. Effect on the duration of mechanical ventilation of identifying patients capable of breathing spontaneously. N Engl J Med 1996; 335:1864–1869.
16. Kollef MH, Shapiro SD, Silver P, et al. A randomized, controlled trial of protocol-directed versus physician-directed weaning from mechanical ventilation. Crit Care Med 1997; 25:567–574.
17. Estaban A, Frutos F, Tobin MJ, Alia I, et al. A comparison of four methods of weaning patients from mechanical ventilation. NEJM 1995; 332:345.
18. Brochard L, Rauss A, Benito S, Conti G, Mancebo J, Rekik N, et al. Comparison of three methods of gradual withdrawal from mechanical ventilatory support during weaning from mechanical ventilation. Am J Respir Crit Care Med 1994; 150:896–903.
19. Knaus WA. Prognosis with mechanical ventilation: the influence of disease, severity of disease, age, and chronic health status on survival from an acute illness. Am Rev Respir Dis 1989; 140:S8–S13.
20. Pontoppidan H, Geffin B, Lowenstein E. Acute respiratory failure in the adult. N Engl J Med 1972; 287:690–698.
21. Seneff MG, Zimmerman JE, Knaus WA, Wagner DP, Draper EA. Predicting the

duration of mechanical ventilation: the importance of disease and patient characteristics. Chest 1996; 110:469–479.

22. Henning RJ, McClish D, Daly B, et al. Clinical characteristics and resource utilization of ICU patients: implications for organization of intensive care. Crit Care Med
1987; 15:264–269.

23. Knaus WA, Wagner DP, Draper EA, et al. The range of intensive care services
today. JAMA 1981; 246:2711.

24. Thibault GE, Mulley AG, Barnett GO, et al. Medical intensive care: indications,
interventions, and outcomes. N Engl J Med 1980; 302:938–942.

25. Wagner DP, Knaus WA, Draper EA. Identification of low-risk monitor admissions
to medical-surgical ICUs. Chest 1987; 92:432.

26. Estaban A, Anzueto A, Alia I, et al. Clinical characteristics of patients receiving
mechanical ventilation. AJRCCM 1999; 159:A47.

27. Estaban A, Anzueto A, Alia I, Tobin MJ, et al. Mortality of patients receiving
mechanical ventilation. Am J Respir Crit Care Med 1999; 159:A47.

28. Cohen IL, Bari N, Strosberg MA, et al. Reduction of duration and cost of mechanical ventilation in an intensive care unit by use of a ventilatory management team.
Crit Care Med 1991; 19:1278–1284.

29. Calvin JE. Clinical trial networks: a unique opportunity for critical care. Crit Care
Med 1998; 26:625–626.

30. Keenan SP, Martin CM. Creation of a critical care research network. Curr Opin
Crit Care 1998; 4:470.

31. Miranda ER, Ryan DW, Schaufeli WB, VF, eds. Organization and Management
of Intensive Care: A Prospective Study in 12 European Countries. Berlin: Springer-
Verlag, 1998.

32. Villar J, Manzano JJ, Blazquez MA, Quintana J. Multiple system organ failure in
acute respiratory failure. J Crit Care 1991; 6:75–80.

33. Ashbaugh DG, Bigelow DB, Petty TL, Levine BE. Acute respiratory distress in
adults. Lancet 1967; ii:319–323.

34. Murray JF, Mathay MA, Luce JM, Flick MR. An expanded definition of the adult
respiratory distress syndrome. Am Rev Respir Dis 1988; 138:720–723.

35. Sloane PJ, Gee MH, Gottlieb JE, Albertine KH, Peters SP, Burns JR, et al. A
multicenter registry of patients with acute respiratory distress syndrome. Am Rev
Respir Dis 1992; 146:419–426.

36. Bernard G, Artigas A, Brigham K, Carlet J, Falke K, Hudson L, et al. The American-European Consensus Conference on ARDS: definitions, mechanism, relevant
outcomes, and clinical trial coordination. AJRCCM 1994; 149:818–824.

37. Petty TL. The adult respiratory distress syndrome (confessions of a ''lumper'').
Am Rev Respir Dis 1975; 111:713.

38. Gattinoni L, Pelosi P, Suter P, Pedoto A, Vercesi P, Lissoni A. Acute respiratory
distress syndrome caused by pulmonary and extrapulmonary disease: different syndromes? AJRCCM 1998; 158:3–11.

39. Garber BG, Hebert PC, Yelle JD, Hodder RV, McGowan J. Adult respiratory distress syndrome: a systematic overview of incidence and risk factors. Crit Care Med
1996; 24:687–695.

40. Respiratory Diseases: Task Force Report on Problems, Research Approaches,

Needs. Washington, DC: National Heart and Lung Institutes, U.S. Government Printing Office, 1972.

41. Villar J, Slutsky AS. The incidence of the adult respiratory distress syndrome. Am Rev Respir Dis 1989; 134:814–816.

42. Webster NR, Cohen AT, Nunn JF. Adult respiratory distress syndrome: how many cases in the UK? Anaesthesia 1988; 43:923–926.

43. Thomsen G, Morris A. Incidence of the adult respiratory distress syndrome in the state of Utah. Am J Respir Crit Care Med 1995; 152:965–971.

44. Lewandowski K, Metz J, Deutschmann C, Preib H, Kuhlen R, Artigas A, et al. Incidence, severity, and mortality of acute respiratory failure in Berlin, Germany. AJRCCM 1995; 151:1125.

45. Valta P, Uusaro A, Nunes S, Ruokonen E, Takala J. Acute respiratory distress syndrome: Frequency, clinical course, and costs of care. Crit Care Med 1999; 27: 2367.

46. Pepe PE, Potkin RT, Reus DH, Hudson LD, Carrico CJ. Clinical predictors of the adult respiratory distress. Am J Surg 1982; 144:124–130.

47. Fowler AA, Hamman RF, Good, Benson KN, Baird M, Eberle DJ, et al. Adult respiratory distress syndrome: risk with common predispositions. Ann Intern Med 1983; 98:593–597.

48. Pittet JF, Mackersie RC, Martin TR, Matthay MA. Biological markers of acute lung injury: Prognostic and pathogenetic significance. AJRCCM 1997; 155:1187.

49. Milberg JA, Davis DR, Steinberg KP, Hudson LD. Improved survival of patients with acute respiratory distress syndrome (ARDS). JAMA 1995; 273:306–309.

50. Krafft P, Fridrich P, Pernerstorfer T, et al. The acute respiratory distress syndrome: definitions, severity and clinical outcome. Intensive Care Med 1996; 22:519.

51. Able SJ, Finney SJ, Brett SJ, Keogh BF, Morgan CJ, Evans TW. Improved survival in association with ARDS. Thorax 1999; 53:292–294.

52. Suchyta MR, Clemmer TP, Elliot CG, Orme JF, Weaver LK. The adult respiratory distress syndrome: a report of survival and modifying factors. Chest 1992; 101: 1074–1079.

53. Zilberberg M, Epstein S. Acute lung injury in the medical ICU: comorbid conditions, age, etiology, and hospital outcome. AJRCCM 1998; 157:1159–1164.

54. Heuser MD, Case LD, Ettinger LM. Mortality in intensive care patients with respiratory disease: Is age important? Arch Intern Med 1992; 152:1683–1688.

55. Monchi M, Bellenfant F, Cariou A, Joly L, Thebert D, Leurent I, et al. Early predictive factors of survival in the acute respiratory distress syndrome: a multivariate analysis. AJRCCM 1998; 158:1076–1081.

56. Bone RC, Balk R, Slotman G, Maunder R, Silverman H, Hyers TM, et al. Adult respiratory distress syndrome: sequence and importance of development of multiple organ failure. Chest 1992; 101:320–326.

57. Villar J, Blazquez MA, Lubillo S, Quintaner J, Mazuno JL. Septic adult respiratory distress syndrome and multiple system failure. Prog Clin Biol Res 1989; 308:57–60.

58. Montgomery AB, Stager MA, Carrico CJ, Hudson LD. Causes of mortality in patients with adult respiratory distress syndrome. Am Rev Respir Dis 1985; 32:485–489.

59. Bell RC, Coalson JJ, Smith JD, Johanson WG. Multiple organ system failure and infection in adult respiratory distress syndrome. Ann Intern Med 1983; 99:293–298.

60. Mancebo J, Artigas A. A clinical study of the adult respiratory distress syndrome. Crit Care Med 1987; 15:243–246.

61. Artigas A, Carlet J, LeGall JR, Chastang C, Blanch L, et al. Clinical presentation, prognostic factors and outcome of ARDS in the European Collaborative Study (1985–1987): a preliminary report. Acute Respir Failure 1990:37–60.

62. Seidenfeld JJ, Pohl DF, Bell RC, Harris GD, Jr JW. Incidence, site, and outcome of infections in patients with the adult respiratory distress syndrome. Am Rev Respir Dis 1986; 134:12–16.

63. Ridley S, Jackson R, Findlay J, Wallace P. Long term survival after intensive care. Br Med J 1990; 301:1127–1130.

64. Stauffer JL, Fayter NA, Graves B, Cromb M, et al. Survival following mechanical ventilation for acute respiratory failure in adult men. Chest 1993; 104:1222–1229.

65. McLean RJ, McIntosh JD, Kung GY, Leung DM, Byrick RJ. Outcome of respiratory intensive care for the elderly. Crit Care Med 1985; 13(8):625–629.

66. Ridley S, PW. Quality of life after intensive care. Anaesthesia 1990; 45:808–813.

67. Ridley S, Crispin P, Scotton H, Rogers J, Lloyd D. Changes in quality of life after intensive care: comparison with normal data. Anaesthesia 1997; 52:195–202.

68. Jacobs C, van der Vliet J, van Roozendaal M, Van der Linden CJ. Mortality and quality of life after intensive care for critical illness. Intensive Care Med 1988; 14:217–220.

69. Goldstein R, Campion W, Thibault G, Mulley A, Skinner E. Functional outcomes following medical intensive care. Crit Care Med 1986; 14(9):783–788.

70. Chelluri L, Pinsky M, Gresnik AL. Outcome of intensive care of the ''oldest-old'' critically ill patients. Crit Care Med 1992; 20(6):757–761.

71. Konopad E, Noseworthy T, Johnston R, Shustack A, Grace M. Quality of life measures before and one year after admission to an intensive care unit. Crit Care Med 1995; 23(10):1653–1659.

72. Bams JL, Miranda DR. Outcome and costs of intensive care. Intensive Care Med 1985; 11:234–241.

73. Mahul P, Perrot D, Tempelhoff G, Gaussorgues P, Jospe R, Ducreux J, et al. Short- and long-term prognosis, functional outcome following ICU for elderly. Intensive Care Med 1991; 17:7–10.

74. Thoner J. Outcome and costs of intensive care. A follow-up study on patients requiring prolonged mechanical ventilation. Anaesthesiol Scand 1987; 31:693–698.

75. Tian Z, Miranda DR. Quality of life after intensive care with the sickness impact profile. Intensive Care Med 1995; 21:422–428.

76. Schelling G, Stoll C, Haller M, Briegel J, et al. Health related quality of life and posttraumatic stress disorder in survivors of the acute respiratory distress syndrome. Crit Care Med 1998; 26:651–659.

77. Davidson TA, Rubenfeld GD, Caldwell ES, Hudson LD, Steinberg KP. The effect of acute respiratory distress syndrome on long-term survival. AJRCCM 1999; 160:1838.

78. Macnaughton PD, Evans TW. Lung function in ARDS. AJRCCM 1995; 150:770–775.
79. Wright PE, Bernard GR. The role of airflow resistance in patients with the adult respiratory distress syndrome. Am Rev Respir Dis 1989; 139:1169–1174.
80. Ghio AJ, Elliott CG, Crapo RO, et al. Impairment after adult respiratory distress syndrome. Am Rev Respir Dis 1989; 139:1158–1162.
81. Elliott CG, Rasmusson BY, Crapo RO, et al. Prediction of pulmonary function abnormalities after adult respiratory distress syndrome. Am Rev Respir Dis 1987; 135:634–638.
82. Suchyta MR, Elliott CG, Colby T, et al. Open lung biopsy does not correlate with pulmonary function after the adult respiratory distress syndrome. Chest 1991; 99: 1232–1237.
83. Hulsebos R, Beltman F, dos Reis Miranda DR, Spangenberg JF. Measuring quality of life with the sickness impact profile: a pilot study. Intensive Care Med 1991; 17:285–288.
84. Kerridge R, Glasziou P, Hillman KM. The use of "quality-adjusted life years" (QALYs) to evaluate treatment in intensive care. Anaesth Intens Care 1995; 23: 322–331.
85. Rogers J, Ridley S, Chrispin P, Scotton H, Lloyd D. Reliability of the next of kins' estimates of critically ill patients' quality of life. Anaesthesia 1997; 52:1137–1143.
86. McHugh LG, Milberg JA, Whitcomb ME, Schoene RB, Maunder RJ, Hudson LD. Recovery of function in survivors of the acute respiratory distress syndrome. AJRCCM 1994; 150:90–94.
87. Weinert CR, Gross CR, Kangas JR, Bury CL, Marinelli WA. Health related quality of life after acute lung injury. AJRCCM 1997; 156:1120–1128.
88. Davidson T, Caldwell ES, Curtis J, Hudson L, Steinberg KP. Reduced quality of life in survivors of acute respiratory distress syndrome compared with critically ill control patients. JAMA 1999; 281(4):254–360.
89. Chen JC, Manino DM. Worldwide epidemiology of chronic obstructive pulmonary disease. Curr Opin Pulm Med 1999; 4:93–99.
90. Morano MA. Current estimates from the National Health Interview Survey. Washington, DC: National Center for Health Statistics, U.S. Government Printing Office, 1994.
91. Ventura SJ, Peters KD, Martin JA, Maurer JD. Births and Deaths, United States. Hyattsville, MD: National Center for Health Statistics, 1996.
92. Morbidity and Mortality: 1996 Chartbook on Cardiovascular, Lung, and Blood Diseases. Bethesda, MD: National Heart, Lung, and Blood Institute, 1996.
93. Bott J, Carroll MP, Conway JH, et al. Randomised controlled trial of nasal ventilation in acute ventilatory failure due to chronic obstructive airways disease. Lancet 1993; 341:1555–1557.
94. Angus RM, Ahmed AA, Fenwick LJ, Peacock AJ. Comparison of the acute effects on gas exchange of nasal ventilation and doxapram in exacerbations of chronic obstructive pulmonary disease. Thorax 1996; 51:1048–1050.
95. Weiss SM, Hudson LD. Outcome from respiratory failure. Crit Care Clin 1994; 10:197–215.

96. Asmundssen T, Kilburn KH. Survival of acute respiratory failure: a study of 239 episodes. Ann Intern Med 1969; 70:471.
97. Bone RC, Pierce AK, Johnson RL. Controlled oxygen administration in acute respiratory failure in chronic obstructive pulmonary disease: a reappraisal. Am J Med 1978; 65:896.
98. Burk RH, George RB. Acute respiratory failure in chronic obstructive pulmonary disease: immediate and long-term prognosis. Arch Intern Med 1973; 132:865.
99. Jeffrey AA, Warren PM, Flenley DC. Acute hypercapnic respiratory failure in patients with chronic obstructive lung disease: risk factors and use of guidelines for management. Thorax 1992; 47:34.
100. Kettel LJ. The management of acute ventilatory failure in chronic obstructive lung disease. Med Clin North Am 1973; 57:781.
101. Martin TR, Lewis SW, Albert RK. The prognosis of patients with chronic obstructive pulmonary disease after hospitalization for acute respiratory failure. Chest 1982; 82:310–314.
102. Moser KM, Shebel EM, Deamon AJ. Acute respiratory failure in obstructive lung disease: long-term survival after treatment in an intensive care unit. JAMA 1973; 225:705.
103. Portier F, Defouilloy C, Muir JF, et al. Determinants of immediate survival among chronic respiratory insufficiency patients admitted to intensive care unit for acute respiratory failure: a prospective multicenter study. Chest 1992; 101:204–210.
104. Seriff NS, Khan F, Lazo BJ. Acute respiratory failure: current concepts of pathophysiology and management. Med Clin North Am 1973; 57:1539.
105. Sluiter HJ, Blokzyl EJ, van Dijl W, et al. Conservative and respiratory treatment of acute respiratory insufficiency in patients with chronic obstructive lung disease: a reappraisal. Am Rev Respir Dis 1972; 105:932.
106. Vandenbergh E, van de Woestijne KP, Gyesin A. Conservative treatment of acute respiratory failure in patients with chronic obstructive lung disease. Am Rev Respir Dis 1968; 98:60.
107. Avdeev SN, Tret'iakov AV, Grigor'iants RA, Kutsenko MA, Churalin AG. Study of the use of noninvasive ventilation of the lungs in acute respiratory insufficiency due to exacerbation of chronic obstructive pulmonary disease. Anesteziol Reanimatol 1998; 3(May-Jun):45–51.
108. Brochard L, Mancebo J, Wysocki M, et al. Noninvasive ventilation for acute exacerbations of chronic obstructive pulmonary disease. N Engl J Med 1995; 333:817–822.
109. Celikel T, Sungur M, Ceyhan B, Karakut S. Comparison of noninvasive positive pressure ventilation with standard medical therapy in hypercapnic acute respiratory failure. Chest 1998; 114:1636–1642.
110. Conners AF, Dawson NV, Thomas C, et al. Outcomes following acute exacerbation of severe chronic obstructive lung disease. Am J Respir Crit Care Med 1996; 154:959–967.
111. Fuso L, Incalzi RA, Pistelli ET, et al. Predicting mortality of patients hospitalized for acutely exacerbated chronic obstructive pulmonary disease. Am J Med 1995; 98:272–277.
112. Kramer N, Meyer TJ, Meharg J, Cece RD, Hill NS. Randomized, prospective trial

of noninvasive positive pressure ventilation in acute respiratory failure. AJRCCM 1995; 151:1799–1806.

113. Menzies R, Gibbons W, Goldberg P. Determinants of weaning and survival among patients with COPD who require mechanical ventilation for acute respiratory failure. Chest 1989; 95:398–405.

114. Rieves RD, Bass D, Carter RR, Griffith JE, Norman JR. Severe COPD and acute respiratory failure: correlates for survival at the time of tracheal intubation. Chest 1993; 104:854–860.

115. Seneff MG, Wagner DP, Wagner RP, Zimmerman JE, Knaus WA. Hospital and 1-year survival of patients admitted to intensive care units with acute exacerbation of chronic obstructive pulmonary disease. JAMA 1995; 274:1852–1857.

116. Vitacca M, Clini E, Porta R, Foglio K, Ambrosino N. Acute exacerbations in patients with COPD: predictors of need for mechanical ventilation. Eur Respir J 1996; 9:1487–1493.

117. Vitacca M, Clini E, Rubini F, Nava S, Foglio K, Ambrosino N. Non-invasive mechanical ventilation in severe chronic obstructive lung disease and acute respiratory failure: short- and long-term prognosis. Intensive Care Med 1996; 22:94–100.

118. Costello R, Deegan P, Fitzpatrick M, McNicholas WT. Reversible hypercapnia in chronic obstructive pulmonary disease: a distinct pattern of respiratory failure with a favorable prognosis. Am J Med 1997; 103:239–244.

119. Gottieb LS, Balchum OJ. Course of chronic obstructive pulmonary disease following first onset of respiratory failure. Chest 1973; 63:5–8.

120. Confalonieri M, Parigi P, Scartabellati A, Aiolfi S, Scorsetti S, Nava S, et al. Noninvasive mechanical ventilation improves the immediate and long-term outcome of COPD patients with acute respiratory failure. Eur Respir J 1996; 9:422–430.

121. Cydulka RK, McFadden ER, Emerman CL, Sivinski LD, Pisanelli W, Rimm AA. Patterns of hospitalization in elderly patients with asthma and chronic obstructive pulmonary disease. Am J Respir Crit Care Med 1997; 157:1418–1422.

122. Seemungal TAR, Donaldson GC, Paul EA, Bestall JC, Jeffries DJ, Wedzicha JA. Effect of exacerbation on quality of life in patients with chronic obstructive pulmonary disease. Am J Respir Crit Care Med 1998; 157:1418–1422.

123. Prendergast TJ, Luce JM. Increasing incidence of withholding and withdrawal of life support from the critically ill. Am J Respir Crit Care Med 1997; 155:15–20.

124. Prendergast TJ, Claessens MT, Luce JM. A national survey of end-of-life care for critically ill patients. Am J Respir Crit Care Med 1998; 158:1163–1167.

125. Keenan SP, Busche KD, Chen LM, Esmail R, Inman KJ, Sibbald WJ. Withdrawal and withholding of life support in the intensive care unit: a comparison of teaching and community hospitals. Crit Care Med 1998; 26:245–251.

126. Sullivan KE, Hebert PC, Logan J, O'Connor AM, McNeely PD. What do physicians tell patients with end-stage COPD about intubation and mechanical ventilation? Chest 1996; 109:258–264.

127. McNeely PD, Hebert PC, Dales RE, O'Connor AM, Wells G, McKim D, et al. Deciding about mechanical ventilation in end-stage chronic obstructive pulmonary disease: how respirologists perceive their role. CMAJ 1997; 156:177–183.

2

Evolution of the Modern Mechanical Ventilator

NEIL MacINTYRE

Duke University
Durham, North Carolina

I. Evolution of the Concepts Underlying Mechanical Ventilation

Since ancient times the movement of air in and out of the chest was known to be necessary for life. Indeed, the concept of mouth-to-mouth resuscitative maneuvers appears in numerous biblical passages (1). The importance of a patent airway to allow air into the chest has also been known for thousands of years, and the concept of a tracheotomy to bypass an upper airway obstruction was recorded in ancient writings as old as 2000 BC (2). One particularly dramatic account is that of Alexander the Great performing a tracheotomy with his sword to save the life of a soldier with an upper airway injury in 400 BC.

An understanding of the physiology of ventilation and respiration, however, did not start to develop until the sixteenth century (3). Vesalius, Servetus, and others first introduced the concept that the air in the lungs exchanged substances with the blood in the lungs (4,5). When Harvey subsequently described blood flow in the seventeenth century, the idea took hold that ventilation eliminated body wastes delivered to the lungs by the blood (6). Malpighii and Borelli followed this with the concept that gaseous substances diffused across the alveolar/capillary interface (2,7).

37

In the eighteenth century, the chemical makeup of ventilated air was discovered. Black first described CO_2 as the body's "waste" gas (2,8,9), and Priestly followed with his description of oxygen as the air substance necessary for life (2,8,10). Lavoisier and LaPlace then equated combustion (oxygen plus substrate yields heat plus CO_2) with body metabolism (2,4,8).

In the nineteenth century, hemoglobin was described as the blood's oxygen transport substance by Hoppe-Seyler (11). With Bert's concept that ventilation was proportional to oxygen and CO_2 transport near the end of the century (10), all of the necessary physiological foundations were in place to permit the development of the modern mechanical ventilator.

II. Devices Used for Resuscitation

Even though respiratory physiology was not well understood, mechanical devices to provide positive lung pressure to prevent lung collapse during animal vivisection were first described in the sixteenth century (12,13). Not long thereafter,

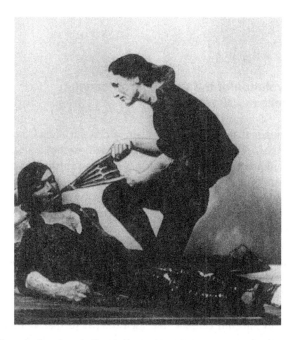

Figure 1   Use of a fireplace bellows to supply positive pressure breaths into the airway in the 16th century. (From the American Heart Association Basic/Advanced Life Support Manual, Dallas, TX.)

mechanical devices to provide ventilation in resuscitative efforts in humans were also described (2,13–16). The earliest devices were bellows systems with simple attachments to insert in the mouth/nose (Fig. 1). By the eighteenth century, however, tracheal intubation was described by Cullen, Chausier, and others, and a variety of positive pressure generators mimicking the normal human ventilatory pattern were being utilized (17,18). Indeed, the Royal Humane Society actually sponsored competitions for novel techniques to resuscitate the drowned (2,19).

In the early nineteenth century, concerns about pneumothorax from positive pressure systems stimulated the development of negative pressure systems. Dalziel first described an air-tight box enclosing the patient up to the neck which could ventilate subjects through a bellows attached to the box (20). This was followed by other box systems with bellows powered by steam engines and even "respirator rooms" by the turn of the twentieth century (Fig. 2) (21,22).

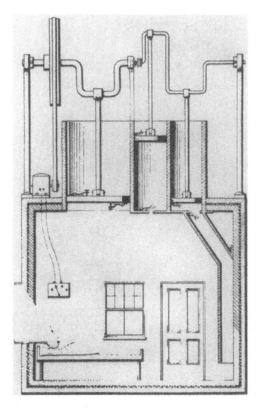

Figure 2 A negative pressure "respirator room" patented by Lord in 1908. (From Ref. 30.)

III. Devices Used for Ventilatory Support of Healthy Lungs

The use of mechanical ventilation for conditions other than merely resuscitation was driven by two developments: the development of anesthesia in the mid-nineteenth century and the polio epidemics of the early twentieth century.

Inhalational anesthesia was introduced in the mid-nineteenth century (23,24), and it immediately became apparent that ventilatory support was going to be needed during deep anesthesia and thoracic surgery. McEwan first used the endotracheal tube to administer anesthesia (25), and subsequently Fell and O'Dwyer developed an endotracheal tube insufflation system for both anesthesia administration and ventilatory support (Fig. 3) (26,27). By the beginning of the twentieth century, cuffed endotracheal tubes were being used and a number of

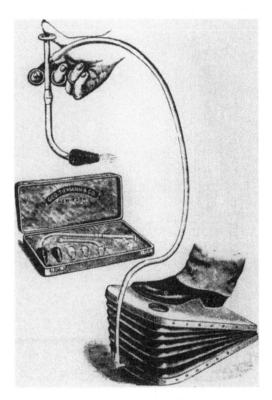

Figure 3 The Fell-O'Dwyer device as modified by Mathas for delivering anesthesia. (Reprinted with permission from Mathas R. Artificial respiration by direct intralaryngeal intubation with a modified O'Dwyer tube and new graduated air pump. Am Med 1902; 3:97–103.)

manual, gas-powered, and electrically powered positive pressure systems that had been developed for animal physiology experiments [e.g., Bowditch's animal positive pressure ventilator (28)] were being adapted for human use in the operating room. In general, these devices attempted to mimic the normal ventilatory pattern and some could supply supplemental oxygen.

Several polio epidemics in the early twentieth century produced a large number of patients with neuromuscular ventilatory failure (29). In many of these patients, it was learned that ventilatory support for various periods of time could "buy time" for the neuromuscular system to recover. Negative pressure systems developed by Drinker, Shaw, and Emerson provided such support and saved countless lives (20–22,30). Positive pressure systems were also employed, although artificial airway management made this approach difficult. Nevertheless, the concept that mechanical devices mimicking the normal ventilatory pattern could support ventilatory function in otherwise normal lungs was now apparent.

IV. Devices Designed for Respiratory Support of Diseased Lungs—The Modern Era

Mechanical support of neuromuscular ventilatory failure had clearly been shown to be effective by the early twentieth century. Over the next 100 years, a number of important developments expanded this capability to support respiratory function in even the most severe forms of respiratory failure. Among the most important milestones are the following:

Early Twentieth Century: In 1909 Emerson introduced the concept of using ventilatory support to manage lung edema (31). Twenty-nine years later, Barach described the use of positive pressure ventilation to treat cardiogenic pulmonary edema (32). These were the first attempts to manage a gas exchange problem as well as a ventilation problem with positive airway pressure. Although not yet fully understood, the concept of using positive airway pressure to provide more than simple ventilation (i.e., alveolar recruitment and manipulation of ventilation distribution to perfused areas) originated in these early twentieth-century experiences.

1940s: Although it had been long known that positive pressure ventilation could impair cardiac performance, it wasn't until Cournand and others demonstrated the importance of elevated intrathoracic pressures in compromising cardiac filling (33) that the physiology of heart-lung interactions was appreciated. Subsequent studies throughout the last half of the twentieth century (34) demonstrated the importance of mean airway pressure, spontaneous breaths (which lower intrathoracic pressures), and fluid resuscitation in monitoring and managing cardiac function during positive pressure ventilation.

Barach and others during World War II developed pneumatic valving systems that could be used for high-altitude combat flight as well as for anesthesia use and ventilatory support (Fig. 4) (35–37). These simple systems, when attached to a high-pressure gas source, subsequently provided life support in countless field hospitals throughout the world. As such, they represented the first mass-produced, easy-to-use, and reliable mechanical ventilator.

1950s: Morch and Engstrom develop the first true volume-targeted ventilators, primarily for operating room use (38,39). These were piston-based devices that guaranteed a certain tidal volume delivery. Clinicians outside the operating room initially welcomed these devices as a way of controlling minute ventilation in patients with respiratory failure. Indeed, manufacturers would advertise the "power" of their machine by quantifying how much pressure it could generate to assure ventilation in even the sickest of lungs. Ironically, it was not until some 40 years later that it became apparent that guaranteeing a minute volume at the expense of very high pressures and volumes may have done more harm than good in some patients (see below).

Astrup and Radford introduced the concept of using arterial blood gases to guide support (40,41). Reliable O_2 and CO_2 electrodes developed by Clark and

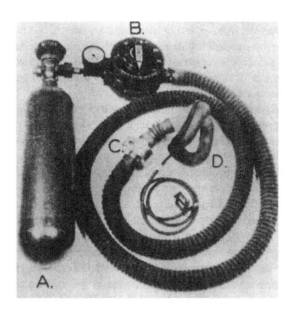

Figure 4 An intermittent positive pressure breathing device used by Motley in 1948. A, oxygen supply; B, regulator; C, exhalation valve; D, mask. (Reprinted with permission from Motley JL, et al. Intermittent positive pressure breathing. JAMA 1948; 137:371–376.)

Severinghaus had only recently been developed (42,43). These could now be used to assess efficacy of support instead of relying simply on clinical observations and assessment of delivered pressure and volume. Indeed, "normalization" of blood gases became an important clinical goal and was the basis for a number of support strategies. As noted above, however, it wasn't until many years later that it became apparent that a "normal" blood gas may not always be desirable if it requires the delivery of excessive pressures or volumes.

Extracorporeal membrane oxygenation (ECMO) was first used for cardiopulmonary bypass during open heart surgery (44). Adaptations of this technique have been tried in severe forms of respiratory failure since the mid-1960s. Outcomes of severe respiratory failure patients treated with ECMO, however, have never been shown to be better than with conventional strategies. Thus, this expensive approach to respiratory support has never been widely adopted (45). An interesting adaptation of ECMO is the intravascular oxygen catheter, introduced during the late 1980s. This device was actually an "intracorporeal membrane oxygenator" with long oxygen-filled fibrils that were implanted into the great veins and provided oxygen through diffusion (46). Technical complications, however, presented the full clinical implementation of the device.

The American Standards Association (later the American National Standards Institute) established the Z79 committee, which is charged with setting performance standards for positive pressure ventilators. This provided a necessary set of engineering definitions and testing protocols to quantify performance capabilities and to assess innovations. The Z79 later evolved into the American Society for Testing Materials F79 committee and was joined by the International Standards Organization in 1967. Definitions and performance standards set by these organizations remain in effect today.

Frumin showed that elevated positive end-expiratory pressure (PEEP) improves oxygenation in infiltrative lung disease (47). This was a critical development because it was the first time that clinicians appreciated the concept that positive pressure could be used to prevent alveolar collapse (derecruitment) at the end of a positive pressure breath. The subsequent description of the acute respiratory distress syndrome by Ashbaugh and Petty in 1967 emphasized the importance of PEEP in maintaining gas exchange in diffuse lung injury (48).

1960s: Munch observed that obstructive as well as infiltrative lung disease could be supported by positive pressure ventilation through an artificial airway (49). Widespread use of positive pressure ventilatory support for asthma and COPD "flares" subsequently followed. Interestingly, it was in this patient population that the concept first developed that a target of a "normal" Pco_2 could be sacrificed if it protected the lung from very high pressures and barotrauma risk ("permissive hypercapnia").

Burton and others emphasized that inspired gases during anesthesia need to be heated and humidified in order to avoid mucosal injury (50). Initially, this was done by active heating/humidification systems that subsequently attempted to bring inspired gases to body temperature with 100% relative humidity. However, by the 1980s simple heat- and moisture-exchange devices that delivered somewhat lower heat and humidity were also shown to be effective in patients requiring short-term support (51).

Suter introduced the concept that optimal ventilator settings ought to be those that produce the best compliance (52). This was an important recognition that lung mechanics could be used to describe when the lung was adequately recruited and not overdistended.

Although the concept of tissue injury from hyperoxia had been appreciated previously (10), the concept of oxygen toxicity in mechanically ventilated patients did not emerge as an important issue until this time (53). Ventilator strategies become focused on reducing oxygen exposure and subsequent controversy developed over the proper balance of Po_2, PEEP, and Fio_2. Even now at the end of the twentieth century, there is still uncertainty as to what a "safe" level of Fio_2 is.

Linton reported that nosocomial pneumonias can be caused by ventilator equipment (54). Indeed, nosocomial pneumonias became recognized as a major complication of mechanical ventilation, responsible for both increased morbidity and prolongation of the need for ventilatory support. Subsequent reports illustrated the importance of handwashing, ventilator circuit integrity, subglottic suctioning, and aggressive weaning in reducing the risk of ventilator associated pneumonia (55).

1970s: The idea of using "nonphysiological" ventilatory patterns in severe respiratory failure emerged on two fronts. First, the idea of using long inspiratory time patterns (i.e., "reverse ratio" ventilation, or IRV) to improve gas mixing and limit maximal airway pressure was introduced (56). Second, the first commercially available high-frequency ventilators (HFV) were introduced (57). HFV generated considerable interest because of its unique nonconvective gas transport mechanism that offers the opportunity to provide lung recruitment at low maximal pressures. HFV was subsequently shown to be beneficial in neonates/pediatric patients at risk for overdistension injury, but adult data are still lacking.

Webb and Tierney dramatically illustrated in an animal model that overdistension and underrecruitment during positive pressure ventilation can produce severe lung injury (Fig. 5) (58). Clinicians began to appreciate the fact that endpoints other than "normal blood gases" (e.g., lung mechanics) may be important in setting up optimal ventilator parameters.

The ability to have patients trigger ventilator breaths through airway pressure sensing was developed. Patients no longer needed to be sedated (or paralyzed) to receive ventilator breaths. The ability to have patients breathe spontaneously between machine breaths (so-called intermittent mandatory ventilation) was also introduced as a way of enhancing patient-ventilator interactions (59).

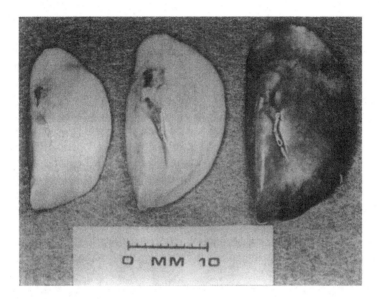

Figure 5 Lung injury induced by excessive ventilatory pressures in a rat model. The lung on the left received normal ventilatory pressures, the lung on the right received ventilatory pressures exceeding normal maximal transpulmonary pressures, the lung in the middle also received excessive ventilatory pressures but also received PEEP. Note the severe injury induced by excessive pressures and how it can be attenuated with PEEP application. (From Ref. 58.)

Surfactant installation through the endotracheal tube was shown to improve the ability of mechanical ventilation to provide safe levels of ventilatory support in the premature neonate with surfactant depletion (60). Surfactant replacement, however, was less successful in adult lung disease (61), perhaps related to problems in delivery of the material and to the fact that surfactant-related proteins are probably needed along with the surface active properties of the phospholipids.

1980s: The concept of synchronizing patient effort and ventilator support throughout inspiration was developed as pressure-targeted variable flow capabilities were introduced to enhance patient-triggered breaths (62). The goal was to improve patient comfort (thereby reducing sedation needs) and normalize muscle loads in patients with spontaneous breathing efforts. Pressure support and pressure assist became widely used, and proportional assist ventilation (a similar concept that utilizes a flow and volume gain setting on sensed effort) was developed during the late 1980s (63).

The microprocessor was widely incorporated into mechanical ventilators. This permitted a number of gas-delivery patterns, patient-ventilator interactive features, and graphical monitoring capabilities. Interest in ventilatory muscle function and the role of partial ventilatory support in managing recovering muscle abnormalities developed as a consequence (64). Interestingly, clinicians today are still grappling with the ideal way to utilize the vast array of management options made available by the microprocessor for both total and partial ventilatory support.

The use of mask positive pressure systems was reintroduced (65). Clinical trials showing success of this noninvasive form of support appeared first for obstructive sleep apnea and later for acute exacerbations of obstructive airway disease. By the 1990s, additional reports suggested utility of mask ventilation in other forms of respiratory failure and perhaps in allowing earlier extubation.

1990s: Several large trials were published addressing the proper way to "wean" patients from the ventilator (66–69). The concept emerged that daily assessments for ventilator withdrawal are important in facilitating this process in patients recovering from respiratory failure. Protocols to allow skilled nonphysicians (e.g., respiratory therapists) to do this routinely show dramatic reductions in ventilator days (70).

A resurgence of interest in ventilator-induced lung injury developed. Numerous animal models underscore the importance of both underrecruitment and overdistension in producing lung injury (71). The potential for an injured lung to liberate inflammatory cytokines into the circulation and cause multiorgan failure is also recognized (71). In 1998, Amato reports a significant reduction in mortality if the ventilator management strategy is aimed at maximizing recruitment and minimizing end inspiratory distension (72). This is followed by the U.S. National Institutes of Health (NIH) ARDS Network reporting a significant reduction in ARDS mortality in 841 patients if the ventilator strategy is aimed at reducing maximal distension (73).

V. Mechanical Ventilation—Current Status

Today there are an estimated 100,000 positive pressure ventilators in use worldwide. In the United States alone, an estimated 1.5–2.5 million patients receive mechanical ventilation outside of the operating room/recovery room per year. In the acute care setting, the average length of mechanical ventilation is 6–8 days, although this is heavily dependent on why mechanical ventilation is required (74).

The costs associated with mechanical ventilation today are substantial. The devices themselves can cost $30,000–$40,000 when fully equipped with a powerful microprocessor, sophisticated valving systems, and extensive monitoring capabilities. Proper maintenance can result in a device life span of 10 years or more. Supplies include circuitry, heat/humidification systems, suction catheters, and aerosol delivery systems. Ventilator management requires well-trained professionals who are most cost-effective when operating under management protocols. Finally, costs of complications (i.e., barotrauma, cardiac compromise, and infection) must be recognized as well.

VI. Mechanical Ventilation—Challenges for the Future

Several trends will emerge in the evolution of the mechanical ventilator over the next decade (74). First, the need for mechanical ventilation is likely to grow substantially. The aging population and the aggressiveness of medical/surgical therapies will create an increasing requirement for mechanical ventilatory support. Second, a greater attention to iatrogenic injury will develop. More focus will be placed on reducing lung injury, improving patient comfort (thereby reducing sedation needs), reducing infections, and shortening unnecessarily prolonged support in the patient recovering from respiratory failure. Third, adjuncts to improve gas exchange and reduce complications are likely to emerge. Possible examples include fluorocarbons for "liquid PEEP," nitric oxide, and antioxidants to reduce lung injury. Fourth, the venue and the personnel required for mechanical ventilation will shift to less costly models. Long-term ventilator units and respiratory care professionals operating under medically directed protocols are already emerging. Finally, the devices themselves are likely to become less costly to own and operate as microprocessor technology improves and computer-driven management algorithms are developed.

Careful and formal assessments of innovations in mechanical ventilation for safety, efficacy, and cost-effectiveness will become increasingly important in the future (75). This is because traditional mechanisms for assessing innovations, so-called market forces, can no longer be considered a reliable way of assessing the complex interactions of efficacy/safety/costs in an increasingly expensive health care system.

Future mechanical ventilation innovations will come both from new engineering designs as well as from new applications of existing designs. Benefits of these innovations will be of three general types or "levels":

1. An engineering benefit means that the innovation improves technical performance, ease of operation, or cost of operation.
2. A physiological benefit means that the innovation improves a physiological parameter such as gas exchange or patient work.
3. An outcome benefit means that the innovation improves an important clinical outcome.

Assessing an engineering benefit is the easiest and cheapest assessment, as it only requires an engineering or a user preference analysis. Assessing a physiological benefit is more costly and usually requires human subjects in the analysis.

| | | Incremental Cost Increase (Payer Issues) | | |
		Minor	Moderate	Major
Incremental	Minor	Level I	Level II	Level III
Risk Increase (Regulatory/	Moderate	Level II	Level II	Level III
Clinician Issues)	Major	Level III	Level III	Level III

Figure 6 Proposed scheme for efficacy assessment based on risk and cost. Level I = engineering endpoints; Level II = physiological (intermediate) endpoints; Level III = clinical outcome endpoints.

The clinical outcome study is the most complex and expensive because it generally requires a large-scale randomized clinical trial.

The type or ''level'' of benefit required of an innovation (and the accompanying assessment requirements) depends on two important factors: the incremental risk of the innovation and the incremental cost of the innovation. Clinicians and regulators are particularly concerned about the incremental risks. Specifically, the higher the potential risk of the innovation, the greater the need for proof of an outcome benefit through an appropriate risk-benefit outcome assessment. On the other hand, payers are particularly concerned about the cost of the innovation. From this perspective, the higher the cost of the innovation, the greater the need for proof of an outcome benefit through an appropriate cost-benefit outcome assessment (Fig. 6) (75). Payers often do not even consider an innovation until risk-benefit issues have been judged favorable. Indeed, it is their subsequent cost-benefit assessment that may well determine the innovation's reimbursement potential and, ultimately, the likelihood that it will be used.

VII. Conclusion

Mechanical ventilation is certainly not a new idea. Indeed, the importance of delivering fresh air to the chest and removing stale air from it has been known since antiquity. However, only over the last 500 years have the physiological principles underlying ventilation, gas exchange, and metabolism been understood. Moreover, it has been primarily during the twentieth century that the modern positive pressure mechanical ventilation has evolved. As we enter the next millennium, a number of important challenges confront us. Innovations in ventilatory/respiratory support are clearly going to be needed, and appropriate processes to evaluate such innovations will be critical.

References

1. Book of Ecclesiastics, St. James version of the Bible.
2. Smith JC. Historical Perspective on the Development of Mechanical Ventilation. In: Tobin M, ed. Principles and Practice of Mechanical Ventilation. Philadelphia: WB Saunders, 1995.
3. Perkins JF. Historical development of respiratory physiology. In: Fenn WO, Rahn H, eds. Handbook of Physiology. Washington, DC: American Physiological Society, 1964: 1–62.
4. Vesalius A. The Epitome. Lind LR, trans. New York: Macmillan, 1949.
5. Servetus M. The Restoration of Christianity. O'Malley CD, trans. Philadelphia: American Philosophical Society, 1953.
6. Harvey W. Anatomical studies on the motion of the heart and blood in animals. Leake CD, trans. Springfield, IL: Charles C Thomas, 1941.
7. Graubard M. Circulation and Respiration. New York: Harcourt, Brace & World, 1964.
8. Astrup P, Severinghaus JW. The History of Blood Gases, Acids and Bases. Copenhagen: Munksgaard, 1986.
9. Boyle R. New pneumatical experiments about respiration. Phil Trans R Soc London 1670; 5:2011–2058.
10. Bert P. Barometric pressure. Hitchcock MA, Hitchcock FA, trans. Columbus, OH: College Book, 1943.
11. Hoppe-Seyler F. Über die Oxidation im lebenden Blute. Med Chem Unters 1866–1871; 132:1–4.
12. Vesalius A. De Humani Corporis Fabrica. Basel: Oporinus, 1543.
13. Baker AB. Artificial respiration, the history of an idea. Med Hist 1971; 15:336–351.
14. Morch ET. History of mechanical ventilation. In: Kirby RR, Smith RA, Desautels DA, eds. Mechanical Ventilation. New York: Churchill Livingstone, 1985:1–58.
15. Highmore N. Corporis Humani Disquisition Anatomica. The Hague: Comitis S Brown, 1651.
16. Fothergill J. Observations on a case published in the last volume of medical essays. Philos Trans R Soc London 1745; 43:378.
17. Cullen W. A letter to Lord Cathcart: concerning the recovery of persons drowned and seemingly dead. Edinburgh: 1776:1–41.
18. McClellan I. Nineteenth century resuscitation apparatus. Anaesthesia 1981; 36:307–311.
19. Lee RV. Cardiopulmonary resuscitation in the eighteenth century. J Hist Med 1972; 27:418–433.

20. Dalzeil J. On sleep and an apparatus for promoting artificial respiration. Br Assoc Adv Sci 1838; 2:127.
21. Woollam CHM. The development of apparatus for intermittent negative pressure respiration 1919–1976. Anaesthesia 1976; 31:666–685.
22. Drinker P, Shaw LA. An apparatus for the prolonged administration of artificial respiration. J Clin Invest 1929; 7:229–247.
23. Warren JC. Inhalation of ethereal vapor for the prevention of pain in surgical operations. Boston Med Surg J 1846; 35:375–379.
24. Gillespie NA. The evolution of endotracheal anesthesia. J Hist Med 1946; 1:583–594.
25. MacEwen W. Clinical observations on the introduction of tracheal tubes by the mouth instead of performing tracheostomy of laryngotomy. Br Med J 1880; 2:122–124, 163–165.
26. Fell GE. Forced respiration. JAMA 1891; 16:325–330.
27. O'Dwyer J. Intubation of the larynx. NY Med J 1885; 42:145.
28. Bowditch HP. Physiological apparatus in use at the Harvard Medical School. J Physiol 1879–1880; 2:202–205.
29. Lassen HCA. A preliminary report on the 1952 epidemic of poliomyelitis in Copenhagen with special reference to the treatment of acute respiratory insufficiency. Lancet 1953; i:37–40.
30. Emerson JH. The Evolution of Iron Lungs. Cambridge: JH Emerson, 1978.
31. Emerson H. Artificial respiration in the treatment of edema of the lungs. Arch Intern Med 1909; 3:368–371.
32. Barach AL, Martin J, Eckman M. Positive pressure respiration and its application to the treatment of acute pulmonary edema. Ann Intern Med 1938; 17:754–795.
33. Cournand A, Motley HL, Werko L, Richards DW. Physiological studies of the effects of intermittent positive pressure breathing on cardiac output in man. Am J Physiol 1947; 152:162–174.
34. Miro AM, Pinsky MR. Heart-lung interactions. In: Tobin M, ed. Principles and Practice of Mechanical Ventilation. New York: McGraw-Hill, 1994:647–672.
35. Barach AL, Fenn WO, Ferris EB, Schmidt CF. The physiology of pressure breathing. J Aviat Med 1947; 18:73–86.
36. Eckman J, Barach B, Fox C, Rumsey CC, Somkin E, Barach AL. An appraisal of intermittent pressure breathing as a method of increasing altitude tolerance. J Aviat Med 1947; 18:565–574.
37. Motley HL, Werko L, Cournand A, Richards DW. Observations on the clinical use of intermittent positive pressure. J Aviat Med 1947; 18:417–435.
38. Morch ET, Saxton GA, Gish G. Artificial respiration via the uncuffed tracheostomy tube. JAMA 1956; 160:864–867.
39. Engstrom CG. Treatment of severe cases of respiratory paralysis by the Engstrom universal respirator. Br Med J 1954; 2:666–669.
40. Astrup P, Gotzche H, Neukirch F. Laboratory investigations during treatment of patients with poliomyelitis and respiratory paralysis. Br Med J 1954; 1:780–786.
41. Radfrod EP, Ferris BG, Kriete BC. Clinical use of a nomogram to estimate proper ventilation during artificial respiration. N Engl J Med 1954; 251:879–883.

42. Clark LC. Monitor and control of blood and tissue oxygen tension. Trans Am Soc Artif Intern Organs 1956; 2:41–50.
43. Severinghaus JW, Bradley AF. Electrodes for PO_2 and PCO_2 determinations. J Appl Physiol 1958; 13:515–525.
44. Gibbon JH. Application of a mechanical heart and lung apparatus to cardiac surgery. Minn Med 1954; 37:171–180.
45. NHLBI-NIH. Extracorporeal Support for Respiratory Insufficiency. Bethesda, MD: Dept. Health Education Welfare, 1980.
46. Mortensen JD, Berry G. Conceptual and design features of a practical, clinically effective intravenous mechanical blood oxygen/carbon dioxide exchange device. Int J Artif Organs 1989; 12:384–389.
47. Frumin MJ, Bergman NA, Holaday DA, Rackow H, Salnitre E. Alveolar-arterial O_2 difference during artificial respiration in man. J Appl Physiol 1959; 14:694–700.
48. Ashbaugh DG, Petty TL, Bigelow DB, Harris TM. Continuous positive-pressure breathing (CPPB) in adult respiratory distress syndrome. J Thorac Cardiovasc Surg 1969; 57:31–41.
49. Munck O, Kristensen HS, Lassen HCA. Mechanical ventilation for acute respiratory failure in diffuse chronic lung disease. Lancet 1961; i:66–67.
50. Burton JDK. Effect of dry anesthesia gases on the respiratory mucous membrane. Lancet 1962; 1:235–238.
51. Wilkes AR. Heat and moisture exchangers. Respir Care Clin North Am 1998; 4: 261–280.
52. Suter PM, Fairley B, Isenberg MD. Optimum end expiratory airway pressure in patients with acute pulmonary failure. N Engl J Med 1975; 292:284–289.
53. Balentine JD. Pathology of Oxygen Toxicity. New York: Academic Press, 1982.
54. Linton RC, Walker FW, Spoerel WE. Respirator care in a general hospital: a five-year survey. Can Anaesth Soc J 1965; 12:450–457.
55. Chastre J, Fagon JY. Pneumonia in the ventilator dependent patient. In: Tobin MJ, ed. Principles and Practice of Mechanical Ventilation. New York: McGraw-Hill, 1994:857–890.
56. Marcy T, Marini J. Inverse ratio ventilation: rationale and implementation. Chest 1991; 100:494–504.
57. Drazen JM, Kamin RD, Slutsky AS. High frequency ventilation. Physiol Rev 1984; 64:505–543.
58. Webb HH, Tierney DF. Experimental pulmonary edema due to intermittent positive pressure ventilation with high inflation pressures. Protection by positive end-expiratory pressure. Am Rev Respir Dis 1974; 110:556–565.
59. Downs JB, Perkins HM, Model JH. Intermittent mandatory ventilation. Arch Surg 1974; 109:519–523.
60. Jobe AH. Pulmonary surfactant therapy. N Engl J Med 1993; 328:861–868.
61. Anzueto A, and the Exosurf ARDS Study Group. Aerosolized surfactant in adults with sepsis induced ARDS. N Engl J Med 1996; 334:1417–1421.
62. MacIntyre NR. Respiratory function during pressure support ventilation. Chest 1986; 89:677–683.
63. Younes M. Proportional assist ventilation, a new approach to ventilatory support. Am Rev Respir Dis 1992; 145:114–120.

64. Tobin JM. The respiratory muscles. Prob Respir Care 1990; 3:257–542.
65. Hill NS, Bach JR. Noninvasive mechanical ventilation. Respir Care Clinics North Am 1996; 2:161–347.
66. Esteban A, Frutos F, Tobin JM, Alia I, Solsona JF, et al. A comparison of four methods of weaning patients from mechanical ventilation. Spanish Lung Failure Collaborative Group. N Engl J Med 1995; 332:345–350.
67. Brochard L, Rauss A, Benito S, Conti G, Mancebo J, et al. Comparison of three methods of gradual withdrawal from ventilatory support during weaning from mechanical ventilation. Am J Respir Crit Care Med 1994; 150:896–903.
68. Manthous CA, Schmidt GA, Hall JB. Liberation from mechanical ventilation: a decade of progress. Chest 1998; 114:886–901.
69. Yang KL, Tobin MJ. A prospective study of indexes predicting the outcome of trials of weaning from mechanical ventilation. N Engl J Med 1991; 324:1445–1450.
70. Ely EW, Baker AM, Dunagan DP, Burke HL, Smith AD, et al. Effect on the duration of mechanical ventilation of identifying patients capable of breathing spontaneously. N Engl J Med 1996; 335:1864–1869.
71. Slutsky AS. Lung injury caused by mechanical ventilation. Chest 1999; 116:9S–15S.
72. Amato MB, Barbas CS, Medeiros DM, Magaldi RB, Schettino GP, et al. Effect of a protective-ventilation strategy on mortality in the acute respiratory distress syndrome. N Engl J Med 1998; 338:347–354.
73. NIH ARDS Network. Results of a randomized trial of mechanical ventilation using either 6 ml/kg or 12 ml/kg tidal volumes. American Thoracic Society Meeting, San Diego, CA, April 1999.
74. MacIntyre NR. Mechanical ventilation—the next 50 years. Respir Care 1998; 43:490–493.
75. American Respiratory Care Foundation. Consensus conference on innovations in mechanical ventilation. Respir Care 1995; 40:928–932.

3

Utilization of Mechanical Ventilation for Critical Care
An International Perspective

ANTONIO ANZUETO

University of Texas Health Science Center
San Antonio, Texas

ANDRES ESTEBAN

Hospital Universitario Getafe
Getafe, Spain

I. Introduction

Mechanical ventilation has become the mainstay therapy for patients with respiratory failure. The use of mechanical ventilation has increased in recent years and constitutes a major therapeutic modality in intensive care units (ICUs) (1). However, remarkably little information is available concerning the frequency or appropriateness of mechanical ventilator use in the ICU. New generations of microcomputer-based mechanical ventilators have become available in recent years (2). The physiological basis for these new ventilatory maneuvers has been developed in animal models and small clinical trials. These newer modes have not yet been shown to improve ventilatory capabilities, enhance the efficacy of weaning, or decrease the morbidity or mortality rate associated with mechanical ventilation. Precise data on how many critically ill patients are actually treated with new modes of mechanical ventilation are not available (5).

A Mechanical Ventilation Consensus Conference was recently held in order to understand the beneficial effects and potential complications of mechanical ventilation (4). The American College of Chest Physicians sponsored this conference, which focused on the treatment of patients with acute ventilatory failure and on the principles of ventilation after the decision to initiate mechanical ventilation had been made (4). Because of the lack of well-controlled clinical trials comparing the efficacy of different ventilator modes and settings, the recommendations of this consensus conference were based on the opinion of "individual experts" rather than on concrete data. Furthermore, the lack of large demographic studies characterizing patients receiving mechanical ventilation limited some of the recommendations.

In this review we will summarize the indications for mechanical ventilation, the characteristics of patients receiving mechanical ventilation, the use of available ventilator mode settings and artificial airways, and the methods employed for discontinuation of mechanical ventilation. We are placing emphasis on the experience obtained from international studies.

II. The Use of Mechanical Ventilation

Several investigators have reported the use of mechanical ventilation in the ICU population. Knaus (5), in a multicenter study of 3884 patients in 12 hospitals that were included in the APACHE II database, found that 1886 (49%) received mechanical ventilation during part or all of their ICU stays. It is important to point out that 64% of the ventilated patients were postoperative patients ventilated for one day or less. The investigators did not report what proportion of nonsurgical patients in the ICU received mechanical ventilation. In 1992, the Spanish Lung Failure Collaborative Group conducted a survey of the use of mechanical ventilation (6). The investigators surveyed all patients residing in 47 multidisciplinary ICUs in Spain on a single day. Of the 630 patients in an ICU at the time, 46% received mechanical ventilation for at least 24 hours. A one-day point utilization review was recently reported by Esteban et al. (7). This study involved 412 medical-surgical ICUs and 4153 patients from 8 countries. Of these, 1638 patients or 39% of the total group were receiving mechanical ventilation. These data suggest that one of the major functions of an intensive care unit is to provide a location for the delivery of mechanical ventilation. Despite the different techniques of these studies, they show that at any given time 39–49% of patients in an ICU are receiving mechanical ventilation.

Little is known about regional differences in patients receiving mechanical ventilation. Table 1 shows the demographic characteristics of patients receiving mechanical ventilation in eight countries. The proportion of patients receiving mechanical ventilation varied considerably. This may reflect differences in ICU criteria between countries as well as ICU characteristics. It is important to note that this utilization review collected data at 11:00 a.m. in order to minimize the influence of patients receiving brief ventilatory support following surgery. Despite the differences in ventilator use observed, the mean patient's age and other demographic characteristics were similar between countries.

Table 1 Characteristics of Intensive Care Units and Patients According to Country

	USA/Canada	Spain	Argentina	Brazil	Chile	Portugal	Uruguay	Total
Number of ICUs	167	79	89	25	27	10	15	412
Patients admitted	1833	1028	680	273	160	90	89	4153
Patients ventilated	747	443	154	122	60	68	44	1638
Ventilation (%)[a]	40 (20,60)	39 (27,60)	17 (0,33)	47 (25,50)	40 (20,50)	75 (50,76)	45 (25,86)	36 (17,58)

Results are shown as median (25th, 75th percentiles) or percentage (95% confidence interval).
[a] Median (25th, 75th percentiles).
Source: Adapted from Ref. 7.

A limitation of a utilization review study is that it provides only a snapshot in time and that, in comparison with incidence studies, it may tend to overestimate the problem. For a survey on this scale, follow-up of all missing data was not feasible. Finally, and perhaps most importantly, this survey by questionnaire was unmonitored in the field and relied on the correct use of the predefined criteria. Despite these limitations, the study of Esteban et al. provided an important insight into the current use of mechanical ventilation not only in the United States, but also in other countries.

III. Duration of Mechanical Ventilation: Effect on Morbidity and Mortality

A greater duration of mechanical ventilation has been associated with an increase in morbidity and mortality (Fig. 1). Pranikoff et al. (8) showed that the mortality rate of patients with acute respiratory failure increased with increasing time of mechanical ventilation. For example, the predicted mortality after 5 days of mechanical ventilation was 50% (8). Analysis of the data did not provide information on the effect of ventilator settings such as the level of ventilatory pressures, fraction of inspired oxygen (FIO_2), or the mode of mechanical ventilation, or the impact of associated complications on survival. Whether newer techniques were applied, such as pressure control, high positive end-expiratory pressure (PEEP), PEEP above the lower infection point, or permissive hypercapnia was not known; however, the care reflected the techniques available at the time of the study.

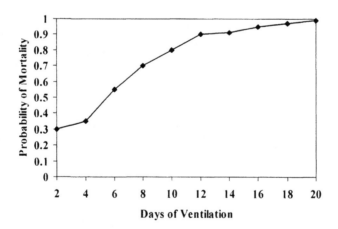

Figure 1   Logistic analysis of probability of mortality during the support with mechanical ventilation. This is from a database of 36 patients who developed acute respiratory failure and was prior to receiving extra life support. (From Ref. 8.)

The underlying condition that precipitates the need for mechanical ventilation may be an important determinant of the duration of ventilation (Fig. 2), and these conditions differ between medical and surgical ICUs. The most frequent reason for the initiation of mechanical ventilation according to Esteban et al. (7) was acute respiratory failure (66%). Acute respiratory failure as a precipitating cause was more common in North America (73%) than in other countries such as Spain, Uruguay, Portugal, and Argentina ($p < 0.001$) (Table 2). Acute respiratory distress syndrome (ARDS) accounted for 12% of patients in acute respiratory failure and 8% of the total study population. The reported incidence by other investigators of ARDS ranges from 1.5 to 8 cases per 100,000 inhabitants (9,10). Of all ICU patients on the day of study, only 3% had ARDS, a rate similar to that of 2% or 3% observed in two retrospective studies (11,12).

Acute exacerbation of chronic lung disease accounted for 13% of all patients receiving mechanical ventilation. The proportion of patients with COPD in this study is markedly higher than in the APACHE III database (13), where only 1% of 17,440 unselected admissions to 42 ICUs received mechanical ventilation because of an acute exacerbation of chronic lung disease. It is important to point out that medical ICUs accounted for only 10% of ICUs in this database (14). Another possible explanation for differences between the databases is that

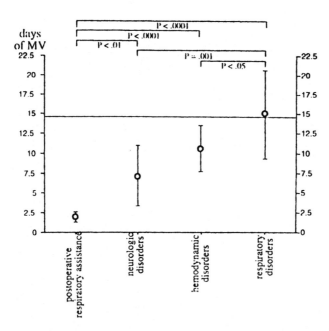

Figure 2 Duration of mechanical ventilation according to etiology. (From Ref. 17.)

Table 2 Indications for the Initiation of Mechanical Ventilation According to Country[a]

	USA/Canada	Spain	Argentina	Brazil	Chile	Portugal	Uruguay	Total
Reason for MV	$n = 747$	$n = 443$	$n = 154$	$n = 122$	$n = 60$	$n = 68$	$n = 44$	$n = 1078$
COPD	16 (13,18)	11 (8,14)	10 (6,16)	9 (5,16)	10 (4,21)	23 (14,36)	5 (1,17)	13 (11,15)
ARF	74 (70,77)	64 (59,68)	50 (42,58)	66 (56,74)	62 (48,74)	47 (35,59)	50 (35,65)	66 (63,68)
Coma	7 (6,9)	20 (17,25)	32 (25,40)	21 (15,30)	15 (7,27)	10 (5,21)	43 (29,59)	15 (13,17)
Neuromuscular	3 (2,5)	4 (3,7)	8 (5,14)	4 (1,10)	13 (6,25)	19 (11,31)	2 (0,13)	5 (4,6)
Cause of ARF	$n = 547$	$n = 283$	$n = 77$	$n = 80$	$n = 37$	$n = 32$	$n = 22$	$n = 1078$
ARDS	9 (7,12)	14 (10,18)	18 (11,29)	11 (6,21)	32 (18,50)	6 (1,22)	14 (4,36)	12 (10,14)
Postoperative	17 (14,21)	13 (10,18)	10 (5,20)	5 (2,13)	5 (1,19)	28 (14,47)	23 (9,46)	15 (13,17)
Heart failure	13 (10,16)	14 (11,19)	16 (9,26)	5 (2,13)	5 (1,19)	16 (6,33)	4 (0,25)	12 (10,14)
Pneumonia	13 (10,16)	18 (13,23)	17 (10,27)	29 (20,40)	19 (3,36)	19 (8,37)	23 (9,46)	16 (14,18)
Sepsis	17 (14,20)	12 (8,16)	19 (12,30)	116 (9,27)	24 (12,42)	12 (4,30)	18 (6,41)	16 (13,18)
Trauma	13 (10,16)	15 (12,20)	3 (0,10)	9 (4,18)	8 (2,23)	12 (4,30)	4 (0,25)	12 (10,14)
Others	16 (13,19)	11 (8,15)	9 (4,18)	16 (9,27)	3 (0,16)	3 (0,18)	—	13 (11,15)

ARF = denotes acute respiratory failure.
[a] Results are shown as percentages (95% confidence interval).
Source: Adapted from Ref. 7.

more patients with acute exacerbation of chronic lung disease are receiving non-invasive ventilation, and mechanical ventilation via an endotracheal tube is the last resource. Neuromuscular disease was an indication for mechanical ventilation in less than 8% of patients in all but two countries (7). The other conditions that led to mechanical ventilation were similar in occurrence between countries (Table 2).

Pathological conditions requiring mechanical ventilation in surgical ICUs differ from those reported in medical ICUs (Table 3). Troche and Moine in France (17) reported that the most frequent reasons that patients in surgical ICUs required postoperative ventilation were the underlying problems of hemodynamic and primary respiratory disorders. It is important to point out that overall duration of ventilatory support was shorter in this patient population.

Several studies have tried to predict the duration of mechanical ventilation. One approach suggested by Ely and collaborators in the United States (15) is the early recognition of reversal of ventilatory failure that may permit prompt discontinuation of mechanical ventilation. These investigators conducted a study of 300 adult patients who received mechanical ventilation in medical and coronary ICUs. In the intervention group, patients underwent daily screening of respiratory function by physicians, respiratory therapists, and nurses to identify those possibly capable of breathing spontaneously. Successful screens were followed by 2-hour trials of spontaneous. Control subjects had a daily screening, but no other interventions. Although the patients randomly assigned to the intervention

Table 3 Pathological Conditions for
Mechanical Ventilation: Surgical ICU

Condition	Number (percentage)
Postoperative ventilation	88 (43%)
Hemodynamic disorders	49 (23%)
Hemorrhagic shock	23
Septic shock	23
Cardiac shock	3
Respiratory disorders	35 (17%)
ARDS	12
Nosocomial pneumonia	8
Fat embolism	6
Pulmonary edema	4
Neurological disorders	31 (15%)
Cerebral ischemia	11
Brain trauma	10
Seizures	5

Source: Adapted from Ref. 17.

group were sicker, they received mechanical ventilation for a median of 4.5 days compared to 6 days in the control group ($p < 0.003$). The investigators concluded that daily screening of respiratory function of those patients receiving mechanical ventilation, followed by a trial of spontaneous breathing in appropriate patients, could reduce the duration of mechanical ventilation and the time of intensive care stay.

Other investigators have looked at easily obtainable parameters that can predict the duration of mechanical ventilation in critically ill patients. Velmahos et al. in the United States (16) prospectively collected data on all critically injured patients receiving mechanical ventilation for more than 2 days in an academic level 1 trauma center. Prolonged mechanical ventilation was defined as the need for mechanical ventilatory support for more than 7 days. Among 119 patients, those requiring prolonged mechanical ventilation had one or more of the following variables: a Swan-Ganz catheter, a severity of injury score of >20, a $Po_2/Fio_2 < 250$, or fluid retention of more than 2 L during the first 48 hours. A score for predicted prolonged mechanical ventilation based on these four variables (0–4 points) was developed. This approach may facilitate planning for personnel allocation as well as important therapeutic procedures if the duration of mechanical ventilation can be accurately predicted.

In another French prospective study on 195 patients in a surgical ICU who had 203 episodes of mechanical ventilation, clinical features, physiological parameters, and other factors present at the time of admission or intubation were evaluated as predictors of the need for more than 15 days of mechanical ventilation (17). Univariate analysis showed that emergent tracheal intubation as opposed to elective intubation; the indication for mechanical ventilation; sepsis score at the time of admission and intubation; lung injury score at the time of admission and intubation; number of organ system failures at the time of admission; and low serum albumin concentration predicted the duration of mechanical ventilation. However, by multivariate analysis, only emergent endotracheal intubation and lung injury score on the day of intubation had predictive value. Primary respiratory disorders were also factors that predicted mechanical ventilation for more than 15 days. This study showed that the mortality increased significantly after 3 days of mechanical ventilation, from 23.9% before to 55.8% after ($p \leq 0.05$). Further, the mortality was higher in the 8- to 14-day group (74.1%) than in the >15-day group (15%), although the difference was not statistically significant.

Baseline respiratory mechanics and oxygenation have also been studied as predictors of duration of mechanical ventilation. In elective cardiac surgery patients, Durand et al. in Belgium (18) reported that vital capacity, FEV_1, and arterial oxygen pressure before surgery predict the duration of postoperative mechanical ventilation. However, this was a retrospective study and regression coefficients were low. Moreover, respiratory parameters cannot be measured before emergent intubation. Kuo et al. in Taiwan (19) analyzed data from 33 premature infants with severe respiratory distress syndrome to determine if the alveolar-arterial oxygen gradient (PA-Pao_2) obtained immediately after intubation could be used as a predictor of intubation duration. A correlation between the Pao_2 and intubation duration ($r = 0.93$; $p < 0.001$) was demonstrated only for surviving infants who had comorbid conditions or complications. Since complications and survival cannot be predicted, Pao_2 is not a practical predictor for duration of mechanical ventilation in a general population.

In patients with ARDS, Heffner and Zamora in the United States (20) reported that on the seventh day of mechanical ventilation, Pao_2/PAo_2 ratio, PEEP, chest radiographic improvement of pulmonary infiltrates (comparing day 7 with day 0), and scoring chest radiograph severity can predict mechanical ventilation duration for more than 14 days. This study demonstrated that these four parameters can determine the likelihood of successful extubation within 7 days with high sensitivity (57–78%) and specificity (80–100%). Problems with this study are that it was retrospective, the sample size was small (24 patients), and only patients with ARDS were studied.

In medical and surgical patients with acute respiratory failure, the duration of mechanical ventilation seems to be related to the underlying condition. Stauffer et al. in the United States (21) have shown that mechanical ventilation was significantly longer in patients with pneumonia (11.4 days) than in other diagnostic groups (3.7–7.9 days). Troché and Moine in France (17) showed that the duration of mechanical ventilation ranges from 2 to 10 days and is based on the patient's underlying condition (Fig. 2). Nonspecific severity scoring systems (SAPS, APACHE II and III, etc.) have been demonstrated to predict survival in a general population, but no data are available to show that these scoring systems can be effective in predicting the duration of mechanical ventilation.

The duration of mechanical ventilation from the Spanish Respiratory Failure study group (6) was 27 days for the overall group of patients. Remarkably little variation in the duration of ventilator support was noted between patients with different disease conditions, with the exception of patients with myocardial infarction (15 days), in whom the duration was significantly shorter ($p \leq 0.05$) (Fig. 3). Patients with neuromuscular disease (40 days) had a longer duration of ventilatory support, but this was not statistically significant. It should be considered that the study design might have predisposed to an overestimation of the duration of mechanical ventilation.

Other investigators in the United States have reported a wide variation in the duration of ventilatory support in the ICU setting. Davis et al. (22) reported a mean duration of ventilatory support of 8.9 days; Gillespie et al. (23) reported a mean duration of 11.8 ± 1.1 days, while Witek et al. (24) noted a mean duration of only 2.3 ± 0.4 days. A likely explanation of this wide variety is that these studies were each conducted at a single institution and were thus subject to biases

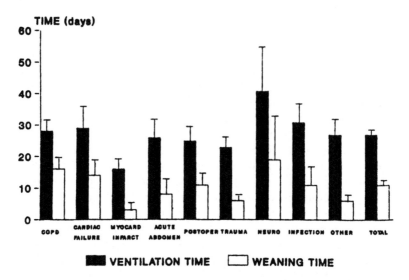

Figure 3 Total duration of mechanical ventilation and weaning: Differences were based on the patient's underlying condition, the total duration of ventilation, and the weaning time. Data are mean ± SEM for each category and the total group of patients. (From Ref. 6.)

in the type of patient admitted to that institution and in physician practice. A study by Esteban et al. (6) was conducted in 47 different hospitals, and no single ICU accounted for more than 6% of total patients. It is interesting to note that the duration of ventilatory support for patients with acute exacerbation of chronic obstructive pulmonary disease in the Spanish Respiratory Failure study group was 27.8 ± 1.4 days. This was similar to that reported by Gillespie et al. (23) for patients with the same conditions at the Mayo Clinic (23.3 ± 4.9 days. Therefore, the patient's underlying condition does not appear to cause major differences in ventilator duration between institutions.

IV. Demographic Characteristics of Patients Who Undergo Mechanical Ventilation

As previously mentioned, most studies that have looked at the outcome of mechanical ventilation have been done at single institutions. Recently, data from the Spanish Respiratory Failure group composed of multiple institutions in a single country reviewed data on 1638 patients requiring mechanical ventilation provided a broader patient population (6,7). The median age of patients undergoing mechanical ventilation was 61 years (25th and 75th percentiles 44 and 71 years, respectively) (Table 4). In recent series on mechanical ventilation, the mean patient age has been approximately 60 years and is similar to the results of the international study (15,25–27). Importantly, there were no age differences between countries. Men predominated in every country, averaging 60% of patients, except in Brazil where the median was 42%. The median APACHE II score on admission to the ICU in the international study was 19 (25th and 75th percentiles 14 and 25, respectively), the median duration of ICU stay was 8 days and of mechanical ventilation was 7 days. An exception was Portugal where the median duration was 12 days (7).

The effect of age on the outcome of mechanical ventilation has been the subject of extensive investigation. In a retrospective study, Dardaine et al. (28) reported data from 110 patients admitted consecutively during a 1-year period and receiving mechanical ventilation for the first time for at least 24 hours. The aim was to determine predictors of mortality during admission to the ICU and at 6, 12, and 18 months after discharge. The mean age was 78 ± 0.5 years (range 70–95 years). Median duration of both hospitalization and artificial ventilation was 12.5 days. Mortality at admission and at 6, 12, and 18 months after discharge was 38, 60, 63, and 67%, respectively. Multivariate analysis revealed that the factors predictive of hospital mortality were the seriousness of the patient's illness on admission and the need for invasive therapy during the hospital stay (dialysis, pulmonary artery catheterization, etc.). The factors predictive of mortality 6 months after discharge and thereafter were impaired health status and marriage status.

Similar results were reported by Meinders et al. (29) in a retrospective study of 181 patients over 70 years old receiving mechanical ventilation for at least 3 days. The authors found that mortality during an intensive care unit stay was associated with cardiac arrest at admission and/or during hospitalization. These investigators also confirmed that the seriousness of the patients' general state on admission, but not age, was a good prognostic factor for patients over 30 years old. Other variables, such as the patients' performance status, affect outcome during the first 6 months after hospital discharge (30).

In a retrospective study on the effect of age on outcomes of mechanical ventilation, Kurek et al. (31) analyzed data from 10,473 hospital discharges from acute-care hospitals in the New York State Medicaid database for 1993. The investigators looked at a diagnosis related group (DRG) code primarily applied to respiratory failure that did not result in tracheotomy (DRG 475). Patients having different disease processes, unified by the primary respiratory diagnosis and the need for mechanical ventilation, were included. This DRG included three procedure codes and was applied to patients undergoing mechanical ventilation for a variable period of time. The distribution of patients by gender and age is shown in Figure 4. Although the overall number of male and female patients was similar,

Table 4 Demographic Characteristics of Mechanical Ventilation Patients

	USA/Canada	Spain	Argentina	Brazil	Chile	Portugal	Uruguay	Total
Age	60 (45,71)	64 (46,71)	59 (40,68)	58 (38,71)	60 (39,69)	66 (50,73)	56 (43,68)	61 (44,71)
APACHE II	19 (15,25)	19 (14,25)	17 (12,24)	19 (14,26)	20 (12,25)	19 (15,26)	17 (12,21)	19 (14,25)
Women (%)	43 (39,46)	35 (30,39)	35 (28,43)	58 (49,67)	38 (26,52)	37 (26,49)	32 (19,48)	40 (38,43)
Days in ICU	8 (3,19)	8 (3,16)	6 (3,12)	8 (4,18)	8 (4,17)	13 (4,46)	7 (2,15)	8 (3,18)
Days of ventilator	7 (3,18)	7 (3,15)	6 (2,10)	7 (3,18)	8 (3,16)	12 (2,47)	5 (2,12)	7 (3,17)

Results are shown as median (25th, 75th percentiles) or percentage (95% confidence interval). Age, APACHE II, and gender refer to patients receiving mechanical ventilation.

a Median (25th, 75th percentiles).
b Percentage (95% confidence interval).
Source: Adapted from Ref. 7.

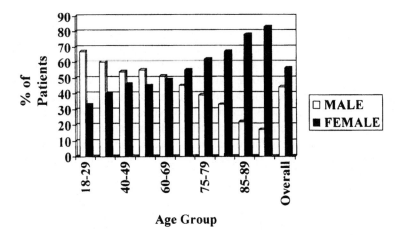

Figure 4 Gender distribution and age of patients on the DGR 478 in New York State in 1993. (From Ref. 31.)

the distribution across the group was not. There was a significant predominance of male subjects in the younger population, while the reverse was true for the older age group. This may reflect the predominance of certain risk factors for mechanical ventilation in young men and a higher life expectancy in women. Figure 5 shows that there was an inverse relationship between survival rate and

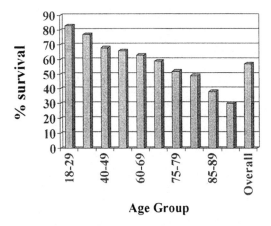

Figure 5 Survival rate for patients under DRG 475 in New York State in 1993. (With permission from Ref. 31.)

age. The data showed that, in the youngest age group (18–29 years), approximately 85% survived hospitalization and 80% of the survivors were discharged directly to the home. By contrast, patients older than 80 years had a hospital discharge rate of less than 40% and approximately 60% of those survivals were discharged directly to the home. Limitations of this study included the inability to clearly determine if a certain condition was present on admission (comorbidity), developed during the hospitalization, or occurred as a consequence of therapy (complication). Furthermore, this database did not provide information on the patients' quality of life or functional status. Prospective studies may provide additional information on the risk factors and underlying conditions that are present in older patients.

Data from Anzueto et al. (32) were arbitrarily divided into two groups based on the patient's age (<75 and >75 years old). (Table 5). No geographic differences between the groups were noted for age distribution, modes of mechanical ventilation, or weaning techniques. Patients > 75 years of age had a significantly shorter time on mechanical ventilation, 15 ± 23 days, compared to 21 ± 107 days in patients < 75 years (p = 0.06). The mean APACHE II score was worse in the >75 year group, 22 ± 8 days, compared to 19 ± 8 days in the <75 year group (p < 0.01). Cardiogenic pulmonary edema was the most common cause of acute respiratory failure in the patients > 75 years, 24% and 10% (p < 0.01) respectively. The frequency of acute exacerbation of chronic lung disease was similar in both age groups. These data suggest that patients >75 years old were sicker and received mechanical ventilation for a shorter period of time, presumably because they have a higher mortality or earlier withdrawal of care. The impact of age on overall morbidity and mortality of mechanical ventilation will need to be addressed in a prospective study.

Another important issue that needs to be addressed in elderly patients undergoing mechanical ventilation is the patients' preference regarding the use of

Table 5 Effect of Age in Mechanically Ventilated Patients

	<75 years	>75 years	p
N	1355	254	
Days ICU	21 ± 107	15 ± 23	0.06
Days—MV	21 ± 110	14 ± 23	0.02
APACHE II	19 ± 8	22 ± 8	<0.001
CPE	87 (10%)	46 (24%)	<0.001
AECOPD	171 (13%)	40 (16%)	NS

Mean ± SD. ARF = Acute respiratory failure; CPE = cardiogenic pulmonary edema; AECOPD = acute exacerbation of chronic obstructive pulmonary disease.
Source: Adapted from Ref. 32.

short- or long-term life support interventions. Murphy and Santilli (33) reported the results of patient interviews by clinicians during routine office visits. Two hundred and eighty-seven elderly persons (mean age 77, range 60–99 years) were interviewed in reference to their preference to use or withhold short-term mechanical ventilation, long-term mechanical ventilation, short-term tube feedings, and long-term tube feedings. Of the total sample, 253 patients (88%) preferred short-term mechanical ventilation, but if the chance of recovery was not very good only 1 patient (3.5%) preferred long-term mechanical ventilation. One hundred and eighty-nine patients (65%) preferred short-term tube feeding, but only 13 patients (4.5%) preferred long-term tube feeding in the case of significant cognitive impairment. This study concluded that most elderly persons would agree to the use of short-term mechanical ventilation or tube feeding if their likelihood of recovery was reasonably good. Only a small minority would opt for long-term mechanical ventilation or tube feeding.

V. Airway Management

Endotracheal intubation remains the most common way of delivering mechanical ventilation. Data from the international study of Esteban et al. (7) showed that an endotracheal tube was used in 75% of patients, tracheostomy in 24%, and facial mask in 1%. There were no significant differences between countries. Of the endotracheal tubes, 96% were passed through the mouth and 4% through the nose. Facial mask and noninvasive ventilation were found in a very small number of patients. This study was not designed to study the use of noninvasive ventilation. Furthermore, the study design included only patients admitted to an intensive care unit and receiving mechanical ventilation. The use of tracheostomy varied based on the underlying condition and the time from initiation of mechanical ventilation. Tracheostomy was performed at a median time of 11 days (25th and 75th percentile 5 and 19, respectively) following intubation. Tracheostomy was present in 39% of patients with neuromuscular disease, 28% with COPD, and 20% with acute respiratory failure. In patients receiving mechanical ventilation for 1–7 days, 16% of patients with neuromuscular disease had a tracheostomy as compared to 5% of patients with acute respiratory failure. In patients receiving mechanical ventilation for more than 21 days, 69% of patients with neuromuscular disease and 65% of patients with acute respiratory failure had tracheostomies.

General recommendations suggest that tracheostomy should be performed when the clinician anticipates the need for prolonged ventilatory support (34). Published data suggest that the underlying condition may be an important determinant of when to perform a tracheostomy in patients who have received mechanical ventilation. Another important factor to consider is that percutaneous techniques are now available that allow tracheostomies to be performed at the patient's bedside. These techniques have been shown to be safe and can be performed by intensivists.

VI. Ventilator Modes and Settings

There are limited data on practitioners' preferences for different modes of mechanical ventilation. Venus et al. (35) reported the results of a United States survey of hospital-based respiratory care departments. A questionnaire was mailed to the technical directors of respiratory therapy departments listed by the American Association for Respiratory Therapy. The objective was to quantitate the use of various techniques and criteria employed to facilitate weaning of patients from mechanical ventilation. Of 3992 questionnaires mailed, 1272 (31.9%) were returned but 149 (11.7%) were excluded because they were improperly filled out. The respondents included data from 50% private practice, 27% nonprivate, and 22% university-affiliated hospitals. Seventy-two percent of the respondents indicated that intermittent mandatory ventilation was the primary mode of ventilatory support used in their institutions. Unfortunately, these investigators did not record the frequency with which other modes were used. A major limitation of the study was that questionnaires were mailed to the technical directors of the respiratory therapy department and the results were based on the "best guess" (or perhaps bias) of the individual filling out the form. Furthermore, the investigators did not obtain information on the use of primary modes of mechanical ventilation other than synchronized intermittent mandatory ventilation (SIMV). Finally, when this survey was conducted during the mid-1980s, most ventilators were not capable of delivering the newer techniques such as pressure control ventilation or pressure support ventilation.

Several years later, Esteban et al. (6) carried out a cross-sectional multicenter study in 47 medical and surgical ICUs in Spain in 290 patients who received mechanical ventilation for at least 24 hours. Relative frequency of different modes was as follows: assist control ventilation in 55%; SIMV in 26%; pressure support ventilation in 8%; SIMV plus pressure support (PS) in 8%; pressure control ventilation in 1%; and continuous positive airway pressure in 2%. In this study, the investigators also obtained information on the capabilities of the ventilator for delivering different modes of support. All the ventilators were capable of delivering controlled mechanical ventilation and assist control ventilation. Most (86%) were capable of delivering SIMV, and fewer were capable of delivering pressure support ventilation. The relative frequency of ventilatory modes actually used in the patients is shown in Figure 6.

Esteban et al. (7) showed in an international study that assist control ventilation was the most common mode of ventilator support used in 47% of patients. An almost equal proportion, 46%, of the overall group was ventilated with SIMV,

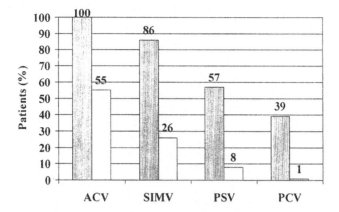

Figure 6 Capability of ventilators to provide different modes of support (light columns) and the proportion of patients ventilated with each mode (dark columns) expressed as a percentage of the total number of patients who received ventilatory support. ACV = Assist controlled ventilation; SIMV = synchronized intermittent mandatory ventilation; PSV = pressure support ventilation; PCV = pressure control ventilation. (From Ref. 6.)

pressure support, or the combination of both. The combination of SIMV and pressure support showed considerable variations among countries ranging from 7% in Argentina to 52% in Uruguay. In North America, this combination was used 34% of the time—the same as assist control. There were substantial differences in ventilator mode use between countries. Several factors may account for these differences, including the availability of ventilators with limited modes capability, tradition, and physician experience. For example, Argentina and other countries in South America rely on ventilators that are locally manufactured, most of which do not have all the different ventilator modes. Regional physician experience and tradition may be the most important factors. Esteban et al. (6) showed in Spain that despite ventilator capability to deliver almost any mode, physicians choose other modes (Fig. 6). Another important factor has been the lack of prospective international studies that have demonstrated the superiority of one mode over another taking into consideration the cause for mechanical ventilation.

It was recently recognized that in ARDS and other forms of acute lung injury, the initial ventilator settings might have important implications for the patient's outcome (25,26). The setting of tidal volume has been controversial and arbitrary in nature; 10–15 mL/kg became conventional in the early 1970s and was until recently routinely used in all patients requiring mechanical ventilation (36). These high tidal volumes were used in patients undergoing general anesthesia in order to prevent the development of atelectasis and hypoxemia. Since the work of Dreyfuss et al. (37), there has been a growing awareness of the potential

Table 6 Ventilator Settings in Patients Receiving Assist-Control Ventilation or Pressure Support Ventilation According to Country[a]

	USA/Canada	Spain	Argentina	Brazil	Chile	Portugal	Uruguay	Total
Assist/Control	$n = 256$	$n = 273$	$n = 105$	$n = 49$	$n = 42$	$n = 30$	$n = 11$	$n = 767$
Tidal volume, mL/kg	8 (7,10)	9 (8,10)	9 (8,10)	8 (7,10)	9 (8,11)	8 (7,0)	10 (9,12)	9 (8,10)
Respiration rate, breaths/min	16 (12,20)	16 (13,18)	14 (12,17)	18 (16,24)	18 (15,20)	20 (16,20)	14 (12,18)	16 (13,20)
Peak pressure, cmH_2O	32 (27,38)	32 (25,40)	27 (20,30)	26 (22,30)	28 (20,32)	22 (20,30)	29 (22,42)	30 (25,37)
PSV	$n = 134$	$n = 51$	$n = 15$	$n = 12$	$n = 3$	$n = 23$	$n = 1$	$n = 239$
Tidal volume, mL/kg	6 (5,8)	9 (7,9)	8 (5,10)	7 (7,10)	—	7 (6,9)	—	7 (5,9)
Respiration rate, breaths/min	23 (20,38)	21 (17,25)	18 (16,24)	21 (17,25)	—	19 (16,24)	—	22 (18,26)
Peak pressure, cmH_2O	18 (13,23)	19 (15,25)	18 (15,22)	21 (15,26)	—	20 (15,25)	—	19 (15,25)
PEEP cmH_2O	5 (5,6)	5 (5,8)	5 (5,7)	5 (4,8)	5 (4,6)	4 (4,5)	5 (4,6)	5 (5,6)

PEEP values were calculated for patients receiving some level of PEEP irrespective of the employed ventilator mode.

[a]Values are shown as median (25th, 75th percentiles).

Source: Adapted from Ref. 7.

for ventilator-induced lung injury (or volutrauma), which culminated in the deliberate use of low tidal volumes (38,39). These data support the theory that tidal volume, PEEP, and other ventilator parameters can have a significant impact on patient morbidity and mortality.

In order to learn the ventilator parameters used by clinicians treating patients with ARDS, Carmichael et al. (40) reported the results of a postal survey completed by nearly 1000 critical care physicians in 1992. This data showed that for initial treatment of ARDS patients, volume-cycled ventilation in the assist-control mode was most common (65%), followed by SIMV (18%) (36). An almost equal number of clinicians used tidal volumes of 10–13 mL/kg and tidal volumes of 5–9 mL/kg. Seventy-nine percent allowed permissive hypercapnia, 62% accepted oxygen saturations in the 86–90% range, and 21% accepted the 91–95% range. The mean maximum level of PEEP was based on a given range of 5–22 cmH$_2$O at F$_{IO_2}$ of 1.0 (40). Amato et al. (38) showed that patients with lower tidal volumes and higher PEEP have significantly less mortality than patients who are ventilated with tidal volumes of 12 mL/kg and lower PEEP (5).

Esteban et al. (7) reported that the median tidal volume setting was 9 mL/kg (25th and 75th percentiles were 8 and 10, respectively) in patients receiving assist control. The median pressure support setting was 18 cmH$_2$O (25th and 75th percentile were 13 and 23, respectively). Sixty-three percent of patients receiving assist control ventilation had tidal volumes of less than 10 mL/kg. The setting of tidal volume was remarkably similar between countries (Table 6).

PEEP is a ventilator setting that not only has an important impact on oxygenation but also has potential adverse events. There have been extensive studies looking at the hemodynamic effects of PEEP (41) and the effect of the small and regional distribution of tidal volume and recruitment, particularly in patients with severe lung injury (42). Esteban et al. (7) showed that the median level of PEEP was 5 cmH$_2$O (25th and 75th percentile were 5 and 6 cmH$_2$O, respectively). These values of PEEP were very similar between countries (Table 6). It is important to point out that in this database, a third of patients (31%) were ventilated without PEEP, and only three patients received PEEP above 15 cmH$_2$O.

VII. Weaning Techniques

Discontinuation of mechanical ventilation is usually an easy task in patients receiving short-term ventilatory support, such as in patients recovering from routine surgery. The discontinuation process can be much more difficult in patients recovering from severe respiratory failure, and weaning such patients constitutes a large portion of the workload in an ICU (43). In the data from the Spanish Respiratory Failure study group (6), weaning was initiated after 18.2 ± 1.3 days (range 1–145 days) on mechanical ventilation, and a further 10.9 ± 1.5 days (range 1–

119 days) passed before the removal of ventilatory support. Thus, 41% of the total time of mechanical ventilation was devoted to weaning. Interestingly, these investigators reported that there are significant differences in weaning time based on the patients' underlying diseases (Fig. 3). Weaning time occupied 57% of the total ventilator time in patients with COPD as opposed to only occupied 19% in patients with myocardial infarction.

Weaning is an aspect of mechanical ventilation that has been subjected to several randomized controlled trials. The data from Venus et al. (35) showed that intermittent mechanical ventilation (IMV) was the most frequent mode of weaning. A multicenter study reported by the Spanish Respiratory Failure study group (6) showed that intermittent spontaneous trials with synchronized intermittent mechanical ventilation (SIMV), pressure support, and T-tube were the most common modes of weaning. In preselected groups of difficult-to-wean patients, Brochard et al. (44) reported no difference in the rate of successful weaning between trials of spontaneous breathing and pressure support. On the other hand, the Spanish Lung Failure Collaborative Group (45,46) reported that a single trial of spontaneous breathing achieved a significant increase in the rate of successful weaning when compared to SIMV and pressure support, respectively.

In the data from Esteban et al. (7), physicians considered 32% of the patients to be in the weaning phase. The methods of weaning varied widely among countries. Overall, the most frequent method of weaning was pressure support, used in 33% of the patients. The combination of SIMV and pressure support was used in 28% of patients but varied widely among countries ranging from 3% in Argentina to 47% in Uruguay. Trials of spontaneous weaning were being used in 46% of the patients in Spain versus only 16% in North American patients. The demonstration of the superiority of spontaneous breathing trials by the Spanish Lung Failure Collaborative Group may account for the almost twofold increase in the use of this approach in Spain (27). Meanwhile, the combination of SIMV plus pressure support was used in 66% of patients in Uruguay versus only 7% of patients in Portugal. This combination was the second most frequently used method of weaning in the United States despite it being the only technique whose efficacy has never been evaluated as a weaning technique. These data suggest that despite the availability of information from randomized, controlled, clinical weaning trials that showed the superiority of daily trail of spontaneous breathing over SIMV plus pressure support, there is no widespread use of these methods in current clinical practice.

VIII. The Economic Impact of Mechanical Ventilation

The impact of mechanical ventilation on both ICU and hospital resources is significant. Knowledge of the financial aspects of mechanical ventilation is becoming increasingly important in the determination of resource allocation among hospitals (47,48). Kurek et al. (31), in an analysis of Medicaid patients treated with mechanical ventilation in New York State, showed that there was a difference between age group and survival depending on Medicaid reimbursement. Although the smallest subset of patients was older than 70 years, their lengths of hospital and ICU stay were the highest. In general, the cost of hospital survival increases with advancing age. Angus et al. (49) reported data from a cohort of ICU patients younger than 65 years requiring prolonged mechanical ventilation. These patients had a significantly higher death rate up to 18 months beyond hospital discharge when compared with actuarial expectations. At 18 months post–hospital discharge, the death rate for these individuals had declined exponentially to a constant rate that approximated the actuarial risk. These data provide strong evidence that the morbidity of critical illness lasts well beyond hospital discharge.

Many other variables have to be taken into consideration when evaluating the overall cost of mechanical ventilation. In a recent report Bach et al. (50) determined whether 118 patients with prolonged critical illness had different outcomes if managed by university-based as compared to community-based intensive care units. Patients on the university-based service were weaned from mechanical ventilation in 32% fewer days ($p = 0.02$) and physicians were more likely to write "do not resuscitate" orders, but there was no detectable difference in survival between the two groups. The estimated reimbursement for community-based physicians ($6,797/patient) was 46% greater than for university-based physicians ($4,651/patient) for discharged patients ($p = 0.03$). The frequency of ventilator circuit changes can also have a significant impact on overall cost (51).

Finally, other modalities of patient support such as noninvasive ventilation can be used in patients with acute respiratory failure. Noninvasive ventilation has been shown to be an effective mode of ventilatory support in such patients, mainly those with chronic lung disease (53). Little information is available on its current use. Both of the Esteban et al. (6,7) studies required at least 24 hours of mechanical ventilation many patients treated with noninvasive ventilation were excluded. Although, it has been suggested that noninvasive ventilation is a time-consuming procedure for medical and paramedical personnel, an Italian study by Nava et al. (54) showed that noninvasive ventilation is not more expensive or time-consuming for medical staff than endotracheal ventilation. Therefore, noninvasive ventilation is a potentially important therapy for patients with acute respiratory failure, but at this time the extent of its use is not known.

IX. Conclusion

Mechanical ventilation is the mainstay therapy in patients with acute respiratory failure. The primary indications for mechanical ventilation and the demographic characteristics of patients who receive this therapy are very similar among different countries. Similar trends have occurred in most countries over time, such as the reduction of tidal volume from 10 to 7 mL/kg and the use of PEEP in patients with ARDS. However, there is great variability between countries in the selection of ventilator modes and weaning procedures despite the fairly similar patient demographics. In spite of the results of randomized controlled trials favoring particular weaning techniques (daily trial of spontaneous breathing vs. pressure support or SIMV), these techniques are not extensively used. This suggests that findings from research on mechanical ventilation and weaning are incorporated into clinical practice at a very slow pace. Prospective studies are needed to further analyze and understand international differences, and by sharing information on outcomes, progress toward optimization of ventilator utilization in critical care settings will be enhanced.

References

1. Snider GL. Historical perspective on mechanical ventilation; from simple life support system to ethical dilemma. Am Rev Respir Dis 1989; 140:52–57.
2. Braun SR, Smith RF, McCarthy TM, et al. Evaluating the changing role of respiratory therapy services at two hospitals. JAMA 1981; 245:2033–2037.
3. Swinburne AJ, Fedullo AJ, Shayne DS. Mechanical ventilation: analysis of increasing use and patient survival. J Intensive Care Med 1988; 3:315–320.
4. Slutsky AS. ACCP consensus conference. Mechanical ventilation. Chest 1993; 104: 1833–1859.
5. Knaus WA. Prognosis with mechanical ventilation: the influence of disease, severity of disease, age, and chronic health status on survival from an acute illness. Am Rev Respir Dis 1989; 140:S8–S13.
6. Esteban A, Alia I, Ibañez J, et al. Modes of mechanical ventilation and weaning. A national survey of Spanish hospitals. Chest 1994; 106:1188–1193.
7. Esteban A, Anzueto A, Alia I, et al. How is mechanical ventilation employed in the intensive care unit? An international utilization review. Am J Respir Crit Care Med 2000; 161:1450–1458.
8. Pranikoff T, Hirschl RB, Steimle CN, et al. Mortality is directly related to the duration of mechanical ventilation before the initiation of extracorporeal life support for severe respiratory failure. Crit Care Med 1997; 25:28–32.
9. Villar J, Slutsky AS. The incidence of the adult respiratory distress syndrome. Am Rev Respir Dis 1989; 140:814–816.
10. Thomsen GE, Morris AH. Incidence of the adult respiratory distress syndrome in the State of Utah. Am J Respir Crit Care Med 1995; 152:965–971.
11. Knaus WA, Sun X, Hakim R, et al. Evaluation of definitions for adult respiratory distress syndrome. Am J Respir Crit Care Med 1994; 150:311–317.
12. Ferring M, Vincent JL. Is outcome from ARDS related to the severity of respiratory failure? Eur Respir J 1997; 10:1297–1300.
13. Seneff MG, Wagner DP, Wagner RP, et al. Hospital and 1-year survival of patients

admitted to intensive care units with acute exacerbation of chronic obstructive pulmonary disease. JAMA 1995; 274:1852–1857.

14. Knaus WA, Wagner DP, Draper EA, et al. The APACHE III prognostic system; risk prediction of hospital mortality for critically ill hospitalized adults. Chest 1991; 100:1619–1636.

15. Ely EW, Baker AM, Dunagan DP, et al. Effect on the duration of mechanical ventilation of identifying patients capable of breathing spontaneously. N Engl J Med 1996; 335:1864–1869.

16. Velmahos GC, Belzberg H, Chan L, et al. Factors predicting prolonged mechanical ventilation in critically injured patients: introducing a simplified quantitative risk score. Am Surg 1997; 63:811–817.

17. Troché G, Moine P. Is the duration of mechanical ventilation predictable? Chest 1997; 112:745–751.

18. Durand M, Combes P, Eisele JH, et al. Pulmonary function tests predict outcome after cardiac surgery. Acta Anaesth Belg 1993; 44:17–23.

19. Kuo CY, Wang JW, Hsich WS, et al. First alveolar-arterial oxygen gradient (AaDO$_2$) in mechanical ventilation as a predictor for duration of intubation in respiratory distress syndrome. J Formos Med Assoc 1993; 92:402–406.

20. Heffner JE, Zamora CA. Clinical predictors of prolonged translaryngeal intubation in patients with the adult respiratory distress syndrome. Chest 1990; 97:447–452.

21. Stauffer JL, Fayter NA, Graves B, et al. Survival following mechanical ventilation for acute respiratory failure in adult men. Chest 1993; 104:1222–1229.

22. Davis HH, Lefrak SS, Miller D, et al. Prolonged mechanically assisted ventilation: an analysis of outcome and charges. JAMA 243:43–45.

23. Gillespie DJ, Marsh HM, Divertie MB, et al. Clinical outcome of respiratory failure in patients requiring prolonged (>24 hours) mechanical ventilation. Chest 1986; 90: 364–369.

24. Witek TJ, Schacter EN, Dean NL, et al. Mechanically assisted ventilation in a community hospital: immediate outcome, hospital charges and follow-up of patients. Arch Intern Med 1985; 145:235–239.

25. Stewart TE, Meade MO, Cook DJ, et al. Evaluation of a ventilation strategy to prevent barotrauma in patients at high risk for acute respiratory distress syndrome. N Engl J Med 1998; 338:355–361.

26. Brochard L, Roudot-Thoraval F, Roupie E, et al. Tidal volume reduction in the adult respiratory distress syndrome. Am J Respir Crit Care Med 1998; 158:1831–1838.

27. Esteban A, Frutos F, Tobin MJ, et al. A comparison of four methods of weaning from mechanical ventilation. N Engl J Med 1995; 332:345–350.

28. Dardaine V, Constans T, Lasfarques G, et al. Outcome of elderly patients requiring ventilatory support in intensive care. Aging Clin Exp Res 1995; 7:221–227.

29. Meinders AJ, Van Der Hoeven JG, Meinders AE. The outcome of prolonged mechanical ventilation in elderly patients: are the efforts worthwhile? Age Ageing 1996; 25:353–356.

30. Mayer-Oakes SA, Oye RK, Leake B. Predictors of mortality in older patients following medical intensive care: the importance of functional status. J Am Geriatr Soc 1991; 39:862–868.

31. Kurek CJ, Dewar D, Lambrinos J, et al. Clinical and economic outcome of mechani-

cal ventilated patients in New York State during 1993. Chest 1998; 114:214–222.

32. Anzueto A, Esteban A, Alia I, et al. International study of mechanical ventilation: effect of age. Chest 1998; 114:357S.

33. Murphy DJ, Santilli S. Elderly patients' preferences for long-term life support. Arch Fam Med 1998; 7:484–488.

34. Heffner JE. timing of tracheostomy in ventilator-dependent patients. Clin Chest Med 1991; 12:611–625.

35. Venus B, Smith RA, Mathru M. National survey of methods and criteria used for weaning from mechanical ventilation. Crit Care Med 1997; 15:530–533.

36. Lutch JS, Murray JF. Continuous positive pressure ventilation: effects of systemic oxygen transport and tissue oxygenation. Ann Intern Med 1972; 76:193–202.

37. Dreyfuss D, Soler P, Basset G, et al. High inflation pressure pulmonary edema: respective effects of high airway pressure, high tidal volume, and positive end-expiratory pressure. Am Rev Respir Dis 1988; 137:1159–1164.

38. Amato MBP, Barbas CSV, Medeiros DM, et al. Effect of a protective-ventilation strategy on mortality in the acute respiratory distress syndrome. N Engl J Med 1998; 338:347–354.

39. Darioli R, Perret C. Mechanical controlled hypoventilation in status asthmaticus. Am Rev Respir Dis 1984; 129:385–387.

40. Carmichael LC, Dorinsky PM, Higginsbetl. Diagnosis and therapy of acute respiratory disstress syndrome in adults: an international survey. J Crit Care 1996; 11:9.

41. Matamis D, Lemaire F, Harf A, et al. Redistribution of pulmonary blood flow induced by positive end-expiratory pressure and dopamine infusion in acute respiratory failure. Am Rev Respir Dis 1984; 129:39–44.

42. Gattinoni L, Pelosi P, Crotti S, et al. Effects of positive end-expiratory pressure on regional distribution of tidal volume and recruitment in adult respiratory distress syndrome. Am J Respir Crit Care Med 1995; 151:1807–1814.

43. Tobin MJ. Weaning from mechanical ventilation. Curr Pulmonol 1990; 11:47–105.

44. Brochard L, Rauss A, Benito S, et al. Comparison of three methods of gradual withdrawal from ventilatory support during weaning from mechanical ventilation. Am J Respir Crit Care Med 1994; 150:896–903.

45. Esteban A, Alia I, Gordo F, et al. Extubation outcome after spontaneous breathing trials with T-tube or pressure support ventilation. Am J Respir Crit Care Med 1997; 156:459–465.

46. Esteban A, Alia I, Tobin MJ, et al. Effect of spontaneous breathing trial duration on outcome of attempts to discontinue mechanical ventilation. Am J Respir Crit Care Med 1999; 159:512–518.

47. Rosen RL, Bone RC. Economics of mechanical ventilation. Clin Chest Med 1990; 9:163–169.

48. Rosen RL, Bone RC. Financial implications of ventilator care. Crit Care Clin 1990; 6:797–805.

49. Angus DC, Linde-Zwirble WT, Sirio CA, et al. Understanding post-discharge mortality after prolonged mechanical ventilation. Crit Care Med 1995; 23:A55.

50. Bach PB, Carson SS, Leff A. Outcomes and resource utilization for patients with

prolonged critical illness managed by university-based or community-based sub-specialists. Am J Respir Crit Care Med 1998; 158:1410–1415.

51. Kotilainen HR, Keroack MA. Cost analysis and clinical impact of weekly ventilator circuit changes in patients in intensive care unit. Am J Inf Con 1997; 25(2):117–120.

52. Brochard L, Mancebo J, Wysocki M, et al. Noninvasive ventilation for acute exacerbation of chronic obstructive pulmonary disease. N Engl J Med 1995; 333:817–822.

53. Kramer N, Meyer TJ, Meharg J, et al. Randomized prospective trial of noninvasive positive pressure ventilation in acute respiratory failure. Am J Respir Crit Care Med 1995; 151:1799–1806.

54. Nava S, Evangelisti I, Rampulla C, et al. Human and financial costs of noninvasive mechanical ventilation in patients affected by COPD and acute respiratory failure. Chest 1997; 111:1631–1638.

4

Costs Associated with Mechanical Ventilation

WILLIAM T. McGEE

Baystate Medical Center
Springfield, Massachusetts
Tufts University
Boston, Massachusetts

I. Introduction

All discussions concerning costs are important for one of two basic reasons: either resources are limited and cost becomes an important overriding economic concern, or the utility of the expenditure is questionable and these dollars could be put to better use through another application. If the goal of health care in the United States is to improve the health of the population, with the best allocation of resources it is unlikely that mechanical ventilation would ever factor into that equation. It is unlikely that formal cost-benefit analysis could ever elevate mechanical ventilation as it is presently used above the potential health benefits of population-based health screening, nutrition, and immunization programs or programs to assure clean air, clean water, abolition of cigarette smoking, automobile safety, and firearm control. The impact that these types of national health programs would ultimately have on the health of the population would be far in excess of those gained from all but the shortest courses of mechanical ventilation. We must further realize that the way the health systems have evolved in the United States resources expenditure takes a much more parochial and individualistic approach that is very dependent on reimbursement patterns. Health outcome relative to other health benefits that may be derived from using these dollars more efficiently has not been a paramount societal agenda primarily related to the way health systems have evolved in this country (1).

Critical care beds account for roughly 10% of all hospital beds and may consume up to one third of hospital budgets (2,3). The dollar amount spent on critical care in the United States has been estimated to be greater than 1% of the gross domestic product (2,3). Ventilator care is a primary driver of intensive care unit (ICU) costs. The minority of patients requiring prolonged mechanical ventilation may account for 40% of an ICU's budget (4,5). Even if the outcome were uniformly excellent for all these patients, which it is not (6,7), formal population-based cost-benefit analysis would still favor less sophisticated population-based screening and health promotion programs (8,9). For this high cost group of critically ill patients, intensive care is expensive and often associated with a poor outcome. Advances in medical technology along with expansion of reimbursement and patients' families' desire for this particular type of care have continued to expand this group. It is important to understand that cost-effectiveness, as the terminology is typically applied to this patient population, considers only this population, examining less costly ways or, more typically, less expensive locations for treatment. It is only through this patient-centered approach, ignoring the population as a whole, that these discussions regarding cost-effectiveness are carried out. The published literature supports this narrow viewpoint when considering cost-effectiveness and the use of mechanical ventilation.

If mechanical ventilation and particularly long-term mechanical ventilation are major cost drivers in the ICU, it is likely that these costs of ICU care and care of the hospitalized patient will continue to grow. ICUs will consume an ever-increasing portion of hospital and therefore national health care expenditures, as long as the population of patients receiving long-term mechanical ventilation increases. It has been our observation that this population has grown steadily and fairly rapidly over the past 10–15 years. There are multiple reasons for this. Medicine has advanced over time, and our understanding of the pathophysiology of multiple disease processes is better. Treatments for these diseases have also improved, leading to an ever-increasing population of patients with either acute medical or surgical illness that can now be treated. Patients are also living longer with chronic diseases. Patients who in the past might have been considered high risk for operative intervention for particular disease processes because of preexisting medical illness are now routinely operated on and typically do well. This is often related to improvements in critical care monitoring and therapies. Better therapies for patients with chronic cardiopulmonary disease have led to a whole new class of patients who use ICUs for brief "tune-ups," so-called frequent flyers. Newly trained physicians are familiar with this concept and the application of mechanical ventilation and may be more apt to use it or recommend it for their patients. Mechanical ventilation, although associated with its own unique complications, is generally regarded as safe and can be used for long periods of time. It is not uncommon for patients on mechanical ventilation to be managed outside of ICUs. This certainly was not the case as recently as 10 years ago. An upward trend in the severity of illness for ICU patients has resulted in a greater percentage of these patients on mechanical ventilation. In fact, it is rare in some ICUs to have a patient who does not require mechanical ventilation along with other problems. Longer survival of patients with impaired host-defense mechanisms has increased the incidence of sepsis and septic shock, which is frequently complicated by adult respiratory distress syndrome (ARDS). ARDS is a particular pulmonary process that often requires long-term mechanical ventilation. Improved management of a wide variety of disease processes has resulted in a population of patients who are chronically critically ill and are often receiving pharmacological support or mechanical replacement for other organ dysfunctions or failures. Ventilator strategies for these populations have only focused on these patients' individual outcomes over the short term. A societal perspective would evaluate the cost relative to the health outcome of the population, not simply the individual (8).

Mechanical ventilation is part of the ICU landscape. A majority of patients require a short course of mechanical ventilation, typically less than 2–3 days, and have excellent health outcomes. For the much smaller group requiring longer-term mechanical ventilation, the issues of location of treatment and outcome become much more important. For the majority of patients with severe acute illness, the development of specialized critical care units has improved outcome. Because of its importance in driving hospital, and therefore national, health care costs, the ICU has become a hot bed of cost-containment efforts. The large role that mechanically ventilated patients play in the ICU, especially considering the increased cost associated with this modality of care, have made the ventilated patients in the ICU the focus of these efforts (10). Widespread application of this technology, which has accelerated in the last 20 years, traces itself back to the poliomyelitis epidemics in Los Angeles in the late 1940s and Copenhagen in 1952 (11). The development of mechanical ventilation related to the Vietnam conflict and a description of the adult respiratory distress syndrome led to a more widespread application of this technique outside of the trauma setting (11,12). The application of mechanical ventilation is now routine in most hospitals throughout the United States.

II. Economic Terminology

Cost-effective analysis, potentially very useful when evaluating medical interventions, is often misapplied or misunderstood. Health benefits or effectiveness usually evaluates a clinical outcome and must be quantitated. Costs must be broken down into their component variables and are not the same as charges, although they can often be related by a mathematical formula. Tracking and quantitating all costs that accrue to achieve any particular outcome is the basis for a cost-effectiveness analysis. This ratio is usually in the format of dollars per outcome. It is then compared with ratios that have been developed for other treatment strategies (8,13). This approach is different than simple cost-saving analysis. Cost savings, often presented to us by nonclinical management, i.e., simply to spend less and save money, does not consider the health outcome impact on the patient. Conversely, costlier interventions are not necessarily less cost-effective as the incremental gain in outcome may exceed the incremental gain in cost. Cost-benefit analysis, cost-utility analysis, and cost-minimization techniques are often used interchangeably with cost-effectiveness analysis but are not the same thing. Cost-minimization techniques represent the most simplistic approach—Can we do less assuming that the outcomes will be the same? No quantitation of the outcome is actually made. Examples of this might be the limitation of blood gases or chest x-rays in the management of a patient with ARDS, the assumption being that the disease outcome will be similar based on management of respiratory failure and the underlying disease independent of monitoring of patient status. Cost-benefit analysis is often used interchangeably with cost-effectiveness analysis, but in its purest sense the benefit is measured in strictly economic terms. Simply, how many dollars of output does one obtain for dollars of input? This is not usually generalizable to health outcomes. Cost-utility analysis can be looked at as a specific type of cost-effectiveness analysis that incorporates quality of the outcome along with the quantity. Quality-adjusted life-years (QALY) is a common effectiveness measure reported. As an example, a 3-month period totally disease-free might be equated to several years of poor functional status in a nursing home, the quality of the outcome, not just survival, being the important parameter in this type of analysis. Several excellent references describe the steps of a cost-effectiveness analysis in detail (8,13). Some of the basic steps are reviewed below. How these steps are applied and the perspective that is taken along with the quantification of outcomes ultimately will determine the cost-effectiveness of any therapy. Although often viewed as hard economic facts, because of the assumptions made in developing these ratios, these analyses rarely have any intrinsic meaning. Their meaning is always relative to an alternative intervention using the same assumptions and achieving the same health outcome. Although a societal viewpoint would likely be the best in terms of health outcomes, this may not be the important perspective of the particular decision maker. A more narrow perspective is typical under the present management and reimbursement systems in place, particularly when it comes to mechanical ventilation. A fair amount of cost shifting is usually an important piece of cost control. Using this technique is useful to those making decisions for a population of patients with a fixed budget. It is not particularly useful to the clinician making individual decisions about a patient for whom he or she has limited fiscal responsibility.

The first step requires a comparison with an alternative method of therapy. Considering mechanical ventilation, this may be the particular mode or type of ventilator used, the location of therapy, ancillary treatments and tests that are done to monitor mechanical ventilation or whether noninvasive positive pressure ventilation in certain circumstances could be compared to mechanical ventilation. Very often the standard of care commonly available in the community is used as a reference. Once it has been determined that a particular course of action improves clinical outcomes with lower resource expenditure, then further analysis is not warranted. Typically, however, improvements in outcomes involve greater costs. This is most important if the decision maker is responsible for prioritizing funding. The cost-utility ratio is probably the most useful in medicine because the outcome or the utility gained is the quality-adjusted year of life, a more important outcome for most patients than just extending life. Typically perfect health is given a value of one, with zero representing death. The entire spectrum of health outcomes can be measured in between. These are by their very nature subjective measures. Once these ratios are developed for similar clinical outcomes, therapies can basically be ranked with those with the lowest ratio taking priority over those with higher ratios (8,13).

Determining the costs involved may be the most difficult part of a cost-effectiveness analysis. Many hospital accounting systems are not designed to measure the true incremental costs of delivering a specific service to a specific patient. Most of the early literature on this topic actually looks at charges and not costs for these patients. Although there is some relationship between costs and changes, it would make any direct comparison problematic. The first step is identification of cost items. Direct cost is the amount of money that is directly paid for products or services related to the treatment being analyzed. These costs may be fixed or variable. Variable costs by definition change in direct proportion to the volume of services. Fixed costs have no relationship to volume. Floor space in the ICU and hospital overhead are examples of fixed costs in the ICU environment. Variable costs for a ventilated patient would relate to therapist time to maintain and adjust the ventilator once in use along with the increase in ancillary services that are anticipated when the patient is on mechanical ventilation. The use of ventilator circuit tubing is an example of this. Indirect costs are often related to outcome and change in productivity. Time lost from work or the reallocation of resources from more worthwhile projects are examples of indirect costs. Finally, other indirect costs may be costs of an adverse event or savings realized as a result of change in health status. Because of the assumptions and modeling techniques that are inherent in cost-effectiveness analyses, sensitivity analysis should be performed. Sensitivity analysis involves varying the values and assumption for the input and outcome variables so that one can see the impact of a change in assumptions.

Finally, societal preferences and ethical considerations may take precedence over these simple economic arguments. Cost-effectiveness analysis has not been rigorously applied to mechanical ventilator support. The comparisons most commonly sited in the literature relate to comparing mechanical ventilation in one setting, i.e., the critical care unit, compared to another site, stepdown unit, or long-term care facility. There are other concerns related to health care that should at least be understood as we attempt to assess the cost of mechanical ventilation. Because of the value judgments and assumptions made in performing cost-effectiveness analyses for health care, this type of analysis is more difficult to quantify and use for absolute comparisons than it might be for a manufacturer of hamburgers.

Some of the outputs of critical care, including death and disability, are not easily quantitated, and inevitably trade-offs, particularly related to length of life and disability as they relate to health expenditures, are made (14). Furthermore, there are significant downstream effects—a lot of cost savings is ultimately cost shifting. Although it often seems otherwise for a patient being treated in a hospital or on a mechanical ventilator, health care dollars are a limited resource, and therefore it is important for us as practitioners to look at costs related to outcomes and at least have some opinion about the cost utility of any modality we employ. It is also important to look at downstream effects of our decision making. Certainly it may be cost saving for us in the ICU to discharge a patient sooner either to a step-down unit or long-term care facility or even to home. However, costs of care in these areas will necessarily increase, and the outcomes potentially are worse with less intensive care. In these scenarios, although our costs have declined, others have increased and patient outcome may suffer directly related to less expensive care. Certainly there are many patients who have done well with ICU-level care that deteriorate within a very short period of time when transferred to a less intensive environment. We should also understand the market issues that led initially to the growth of mechanical ventilation based on cost reimbursement and the implementation of the Medicare program in the late 1960s and early 1970s. These environmental influences resulted in exponential growth of ventilated patients, initially in ICUs. More recent changes in Health Care Financing Administration (HCFA) funding for chronic ventilator facilities have created a market for these types of patients and facilities. External market forces and economics, not simply patient preferences or expansion of medical knowledge, has led to an explosion in the numbers of ventilated patients throughout the United States. Economics, coupled with the desires of patients and their often inaccurate perceptions about what their own outcomes might be, have both led to an increase in the use of this modality (15,16). The difficulties that policy makers and health economists have had regarding the health care marketplace relate to the simple fact that the basic economic tenet of supply and demand does not apply. Cost of mechanical ventilation through the early years of its proliferation in hospitals and intensive care units throughout the country was simply not considered as

Table 1 Comparison of Length of Stay and Financial Data on DRG 87 Patients by Mortality Status

| | Institution | | | | |
	1	2	3	4	Combined
No. cases	62	23	26	39	150
% Male	54.8	60.9	42.3	71.8	58.0
Age: mean	76.6	70.0	69.8	72.1	73.2
% Surgery	50.0	52.2	76.9	69.2	60.0
% Mortality	62.9	56.5	42.3	33.3	50.7
Ventilator days: mean	16.0	7.5	12.2	12.1	13.0
Length of stay: mean (days)	31.4	24.6	33.5	23.5	28.7
Charge: mean ($)	63,180	38,665	42,739	30,538	47,391
Cost: mean ($)	31,617	23,903	41,178	30,865	31,896
Payment: mean ($)	11,825	9,282	9,674	11,508	10,981

Source: Ref. 18.

long as cost-based reimbursement assured providers that their costs were covered and profits could be made on these patients. Revenue stream actually would grow significantly in direct proportion to the number of patients on mechanical ventilation. The implementation of the diagnosis-related group (DRG) system in 1983 changed this paradigm. The DRG system did not use mechanical ventilation as a specific modifier for most diseases, and these patients quickly became big money losers for the hospital and a large area of concern for doctors and administrators (17,18) (Table 1). Table 1 provides descriptive information on 150 Medicare patients with greater than 48 hours of mechanical ventilation. Average loss per patient was approximately $21,000 (18). Multiple publications related to the cost of care of patients on mechanical ventilation now appeared in the literature (3,4,17–25). Prior to the implementation of this program, few publications voiced specific concerns regarding this issue. Further restriction of payments from Medicare and third parties has only heightened this issue for hospitals.

III. Cost of Mechanical Ventilation in Critical Care

The data on the cost of caring for the patient on mechanical ventilation are often difficult to interpret. Cost directly related to mechanical ventilation are difficult to dissect from those related to severe acute illness. In general, patients requiring mechanical ventilation are sicker than those without (26) and would be expected, independent of mechanical ventilation, to have increased costs. Davis and Lefrak studied patients receiving mechanical ventilatory support for greater than 48 hours during 1975 and 1976 (24). Patients were evaluated for charges and outcome. These patients were also compared to all other patients hospitalized during the same 12-month period. Total charges were analyzed along with the percentage of hospital charges for the group related to respiratory care. The mean charge for these patients using 1975 dollars was $12,300 compared to $1,600 for all other hospitalized patients. Mortality prior to discharge was 56% for this population and increased to 72% after 2 years. Respiratory care charges amounted to approximately 17% of these charges (24). A similar study, conducted in a community hospital, of mechanically ventilated patients in 1983–1984 with length of mechanical ventilation varying from one hour to 28 days found charges averaged approximately $11,000 per patient and respiratory therapy accounted for 20% of the overall hospital charge (20). The average length of mechanical ventilation was 14.2 days and the average loss per patient was $23,129 for 95 nonsurgical Medicare patients who required more than 3 days of mechanical ventilator support during 1983 and 1984. Under the DRG reimbursement system, patients with a similar diagnosis but outside of the ICU and not on a mechanical ventilator would be reimbursed the same rate as those who required intensive care. The lack of severity adjustment probably accounts for most of the cost differential. Of this entire population, only 35% of the patients were discharged alive. The cost calculation in this study used similar methodology to Medicare cost reporting but included more detailed cost-to-charge ratios (20). Several other studies (17,25,27) using various cost-accounting measures reported similar losses per patient. Wagner's study (5) of patients ventilated for 7 or more days who were part of the APACHE II validation group at 12 major teaching hospitals revealed worse losses. These costs were estimated based on an estimated cost of $113 per TISS point using 1985 prices and the total number of TISS points received by the 227 patients ventilated for more than 7 days. Reimbursement data in this study were based on Blue Cross rates using 30% discount from published charges. The average loss per patient ventilated for more than 7 days was estimated to be $50,000. For patients ventilated for between 1 and 7 days, the average loss was estimated to be $13,000 per patient. Less than half of these high-cost patients actually survived to hospital discharge. In response to concerns over significant economic losses to hospitals for this patient population, the health care financing administration created two new DRGs in 1987 for patients requiring more than 48 hours of mechanical ventilation (17). These DRGs were created to increase reimbursement to hospitals for this group.

Several outcome and economic analyses have been published since the institution of mechanical ventilation DRGs in 1987. A report by Cohen and Lambrinos (21) examined the effect of age on outcome in 41,848 patients from a statewide database in New York who required mechanical ventilation. The economic impact of this patient group was substantial. From the original dataset of approximately 42,000 patients, 15,527 were identified who spent time in the ICU and whose number of ICU days could be calculated. For patients over the age of 70, mortality rates increased significantly. More importantly, a minority of these patients were actually discharged to home. Hospital mortality for the 70- to 74-year age group was 51%, quickly rising to 75% for those over the age of 90. The data looking at discharge to home is even more compelling. For the 70- to 74-year age group, only 31% of patients were discharged to home. In the oldest group, this number dropped to 10%. Specific principal diagnoses, infections, and neoplasm, especially in the older age groups, are even more likely to result in death. These data on poor outcomes specifically related to age may guide patients considering use of this expensive technology (21).

In pursuing this theme, the same group of investigators evaluated the clinical and economic outcome of patients undergoing tracheostomy in New York State during 1993. In this study 6353 cases discharged under DRG 483 "tracheostomy for indication other than face, mouth, or neck diagnosis" were analyzed (28). Average reimbursement for these patients was $107,498. The disposition of the oldest patients again showed high mortality ranging from 55% in the 70- to 74-year age group to 78% in the >90-year age group compared to an overall mortality for the entire population of 48.5%. Of those patients surviving in these older groups, the minority would be discharged to home without home care, dropping from 22.5% in the 70- to 74-year age group to <2½% in the category over the age of 90. An increasing majority of patients in these older age groups who did survive were discharged to a residential health care facility. The costs per survivor were significantly above Medicare reimbursement for all groups ranging from $132,713 in the youngest group, those aged 18–29 years, to $488,627 for those over the age of 90. Length of stay increased with age, the average for the youngest patients being 49 ± 86 days to >72 days for all age groups over the age of 70. The cost to the state for patients with this DRG in 1993 was estimated to be greater than $650 million. The authors suggested that a more rigorous cost-effectiveness analysis considering the diminished quality of life, shortened life expectancy, and long-term care costs for this group be analyzed so that the social and economic impact of this diagnosis could be fully understood (28) (Table 2). To further this theme, investigators from the same group looked at patients in DRG 475 who had respiratory failure that did not result in a tracheostomy (7). From their database, 10,473 patients over the age of 18 were discharged from hospitals in New York State with this diagnosis. The average reimbursement for this discharge was $21,578. They examined the relationship between age, outcome, and economic impact of this diagnosis. The majority of these patients (~55%) were over the age of 70. The average cost per survivor in this group was in the neighborhood of $50,000, with the length of stay averaging slightly less than 3 weeks. The outcomes for these patients was slightly better than in

Table 2 Age Distribution of Patients Under Diagnosis-Related Group 483 and Cost Per Survivor[a]

Age (yr)	Number of patients	Hospital LOS (days)	Cost ($)/survivor
18–29	326	49 ± 86	132,713
30–39	334	61 ± 81	143,330
40–49	454	66 ± 81	158,085
50–59	644	68 ± 72	176,226
60–69	1,339	71 ± 79	210,780
70–74	964	77 ± 79	244,313
75–79	943	77 ± 72	286,661
80–84	720	77 ± 76	318,041
85–89	426	79 ± 111	443,459
90+	203	72 + 61	488,627
Total	6,353	69.7	221,645

LOS = Length of stay.
[a] Average reimbursement was $107,498.
Source: Ref. 28.

those patients receiving tracheostomy. Approximately 60% of the group age 70–74 years decreasing to 30% in the group over the age of 90 survived their hospital stay. Overall, survival was 57%. Significantly greater percentages of these patients were discharged home without home care than those patients receiving tracheostomies. Whereas few of the patients under the age of 70 were discharged to a residential health care facility, in the aggregate for those over the age of 70, roughly 25% had this type of disposition (7).

These studies provide a guide for clinicians caring for this population. Prolonged mechanical ventilation as a diagnosis interpreted under these codes is primarily an affliction of the elderly, with more than 50% of the patients with these diagnoses being over the age of 70 (7,21,28). In younger age groups (<70 years) outcomes were uniformly better and achieved at lower cost, although the cost per survivor in all groups was greater than reimbursement. In the group over the age of 70, the likelihood of independent function at home was small and the costs were high (7,21,28).

A more detailed cost-effectiveness analysis of patients over the age of 80 requiring 3 or more days of mechanical ventilation was performed (29). During a 1½-year time period, 45 patients who met these criteria and also had complete billing records were found. Only 10 of these patients survived hospitalization. Of these 10 patients, after approximately 4 years of follow-up, 7 were still alive. For those patients whose age plus length of mechanical ventilation exceeded 100, this being 22 of the entire group of 45 patients, only 2 survived hospitalization and none were alive at follow-up. Of these 2, one survived 2 months and the

Table 3 Incremental Charges and Benefits Assessed in 45 Patients Over the Age of 80 Requiring >3 Days of Mechanical Ventilation

Sample	No. of patients	Lives saved	Charge per life, ($)	Years of life saved	Charge per year of life saved ($)
All patients					
Lower limit	44	9	305,940	22.1	123,899
Upper limit	45	10	279,623	32.5	86,038
A + D ≥ 100[a]	22	2	721,895	4.8	300,790

1992 dollars were obtained by using the hospital component of the medical care price index from the *Consumer Price Index Detailed Report, January 1992,* U.S. Bureau of Labor Statistics, p. 91, Table 26.
Upper limit uses actuarial data for life expectancy for remaining three survivors. Actual survival will likely be less. Lower limit is actual survival of remaining two patients (one patient could not be located, but was counted as survivor for upper limit analysis).
[a] Age plus days on mechanical ventilation ≥100.
Source: Ref. 29.

other patient survived either in a nursing home or back on the ventilator in the hospital for 56 months. For the entire population, the charge for year of life saved ranged from $51,854 to $75,090. For that subset with age plus length of time on mechanical ventilation greater than 100, which represents fully half the patients in the study, the charge for year of life saved ranged between $181,308 and $300,790 using 1987 dollars (29) (Table 3). The adjusted charge per QALY for the two patients in the latter group considering their outcome, although not calculated in this study based on limitations of the data, would be expected to be significantly greater.

IV. Effects of Specific Diagnoses on Costs and Outcomes of Mechanical Ventilation

Although the age of the patient is significantly associated with the risk of requiring prolonged mechanical ventilation in the hospital, other specific disease states have been studied relative to their outcomes and length of stay. Seneff et al. (30) report on 362 admissions for COPD exacerbation selected from the APACHE III database. Of those patients greater than 65 years old, which in this study was slightly less than one half, 30% died while in the hospital. Approximately one-half were dead by 6 months and 59% in one year. The hospital mortality was significantly associated with age and severity of organ dysfunction. After controlling for severity of illness, mechanical ventilation at admission to the ICU was not associated with either hospital or subsequent survival. Although the need for mechanical ventilation was not independently associated with outcome, patients requiring mechanical ventilation at admission to the ICU were significantly more ill based on APACHE III and acute physiology scoring. The mean hospital length of stay in this group was 30 days, 50% greater than for those not ventilated. The ICU length of stay was 11 days, almost three times that of the nonventilated group (30). Although economic data are not reported in this study, it is clear that longer lengths of stay in the ICU and hospital are associated with increased cost.

Numerous other studies have looked at specific disease categories and the outcome of mechanical ventilation. Those patients with easily reversible disease such as asthma or drug overdose consistently have the best outcome (22). Patients with malignancy uniformly do poorly, and for other diagnostic categories survival is intermediate (6,22). Economic data on the cost-effectiveness of patients mechanically ventilated in an ICU for *Pneumocystis carinii* pneumonia reveals significant change over time. A study published by Wachter and coworkers in 1995 (31) emphasizes that as our understanding of a disease process and its treatment improve, cost-effectiveness ratios related to the treatments are widely variable. They evaluated 113 patients with HIV disease who were ventilated for respiratory failure secondary to pneumocystis pneumonia from 1981 through 1991. These patients were divided into three groups related to the year of admission to the hospital. For patients admitted early during the HIV epidemic (1981–1985), only 14% survived to hospital discharge, with a cost per year of life saved of $305,795. For patients admitted between 1986 through 1988, survival increased to 39%, with a significant decrease in cost per year of life saved, which averaged $94,528.

Table 4 Summary of Cost-Effectiveness of Various Interventions

Strategy	Cost ($)[a]
Propranolol for moderate hypertension[b]	11,000
Bone marrow transplantation in acute nonlymphocytic leukemia	62,500
Early intervention for HIV infection with zidovudine[b]	7,000–70,000
ICU care for patients with hematologic malignancies[b]	189,339
ICU care for patients with AIDS, PCP, and respiratory failure 1986–1988[a]	94,528
Mechanical ventilation for elderly ICU patients[c]	86,600–300,790
t-PA compared with streptokinase for MI: quality-adjusted life year[c]	30,300
CPR per survivor[c]	110,270
Monoclonal antibodies for gram-negative sepsis[c]	5,200–110,000

[a] Per year of life saved except where noted.
[b] From Ref. 31.
[c] From Ref. 13.

In the final time period evaluating patients admitted between 1989 and 1991, the cost per year of life saved averaged $215,233 (31). For this group the strongest predictors of mortality were low CD4 cell count and the development of pneumothorax during mechanical ventilation. Although the cost-effectiveness of intensive care for patients with respiratory failure related to PCP improved during the first 8 years of the AIDS epidemic, it is now below that of many accepted medical interventions (31) (Table 4). This study reminds us that as our understanding and treatments of disease change, the cost and outcomes of caring for these patients in any particular situation are also subject to change. For the majority of patients weaned off the ventilator within 48 hours, these cost concerns are less important.

V. Economics and Outcomes of Patients Transferred Out of the ICU to Less Acute Settings

The Health Care Financing Administration created a long-term care exemption from Medicare prospective payments. As a result of this, the growth in long-term acute care hospitals has been significant. These hospitals generated revenues of over $3 billion in 1997. The outcome of 133 consecutively admitted patients transferred from an ICU while being mechanically ventilated to an urban long-term care hospital were evaluated. Patient-specific variables were used to develop a model predictive of survival (32). Fifty percent of the patients died prior to discharge from a long-term acute care facility. Of the discharged patients, the majority (70%) had been weaned from mechanical ventilation. One year after admission to a long-term acute care hospital, 77% of the original 133 patients had expired, typically spending the majority of their days in acute care or long-term care facilities. Only 11 patients surviving one year were fully functional. This represents 8% of the original group of 133 patients. For those patients either older than 74 years of age or 65 years and older and not functionally independent before admission, the one year mortality was 95% (CI = 84–99%). In those patients without these characteristics, one-year mortality was 56% (32) (Table 5). Although costs are anticipated to be significantly less in the long-term acute care facility than in intensive care, these easily identifiable clinical parameters predict poor outcome with a high degree of certainty. It is unknown what the outcome for these patients would have been had they stayed in the ICU. Prior data as reported in this chapter consistently showed poor outcomes for the elderly population receiving long-term mechanical ventilation in the ICU. Cost shifting is one way to decrease the negative financial impact of prolonged mechanical ventilation for patients in the ICU.

A report analyzing 1123 patients at a regional weaning center suggests that cost shifting is occurring to an increasing degree, largely because of economic pressures and the availability of mechanical ventilation at long-term acute care

Table 5   One-Year Mortality for Cohort of Mechanically Ventilated Patients
Admitted to an Urban Long-Term Acute Care Hospital, Stratified by Both Age Group
and Functional Status Prior to Admission[a]

Prior function	Age group (yr)		
	25–64	65–74	75–100
Independent	**44% (8/18)**	**62% (13/21)**	93% (14/15)
Dependent	**67% (6/9)**	100% (12/12)	94% (15/16)

Boldface refers to group with 56% likelihood of surviving 1 year.
$n = 91$; confidence interval = 41–71%.
Source: Ref. 32.

hospitals or regional weaning centers (33). Patients are being transferred sicker
and quicker from ICUs. These transfers will have significant economic impact
on the ICUs that have this option available. Societal impact is unknown. Daily
costs are expected to be less at regional weaning centers, but the length of time
that the patient stays there along with the outcomes when compared to similar
treatment in an acute care setting is not known. These 1123 patients admitted
over an 8-year period had similar APACHE III scores on admission to the regional weaning center as other patients remaining in ICU. The existence of pressure ulceration had increased over the 8-year study period. Patients were found
to have poor nutritional status and worse pulmonary disease at the time of transfer. One year survival for this patient population improved from 29% in 1988
through 1991 to 45% after 1992. For those patients transferred to the regional
weaning center after 1992, the prior duration of mechanical ventilation was significantly shorter at approximate 28 days as compared to 48 days for the earlier
time period (33).

The best outcome data for patients transferred from an ICU to a weaning
center comes from the Mayo Clinic (34). This unit, which is hospital based,
encompasses a multispecialty team employing a holistic management approach
for the care of long-term ventilated patients. Two hundred and six patients were
admitted to the unit during the study period of 1990–1994. The outcomes of
these patients were compared to a group of historical controls. The data reported
in this group are significantly better than those of the two prior studies. The
reasons for this are not clear and may be related to severity of illness and length
of prior mechanical ventilation. In any event, these data provide at least some
encouragement that a ventilator-dependent rehabilitation unit may provide beneficial therapy to patients requiring long-term mechanical ventilation and do it at
lower cost. The study group included patients ventilated for more than 21 days

who had at least two attempts to remove the endotracheal tube without success. The mean age of the patients was 65, and the median number of weaning center ventilator days was 44. Of the 206 patients, 16 died prior to discharge, leaving 190 who were successfully discharged from the ventilator-dependent rehabilitation unit. Eighty percent of these patients were completely liberated from mechanical ventilation. Of the 37 patients still requiring mechanical ventilation, 27 received ventilation only at night, 24 of which were able to go home. After four years, 53% of the patients were still alive (34). The difference in daily care costs between the ventilator-dependent rehab unit and the intensive care unit was more than $200 per day. The potential savings per year to a hospital with a 10-bed ventilator-dependent unit was calculated to be approximately $730,000. The reasons for these improved survival data in this cohort of patients are unclear and cannot be determined from the data presented. However, only 12% of the total population had previous lung disease as the major cause of ventilator dependence, and fully 60% of the group were postoperative. Although it does not state in this report what percentage of these patients were emergent or elective operation, certainly the expectation for an elective operation would be that the patient would ultimately be weaned from the ventilator (34).

Other data have shown similar benefits by using less expensive alternatives to the ICU for mechanically ventilated hospitalized patients. Kreiger et al.'s report of their initial experience with a central respiratory monitoring unit reported significant cost savings for long-term ventilator patients when compared to ICU care (35). Their data are based on average cost to the hospital using 1986 data. They calculated cost savings per patient per day at $203. They also found that the noninvasive monitoring unit was also less costly than a regular room, primarily because of extra personnel that would be required in a regular patient room. They further hypothesized that if four ICU beds at their institution were converted to four noninvasive monitoring unit beds that the estimated cost reduction for their institution would have been $106,000 (35). Elpern et al. reported on their experience with 107 mechanically ventilated patients also treated in a noninvasive respiratory care unit (36). Although reported outcomes were poor, with greater than 50% of the patients dying and only a third discharged to home, the loss per patient was significantly less when compared to the cost of ventilating the patient in the medical ICU. In this study, hospital costs were obtained by multiplying charges by cost-to-charge ratios. Using these data, the average cost per ventilator day was $1,976 less than the average daily cost of care in the ICU. Despite this, their analysis revealed the average cost per ventilated patient exceeded payments from Medicare or Medicaid by approximately $730 per day (36). The savings related to the noninvasive unit were calculated from the number of days on mechanical ventilation resulting in a projected savings for this population of $20,000 per patient. Outcome data were not directly compared to patients treated in an

ICU, although time outside the ICU is significantly less costly than caring for patients in the intensive care unit. Further experience with a less intensive setting for mechanically ventilated patients was reported by Latriano et al. in 1996 (37). Hemodynamically stable, mechanically ventilated patients were treated on a non-monitored respiratory care floor. Other than occasional use of pulse oximetry and capnography, no other monitoring devices were used. The 1:3 nurse-to-patient ratio reported on the respiratory care floor is similar to that of many ICUs. Seventy-two percent of patients had a tracheostomy at the time of transfer to the respiratory care unit. Overall survival was 50%, and 94% of the surviving group were successfully weaned from mechanical ventilation. However, only 40% of the survivors were discharged home, with a third going to a rehabilitation unit and 24% discharged to a skilled nursing facility. Only 20% of the patients had chronic lung disease as a primary diagnosis. Although cost-accounting methods were not specifically described, similar techniques were used for patients within the ICU or the respiratory care unit. Using these data resulted in a cost savings per day of $376 to treat a patient in the respiratory care unit versus the intensive care unit. For their population requiring a total of 10,891 ventilator days on the respiratory care unit, they calculated a savings of over $4 million (37). Outcomes in these groups were not directly compared to a controlled group continuing care in the ICU. These data are not significantly different than what has been obtained with similar populations.

Concern has been raised about intermediate care units (38), particularly since the major motivation for transferring patients to these units is overwhelmingly economic. Concern for this bias considering resource allocation is clearly warranted. The high mortality in this population along with the poor functional status of many of those who do survive only heightens concern over this issue. Similar concerns, however, may be true of any patient transferred from the ICU to an intermediate care unit, a rehab facility, or the medical and surgical wards. Those working in the ICU can easily recall instances where patients transferred out of the unit who should have done well, do not. Concerns over the adequacy of monitoring, nursing, and physician care outside the protective environment of the typical critical care unit are appropriately considered by practitioners and family alike in these instances. Unfortunately, health care dollars are a limited resource, and perhaps we should realize that society has already placed economic limits on what they are willing to pay for certain types of care. Based on the data presented looking at reimbursement versus cost for longer term mechanically ventilated patients, either within or outside the ICU, payors have already clearly made this decision. Data from prospective scientific experiments regarding outcome of these patients treated in ICUs or elsewhere will never be answered. Considering the present reimbursement situation for this population, these answers will remain elusive and cost-containment pressure will favor less expensive settings for ongoing management.

VI. Outcome Prediction and the Decision to Use Mechanical Ventilation

Anticipated outcomes will be useful to physicians and families when making decisions about continuing mechanical ventilation. A fairly comprehensive assessment of outcome probability for mechanically ventilated medical patients was performed using the validation set for the APACHE II scoring system (6). Thirteen large teaching hospitals provided the patients for this study. The APACHE II system has been reported elsewhere but includes acute physiology and chronic disability (26). For this study, 571 consecutive nonoperative ventilated ICU admissions were included. Using disease information alone, patients with a high risk of death on admission could be identified. Patients requiring mechanical ventilation for respiratory failure and cancer, cardiac arrest, intracranial hemorrhage or septic shock had a 67–75% chance of dying in the hospital. Interestingly, for these and the other major diagnoses studied—gastrointestinal (GI) bleeding, pneumonia, ARDS, respiratory arrest, chronic obstructive pulmonary disease (COPD) and congestive heart failure—the length of time of mechanical ventilation out to seven days did not influence outcome. Using the APACHE II severity score and including those with a score of 26 or greater on admission, >75% mortality in all diagnosis categories except respiratory arrest, COPD, and congestive heart failure was predicted. Sequential data in this population significantly increased the potential accuracy of outcome prediction. For those patients whose day 4 APACHE II score remained 26 or greater, the hospital mortality rate was 97%, producing a single survivor of the 39 patients in this category. For the 16 patients remaining ventilated on day 7 whose APACHE scores were 26 or greater, there were no survivors. Although the numbers of patients were small, especially on days 4 and 7, the predictive power of acute physiology scoring was significant (6). These types of data regarding prognosis should be useful to clinicians, patients, and families when used in conjunction with patient preferences for treatments and attitudes about quality of life. An enlarged data base prospectively validated to evaluate outcomes for this high-risk group of patients has the potential to eliminate care that only prolongs the dying process. Although an individual patient's probability cannot be accurately estimated, the population-based data are useful to patients considering decisions about a prolonged course of mechanical ventilation.

VII. Noninvasive Positive Pressure Ventilation as a Cost-Saving Technique

Multiple other techniques have been used in an attempt to decrease costs for this expensive group of patients. Several studies have addressed the alternative of positive pressure ventilation using a mask instead of an endotracheal tube for patients admitted with impending respiratory failure. Attempting to treat patients this way has obvious nonmonetary benefits to the patient. Although in the aggregate, the proportion of ventilated patients to whom this may ultimately apply, when considering days of mechanical ventilation, is small, the economic savings can be significant. A study by Holt using a fairly comprehensive costing methodology showed a significant reduction in the use of mechanical ventilation for patients treated with mask continuous positive airway pressure (CPAP), yielding significant cost savings (39). Patients who had severe cardiogenic pulmonary edema and did not respond to oxygen, furosemide, and nitrates were entered into this study. These patients were then treated with mask CPAP. Interestingly, the need for mechanical ventilation was reduced to 0 from a historical proportion of 35%. Using this approach, however, roughly tripled the number of admissions to the ICU with this diagnosis because all the patients receiving mask CPAP were admitted to the intensive care unit. Despite this, overall cost even for this increased number of patients was significantly less than projected for ventilating approximately one-third of them. Patients were typically treated with mask CPAP for approximately 1.2 days with a mean cost of $1156 compared to those patients who were ventilated and remained on the ventilator for an average of 4.2 days at a cost of $5055. Major contributors to cost in both these groups were physician fees, nursing salaries, and hospital overhead. The cost for the patients on CPAP was even less than for those patients who did not require mechanical ventilation. The reason for this is that patients who were admitted to the ICU and not ventilated or placed on mask CPAP had longer lengths of stay than patients treated with CPAP alone (39) (Table 6). Although not a randomized, prospective experiment, this study does show a profound difference in cost for those patients who can be managed with mask CPAP compared to mechanical ventilation (39). These data should encourage clinicians to at least institute a trial of mask CPAP for this diagnosis.

Cost savings related to noninvasive positive pressure ventilation for other diagnoses, however, may not be significant (40). This study looked at the economics of noninvasive positive pressure ventilation in 27 patients with severe COPD or restrictive lung disease. These patients were all hypercapnic at the time of hospital admission and had poor functional status. Patients were treated either initially in the ICU or admitted directly to the ventilator rehabilitation unit (40). Eleven patients were admitted with DRG 475 (respiratory system diagnosis with ventilation support), with the remainder being admitted across five different DRG codes with average reimbursement rates ranging from $2,673 to $4,215. The reimbursement rate for DRG 475 was $11,149. Including outlier reimbursement, a total deficit of $261,948 or an average deficit of $9,701 per patient was recorded. Eighty-two percent of the patients treated with noninvasive positive pressure ventilation in this study incurred significant financial losses. Although

Table 6 Cost Components of Average ICU Episode for Patients with Respiratory Failure and Pulmonary Edema: An Initial Approach Using CPAP Instead of Mechanical Ventilation Lowered Costs Substantially

	CPAP $ (%)	Oxygen alone	
		Nonventilated, $ (%)	Ventilated, $ (%)
Nursing salaries/wages	324 (28)	459 (30)	2,187 (43)
Medical salaries/wages	161 (14)	228 (15)	563 (11)
Drug supplies	12 (1)	13 (1)	158 (3)
Med/surg consumables	44 (4)	21 (1.5)	275 (5.5)
Other costs	41 (3.5)	59 (4)	145 (3)
Allied health	0 (0)	0 (0)	20 (0.5)
Pathology	120 (10)	129 (8)	185 (4)
Radiology	66 (5.5)	79 (5)	165 (3)
Hospital overhead	388 (34)	549 (35.5)	1,357 (27)
Average total:			
Episode cost	$1,156	$1,537	$5,055
Average daily cost	$ 963	$ 904	$1,204

Source: Ref. 39.

there is no comparison with the cost of invasive ventilation for these patients, it does point out that this type of therapy is very labor intensive (40). Sixty-three percent of direct costs for these patients are related to nursing and respiratory therapy activities. Prior data showed that 95% of one ICU nurse's time is required to deliver noninvasive ventilation effectively (41). For those patients with more chronic respiratory ailments, although noninvasive positive pressure ventilation may enable them to avoid intubation and mechanical ventilation, this therapy is time consuming and costly. Average length of stay for the entire group was 29 days (40). A prospective trial comparing 10 consecutive patients with COPD treated with noninvasive mechanical ventilation was compared to a group of six patients receiving invasive mechanical ventilation (42). Daily costs and time spent by doctors, therapists, and nurses were recorded during the first 48 hours of ventilation. These groups were similar in terms of degree of hypercapnia and admission pH. During the first 48 hours of ventilation, there was no significant difference in the amount of time spent by nurses, doctors, or therapists at the bedside of patients receiving noninvasive mechanical ventilation compared to those receiving invasive mechanical ventilation. Interestingly, the total costs for these patients during this time period were also not significantly different, averaging $806 in the noninvasive group versus $864 in the invasive group. After the initial 40% of total ventilator time, the physician and nursing workload was significantly greater for those patients on a ventilator compared to those receiving noninvasive mechanical ventilation. Costs beyond the first 48 hours were not assessed (42).

These and other data have shown that noninvasive positive pressure ventilation is a reasonable initial approach for a significant percentage of patients presenting with a diagnosis of respiratory failure. Although the cost savings may be variable, especially for those patients with acute disease, this approach is likely to result in shorter ICU lengths of stay and less complications.

As has been pointed out in this chapter, the bulk of money expended on these patients is particularly associated with longer length of stay, older age, and poor prognosis. Elimination of these groups from the ICU, although a laudable economic goal and possibly a reasonable health outcome goal, is not likely in the foreseeable future. Rapid stabilization and placement of these patients in less acute settings than the ICU does result in measurable cost savings with uncertain benefits on health outcome. This type of cost shifting with poorly quantitated patient benefit or risk probably represents some of our best efforts to date on minimizing cost for this expensive group of patients.

VIII. Ancillary Approaches to Decrease Cost for Mechanical Ventilation of ICU Patients

A significant number of patients who present with severe acute medical or surgical problems and are not previously afflicted with poor functional status or chronic health problems may require mechanical ventilation for extended periods of time in the ICU. These patients often have complete recovery and are able to return to previously productive lives. There is great potential in this population to minimize cost during their ICU stay without affecting quality of care. How we manage these patients while on the ventilator specifically with regards to management of pain and sedation, number of x-ray, lab, and ancillary tests that are performed, ventilator circuit changes, protocol-driven weaning, and pharmacy intervention have all been identified as significant cost savers. In specific populations of critically ill patients, length of stay is the primary driver of costs and outcome has been positively influenced by the use of full-time critical care specialists. The effects of these interventions and ideas on furthering these applications in mechanically ventilated patients in the ICU will be presented in the next sections.

Multiple aspects of care of patients on mechanical ventilators have been studied with the specific goal of reducing costs to this patient population. A series of studies looking at ventilator circuit changes has been published in the last several years.

Prior data have shown that changing ventilator circuits every 24 hours rather than every 48 hours was an independent risk factor for nosocomial pneumonia (43). The reason for this increased incidence of pneumonia with more frequent circuit changes was not clear, but it was speculated to be simply related to increased intervention. Considering the expense of the circuit and therapists' time necessary to perform circuit changes, several investigators have evaluated a more prolonged protocol for ventilator circuit changes. Two studies evaluated the cost and outcome of prolonging circuit changes out to 7 days. The first study by Hess et al. (44) compared changing circuits at either 48-hour or 7-day intervals. Nosocomial pneumonia was diagnosed using Centers for Disease Control and Prevention (CDC) criteria and the annual cost difference was calculated using total ventilator days. In the control group, 9858 ventilator days were evaluated with a pneumonia rate of 9.64 per 1000. Compared to the 48-hour circuit change, there was no difference when ventilator circuits were changed at one-week intervals: 9160 ventilator days were evaluated with 8.62 pneumonias per 1000 ventilator days. The relative odds of developing pneumonia with the one week change frequency was 0.82 ($p = 0.22$). Ventilator-associated pneumonia occurred earlier in the course of patients using the 48-hour circuit change with a median of 5 days compared to those patients using the 7-day circuit change where the median was 7 days ($p = 0.26$). A cost estimate included an average amount of time to change a circuit of 15 minutes and an hourly salary for respiratory therapy of approximately \$14.50. The cost of the circuit was determined to be \$17.26. In both 6-month periods studied, approximately 1700 patients were mechanically ventilated at the Massachusetts General Hospital. The calculated annualized cost savings in materials and salaries for the 7-day circuit changes was \$11,530. This represented a 77% cost reduction using the 7-day strategy. Further extrapolating their cost data to all patients in the United States undergoing mechanical ventilation, they estimated an \$18,621,000 cost savings and personnel time savings of 107 full-time equivalents.

Kotilainen and Keroack performed a similar study looking at the clinical and cost impact of a 72-hour versus 7-day interval (45). They noted a more frequent occurrence of pneumonia in those patients with a 72-hour circuit change, 9.1%, vs. 6.2% for those with the weekly changes ($p = 0.44$). Weekly changes also significantly reduced the number of circuits used with an annualized cost savings of \$20,246 for their two intensive care units with a total of 17 beds. Although the number of patients diagnosed with ventilator-associated pneumonia was small, they found no correlation with the pathogen causing pneumonia to the corresponding culture from the ventilator circuit.

Kollef and coworkers extended this out and looked at 147 patients randomly assigned to receive no ventilator circuit changes compared to 153 patients receiving circuit changes every 7 days (46). Ventilator-associated pneumonia in this study was significantly greater than the prior studies reported: 24.5% in those patients receiving no routine changes and 28.8% in those patients receiving changes every 7 days. (Relative risk = 0.85; 95% CI = 0.55–1.17.) Patients were not included in this study unless they required mechanical ventilation for greater than 5 days. This factor alone probably accounts for the increase incidence of pneumonia in this study. In terms of important clinical outcomes—mortality of patients either in the ICU or hospital or duration of mechanical ventilation— there were no significant differences between the two treatment groups. The patients receiving circuit changes every 7 days had an approximate 20-fold increase in costs related to 247 circuit changes for these 153 patients compared to 11 circuit changes for 147 patients assigned to no ventilator circuit changes. In this well-designed study, for those expensive patients requiring long-term mechanical ventilation, elimination of routine ventilator circuit changes can significantly reduce medical care costs without adverse clinical consequences (46).

Other interventions related to disposable components necessary for mechanical ventilation have been studied with regard to their impact on economic and clinical parameters. A significant cost savings can be realized with less frequent changes of in-line suction catheters. Kollef, continuing his cost-saving work, looked at daily versus no changes in in-line suction catheters (47). He similarly found a significant cost savings for those patients who had no routine in-line suction catheter changes without a difference in important clinical outcome measures. Approximately four to five catheter changes per patient could be avoided at a cost of approximately $9/catheter change. There were approximately 260 patients in each group whose average duration of mechanical ventilation was $5^{1}/_{2}$ days. For this patient group, ventilated for a relatively short period of time, not changing in-line suction catheters routinely resulted in significant cost savings.

Kirton and coworkers looked at the use of different types of heat and moisture exchange humidifiers on the incidence of ventilator associated pneumonia and the rate of endotracheal tube occlusion (48). Their study of similarly ill trauma patients using an in-line heat moisture exchange filter found significantly decreased rates of ventilator-associated pneumonia compared to a conventional heated wire humidifier. Length of stay and cost was significantly greater for patients who developed pneumonia. An average savings of approximately $10 per patient was also realized using the heat moisture exchanging filter. Concern about adequate tracheobronchial humidification and consequent endotracheal tube occlusion related to these in-line exchange filters was not borne out by this study.

Other cost-modification efforts not directly related to mechanical ventilation but associated with it have been applied in a critical care setting. The more important features of many of these topics will be discussed in more detail in other chapters, but several major themes emerge in view of these data. Protocol development for drug use particularly related to sedatives, analgesics, and neuromuscular blocking agents, especially with the help of full-time pharmacists rounding in the unit may have significant economic impact on the care of these patients. Marx and DeMaintenon were able to show a 75% reduction in cost of neuromuscular blocking drugs along with a 35% decrease in ventilator hours following institution of a protocol for the appropriate use of neuromuscular blocking agents (49). Devlin et al. (50) reported a 75% decrease in sedation drug costs without adverse effect on weaning from mechanical ventilation after institution of ICU sedation guidelines promoting lorazepam rather than midazolam or propofol in mechanically ventilated patients. Simple interventions including the elimination of standing orders, especially for chest x-rays and arterial blood gases, have also shown a significant impact on cost (51). One interesting study, although not a true economic analysis, did report that routine chest x-rays resulted in a mean savings of $98 per patient (52). This estimated cost savings was the result of multiple assumptions and is not proven as an outcome of this study itself.

Incredible amounts of money can be used sedating patients on mechanical ventilation as shown in a study by Barrientos-Vega et al. (53). This study looked at the impact on weaning and overall cost of patients relative to the sedating agent used—either propofol or midazolam in this study. Cost for propofol despite the patients being weaned more quickly was approximately three times that for midazolam: $1,047 versus $378. Despite this, cost per patient was higher with midazolam and directly related to the difference in weaning time between these groups. Overall cost per patient was $10,828 in the midazolam group compared to $9,466 in the propofol group—a difference of $1,362. There was an approximate 2½-day difference in weaning time. A significantly longer time to wean patients who had been sedated with midazolam accounted for most of the cost difference.

IX. Organizational Issues and Optimal Management of Mechanical Ventilation

Optimal management of the clinical diagnosis requiring mechanical ventilation along with other aspects of care related to critically ill patients is probably the single most important determinant of length of time on mechanical ventilation, cost, and outcome. Unfortunately, these paramount treatment issues have not been adequately assessed in prospective randomized trials to allow thoughtful consideration of best medical practice. Ultimately, optimally managing a patient's clinical disease will have the greatest impact on cost-effectiveness. Subsequent chapters in this book will address optimal ventilator management strategies for patients with asthma, COPD, ARDS, and ventilator-associated pneumonia. Prevention of ventilator-associated lung injury or other complications related to ICU treatment will likely have a significant impact on patient outcome and cost.

As outlined earlier in this chapter, high-cost mechanically ventilated patients are typically those requiring prolonged mechanical ventilation. Often these patients have severe pulmonary disease requiring initial ICU admission or as complication of severe medical or surgical illness. Several studies have evaluated the impact of early extubation on patients undergoing coronary artery bypass surgery without significant acute lung disease. These studies have typically shown shortened length of stay and reduced expenditures for those patients who were successfully extubated early (54–58). For this patient population and patients arriving in the ICU intubated as a consequence of anesthesia rather than acute lung disease, the trend has been toward earlier extubation and overall decreased use of ICU resources.

The organization of the ICU has particular impact on outcome and length of stay. Several studies have looked at either a specific ventilatory management team or protocol-directed weaning. A retrospective review compared an historical control of 198 patients whose ventilatory management occurred before the institution of a specific ventilatory management team with the outcomes of 165 patients who were managed by the team (59). The team consisted of an ICU attending, a nurse, and a respiratory therapist, who rounded on the patients and supervised the ventilatory management. In the group managed by this team, there was a significant reduction of resource use. Days on mechanical ventilation decreased by three as did days in the ICU. There was a significant reduction in the number of arterial blood gases and indwelling arterial catheters used. The estimated cost savings were $1303 per episode of mechanical ventilation (59) (Table 7) Using the ventilatory management team expedited the weaning process with significant cost savings. Formalizing the interactive process between nurses, physicians, and respiratory therapists regarding the overall management of weaning in these patients was thought to be the major intervention resulting in improved outcomes. This type of protocol-directed weaning has been instituted on a significantly larger scale with similar good results (60). Investigators at Wake Forest University reported on 1067 patients requiring over 9000 days of mechanical ventilation following the introduction of a validated protocol including a daily screen along with a spontaneous breathing trial. This therapist-driven protocol did not involve physician input or a weaning team. The frequency at which patients who pass a daily screen underwent spontaneous breathing trials increased throughout the implementation process. Although passing this daily screen did lead to an increase in the number of patients undergoing spontaneous breathing trials, ordering of this trial was variable, ranging from 63% in surgical patients to 81% in medical patients (60).

Horst et al. were able to show significant cost savings and decrease in ventilation time using a standardized weaning process (61). Using an historic control and number of ventilator hours per year as the outcome, these investigators were able to show a decrease in the number of ventilator hours from 64,488 hours in 378 patients who underwent physician directed weaning to 57,796 ventilator hours in 515 patients in the protocol-guided pathway. Mean hours of ventila-

Table 7 Monetary Savings Associated with a 3.9-Day Reduction in Time on the Ventilator in ICU[a] for 165 Patients Managed by a Ventilatory Management Team Compared to 198 Historical Controls

	Savings per day ($)	Savings per 3.9 days ($)
Respiratory therapy[b]	75	293
Nursing at $13 per hour[c]	104	406
ABG at $11 each[d]	59	230
Caths at $175 each including physician fee[e]	46	179
Miscellaneous	50	195
Total	334	1303

ABG, arterial blood gas measurements; caths, arterial catheters.

[a] Assumes no reduction in overall length of stay.

[b] Includes equipment and therapist time.

[c] Based on a difference between a 1:2 nurse-to-patient ratio in the ICU and a 1:6 nurse-to-patient ratio on the regular floor. Excludes benefits.

[d] Based on a reduction of an average 5.4 arterial blood gas measurements per day (21.2 ABG reduction over a 3.9-day period).

[e] Based on a reduction of an average of 0.26 catheters per day (1.02 cath reduction over a 3.9-day period).

Source: Ref. 59.

tion decreased by 58, a 46% decrease; hospital length of stay was also decreased by 1.77 days. Severity modeling using APACHE III scoring was unchanged over the two time periods. The number of reintubations was the same, and the marginal cost savings was $603,580 (61). Others have also shown that employing a more standardized approach to weaning patients from mechanical ventilation can result in decreased time on mechanical ventilation and shorter ICU stays (62–64).

Kollef et al. (65) furthered this practice by instituting a protocol-directed weaning pathway run primarily by nurses and respiratory therapists compared to more traditional physician-directed weaning attempts. Those patients randomized to protocol-directed weaning had significantly shorter duration of mechanical ventilation and greater rates of successful weaning compared to those patients receiving physician-directed weaning. Hospital mortality rates for the two treatment groups were similar: 22.3% for protocol patients versus 23.6% for physician-directed patients. The cost savings for the patients in the protocol-directed group amounted to $42,960 for the 4-month time period studied, encompassing 357 patients requiring mechanical ventilation. Using protocol-directed weaning, patients were identified sooner during their course of mechanical ventilation—39.6 hours versus 58.3 hours ($p = 0.016$) for initiation of weaning—and required only about 70% of the time to be extubated compared to the physician directed group—69.4 versus 102 hours ($p = 0.029$) of total ventilation. There was a trend for a decreased number of patients requiring mechanical ventilation for greater than 7 days—11.7% versus 17.4%—but this was not statistically significant. Interestingly, there was no difference in hospital length of stay—12.7 days versus 14.2 days ($p = 0.517$). Also, there was no significant difference in the type of weaning strategy employed in either group (65) (Table 8) Patients were variably weaned on intermediate mandatory ventilation (IMV), pressure support ventilation (PSV), or spontaneous weaning trials. An interesting observation of this study was that the success of the intervention seemed to be related to the organizational structure of the ICU in which it was employed. This strategy had the least impact in the unit that lacked a full-time medical director, suggesting that the organizational characteristics of the ICU may play a significant role in the outcome of patients treated there.

Multiple studies have looked at the impact of an ICU specialist on mortality and length of stay of critically ill patients. Two recent articles can be used to highlight these findings (66,67). Hanson et al.'s study (66) compared simultaneously admitted patients to the surgical ICU. One group was cared for by the on-site critical care team supervised by an intensivist with the control group cared for by a team with multiple care responsibilities outside the ICU and supervised by a general surgeon. Patients managed by the critical care team had more severe illness as measured by APACHE scoring but spent less time in the ICU, used

Table 8 Weaning Strategy: Patients Having Protocol Directed Weaning Were Identified Sooner 39.6 vs. 58.3 Hours and Required Less Total Time on Mechanical Ventilation 69.4 vs. 102 Hours Than Physician-Directed Weaning[a]

Variable	Protocol-directed weaning ($n = 179$)	Physician-directed weaning ($n = 178$)
Pao_2/Fio_2 ratio	273 ± 131	272 ± 124
Maximum inspiratory pressure (cm H_2O)	43.6 ± 15.4 [106]	40.1 ± 12.9 [67]
Tidal volume (mL)	422 ± 207 [103]	442 ± 165 [67]
Respiratory frequency (breaths/min)	22.0 ± 8.5 [104]	21.0 ± 4.8 [67]
Mode of mechanical ventilation, n (%)		
Intermittent mandatory	45 (25.1)	48 (27.0)
Pressure-support	56 (31.3)	41 (23.0)
Assist-control	78 (43.6)	89 (50.0)
Weaning strategy, n (%)		
Intermittent mandatory ventilation	48 (30.6)	55 (35.7)
Pressure-support ventilation	70 (44.6)	57 (37.0)
Spontaneous breathing trials	39 (24.8) [157]	42 (27.3) [154]

[a] Weaning strategies were similar. Numbers in brackets represent the number of patients for which dates were available. Numbers in parentheses are percentages.
Source: Ref. 65.

fewer resources, and had fewer complications along with significantly lower total hospital charges. These differences were most evident in those patients with the worst APACHE II scores. ICU length of stay was approximately 1 day shorter and hospital length of stay 3 days shorter for those patients managed by the critical care service. Overall Medicare adjusted charges were only 60% as great, $34,500 compared to $47,500, for patients who were not managed by an intensivist-led team. Days of ventilation, 0.7 versus 1.2 ($p < 0.01$), and arterial blood gases, 3.0 versus 6.0 ($p < 0.01$), were significantly less for patients managed by the critical care service (66).

Pronovost et al.'s study (67) looked at all Maryland hospitals that performed abdominal aortic surgery from 1994 to 1996. Approximately 3000 patients were studied. In-hospital mortality and hospital length of stay were the main outcome measures evaluated. There was large mortality variation, from 0 to 66%. In multivariate analysis adjusted for comorbidity, severity, hospital and surgeon volume, and hospital characteristics, not having daily rounds by an ICU physician was associated with a threefold increase in in-hospital mortality (OR 3.0; 95% CI 1.9–4.9). The likelihood of reintubation was twice as great in those patients treated in ICUs without daily rounds by an ICU physician (OR 2.0; 95% CI 1–4.1). Not having daily rounds by an ICU physician was associated with increased resource use. In multivariate analysis, not having daily rounds by an ICU physician was associated with an increased ICU length of stay of 83% (95% CI 48–126% increase) (67). The care model, especially when led by a physician who has a qualified interest in the costs and outcomes of patients admitted to his or her unit, may be the most significant independent predictor of these variables when analyzing costs and outcomes of patients admitted to ICUs.

X. Conclusion

For the majority of patients requiring mechanical ventilation in the intensive care unit with short lengths of stay and brief episodes of mechanical ventilation, significant cost savings are possible related to how these episodes are managed. An integrated weaning team with a fair degree of autonomy following validated weaning protocols can significantly shorten length of time on the ventilator. Evidence-based protocols regarding the use of disposable equipment along with noninvasive monitoring of ventilation and oxygenation and judicious use of chest x-rays and arterial blood gases (ABGs) will also yield savings. Avoidance of paralysis when possible and close monitoring of sedation will shorten ventilatory times and minimize complications. In those patients with good functional status prior to admission and severe acute illness requiring prolonged mechanical ventilation, transfer to a specialized weaning center either within or outside the hospital once other acute issues are resolved will probably result in the greatest cost savings. Considering the large group of patients with prolonged mechanical ventilation and previously poor functional status and chronic health problems, most of whom are elderly, minimizing time in the intensive care unit and the hospital will result in the greatest cost benefit as outcomes in this population are uniformly poor. Using more realistic outcome probabilities for this group of stable yet very sick patients may result in a less aggressive approach in some. Global budgeting for health services which maximizes the incremental utility of health expenditures has the potential to lead to the best health outcomes for the population when considering limited economic resources.

References

1. Starr P. The Social Transformation of American Medicine. New York: Basic Books, Inc., 1982.
2. Detsky AS, Stricker SC, Malley AG, Thibault GE. Prognosis, survival and the expenditures of hospital resources for patients in an intensive care unit. N Engl J Med 1981; 305:667–672.
3. Spivack D. The high cost of acute health care: a review of escalating costs and limitations of such exposure in intensive care units. Am Rev Respir Dis 1987; 36: 1007–1011.
4. Rosen RI, Bone RC. Economics of mechanical ventilation. Clin Chest Med 1988; 9:163–169.
5. Wagner DP. Economics of prolonged mechanical ventilation. Am Rev Respir 1989; 140:S14–S18.
6. Knaus WA. Prognosis with mechanical ventilation: the influence of disease, severity of disease, age and chronic health status on survival from an acute illness. Am Rev Respir Dis 1989; 140:S8–S13.
7. Kurek CJ, Dewar D, Lambrinos J, et al. Clinical and economic outcome of mechanically ventilated patients in New York State during 1993. Analysis of 10,473 cases under DRG 475. Chest 1998; 114:214–222.
8. Weinstein MC, Stason WB. Foundations of cost-effectiveness analysis for health and medical practices. N Engl J Med 1977; 296:716–721.
9. Detsky AS, Naglie GI. A physician's guide to cost effectiveness analysis. Ann Int Med 1990; 113:147–54.
10. Snider GL. Historical perspective on mechanical ventilation from simple life support systems to ethical dilemma. Am Rev Respir Dis 1989; 140:S2–S7.
11. Petty TL. A historical perspective of mechanical ventilation. Crit Care Med 1990; 6:489–504.
12. Ashbaugh DG, Bigelow DB, Petty TL, Levine BE. Acute respiratory distress in adults. Lancet 1967; 2:219–223.
13. Chalfin DB. Analysis of cost-effectiveness in intensive care: an overview of methods and a review of applications to problems in critical care medicine. Curr Opin Anesthesiol 1996; 9:129–133.
14. Doubilet P, Weinstein MC, McNeil BJ. Use and misuse of the term "cost effective" in medicine. N Engl J Med 1986; 314:253–256.

15. Chan L, Koepsell TD, Deyo RA, Esselman PC, Haselkorn JK, Lowery JK, Stolov WC. The effect of Medicare's payment system for rehabilitation hospitals on length of stay, charges, and total payments. N Engl J Med 1997; 337:978–985.

16. Weeks JC, Cook F, O'Day SJ, Peterson LM, Wenger N, Reding D, Harrell FE, Kussin P, Dawson NV, Connors AF, Lynn J, Phillips RS. Relationship between cancer patients' predictions of prognosis and their treatment preferences. JAMA 1998; 279:1709–1714.

17. Douglass PS, Rosen RL, Butler PW, Bone RC. DRG payment for long-term ventilator patients. Implications and recommendations. Chest 1987; 91:413–417.

18. Gracey DR, Gillespie D, Nobrega F, Naessens JM, Iqbal Krishan. Financial implications of prolonged ventilator care of Medicare patients under the prospective payment system. A multicenter study. Chest 1987; 91:425–427.

19. Schmidt CD, Elliott CG, Carmelli D, et al. Prolonged mechanical ventilation for respiratory failure: A cost-benefit analysis. Crit Care Med 1983; 11:407–411.

20. Witek TJ, Schachter EN, Dean NL, Beck GJ. Mechanically assisted ventilation in a community hospital. Immediate outcome, hospital charges, and follow-up of patients. Arch Intern Med 1985; 145:235–239.

21. Cohen IL, Lambrinos J. Investigating the impact of age on outcome of mechanical ventilation using a population of 41,848 patients from a statewide database. Chest 1995; 107:1673–1680.

22. Krieger BP. Economics of ventilator care. In: Tobin MJ, ed. Principles and Practice of Mechanical Ventilation. New York: McGraw-Hill, 1994:1221–1232.

23. Oye RK, Bellamy PE: Patterns of resource consumption in medical intensive care. Chest 1991; 99:685–89.

24. Davis H, Lefrak SS, Miller D, Matt S. Prolonged mechanically assisted ventilation. An analysis of outcome and charges. JAMA 1980; 243:43–45.

25. Butler PW, Bone RC, Field T. Technology under Medicare diagnosis-related groups prospective payment. Implications for medical intensive care. Chest 1985; 87:229–234.

26. Knaus WA, Draper EA, Wagner DP, et al. APACHE II: A severity of disease classification system. Crit Care Med 1985; 13:818–829.

27. Edbrooke DL, Stevens VG, Hibbert CL, et al. A new method of accurately identifying costs of individual patients in intensive care: the initial results. Inten Care Med 1997; 23:645–650.

28. Kurek CJ, Cohen IL, Lambrinos J, et al. Clinical and economic outcome of patients undergoing tracheostomy for prolonged mechanical ventilation in New York State during 1993: analysis of 6,353 cases under diagnosis-related group 483. Crit Care Med 1997; 25:983–988.

29. Cohen IL, Lambrinos J, Fein IA. Mechanical ventilation for the elderly patient in intensive care. JAMA 1993; 269:1025–1029.

30. Seneff MG, Wagner DP, Wagner RP, Zimmerman JE, Knaus WA. Hospital and one year survival of patients admitted to intensive care units with acute exacerbations of chronic obstructive pulmonary disease. JAMA 1995; 127:1852–1857.

31. Wachter RM, Luce JM, Safrin S, et al. Cost and outcome of intensive care for patients with AIDS, *Pneumocystis carinii* pneumonia, and severe respiratory failure. JAMA 1995; 273:230–235.

32. Carson SS, Bach PB, Brzozowski L, Leff A. Outcomes after long-term acute care. An analysis of 133 mechanically ventilated patients. Am J Respir Crit Care Med 1999; 159:1568–1573.

33. Sheinhorn DJ, Chao DC, Stearn-Hassenpflug M, LaBree LD, Heltsley DJ. Post ICU mechanical ventilation. Treatment of 1,123 patients at a regional weaning center. CHEST 1997; 111:1654–1659.

34. Gracey DR, Hardy DC, Naessens JM, et al. The Mayo ventilator-dependent rehabilitation unit: a 5-year experience. Mayo Clin Proc 1997; 72:13–19.

35. Krieger BP, Ershowsky P, Spivak D, et al. Initial experience with a central respiratory monitoring unit as a cost-saving alternative to the intensive care unit for Medicare patients who require long-term ventilator support. Chest 1988; 93:395–397.

36. Elpern EH, Silver MR, Rosen RL, Bone RC. The noninvasive respiratory care unit. Patterns of use and financial implications. Chest 1991; 99:205–208.

37. Latriano B, McCauley P, Astiz ME, et al. Non-ICU care of hemodynamically stable mechanically ventilated patients. Chest 1996; 109:1591–1596.

38. Popovich JJ. Intermediate care units. Graded care options. Chest 1991; 99:4–5.

39. Holt AW, Bersten AD, Fuller S, et al. Intensive care costing methodology: cost benefit analysis of mask continuous positive airway pressure for severe cardiogenic pulmonary edema. Anaesth Intens Care 1994; 22:170–174.

40. Criner GJ, Kreimer DT, Tomaselli M, et al. Financial implications of non-invasive positive pressure ventilation (NPPV). Chest 1995; 108:475–481.

41. Chevrolet JC, Joilet P, et al. Nasal positive pressure ventilation in patients with acute respiratory failure: Difficult and time consuming procedure for nurses. Chest 1991; 100:775–782.

42. Nava S, Evangelisti I, Rampalla C, et al. Human and financial costs of noninvasive mechanical ventilation in patients affected by COPD and acute respiratory failure. Chest 1997; 111:1631–1638.

43. Craven DE, Kunshes LM, Kilinsky V, Lichtenberg DA, Make BJ, McCabe WR. Risk factors for pneumonia and fatality in patients receiving continuous mechanical ventilation. Am Rev Respir Dis 1986; 133:792–796.

44. Hess D, Burns E, Romagnoli D, Kacmarek RM. Weekly ventilator circuit change. A strategy to reduce costs without affecting pneumonia rates. Anesthesiology 1995; 82:903–911.

45. Kotilainen HR, Keroack MA. Cost analysis and clinical impact of weekly ventilator circuit changes in patients in intensive care unit. Am J Infect Control 1997; 25:117–120.

46. Kollef MH, Shapiro SD, Fraser VJ, Silver P, Murphy DM, Trovillion E, Hearns ML, Richards RD, Cracchilo L, Hossin L. Mechanical ventilation with or without 7-day circuit changes. A randomized controlled trial. Ann Intern Med 1995; 123: 168–174.

47. Kollef MH, Prentice D, Shapiro SD, Fraser VJ, Silver P, Trovillion E, Weilitz P. Von Harz B, St. John R. Mechanical ventilation with or without daily changes of in-line suction catheters. Am J Respir Crit Care Med 1997; 156:466–472.

48. Kirton OC, DeHaven CB, Hudson-Civetta JA, Morgan JP, Windsor J, Civetta JM. Re-engineering ventilatory support to decrease days and improve resource utilization. Ann Surg 1996; 224:396–402.

49. Marx WH, DeMaintenon NL, Mooney KF, Mascia ML, Medicis J, Franklin PD, Sivak E, Rotello J. Cost reduction and outcome improvement in the intensive care unit. J Trauma Injury Infect Crit Care 1999; 46:625–630.

50. Devlin JW, Holbrook AM, Fuller HD. The effect of ICU sedation guidelines and pharmacist interventions on clinical outcomes and drug cost. Ann Pharamcother 1997; 31:689–695.

51. Civetta JM, Hudson-Civetta JA. Maintaining quality of care while reducing charges in the ICU. Ten ways. Ann Surg 1985; 202:524–532.

52. Brainsky A, Fletcher RH, Glick HA, Lanken PN, Williams SV, Kindel HL. Routine portable chest radiographs in the medical intensive care unit: effects and costs. Crit Care Med 1997; 25:801–805.

53. Barrientos-Vega R, Sanchez-Soria MM, Morales-Garcia C, Robas-Gomez A, Cuena-Boy R, Rincon-Ayensa A. Prolonged sedation of critically ill patients with midazolam or propofol: Impact on weaning and costs. Crit Care Med 1997; 25:33–40.

54. Cheng DCH. Early extubation after cardiac surgery decreases intensive care unit stay and cost. Pro: Early extubation after cardiac surgery decreases intensive care unit stay and cost. J Cardiothoracic Vasc Anesth 1995; 9:460–464.

55. Cheng DCH, Karski J, Peniston C, et al. A prospective randomized controlled study of early versus conventional tracheal extubation following coronary artery bypass graft (CABG) surgery: post operative complications with ICU and hospital discharge. Anesthesiology 1994; 81:A145.

56. Cheng DCH, Karski J, Peniston C, et al. Cost analysis of early vs conventional extubation post coronary artery bypass graft (CABG) surgery: a prospective randomized controlled study. Anesth Analg 1995; 80:S73.

57. Cheng DCH, Karski J, Peniston C, Pavcendran G, Asokumar B, Carroll J, David T, Sandler A. Early tracheal extubation after coronary artery bypass graft surgery reduces costs and improves resource use. A prospective, randomized, controlled trial. Anesthesiology 1996; 85:1300–1310.

58. Heinle JS, Diaz LK, Fox LS. Early extubation after cardiac operations in neonates and young infants. J Thorac Cardiovasc Surg 1997; 114:413–418.

59. Cohen II, Bari N, Strosberg MA, Weinberg PF, Wacksman RM, Millstein BH, Fein IA. Reduction of duration and cost of mechanical ventilation in an intensive care unit by use of a ventilatory management team. Crit Care Med 1991; 19:1278–1284.

60. Ely EW, Bennett PA, Bowton DL, Murphy SM, Florance AM, Haponik EF. Large scale implementation of a respiratory therapist-driven protocol for ventilator weaning. Am J Respir Crit Care Med 1999; 159:439–446.

61. Horst HM, Mouro D, Hall-Jenssens RA, Pamukov N: Decrease in ventilation time with standardized weaning process. Arch Surg 1998; 133:483–488.

62. Knebel AR. Ventilator weaning protocols and techniques: getting the job done. AACN Clin Issues 1996; 7:550–559.

63. Kollef MH, Horst HM, Prang L, Brock WA. Reducing the duration of mechanical ventilation: three examples of change in the intensive care unit. New Horizons 1998; 6:52–60.

64. Saura P, Blanch L, Mestre J, Valles J, Artigas A, Fernandez R. Clinical consequences of the implementation of a weaning protocol. Intens Care Med 1996; 22:1052–1056.

65. Kollef MH, Shapiro SD, Silver P, St John RE, Prentice D, Sauer S, Ahrens TS, Shannon W, Baker-Clinkscale D. A randomized, controlled trial of protocol-directed versus physician-directed weaning from mechanical ventilation. Crit Care Med 1997; 25:567–574.
66. Hanson CW, Deutschman CS, Anderson HL, Reilly PM, Behringer EC, Schwab CW, Price J. Effects of an organized critical care service on outcomes and resource utilization: a cohort study. Crit Care Med 1999; 27:270–274.
67. Pronovost PJ, Jenckes MW, Dorman T, Garrett E, Breslow MJ, Rosenfeld BA, Lipsett PA, Bass E. Organizational characteristics of intensive care units related to outcomes of abdominal aortic surgery. JAMA 1999; 281:1310–1317.

5

Mechanical Ventilation
Protocol-Driven Strategies

MARIN H. KOLLEF

Washington University School of Medicine
St. Louis, Missouri

I. Introduction

Positive-pressure ventilation is a technique of providing ventilatory support usually applied through an artificial airway. The increasing use of mechanical ventilation over the past 40 years has paralleled the development of modern intensive care units (ICUs). Although positive-pressure ventilation can be administered via a facemask, this chapter will focus on ventilatory support delivered via an endotracheal tube or tracheostomy tube. The importance of tracheal intubation and mechanical ventilation are that they allow specific surgical procedures to be carried out (e.g., thoracic or abdominal surgery), they offer a transition therapy for patients awaiting more definitive treatment of their underlying disease process (e.g., lung transplantation), they provide replacement therapy of the diseased pulmonary system in selected patients (e.g., patients with neuromuscular disorders including the muscular dystrophies and amyotrophic lateral sclerosis), and they serve as a life support mode during acute illnesses while specific therapies directed at the underlying disease process are given an opportunity to reverse the patient's medical condition (e.g., antibiotic therapy for severe community-acquired pneumonia) (1).

Although it is difficult to identify specific studies demonstrating the benefits of mechanical ventilation in terms of patient outcomes, several clinical investigations support the hypothesis that ventilatory support can improve selected patients' survival. Mechanical ventilation was demonstrated to save lives during the poliomyelitis epidemics of the 1950s (2). More recently, several reports have suggested that mortality of specific disorders requiring mechanical ventilation have improved over the last two decades. These disorders include the acute respiratory distress syndrome (3–5), lung transplantation (6,7), cystic fibrosis (8,9), and burn-injured patients (10). These reports support the premise that the appropriate application of mechanical ventilation can help to save lives. However, the application of mechanical ventilation can also result in injury to patients both as a direct influence of having positive pressure delivered into the lung (11,12) and as a result of complications associated with the application of mechanical ventilation. These secondary complications include ventilator-associated pneumonia (13,14), barotrauma (15), airway complications including tracheal stenosis and ulceration (16), unanticipated extubation with resultant arterial oxygen desaturation (17), muscle weakness (18), and other nosocomial infections (19,20). Therefore, the clinical application of mechanical ventilation due to its complexity and inherent risks lends itself to being managed, at least in part, by a systematic approach aimed at optimizing patient outcomes and avoiding iatrogenic and nosocomial complications.

It is the goal of this chapter to provide a balanced discussion of the benefits and limitations of employing standardized protocols and/or guidelines for the management of mechanical ventilation. First, a conceptual overview of the topic of protocol development and protocol implementation will be provided using a series of hypothetical questions. This will be followed by a more specific discussion of the use of protocols for the management of mechanical ventilation. Finally, several examples of treatment protocols or guidelines will be provided. These are not meant to serve as ironclad examples that should be applied in all institutions and all patient groups. Rather, they are meant to demonstrate examples of final products developed through the process of institutional protocol development. It is this process of multidisciplinary cooperation aimed at identifying best clinical practices for patient care that is the engine necessary to drive successful development and implementation of treatment protocols.

II. Why Use Protocols and Guidelines?

Health care providers currently work in an "information age," in which much of the clinical data is presented in numerical format, with alarms (both visual and auditory), using dichotomous outputs (e.g., positive vs. negative culture results), and with written reports (e.g., pathological tissue examinations, medication dosing instructions, radiological interpretations). Synthesizing this information, particularly in the ICU setting, is an important task carried out by patients' health care providers. This synthesis of data allows clinical decisions to be made, often on a moment-to-moment basis, if necessary, in order to optimize the treatment of the patient's underlying medical problems. Unfortunately, such a plethora of data can result in "information overload" and a malutilization or inefficient utilization of the available clinical data. The everyday occurrence of information overload is supported by clinical studies demonstrating that significant misadventures occur in the management of patients due to medication errors (21,22), inadequate treatment of underlying infections (23,24), an increased incidence of iatrogenic events or nosocomial infections (25–27), and potentially unnecessary prolongation of the duration of mechanical ventilation (28). In theory, most of these undesired events could be avoided if clinicians possessed a streamlined mechanism for the identification of important tasks needing to be carried out in a timely manner (e.g., medication checks, weaning trials, early removal of tubes and catheters). However, at the present time such tasks are usually identified and carried out according to the inclinations and judgments of bedside health care providers regardless of their experience, resource availability, and workloads.

One variable that appears to be important in the occurrence of undesired iatrogenic or nosocomial events is the relationship of the number of health care providers, particularly nurses, to the number and severity of illness of the patients they are caring for (25,26,28). As we are entering further into the managed care era, there is a tendency to try and do more with less (29), in other words, attempt to provide improved efficiency of medical care so that fewer health care providers (e.g., nurses, respiratory therapist, pharmacists) are needed to care for the same number of patients. This philosophy of health care can potentially increase the likelihood for adverse or unintentional outcomes to occur, despite the presence of protocols or guidelines aimed at preventing such unwanted events (e.g., nosocomial infections, prolongation of mechanical ventilation) (26,28). Nevertheless, protocols and guidelines, if properly employed, offer a means for providing a minimum level of standardized care to patients. These management tools can be viewed as safeguards ensuring that certain procedures or practices are carried out in an expeditious manner. However, such tools will inherently lose their effectiveness if the necessary administrative support for their acceptance, including adequate staffing, is lacking. Currently, clinical data describing the impact of nurse staffing ratios on the successful utilization of ICU protocols are lacking (30). Therefore, clinicians and hospital administrators should understand that the most successfully developed protocols, like readily accepted ideal medical practices (e.g., hand washing between each patient contact), are likely to fail unless providing the best possible medical care is viewed as the primary goal of the health care staff. Reducing medical care costs and improving the efficiency with which medical care is provided should not be the primary goal, yet such outcomes are

Table 1 Potential Benefits and Disadvantages of Employing Treatment Protocols

Benefits	Disadvantages
Standardization of medical practices	Loss of clinical autonomy
Aid in the measurement of clinical outcomes	Costs associated with protocol development and implementation
Facilitate quality improvement efforts	Interference with trainee (e.g., house officers, fellows) education
Focus the efforts of bedside caregivers	Need for regular review, updating, and assessment of compliance with the protocol
Increase health care provider accountability	Requirement for new skill sets (e.g., database management, clinical data collection)
Serve as an educational tool identifying best practices	

almost always associated with the implementation of best medical practices (31,32). Table 1 summarizes the potential benefits and disadvantages of employing rigorously developed protocols for patient care.

III. How Do Protocols and Guidelines Work?

The goal of protocols and guidelines is to influence some aspect of patient care through modification of clinician behavior. However, the mere presence of a protocol will not ensure that it is followed (33). Indeed, it is often difficult to measure compliance with clinical protocols unless they are automated (34). Optimal practice guidelines and protocols require the integration of medical knowledge, experience, patient preferences, and an organized system for their implementation (35). Few institutions can acknowledge the successful implementation of protocols within their ICUs due to lack of familiarity with protocol development, implementation, and monitoring. Therefore, medical institutions must be willing to invest long term in the process of protocol development as a means of achieving desired outcomes (e.g., improved patient-specific outcomes, reduced medical care costs).

For many years physicians working in ICUs have practiced medicine according to their individual biases, which are in part determined by their training and past experiences (36). This has allowed variations in medical practices to occur within and outside of the ICU setting. On a larger scale, such variations have been demonstrated to occur on a regional basis, with wide disparity in the use of specific medical practices or surgical procedures between different areas of the country (37,38). The presence of such differences in practice styles has allowed natural experiments to occur that have offered valuable insights into the relative merits and limitations of various medical practices (39). Standardized protocols and medical treatment guidelines offer a systematic approach for providing less variable or "chaotic" medical care. These are usually developed using the best available medical knowledge from peer-reviewed investigations and expert opinion in order to decrease errors in management, improve the effectiveness of available medical treatments, increase the accountability of medical providers, and provide a reference of measure in order to assess future refinements or upgrades in the treatment protocol (36,39).

Unfortunately, well-developed protocols may not always translate into widely accepted treatment algorithms. Some deviation from treatment protocols is always expected to occur since medical decision making should always be guided by each patient's unique characteristics and the judgment and experience of the caregivers. Moreover, local health care delivery issues may determine protocol utilization, particularly if the protocol requires changing the use of a specific resource such as ICU beds or certain classes of medications (40–42). Additionally, individual physician attitudes often form barriers to the successful implementation of protocols and guidelines due to fears concerning loss of clinical autonomy as well as lack of local data supporting their effectiveness (43). Therefore, locally developed protocols often have the best chance of being successfully implemented due to local health care team member acceptance (44,45). It should be recognized, however, that the way in which a protocol is introduced into a specific medical environment may be as important as the steps that went into its development in order to ensure its success.

By standardizing clinical practices, their association with patient-specific outcomes (e.g., hospital mortality, length of stay, medical care costs, complication rates) can be more easily monitored. Indeed, such standardization of practices has been used to tightly control for the effects of potential confounding variables in the performance of unblinded randomized trials examining different ICU practices (46,47). Similarly, the use of protocols serves as a method for assessing the influence of future practice changes on clinical outcomes. This type of real-time performance assessment can typically be performed using relatively simple data collection methods and data recording procedures (48). However, evaluating such data will help to determine whether practice changes, especially those associated with increased health care costs or patient complications, are producing the desired outcomes compared to previous standards of practice. If so, the new practice can be incorporated into the preexisting treatment protocol. This also represents a method for updating protocols based on the development of new technologies, availability of new medical information, or changes in local patient characteristics (49).

IV. How Do You Successfully Develop and Implement a Protocol or Guideline?

Table 2 offers a step-by-step approach to the development and implementation of a practice guideline or protocol. It is crucial to understand that, in order to be successful, guidelines and protocols should foster a collaborative effort among health care providers with the key aim being to improve relationships so as to achieve the desired clinical outcome. Building better relationships among health care workers is recognized as one of the keys to successful clinical quality improvement (50). Additionally, successful protocols and guidelines allow accelerated improvements in medical processes to occur only by employing rigorous but parsimonious use of measurement (51). Data collection and measurement should not be allowed to become an impediment to the use of treatment protocols. Since some protocols and guidelines may not result in improved outcomes, physicians and others are correct in asking for evidence that these local adaptions are efficacious. Indeed, such evidence can be a powerful tool for overcoming obstacles to the treatment protocol set forth by individuals who are unwilling to participate in the improvement process (52,53). However, clinicians must be careful to focus on the main goal of protocol implementation, which is to achieve a desired practice change or improvement in clinical outcome. Data collection should not be so difficult and time consuming that it takes valuable resources away from patient care. Therefore, the minimum clinical and financial data should be collected and analyzed, which will allow a determination of the success or failure of the protocol.

It would be unwise and impractical to insist that every change in practice be a result of a blinded randomized trial with a concurrent control group (52). The uncertainty over appropriate study design often slows the pace of improvement and pits scientifically based physicians against those who would act with no quantitative data. This slow pace contrasts with the pressing social demand for change in health care. A pragmatic application of the scientific method has been developed that attempts to strike a balance between the need for action and the need for evidence that the action represents an improvement (52). This pragmatic approach involves the use of an improvement model with four basic elements: Plan-Do-Study-Act (PDSA) cycles (54,55). Examples of how PDSA cycles can be successfully employed to test guidelines and protocols implemented at the institutional level are readily available (54,56). Additionally, primers on how to optimize the overall use of protocols within the ICU setting are also increasingly accessible (57–59).

Clinicians should always consider the attributes of an effective protocol when developing and implementing such instruments (59). Protocols should be clinically relevant and applicable to patients' and practitioners' needs (60–63). They should be reliable and sophisticated enough to meet the needs of most

Table 2 Steps Necessary for the Successful Development and Implementation of a Treatment Protocol or Practice Guideline

Step 1	Identify a high-priority medical process or task to be addressed by the guideline/protocol. High-priority designation is determined at the local level due to the potential impact of the process or task on patient outcomes, medical care costs, or both.
Step 2	Assemble key individuals, from the local medical community, as well as out-of-house consultants, for the development of the guideline/protocol. Hospital administrative support is also required at an early point in the process.
Step 3	Establish a draft guideline/protocol based on the existing medical evidence, similar guidelines/protocols at other institutions, local and outside expert opinion, and the local availability of resources.
Step 4	Establish ownership of the guideline/program, by a single individual or a group of individuals, to ensure that it is regularly updated and for accountability purposes regarding its acceptance.
Step 5	Provide hospital staff and admitting physicians with a summary of the guideline/protocol. Organize educational/informational inservices for hospital personnel impacted by the guideline/protocol.
Step 6	Establish parameters to judge the success or failure of the guideline/ protocol (e.g., to reduce the use of routine chest radiographs by 25%; to decrease the occurrence of unplanned patient extubations by 33%).
Step 7	Prior to implementation of the guideline/protocol, collect the *minimum* baseline data necessary to establish a reference point for comparison.
Step 8	Develop a tracking mechanism to collect the *minimum* clinical and financial data necessary to establish the success or failure of the guideline/ protocol.
Step 9	Implement the guideline/protocol on a limited basis and increase its penetration into the eligible clinical area as confidence in its utilization develops.
Step 10	Review the progress of the guideline/protocol at regularly scheduled meetings of key individuals involved with its development/ implementation.
Step 11	Establish a mechanism for informing the hospital staff and the admitting physicians about the successes and failures of the guideline/protocol as well as about future refinements of the guideline/protocol (e.g., posters, mailings, conferences).
Step 12	Update the guideline/protocol based on the availability and analysis of the collected data, new available technologies, changing local disease patterns and patient populations, or alternative procedures identified in the medical literature.

clinical situations. A weaning protocol applicable to only 10% of patients in a given ICU would not meet this attribute. The protocol development team should include representation from all groups impacted by the protocol to maximize its wide acceptance (60,61). This would include representation from attending physicians who admit patients to a given ICU. Such inclusion may avoid nonacceptance of the protocol due to fears about loss of clinical autonomy and individual revenues. The protocols should be explicit, clear, and unambiguous so as to foster their acceptance and utilization. Finally, a mechanism must be clearly in place to review and modify the protocol on a regular basis as experience with its implementation is gained. It should also be recognized that protocols that improve the efficiency or effectiveness of clinical practices, in addition to improving medical care, add value to the medical system, which may allow for system resources to be utilized for their implementation (59).

Various implementation strategies for successful protocol utilization have been developed (59). Acceptance of a protocol by clinicians seems to be greater when they perceive that they have some control over the process and ability to modify it (64). Additionally, it appears that feedback to health care providers on their performance is a more powerful stimulus for quality improvement, including the acceptance and implementation of protocols and guidelines, than is simple knowledge of the available quality improvement projects (64). Seeking early feedback on the development of protocols by the practitioners also appears to enlist their ownership of the process and improve the likelihood of its successful implementation (65). This will require the development of a readily defined individual or group of individuals responsible for gaining acceptance of the protocol at the institutional level. These individuals, especially if they are drawn from the major interest groups within the ICU (e.g., attending physicians, nursing staff, hospital administration), can usually identify the best mechanisms for gaining local protocol acceptance (e.g., professional detailing, inservices, local reporting of protocol results to include performance of patients on protocol compared to patients managed off protocol).

Professional detailing is an important mechanism for ensuring the successful implementation of a protocol. One-on-one discussion has been shown to be an effective tool for modifying behaviors, especially when it is done on the local level in an atmosphere of trust and mutual respect (66,67). The use of small group consensus conferences combined with individual instruction, follow-up of individual performance, ongoing peer review of the improvement process, and regular feedback to practitioners to reinforce the concepts of the improvement process is more likely to successfully alter behaviors (63). Identifying an important opinion setter in the local medical community can also be helpful in establishing the credibility of the process in both face-to-face discussions and small group consensus conferences. The opinion setter should be a clinically competent individual who is well respected by his or her peers. Additionally, they must be perceived as championing the improvement process for the right reasons and not for personal gain so as to generate trust and confidence in others for the process (59). Finally, computer-assisted systems can be employed to facilitate the implementation of protocols and guidelines. The use of computers must be seen as adding value to the system, otherwise they may distract from the goals of the protocol or guideline (68,69). Unfortunately, automated systems for monitoring performance in the ICU setting are only now being developed. Most clinicians will have to rely on traditional methods for the implementation of treatment protocols and the recording of data to assess their effectiveness. This usually means having an individual or group of individuals track data on a real-time basis or perform this task retrospectively.

V. Using Formal Multidisciplinary Teams for the Management of Mechanical Ventilation

For many years physicians working in the ICU, as well as elsewhere in the hospital, have practiced medicine according to their individual training experiences and their inherent biases (36). This approach is represented by the "open" ICU model, where patients are admitted to the ICU, often without formal triage, and cared for by their primary care physician. In such ICUs the level of critical care input is variable. This type of model allows for variations in medical practices to occur because each patient receiving mechanical ventilation could potentially have a different attending physician, with different practice styles, managing their ventilator care. Such variations in practices are inherently inefficient since they require direct and open lines of communication between the patient's treating physician and the patient's bedside attendants (e.g., nurses, respiratory therapists). Establishing continuous open communications can be difficult especially when treating physicians spend much of their time outside of the ICU setting. Additionally, the large variability in practice styles among physicians results in added "stressors" for the ICU nursing staff, who must try to remember each physician's treatment nuances.

In an attempt to provide a more systematic approach to the care of critically ill patients, the use of multidisciplinary teams for patient care have been developed and implemented. These "team" approaches have taken one of two strategies: the use of multidisciplinary teams aimed at the entire management of the critically ill patient and smaller teams or individuals focused on a specific problem or issue like ventilator management. The team approach to quality improvement and medical process change has been employed in both open and closed models of ICU care. An inherent principle in the application of such teams is that variability in medical practices is diminished by their implementation. Therefore, such teams function, in part, like a living protocol or guideline due to their ability to reduce or eliminate practice variations.

Mutlz and coworkers (70) evaluated the impact of a change in ICU organization from an "open" to a "closed" model of care. The closed model included the use of a multidisciplinary team. These investigators found that the duration of mechanical ventilation was significantly reduced for patients treated during the closed ICU format compared to the open ICU format. Similarly, other investigators have found improvement in patient outcomes, including reduced ICU lengths of stay and hospital mortality, from going to a closed ICU organizational plan from an open format (71–73). Carson and colleagues demonstrated that a closed ICU format improved clinical outcomes, and, despite greater severity of illness, mechanically ventilated patients did not require increased resource utilization compared to patients cared for during the open ICU format (74). These types of data support the use of a closed ICU organizational format, especially when timely critical care physician management is not available with an open system. Similarly, teaching hospitals typically employ multidisciplinary teams in closed ICU models. It is likely that the beneficial influence of teaching hospitals on clinical outcomes is, at least partly, due to such organizational differences in critical care as compared with nonteaching hospitals (75).

The use of smaller specialized teams that focus on mechanical ventilation has also been shown to improve clinical outcomes. Such teams often carry out or oversee the implementation of specific guidelines or protocols. Cohen and colleagues demonstrated that a ventilator management team consisting of an ICU attending physician, a nurse, and a respiratory therapist could improve the outcomes of patients requiring mechanical ventilation in the medical-surgical ICU of a community teaching hospital (76). The number of days of mechanical ventilation was reduced by 3.9 days per episode of mechanical ventilation (95% confidence interval 0.3 to 7.5 days), and the use of ancillary procedures such as arterial blood gases and arterial lines was also reduced without any adverse effects on patient outcomes. Similar use of quality improvement teams aimed at reducing the duration of mechanical ventilation and improving patient outcomes have been demonstrated to be successful (77,78). Inherent in the successful implementation of such task-oriented teams is that they are not impeded by geographic barriers. In other words, they should have access to all patients requiring mechanical ventilation regardless of their location in the hospital.

Weaning the patient from ventilatory support seems to be an important and complex task, which may benefit from focused clinical efforts. In addition to the examples noted above, individual nurse-initiated weaning of supplemental oxygen and multidisciplinary team weaning of long-term ventilator-dependent patients have been shown to be successful (79,80). Ely and colleagues found that the duration of mechanical ventilation could be significantly reduced by using a

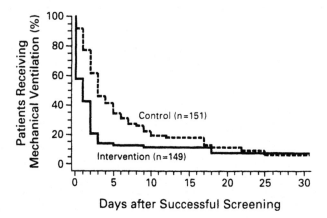

Figure 1 Kaplan-Meier curves of the duration of mechanical ventilation for patients evaluated with an intervention to assess readiness to be liberated from mechanical ventilation compared to standard medical care for the control subjects. (From Ref. 81.)

formalized team approach to the assessment of weaning readiness (81). These investigators randomly assigned 300 mechanically ventilated patients to receive either standard medical therapy alone or standard medical therapy plus the study intervention. The intervention consisted of having patients undergo a daily screening of respiratory function performed by physicians, respiratory therapists, and nurses in order to identify those individuals capable of breathing spontaneously. The patient's attending physician was notified verbally, and a preprinted message was placed in the patient's medical record signifying that they had successfully completed a 2-hour trial of spontaneous breathing. Kaplan-Meier analysis, adjusting for severity of illness at baseline, demonstrated that patients randomized to the intervention group had mechanical ventilation successfully discontinued more rapidly compared with the control group (Fig. 1). Additionally, patients in the intervention group had significantly fewer complications compared with the controls, including fewer reintubations and fewer patients requiring mechanical ventilation for greater than 21 days. Although the costs for the entire hospitalization did not differ between the two study groups, the costs for providing medical care in the ICU was significantly less for the intervention group.

VI. Protocol-Guided Management of Mechanical Ventilation

Due to the complexity of mechanical ventilation and the greater availability of computers in the ICU, protocolized decision-making processes have increasingly been explored as a tool for the management of this clinical technology. The nature of these protocols has varied from fully automated complex systems guiding nearly every aspect of mechanical ventilation to paper-driven protocols dealing with specific aspects of mechanical ventilation (e.g., weaning, arterial blood gas monitoring). The Pulmonary/Critical Care Medicine group at LDS Hospital in Salt Lake City has been a leader in the development and implementation of protocols for the management of mechanical ventilation (69,82). These explicit protocols ensure uniformity of care, with equal frequency of monitoring, consistent decision-making logic for the management of arterial oxygenation, and common Pao_2 endpoints for all patients from the time of initiation of mechanical ventilation to extubation or death (83). For example, the ARDS protocols at LDS Hospital automatically reduce FIO_2 and PEEP to the minimum levels necessary to maintain Pao_2 either between 55 and 60 mmHg when barotrauma is present or between 60 and 68 mmHg in the absence of barotrauma (46). Protocolized therapy is generally increased rapidly and vigorously but decreased slowly and conservatively (increase in FIO_2 and PEEP that followed decreased P_aO_2 were rapid and larger than decreases in FIO_2 and PEEP that followed increased P_aO_2). The use of such protocols has also proven useful for the systematic study of patient outcomes where only one specific variable in the protocol is manipulated to determine its impact on patient outcomes (e.g., low tidal volumes versus high tidal volumes in ARDS) (34).

Unfortunately, with very few exceptions, most intensive care units do not possess the level of computerization and programming expertise necessary to routinely develop and implement broad-scoped protocols for the management of mechanical ventilation. Nevertheless, protocols dealing with specific aspects of care related to mechanical ventilation, usually not requiring computer support, have been demonstrated to be successful. Table 3 gives an overview of several aspects of mechanical ventilation management that have been successfully subjected to protocol management (45,80,84–88). Among these processes, weaning from mechanical ventilation appears to be the one most rigorously evaluated and most popular due to its potential for reducing the duration of mechanical ventilation.

Kollef and coworkers performed a randomized controlled trial of protocol-directed weaning of mechanical ventilation in four ICUs (two medical and two surgical) at an academic medical center (89). Each ICU developed its own weaning protocol in order to gain physician acceptance. Patients were randomly assigned to receive either protocol-directed weaning (n = 179), carried out by nurses and respiratory therapists, or physician-directed weaning (n = 178). The median duration of mechanical ventilation was 35 hours for the protocol-directed group (first quartile 15 hours, third quartile 114 hours) compared with 44 hours for the physician-directed group (first quartile 21 hours, third quartile 209 hours).

Table 3 Components of Mechanical Ventilation Management Evaluated Using Protocol Decision Strategies

Component investigated	Study design	Main finding(s)	Ref.
ABG utilization	Before-after study	A protocol for ABG utilization decreased costs while increasing the appropriateness of ABG use.	45
Weaning F_{IO_2}	Cohort study	Nurse-directed weaning of F_{IO_2} reduced need for ABGs and exposure to toxic levels of F_{IO_2}.	80
Sedation	Before-after study	A sedation guideline reduced sedation costs without any adverse influence on the duration of mechanical ventilation.	84
Sedation	Cohort study	Protocol-guided continuous infusion of benzodiazepine and morphine could control respiratory effort in patients with severe respiratory failure.	85
VAP prevention	Before-after study	A VAP prevention protocol resulted in a reduction of VAP rates and was associated with cost savings.	86
VAP prevention	Before-after study	A VAP prevention protocol reduced VAP rates and their associated medical costs.	87
Weaning mechanical ventilation	Before-after study	Duration of mechanical ventilation was shorter in the protocol group as compared with the control group (10.4 ± 11.6 days vs. 14.4 ± 10.3 days; $p < 0.05$).	88

ABG = Arterial blood gas; F_{IO_2} = fraction of inspired oxygen; VAP = ventilator-associated pneumonia.

Kaplan-Meier analysis demonstrated that the patients randomized to protocol-directed weaning had significantly shorter durations of mechanical ventilation as compared with patients randomized to receive physician-directed weaning (Fig. 2). Hospital costs for patients in the protocol-directed group were $42,960 less than hospital costs for patients in the physician-directed group. No significant differences in hospital mortality, reintubation, or the requirement for prolonged mechanical ventilation were observed between the two study groups. Interestingly, the observed reduction in the duration of mechanical ventilation was simi-

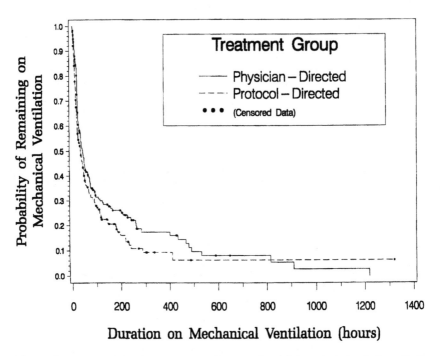

Figure 2 Kaplan-Meier curves of the probability of remaining on mechanical ventilation over time between patients receiving protocol-directed weaning versus physician-directed weaning. (From Ref. 89.)

lar to that observed in the weaning study performed by Ely and coworkers employing a focused weaning team (81).

More recently, protocols aimed at reducing the duration of mechanical ventilation have been examined outside of the strict research setting. Horst and colleagues performed a before-after study comparing historic ventilation times with physician-directed weaning to those obtained with protocol-guided weaning performed by respiratory therapists (90). They were able to decrease their average duration of mechanical ventilation by 58 hours, a 46% decrease ($p < 0.001$) (Fig. 3). The length of hospitalization also decreased by 1.77 days (29% change) for patients weaned by respiratory therapists. Overall, the marginal cost savings was $603,580 with the respiratory therapist–directed protocol. Similarly, the ICUs at Nash General Hospital (Rocky Mount, NC) and Phoebe Putney Hospital (Albany, GA) developed weaning protocols through their participation in the Institute for Healthcare Improvement (IHI), a nonprofit organization designed to be a major force for integrative and collaborative efforts to accelerate improvement in the health care systems of the United States and Canada (91,92). Using PDSA cycles

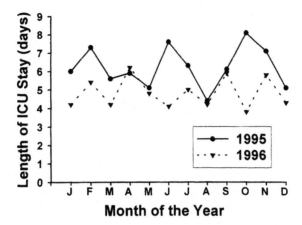

Figure 3 Length of ICU stay by month for the years prior to (1995) and after (1996) the implementation of a formal respiratory therapist initiated weaning protocol. (From Ref. 90.)

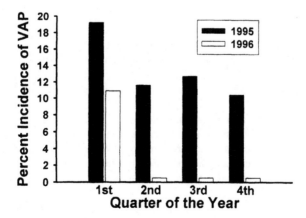

Figure 4 Occurrence of ventilator-associated pneumonia (VAP) by quarter for the years prior to (1995) and after (1996) the introduction of a formal weaning protocol. (From Ref. 92.)

to implement process changes, both institutions achieved reductions in their duration of mechanical ventilation and associated cost savings, while the ICU at Nash Hospital also achieved a dramatic reduction in the occurrence of ventilator-associated pneumonia with its accelerated weaning program (92) (Fig. 4).

VII. Protocol Management of Innovative Mechanical Ventilation Strategies

Clinical advances are continuing to be made in the area of ventilatory support for patients with respiratory failure. Protocols and guidelines hold the promise of offering a means to translate some of the benefits demonstrated in clinical trials to routine patient management at the beside. For example, several investigations have found beneficial patient outcomes with the use of a lung-protective strategy of mechanical ventilation for patients with the acute respiratory distress syndrome (ARDS) (93,94). Applying such ventilatory techniques on a wider scale could be facilitated by the use of protocols or guidelines outlining the necessary ventilator adjustments needed to achieve the targeted airway pressure endpoints. However, due to the presence of contradictory studies using different ventilation strategies, such protocols need to be carefully developed, applicable patients should be clearly defined, and appropriate patient outcomes monitored (95,96). Similarly, more widespread application of validated infection-control methods could be accomplished with the use of clinical protocols. The success of such

Table 4 Guideline for the Prevention of Ventilator-Associated Pneumonia[a]

1. Liberate patient from mechanical ventilation as soon as clinically feasible.
2. Adequate handwashing before all patient contacts.
3. Maintain the patient in a semirecumbent position.
4. Provide scheduled oral hygiene.
5. Avoid self-extubation and resultant reintubation using appropriate chemical and physical restraints.
6. Provide oral (nonnasal) airway intubation.
7. Regular drainage of ventilator circuit condensate.
8. Monitor endotracheal tube cuff pressures to provide an adequate seal between the endotracheal tube cuff and the wall of the trachea.
9. Nutritional supplementation to avoid calorie, protein, vitamin, and macronutrient deficiencies.
10. Avoid ventilator circuit changes unless visibly soiled or mechanically defective.
11. Early patient mobilization to strengthen respiratory muscles and to improve patient endurance.

[a] See Ref. 105 for evidence in support of these recommendations.

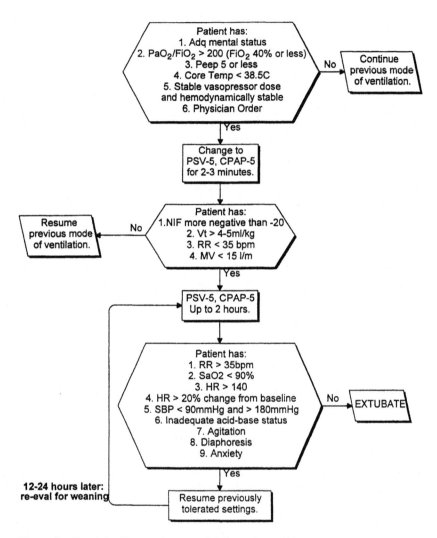

Figure 5 Example of a weaning protocol for patients with acute respiratory failure utilized in the medical intensive care of Barnes-Jewish Hospital. (From Ref. 89.)

interventions has already been demonstrated at the local level (86,87). Last, protocols can be used to implement and test the effectiveness of new ventilation strategies to determine whether they should be accepted at the local hospital level. The use of noninvasive ventilation as a replacement therapy for conventional mechanical ventilation with tracheal intubation represents one such strategy.

The merits and pitfalls of noninvasive mechanical ventilation for the management of acute respiratory failure have been recently reviewed (97). However, several recent clinical studies suggest that the application of noninvasive mechanical ventilation for patients with COPD (98) and hypoxic respiratory failure (99) can reduce the need for tracheal intubation and mechanical ventilation. These investigations also demonstrated a decreased occurrence of adverse events such as the development of ventilator-associated pneumonia for patients managed with noninvasive ventilation. The application of noninvasive ventilation can be problematic since it usually requires skilled respiratory therapists familiar with its use in order to optimize its success. The use of protocols or guidelines represents one approach for educating respiratory therapists, and other health care providers, on the appropriate indications and application of noninvasive ventilation (100). Indeed, several protocols or guidelines for the use of noninvasive mechanical ventilation are readily available (101,102). However, the use of this strategy should be carefully monitored to ensure that the desired outcomes are being achieved. If this is not systematically performed, then undesired outcomes may occur due to unique local practices or patient profiles (103).

VIII. Summary

Protocols and guidelines for the management of mechanical ventilation should be viewed as available clinical tools, similar to other treatments and medical processes accessible to patients with respiratory failure (e.g., nutritional support, physical therapy, weaning parameters, ventilator alarms), which can be employed to optimized patient outcomes. However, the successful application of protocols and guidelines targeting mechanical ventilation requires a dedicated multidisciplinary effort on the part of the ICU team. For institutions lacking experience with the development and application of ventilator management protocols, initial efforts at protocol utilization should target specific tasks or processes with minimal associated controversy (e.g., weaning of inspired oxygen concentration, use of arterial blood gases) (45,80). As successful experience with the use of these protocols is attained, more complicated processes such as the weaning of mechanical ventilation can be addressed. Achieving gradual but steady success in protocol utilization will be facilitated by organizing an institutional process for development and review (Table 2). Only by focusing clinical efforts on specific medical processes and clinical problems, like mechanical ventilation and its associated complications, can we expect to achieve improvements in patient outcomes, health care costs, or both. Table 4 outlines an example of a simple guideline for the prevention of ventilator-associated pneumonia based on the available medical evidence (104,105). Figure 5 is a representative example of a protocol for the weaning of mechanical ventilation (89). These examples should simply be viewed as outlines and products of a systematic approach aimed at improving the quality of medical care for patients requiring ventilatory support.

References

1. Tobin MJ. Mechanical ventilation. N Engl J Med 1994; 330:1056–1061.
2. Ibsen B. The anaesthetist's viewpoint on the treatment of respiratory complications in poliomyelitis during the epidemic in Copenhagen, 1952. Proc R Soc Med 1954; 47:72–74.
3. Schuster DP. What is acute lung injury? What is ARDS? Chest 1995; 107:1721–1726.
4. Milberg JA, Davis DR, Steinberg KP, Hudson LD. Improved survival of patients with acute respiratory distress syndrome (ARDS): 1983–1993. JAMA 1995; 273: 306–309.
5. Suchyta MR, Clemmer TP, Elliott CG, Orme Jr JF, Weaver LK. The adult respiratory distress syndrome. A report of survival and modifying factors. Chest 1992; 101:1074–1079.
6. Grover FL, Fullerton DA, Zamora MR, Mills C, Ackerman B, Badesch D, Brown JM, Campbell DN, Chetham P, Dhaliwal A, Diercks M, Kinnard T, Niejadlik K, Ochs M. The past, present, and future of lung transplantation. Am J Surg 1997; 173:523–533.
7. Williams TJ, Snell GI. Early and long-term functional outcomes in unilateral, bilateral, and living-related transplant recipients. Clin Chest Med 1997; 18:245–257.
8. Rosenstein BJ, Zeitlin PL. Prognosis in cystic fibrosis. Curr Opinion Pulm Med 1995; 1:444–449.
9. Flume PA, Egan TM, Westerman JH, Paradowski LJ, Yankaskas JR, Detterbeck FC, Mill MR. Lung transplantation for mechanically ventilated patients. J Heart Lung Transplant 1994; 13:15–21.
10. Ryan CM, Schoenfeld DA, Thorpe WP, Sheridan RL, Cassem EH, Tompkins RG. Objective estimates of the probability of death from burn injuries. N Engl J Med 1998; 338:362–366.
11. Dreyfuss D, Saumon G. Ventilator-induced lung injury: lessons from experimental studies. Am J Respir Crit Care Med 1998; 157:294–323.
12. Levy BD, Kitch B, Fanta CH. Medical and ventilatory management of status asthmaticus. Intensive Care Med 1998; 24:105–117.
13. Torres A, Aznar R, Gatell JM, Jimenez P, Gonzalez J, Ferrer A, Celis R, Rodriquez-Rosin R. Incidence, risk, and prognosis factors of nosocomial pneumonia in mechanically ventilated patients. Am Rev Respir Dis 1990; 142:523–528.
14. Craven DE, Steger KA. Epidemiology of nosocomial pneumonia. New perspectives on an old disease. Chest 1995; 108:1S–16S.
15. Schnapp LM, Chin DP, Szaflarski N, Matthay MA. Frequency and importance of barotrauma in 100 patients with acute lung injury. Crit Care Med 1995; 23:272–278.
16. Colice GL, Stukel TA, Dain B. Laryngeal complications of prolonged intubation. Chest 1989; 96:877–884.

17. Whelan J, Simpson SQ, Levy H. Unplanned extubation. Predictors of successful termination of mechanical ventilatory support. Chest 1994; 105:1808–1812.

18. Leatherman JW, Fluegel WL, David WS, Davies SF, Iber C. Muscle weakness in mechanically ventilated patients with severe asthma. Am J Respir Crit Care Med 1996; 153:1686–1690.

19. Rouby JJ, Laurent P, Gosnach M, Cambau E, Lamas G, Zouaoui A, Leguillou JL, Bodin L, Khac TD, Marsault C. Risk factors and clinical relevance of nosocomial maxillary sinusitis in the critically ill. Am J Respir Crit Care Med 1994; 150:776–783.

20. Vincent JL, Bihari DJ, Suter PM, Bruining HA, White J, Nicolas-Chanoin MH, Wolff M, Spencer RC, Hemmer M. The prevalence of nosocomial infection in intensive care units in Europe: results of the European Prevalence of Infection in Intensive Care (EPIC) Study; EPIC International Advisory Committee. JAMA 1995; 274:639–644.

21. Lesar TS, Briceland L, Stein DS. Factors related to errors in medication prescribing. JAMA 1997; 277:312–317.

22. Classen DC, Pestotnik SL, Evans RS, Lloyd JF, Burke JP. Adverse drug events in hospitalized patients. Excess length of stay, extra costs, and attributable mortality. JAMA 1997; 277:301–306.

23. Romero-Vivas J, Rubio M, Fernandez C, Picazo JJ. Mortality associated with nosocomial bacteremia due to methicillin-resistant Staphylococcus aureus. Clin Infect Dis 1995; 21:1417–1423.

24. Kollef MH, Sherman G, Ward S, Fraser VJ. Inadequate antimicrobial treatment of infections: a risk factor for hospital mortality among critically ill patients. Chest 1999; 115:462–474.

25. Archibald LK, Manning ML, Bell LM, Banerjee S, Jarvis WR. Patient density, nurse-to-patient ratio and nosocomial infection risk in a pediatric cardiac intensive care unit. Ped Infect Dis J 1997; 16:1045–1048.

26. Fridkin SK, Pear SM, Williamson TH, Galgiani JN, Jarvis WR. The role of understaffing in central venous catheter-associated bloodstream infections. Infect Control Hosp Epidemiol 1996; 17:150–158.

27. Giraud T, Dhainaut JF, Vaxelaire JF, Joseph T, Journois D, Bleichner G, Sollet JP, Chevret S, Monsallier JF. Iatrogenic complications in adult intensive care units: a prospective two-center study. Crit Care Med 1993; 21:40–51.

28. Thoren J-B, Kaelin RM, Jolliet P, Chevrolet JC. Influence of the quality of nursing on the duration of weaning from mechanical ventilation in patients with chronic obstructive pulmonary disease. Crit Care Med 1995; 23:1807–1815.

29. Anderson GF. In search of value: an international comparison of cost, access, and outcomes. Health Affairs 1997; 16:163–171.

30. Shamian J, Lightstone EY. Hospital restructuring initiatives in Canada. Med Care 1997; 35:OS62–OS69.

31. Rubenfeld GD. Cost-effectiveness considerations in critical care. New Horizons 1998; 6:33–40.

32. Kirton OC, Civetta JM, Hudson-Civetta J. Cost-effectiveness in the intensive care unit. Surg Clin North Am 1996; 76:175–200.

33. Lomas J, Anderson GM, Domnick-Pierre K, Vayda E, Enkin MW, Hannah WJ.

Do practice guidelines guide practice? The effect of a consensus statement on the practice of physicians. N Engl J Med 1989; 321:1306–1311.

34. Morris AH, East TD, Wallace CJ, Franklin M, Heerman L, Kinder T, Sailor M, Carlson D, Bradshaw R. Standardization of clinical decision making for the conduct of credible clinical research in complicated medical environments. Proc/AMIA Annual Fall Symp 1996:418–422.

35. Peterson WL, Cook DJ. Using a practice guideline for safely shortening hospital stay for upper gastrointestinal tract hemorrhage. JAMA 1997; 278:2186–2187.

36. Luce JM. Reducing the use of mechanical ventilation. N Engl J Med 1996; 335: 1916–1917.

37. Wennberg JE, Freeman JL, Shelton RM. Hospital use and mortality among medicare beneficiaries in Boston and New Haven. N Engl J Med 1989; 321:1168–1173.

38. Knaus WA, Wagner DP, Zimmerman JE, Draper EA. Variations in mortality and length of stay in intensive care units. Ann Intern Med 1993; 118:753–761.

39. Kollef MH, Schuster DP. Predicting intensive care unit outcome with scoring systems. Crit Care Clin 1994; 10:1–18.

40. Katz DA, Griffith JL, Beshansky JR, Selker HP. The use of empiric clinical data in the evaluation of practice guidelines for unstable angina. JAMA 1996; 276: 1568–1574.

41. Gleason PP, Kapoor WN, Stone RA, Lave JR, Obrosky DS, Schulz R, Singer DE, Coley CM, Marrie TJ, Fine MJ. Medical outcomes and antimicrobial costs with the use of the American Thoracic Society guidelines for outpatients with community-acquired pneumonia. JAMA 1997; 278:32–39.

42. Curtis JR, Bennett CL, Horner RD, Rubenfeld GD, DeHovitz JA, Weinstein RA. Variations in intensive care unit utilization for patients with human immunodeficiency virus-related *Pneumocystis carinii* pneumonia: importance of hospital characteristics and geographic location. Crit Care Med 1998; 26:668–675.

43. Langley C, Faulkner A, Watkins C, Gray S, Harvey I. Use of guidelines in primary care—practitioners' perspectives. Family Practice 1998; 15:105–111.

44. Hay JA, Maldonado L, Weingarten SR, Ellrodt AG. Prospective evaluation of a clinical guideline recommending hospital length of stay in upper gastrointestinal tract hemorrhage. JAMA 1997; 278:2151–2156.

45. Pilon CS, Leathley M, London R, McLean S, Phang PT, Priestley R, Rosenberg FM, Singer J, Anis AH, Dodek PM. Practice guideline for arterial blood gas measurement in the intensive care unit decreases numbers and increases appropriateness of tests. Crit Care Med 1997; 25:1308–1313.

46. Morris AH, Wallace CJ, Menlove RL, Clemmer TP, Orme Jr JF, Weaver LK, Dean NC, Thomas F, East TD, Pace NL. Randomized clinical trial of pressure-controlled inverse ratio ventilation and extracorporeal CO_2 removal for adult respiratory distress syndrome. Am J Respir Crit Care Med 1994; 149:295–305.

47. Valentine RJ, Duke ML, Inman MH, Grayburn PA, Hagino RT, Kakish HB, Glagett GP. Effectiveness of pulmonary artery catheters in aortic surgery: a randomized trial. J Vasc Surg 1998; 27:203–211.

48. Bradley EH, Besdine R. Outcomes-based quality improvement: reducing the data collection burden. J Am Geriatr Soc 1998; 46:534–535.

49. Littenberg B. A practice guideline revisited: screening for hypertension. Ann Intern Med 1995; 122:937–939.
50. Clemmer TP, Spuhler VJ, Berwick DM, Nolan TW. Cooperation: the foundation of improvement. Ann Intern Med 1998; 128:1004–1009.
51. Kilo CM, Kabcenell A, Berwick DM. Beyond survival: Toward continuous improvement in medical care. New Horizons 1998; 6:3–11.
52. Brock WA, Nolan K, Nolan T. Pragmatic Science: accelerating the improvement of critical care. New Horizons 1998; 6:61–68.
53. Hanchak NA. Managed care, accountability, and the physician. Med Clin North Am 1996; 80:245–261.
54. Langley G, Nolan K, Nolan T. The foundation of improvement. Quality Progress 1994; (June):81–86.
55. Moen R, Nolan T. Process improvement. Quality Progress 1987; (Sept):62–68.
56. Reducing costs and improving outcomes in adult intensive care. In: Rainey TG, Kabcenell A, Berwick DM, Roessner J, eds. Institute for Healthcare Improvement 1998:28–39.
57. Cook DJ, Ellrodt G, Calvin J, Levy MM. How to use practice guidelines in the intensive care unit: diagnosis and management of unstable angina. Crit Care Med 1998; 26:599–606.
58. Grimshaw J, Freemantle N, Wallace S, Russell I, Hurwitz B, Watt I, Long A, Sheldon T. Developing and implementing clinical practice guidelines. Qual Health Care 1995; 4:55–64.
59. Clemmer TP, Spuhler VJ. Developing and gaining acceptance for patient care protocols. New Horizons 1998; 6:12–19.
60. Duff LA, Kitson AL, Seers K, Humphries D. Clinical guidelines: an introduction to their development and implementation. J Adv Nurs 1996; 23:887–895.
61. Grimshaw JM. Clinical practice guidelines—Do they enhance value for money in health care? Br Med Bulletin 1995; 51:927–940.
62. Harris JS. Development, use and evaluation of clinical practice guidelines. J Occup Environ Med 1997; 39:23–34.
63. Karuza J, Calkins E, Feather J, Hershey CO, Katz L, Majeroni B. Enhancing physician adoption of practice guidelines. Arch Intern Med 1995; 155:625–632.
64. Palmer RH, Louis TA, Peterson HF, Rothrock JK, Strain R, Wright EA. What makes quality assurance effective? Results from a randomized controlled trial in sixteen primary care group practices. Med Care 1996; 36 (suppl):SS29–SS39.
65. Hoyt DB. Clinical practice guidelines. Am J Surg 1997; 173:32–36.
66. Conroy M, Shannon W. Clinical practice guidelines: their implementation in general practice. Br J Gen Pract 1995; 45:371–375.
67. Axelrod R. The Evolution of Cooperation. New York: Basic Books, 1984.
68. McDonald CJ. Protocol-based computer reminders, the quality of care and the non-perfectibility of man. N Engl J Med 1976; 295:1351–1355.
69. East TD, Bohm SH, Wallace CJ, Clemmer TP, Weaver LK, Orme Jr JF, Morris AH. A successful computerized protocol for clinical management of pressure control inverse ratio ventilation in ARDS patients. Chest 1992; 101:697–710.
70. Multz AS, Chalfin DB, Samson IM, Dantzker DR, Fein AM, Steinberg HN, Niederman MS, Scharf SM. A "closed" medical intensive care unit (MICU) improves

resource utilization when compared to an "open" MICU. Am J Respir Crit Care Med 1998; 157:1468–1473.

71. Manthous CA, Amoateng-Adjepong Y, Al-Kharrat T, Jacob B, Alnuaimat HM, Chatila W, Hall JB. Effects of a medical intensivist on patient care in a community teaching hospital. Mayo Clin Proc 1997; 72:391–399.

72. Pollack MM, Katz RW, Ruttimann UE, Getson PR. Improving the outcome and efficiency of intensive care: the impact of an intensivist. Crit Care Med 1988; 16:11–17.

73. Li TCM, Phillip MC, Shaw L, Cook EF, Natanson C, Goldman L. On site physician staffing in a community hospital intensive care unit. JAMA 1984; 252:2023–2027.

74. Carson SS, Stocking C, Podsadecki T, Christenson J, Pohlman A, MacRae S, Jordan J, Humphrey H, Siegler M, Hall J. Effects of organizational change in the medical intensive care unit of a teaching hospital: a comparison of "open" and "closed" formats. JAMA 1996; 276:322–328.

75. Rosenthal GE, Harper DL, Quinn LM, Cooper GS. Severity-adjusted mortality and length of stay in teaching and nonteaching hospitals. Results of a regional study. JAMA 1997; 278:485–490.

76. Cohen IL, Bari N, Strosberg MA, Weinberg PF, Wacksman RM, Millstein BH, Fine IA. Reduction of duration and cost of mechanical ventilation in an intensive care unit by use of a ventilatory management team. Crit Care Med 1991; 19:1278–1284.

77. Frommater D, Marshall D, Halford G, Rimmasch H, Coons MC. How a three-campus heart service line improves clinical processes and outcomes. Joint Commission J Qual Improvement 1995; 21:263–276.

78. Griffith D, Hampton D, Switzer M, Daniels J. Facilitating the recovery of open heart surgery patients through quality improvement efforts and Care MAP implementation. Am J Crit Care 1996; 5:346–352.

79. Scheinhorn DJ, Chao DC, Stearn-Hassenpflug M, LaBree LD, Heltsley DJ. Post-ICU mechanical ventilation: treatment of 1,123 patients at a regional weaning center. Chest 1997; 111:1654–1659.

80. Rotello LC, Warren J, Jastremski MS, Milewski A. A nurse-directed protocol using pulse oximetry to wean mechanically ventilated patients from toxic oxygen concentrations. Chest 1992; 102:1833–1835.

81. Ely EW, Baker AM, Dunagan DP, Burke HL, Smith AC, Kelley PT, Johnson MM, Browder RW, Bowton DL, Haponik EF. Effect on the duration of mechanical ventilation of identifying patients capable of breathing spontaneously. N Engl J Med 1996; 335:1864–1869.

82. East TD, Morris AH, Wallace CJ, Clemmer TP, Orme Jr JF, Weaver LK, Henderson S, Sittig DF. A strategy for development of computerized critical care decision support systems. Int J Clin Monit Comput 1992; 8:263–269.

83. Henderson S, Crapo RD, Wallace CJ, East TD, Morris AH, Gardner RM. Performance of computerized protocols for the management of arterial oxygenation in an intensive care unit. Int J Monit Comput 1992; 8:271–280.

84. Devlin JW, Holbrook AM, Fuller HD. The effect of ICU sedation guidelines and pharmacist interventions on clinical outcomes and drug cost. Ann Pharmacother 1997; 31:689–695.

85. Watling SM, Johnson M, Yanos J. A method to produce sedation in critically ill patients. Ann Pharmacother 1996; 30:1227–1231.

86. Joiner GA, Salisbury D, Bollin GE. Utilizing quality assurance as a tool for reducing the risk of nosocomial ventilator-associated pneumonia. Am J Med Qual 1996; 11:100–103.

87. Kelleghan SI, Salemi C, Padilla S, McCord M, Mermilliod G, Canola T, Becker L. An effective continuous quality improvement approach to the prevention of ventilator-associated pneumonia. Am J Infect Control 1993; 21:322–330.

88. Saura P, Blanch L, Mestre J, Valles J, Artigas A, Fernandez R. Clinical consequences of the implementation of a weaning protocol. Intensive Care Med 1996; 22:1052–1056.

89. Kollef MH, Shapiro SD, Silver P, St. John RE, Prentice D, Sauer S, Ahrens TS, Shannon W, Baker-Clinkscale D. A randomized, controlled trial of protocol-directed versus physician-directed weaning from mechanical ventilation. Crit Care Med 1997; 25:567–574.

90. Horst HM, Mouro D, Hall-Jenssens R, Pamukov N. Decrease in ventilation time with a standardized weaning process. Arch Surg 1998; 133:483–489.

91. Davidoff F. The 10th National Forum on Quality Improvement in Healthcare. Ann Intern Med 1998; 129:585.

92. Kollef MH, Horst HM, Prang L, Brock WA. Reducing the duration of mechanical ventilation: three examples of change in the ICU. New Horizons 1998; 6:52–60.

93. Amato MB, Barbas CS, Medeiros DM, Magaldi RB, Schettino GP, Lorenzi-Filho G, Kairalla RA, Deheinzelin D, Munoz C, Oliveira R, Takagaki TY, Carvalho CR. Effect of a protective-ventilation strategy on mortality in the acute respiratory distress syndrome. N Engl J Med 1998; 338:347–354.

94. Hickling KG, Walsh J, Henderson S, Jackson R. Low mortality rate in adult respiratory distress syndrome using low-volume, pressure-limited ventilation with permissive hypercapnia: a prospective study. Crit Care Med 1994; 22:1568–1578.

95. Stewart TE, Meade MO, Cook DJ, Granton JT, Hodder RV, Lapinsky SE, Mazer CD, McLean RF, Rogovein TS, Schouten BD, Todd TR, Slutsky AS. Evaluation of a ventilation strategy to prevent barotrauma in patients at high risk for acute respiratory distress syndrome. Pressure- and volume-limited ventilation strategy group. N Engl J Med 1998; 338:355–361.

96. Hudson LD. Protective ventilation for patients with acute respiratory distress syndrome. N Engl J Med 1998; 338:385–387.

97. Jasmer RM, Luce JM, Matthay MA. Noninvasive positive pressure ventilation for acute respiratory failure: underutilized or overrated? Chest 1997; 111:1672–1678.

98. Nava S, Ambrosino N, Clini E, Prato M, Orlando G, Vitacca M, Brigada P, Fracchia C, Rubini F. Noninvasive mechanical ventilation in the weaning of patients with respiratory failure due to chronic obstructive pulmonary disease. A randomized, controlled trial. Ann Intern Med 1998; 128:721–728.

99. Antonelli M, Conti G, Rocco M, Bufi M, DeBlasi RA, Vivino G, Gasparetto A, Meduri GV. A comparison of noninvasive positive-pressure ventilation and conventional mechanical ventilation in patients with acute respiratory failure. N Engl J Med 1998; 339:429–435.

100. Meduri GU, Turner RE, Abou-Shala N, Wunderink R, Tolley E. Noninvasive posi-

tive pressure ventilation via face mask. First-line intervention in patients with acute hypercapnic and hypoxemic respiratory failure. Chest 1996; 109:179–193.

101. Brochard L, Mancebo J, Wysocki M, Lofaso F, Conti G, Rauss A, Simonneau G, Benito S, Gasparetto A, Lemaire F. Non-invasive ventilation for acute exacerbations of chronic obstructive pulmonary disease. N Engl J Med 1995; 333:817–822.

102. Kramer N, Meyer TJ, Meharg J, Cece RD, Hill NS. Randomized, prospective trial of noninvasive positive pressure ventilation in acute respiratory failure. Am J Respir Crit Care Med 1995; 151:1799–1806.

103. Wood KA, Lewis L, Von Harz B, Kollef MH. The use of noninvasive positive pressure ventilation (NPPV) in the emergency department: Results of a randomized clinical trial. Chest 1998; 113:1339–1346.

104. Tablan OC, Anderson LJ, Arden NH, Breiman RF, Butler JC, McNeil MM. Guideline for prevention of nosocomial pneumonia. The Hospital Infection Control Practices Advisory Committee, Centers for Disease Control and Prevention. Infect Control Hosp Epidemiol 1994; 15:587–627.

105. Kollef MH. The prevention of bacterial ventilator-associated pneumonia. N Engl J Med 1999; 340:627–634.

6

Noninvasive Ventilation

A Strategy to Improve Outcomes and Resource Utilization
in Critical Care

NICHOLAS S. HILL

Miriam Hospital
Rhode Island Hospital
and Brown University School of Medicine
Providence, Rhode Island

DENIS LIN

Brown University School of Medicine
Providence, Rhode Island

I. Introduction

Noninvasive ventilation refers to the delivery of mechanical ventilatory assistance
without the need for an invasive artificial airway. Noninvasive ventilatory techniques have been available for many decades, mainly in the form of negative
pressure ventilators, such as the "iron lung," that were used extensively during
the polio epidemics (1). With the advent of increasingly sophisticated mechanical
ventilators, intensive care units, and blood gas machines, negative pressure ventilation fell out of favor and invasive positive pressure ventilation became the preferred ventilator modality for therapy of acute respiratory failure in critical care
units worldwide.

However, the past decade has witnessed a resurgence of noninvasive ventilatory techniques. Following the widespread application of nasal nocturnal ventilation to patients with chronic respiratory failure during the late 1980s (2,3),
reports appeared of successful application of this technique to selected patients
with acute respiratory failure (ARF) (4). With the publication of randomized
controlled trials evaluating noninvasive positive pressure ventilation in acute respiratory failure over the past decade (5–7), more and more patients with acute

respiratory failure are being treated with this technique. Although the technique is still underutilized in many, if not most centers, it offers the potential of improving the efficiency of patient care as well as patient outcomes. Thus chapter will briefly review the rationale for the use of NPPV, appropriate indications for NPPV in the acute care setting, acute application, and evidence that outcomes and resource utilization may be enhanced by the proper application of NPPV.

II. Rationale

The resurgence in the use of noninvasive ventilation has been fueled by the desire to minimize the complications of invasive mechanical ventilation. Increasingly over the past decade, it has become apparent that although invasive mechanical ventilation is highly effective at assisting ventilation in patients with acute respiratory failure, its use poses a substantial risk for complications (8,9). The insertion of an artificial airway, particularly under emergency circumstances, may traumatize the upper airway. Lacerations of the trachea or esophagus may lead to hemorrhage or subsequent abscess formation. Once initiated, invasive ventilation may cause barotrauma or ventilator-induced lung injury (9). The artificial airway also provides a direct conduit for foreign material to enter the lower airways and interferes with upper airway drainage, thereby increasing the risk of infectious complications such as nosocomial pneumonia and sinusitis. Finally, and perhaps of most concern to the patient, a translaryngeal endotracheal tube interferes with communication and feeding, is uncomfortable, and requires the use of sedation that may impede the weaning process.

By avoiding these problems, noninvasive ventilation offers the potential of providing mechanical ventilatory assistance with fewer complications. Trauma to the upper airway is reduced, the airway defense system remains intact, inflation pressures are lower, lessening the risk of barotrauma, and patient discomfort is alleviated. Further, if the weaning processes can be facilitated, patients may be liberated from mechanical ventilation earlier, avoiding complications of prolonged intubation and thus potentially improving the efficiency of hospital utilization. However, there are important caveats with regard to the use of noninvasive ventilation. Direct access to the airway is sacrificed, so patient recipients of noninvasive ventilation must have the capability of adequately protecting their airway. In addition, patient cooperation is mandatory. Appropriate patients must be carefully selected if the modality is to be used optimally.

III. General Considerations for Patient Selection in the Acute Setting

Specific indications for noninvasive positive pressure ventilation (NPPV) in patients with acute respiratory failure are discussed in detail in several other chapters in this volume. In the following, general principles of patient selection will be discussed and a list of appropriate clinical settings will be given.

Noninvasive positive pressure ventilation aims to assist patients with ventilatory insufficiency or oxygenation defects, providing a ''crutch'' while other therapies are given time to work. In this regard, NPPV may be seen as a form of partial ventilatory assistance, the goal of which is to provide temporary support. The modality should be perceived as a means of avoiding intubation, but not as a substitute for invasive mechanical ventilation. Accordingly, good candidates for NPPV have respiratory failure that is anticipated to be reversible within hours to days. Some patients with acute on chronic respiratory failure may continue to use NPPV nocturnally after stabilization of the acute process. However, patients anticipated to have prolonged bouts with respiratory failure who require continuous support with sophisticated ventilator modes, such as those with severe pneumonias or acute respiratory distress syndrome (ARDS) are poor candidates.

Good candidates for noninvasive ventilation should also have respiratory insufficiency that is neither too mild nor too severe (Table 1). Patients with only mild respiratory distress are probably not in need of ventilatory assistance, and the outcome is likely to be good whether NPPV is used or not. On the other hand, patients with very severe distress and advanced respiratory failure are more apt to fail because of the difficulty they have cooperating and the limited time for adaptation (10). Thus, the optimal time for initiation of NPPV may be seen

Table 1 Guidelines for Selection of Patients with Acute Respiratory Failure to Receive Noninvasive Ventilation

Clinical Criteria
   Moderate to severe respiratory distress
   Tachypnea (>24–30/min)[a]
   Accessory muscle use or abdominal paradox
Gas Exchange Criteria
   $Paco_2 > 45$ mmHg, pH < 7.35; > 7.10
   $Pao_2/Fio_2 \leq 200$
Exclusion Criteria
   Respiratory arrest or immediate need for intubation
   Medically unstable
     Acute myocardial infarction, uncontrolled arrhythmias, cardiac ischemia or upper
     GI bleeding, or hypotensive shock
   Unable to protect airway
     Impaired swallowing or cough
     Excessive secretions
   Agitated or uncooperative
   Recent upper airway or esophageal surgery
   Unable to fit mask

[a] Depends on cause of respiratory failure.

as a "window of opportunity," which opens with the development of moderate to severe respiratory distress and closes when a terminal crisis occurs. As summarized in Table 1, patients are identified using clinical criteria indicative of moderate to severe respiratory distress. These may have to be modified depending on the specific disease entity. For instance, a respiratory rate exceeding 24 per minute may be seen with moderate to severe respiratory distress in patients with severe chronic obstructive pulmonary disease (COPD), but patients with acute pulmonary edema may not have moderate to severe distress before the respiratory rate exceeds 30/min. Suggested gas exchange criteria include acute or acute on chronic hypercapnia with a pH of <7.35 but >7.10 or severe hypoxemia. It is important to recall that these are guidelines only and have not been validated in prospective controlled trials.

The exclusion of inappropriate candidates for NPPV is equally important in the selection process (Table 1). This requires skill and experience because a number of the exclusion criteria are qualitative and require judgment on the part of the clinician. NPPV requires a spontaneously breathing patient, and it takes at least several minutes to apply the mask. Thus, patients with a respiratory arrest or the need for immediate intubation are poor candidates. Patients who are medically unstable, i.e., those with uncontrolled cardiac ischemia or arrhythmias, hypotensive shock, or upper GI bleeding, should also be promptly intubated. Because control of the upper airway is sacrificed by use of NPPV, patients who are unable to protect their upper airway by virtue of swallowing or coughing impairment should be excluded. This is a relative contraindication, however, and many patients with some impairment in cough or swallowing succeed with NPPV. Likewise, the presence of excessive airway secretions is a contraindication, but judgment is required in deciding what is excessive. Patient cooperation is essential for the successful application of NPPV, so agitated or uncooperative patients are poor candidates. Some of these patients may be rendered sufficiently cooperative by judicious use of sedation, however. Finally, obvious contraindications include the inability to fit a mask due to facial trauma or recent upper airway or esophageal surgery. By carefully selecting patients with reversible disease who are sufficiently ill to require ventilatory assistance but not so severely ill as to be unsafe candidates for NPPV, the clinician can maximize the likelihood of successful application.

IV. Appropriate Recipients of NPPV

A. Disease Categories

The evidence supporting the use of NPPV for specific etiologies of acute respiratory failure is discussed in more detail in Chapters 11 to 14. The following will briefly discuss applications of NPPV in specific disease categories for which there is some supporting evidence.

Obstructive Diseases

As listed in Table 2, successful treatment with NPPV has been reported for acute exacerbations of obstructive diseases including COPD (5–7,11), asthma (12), cystic fibrosis (13), upper airway obstruction (14), and obstructive sleep apnea (15). The only application supported by randomized controlled studies is that for COPD (see Chap. 12), and a meta-analysis has concluded that NPPV is effective at reducing the need for intubation and mortality in selected patients (16). Acute respiratory failure due to COPD exacerbation is the only application of NPPV that is supported by multiple randomized controlled trials. Accordingly, NPPV is considered the ventilator mode of first choice in appropriately selected COPD patients. For other diagnoses, evidence derives from small case series, sometimes included in larger series comprised of mixtures of diagnoses. For these, NPPV may be tried in patients meeting selection guidelines, but clinical judgment is necessary in selection as well as in deciding when a trial has failed and intubation is required.

Nonobstructive Diseases

Acute Pulmonary Edema

Acute pulmonary edema is one of the most common indications for the application of noninvasive positive pressure techniques (see Chap. 14). However, randomized controlled trials have shown that CPAP alone (10-12.5 cm H_2O) rapidly

Table 2 Specific Disease Categories Reported to Be Successfully Treated with Noninvasive Ventilation

Obstructive Diseases
  COPD exacerbations
  Acute asthma
  Cystic fibrosis
  Upper airway obstruction
  Obstructive sleep apnea
Nonobstructive Diseases
  Acute pulmonary edema
  Pneumonia
    Community acquired
    Immunocompromised
  ARDS
Restrictive Lung Diseases
  Kyphoscoliosis
  Neuromuscular diseases
  Obesity–hypoventilation syndrome

improves oxygenation and vital signs while drastically reducing the need for intubation (17–19). One recent controlled trial that compared CPAP directly with NPPV detected an unexplained increase in the incidence of myocardial infarctions in patients receiving NPPV, while showing comparable intubation rates (20). Thus, CPAP alone is considered the initial ventilatory therapy of choice for selected patients with acute pulmonary edema, and NPPV is recommended for those with persisting dyspnea or marked CO_2 retention.

Pneumonia

Early uncontrolled studies suggested that patients with acute pneumonia had higher failure rates while using NPPV than appropriate candidates with acute respiratory failure but no pneumonia (10). Recently, Confalonieri et al. (21) performed a controlled trial demonstrating that NPPV avoided intubation and shortened length of ICU stay in patients with severe community acquired pneumonia. In the subgroup of patients with COPD, there was also an improvement in survival at 2 months (89 vs. 38%, $p = 0.05$). In addition, immunocompromised patients consisting of HIV positive or post-transplant patients, are particularly attractive recipients of NPPV because of the potential to lower rates of nosocomial infection. A recent controlled study reported significant reductions in the need for intubation (20 vs. 50%), length of ICU stay among survivors (5.5 vs. 9 days), and ICU mortality (20 vs. 50%) among noninvasive ventilation-treated patients compared to controls, although hospital morbidity did not differ (22). Thus, some controlled studies now support the use of NPPV in patients with acute pneumonias. However, selection guidelines have not been clearly established in these trials, and clinicians are cautioned to pay particular attention to the quantity of secretions and the severity of cough impairment when selecting patients.

ARDS

No controlled trials have been published on the use of NPPV in ARDS exclusively. A recent small uncontrolled series reported success in 50% of ARDS patients treated with NPPV (23), and earlier studies that included small numbers of ARDS patients within the context of larger trials reported higher failure rates (14). Although it could be argued that avoiding intubation in up to 50% of ARDS patients may ultimately decrease morbidity and mortality, this has not been established. Until controlled trials provide better evidence of effectiveness and clarify the selection process, NPPV should be used only with great caution in ARDS patients. Those with relatively mild disease and single organ system failure might be considered for a trial, but those with severe oxygenation defects and multiorgan system dysfunction who are likely to require prolonged support with high levels of positive end-expiratory pressure (PEEP) should still be intubated.

Restrictive Lung Diseases

Case series have demonstrated successful application of NPPV in patients with severe kyphoscoliosis (24), but in contrast to the situation among outpatients, those with restrictive thoracic diseases are relatively uncommon among recipients of NPPV in acute care hospitals. In the series of 158 patients treated with NPPV in a critical care by Meduri et al. (14), only 3 had restrictive diseases. This may be partly explained by the use of management protocols aimed at preventing hospitalization in neuromuscular patients already using NPPV at home (25). These patients are instructed to go on continuous NPPV for several days during respiratory infections and to use manually assisted coughing devices like the cough inexsufflator to enhance secretion removal. Such patients are only hospitalized if this more intensive regimen fails, and if so, intubation is usually necessary. Use of NPPV in patients with acute respiratory failure due to pulmonary fibrosis has not been reported in case series, but limited effectiveness would be expected considering that severe oxygenation defects are typical and when severe respiratory failure ensues, many of these patients are considered terminal.

B. Patient Subgroups That May Respond Favorably to NPPV (Table 3)

Hypoxemic Respiratory Failure

The term hypoxemic respiratory failure refers to a group of patients with non-COPD causes of respiratory failure who have severe respiratory distress, are very tachypneic (RR > 35/min), and have Pao_2/Fio_2 ratios of <200. In addition, they have acute pneumonia, ARDS, acute pulmonary edema, or trauma (26). An earlier controlled trial on such patients suggested that unless patients were hypercapnic in addition to their hypoxemia, success with NPPV was unlikely (27). However, more recent randomized controlled trials indicate that NPPV reduces the need for intubation (26,28) and is as effective as invasive ventilation in improving oxygenation. In addition, evidence suggests that NPPV avoids nosocomial pneumonia and has a tendency to reduce intensive care unit (ICU) stays and mortality rates (26). These studies demonstrate that NPPV may be effective in supporting patients with hypoxemic respiratory failure, but the diagnostic category is so broad it is difficult to apply these data to individual patients. The same cautions raised above with regard to patients with acute pneumonia or ARDS apply to those within this larger subgroup of patients.

Table 3 Subgroups of Patients That May Respond Favorably to Noninvasive Ventilation

---

Hypoxemic respiratory failure
Postoperative and trauma patients
Do-not-intubate patients
Slow or difficult-to-wean patients
Extubation failure patients

Postoperative and Trauma Patients

Uncontrolled trials have reported the successful application of NPPV in patients
who develop respiratory insufficiency after surgery (29,30). In these studies, oxygenation was improved while $Paco_2$ fell. In addition, several short-term controlled
trials have demonstrated improved oxygenation or pulmonary functions after use
of NPPV in specific types of postoperative patients such as lung resection (31)
or gastroplasty (32). However, improvement in outcomes such as morbidity, mortality, and lengths of stay has not been demonstrated. Nonetheless, use of NPPV
in carefully selected postoperative patients is indicated to avoid the need for reintubation. Success with NPPV has also been reported in uncontrolled trials in
patients after major trauma, associated with improved gas exchange and low intubation rates (33).

Do-Not-Intubate Patients

Uncontrolled series have reported success rates averaging approximately 60% in
patients who develop acute respiratory failure and decline intubation (34,35). In
general, patients with COPD and congestive heart failure are most apt to succeed
in this category. Patients with end-stage terminal diseases such as malignancy
or severe sepsis are much less likely to respond favorably. This application appears to be justified as long as there is a reasonable expectation of reversibility
in the near term and the patient understands that NPPV is being used as a form
of life support, albeit noninvasive.

NPPV to Facilitate Weaning

NPPV to facilitate weaning is discussed in detail in Chapter 17. Studies suggest
that NPPV can be used to reduce the duration of invasive mechanical ventilation,
at least in patients with COPD (36,37), who would not otherwise meet standard
extubation criteria. However, it is unclear whether this approach should be used
in patients with other diagnoses, and extreme caution is advised if it is to be
applied in marginal candidates, particularly those who were difficult to intubate
in the first place. An appropriate application for NPPV in the weaning process,
however, is to attempt to avoid reintubation in patients who have failed extubation
(38). Although this latter application has not been tested in randomized controlled
trials, empiric use seems justified as long as standard patient selection criteria
are applied.

V. Practical Application of NPPV in the Critical Care Setting

Although application of NPPV for patients with acute respiratory failure is in
principle a simple process, in practice it tests the skills and determination of

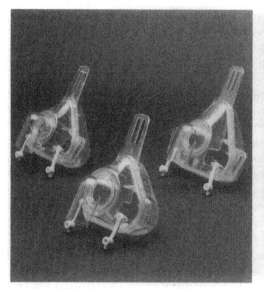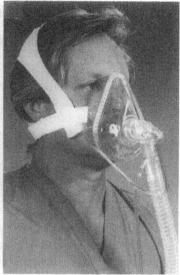

Figure 1 Disposable nasal masks in different sizes (left panel) and oronasal mask (right panel) commonly used for noninvasive positive pressure ventilation.

physicians, nurses, and respiratory therapists alike. Success requires experience and judgment in selecting appropriate patients using the guidelines previously discussed. Once an appropriate recipient of noninvasive ventilation has been identified, the clinician must promptly select an interface (or mask) and a ventilator to deliver pressurized gas through the upper airway. These selections, particularly that of the interface, are critical to success, because an uncomfortable or frightened patient is much more likely to fail. Selection of a ventilator mode, initial settings, and appropriate adjunctive therapies, such as oxygen or humidification, may also contribute to the successful application of NPPV. Although little scientific evidence is available to guide these selections, the following presents a framework for the successful implementation of noninvasive ventilation, with evidence cited when available and opinion given when necessary.

A. Selection of an Interface

Perhaps the most important aspect of NPPV initiation after selection of an appropriate patient is choosing an interface. Either nasal masks (that cover the nose or nares only) or oronasal (or full face) masks (that cover the nose and mouth) may be selected for initiation of NPPV (Fig. 1). Mouthpieces are used at some centers to facilitate initiation, and then patients are quickly switched to more stable masks (39). Nasal mask proponents stress the benefits of the reduced likelihood of claustrophobic reactions, ease of communication and expectoration, possibility of oral intake, and improved sense of comfort by patients. In addition, nasal masks have less dead space and cause less rebreathing of exhaled air than oronasal masks.

Proponents of the oronasal masks argue that dyspneic patients are usually mouth breathers and may adapt more readily to oronasal masks. Also, oronasal masks are more effective in the face of large air leaks through the mouth that are quite common with nasal ventilation. On the other hand, oronasal masks interfere more with speech and expectoration, and rebreathing may be a concern, particularly with large volume oronasal masks. There is also a theoretical risk of aspiration if vomiting occurs or of asphyxiation if ventilator failure occurs and the patient is unable to remove the mask. The incorporation of antiasphyxia valves and rapid release straps into some oronasal masks may reduce these risks. No randomized controlled trial comparing the two types of masks has yet been published, and success rates among studies that have used one mask or the other are similar. Nonetheless, recent advances in oronasal mask design and cost reductions have led to the predominant use of oronasal as opposed to nasal masks at most centers. Some advocate use of both mask types, starting with oronasal masks and switching to nasal masks for enhanced comfort if prolonged use is contemplated. Thus, either mask may be selected initially, with consideration of using an alternative interface if leaks or intolerance is observed.

In the acute setting where disposable masks are often used, cost is an important consideration. For this reason, masks that incorporate gel seals that have facilitated NPPV acceptance in some chronic NPPV users are not practical options for the acute setting. However, a number of manufacturers have recently introduced inexpensive disposable masks for acute applications that are reasonably comfortable and incorporate desirable safety features as discussed above (Spectrum™ Respironics, and Mirage disposable, Resmed, Inc., San Diego, CA).

B. Selection of a Ventilator

Either "critical care" ventilators that were designed with invasive ventilation in mind or less sophisticated ventilators designed for out-of-hospital noninvasive applications may be used for the acute administration of NPPV. In general, critical care ventilators have more sophisticated alarm and monitoring systems, but no direct clinical comparisons between the two ventilator types have been done. Studies that have used one type or the other have observed similar success rates. Critical care ventilators may be preferred when accurate monitoring of tidal or minute volume is desired or when patients have critical oxygenation defects that are better managed with high inspiratory fractions of oxygen. In contrast, noninvasive ventilators, often referred to as "bilevel" ventilators, tend to be more leak tolerant than critical care ventilators and are less apt to generate nuisance alarms that may contribute to patient and clinician anxiety. Although strong opinions are often expressed about the desirability of one ventilator type over the other, this choice during initiation is probably not as important as the type of interface or ventilator settings chosen. Also, it should be borne in mind that recent developments in ventilator technology are blurring the distinction between the two ventilator types as manufacturers introduce noninvasive ventilators with alarm and monitoring capabilities that match those of "critical care" ventilators (i.e., Vision™, Respironics).

C. Selection of a Ventilator Mode and Settings

Once a ventilator/interface combination has been chosen, a ventilator mode and initial settings must be selected, and these strongly influence patient tolerance of NPPV. Available evidence suggests that volume- and pressure-limited ventilator modes are equally effective at assisting ventilation and averting intubation, at least in patients with COPD exacerbations (40). However, pressure-limited ventilation is perceived by patients as more comfortable than volume-limited ventilation (41), and practitioners rate patients as more "compliant" during pressure support ventilation (42). Thus, pressure-limited modes such as pressure support with a back-up rate (such as the S/T mode on the BiPAP ventilator, Respironics, Inc.) are most often chosen for acute applications of NPPV.

Compared with most portable volume-limited ventilators, the pressure-limited "bilevel" ventilators are smaller, lighter, less expensive, and capable of compensating for leaks by adjusting airflow breath by breath to maintain mask pressure. Some devices offer adjustable "rise times," i.e., the rapidity with which target pressure is reached, whereas others offer adjustable triggering and cycling capabilities. Still others may offer pressure control modes in addition to pressure support. These attributes may permit enhanced synchrony and comfort when patients are having problems adapting to NPPV. Limitations of these ventilators include lower maximal pressure generating capabilities (20–35 cm H_2O), the lack of an oxygen blender, and fewer alarms than "critical care" ventilators. These preclude the use of pressure-limited ventilators in critically ill patients who require high inflation pressures of FIO_2s or continuous ventilation unless adequate monitors and alarms are applied. Despite these limitations, the use of pressure-limited ventilation has become the dominant form of noninvasive ventilation. Thus, the remainder of the discussion will focus on pressure-limited ventilators.

With regard to setting initial pressures, studies using pressure support ventilation have used inspiratory positive airway pressures (IPAP) of 8–20 cm H_2O with expiratory positive airway pressures (EPAP or PEEP) of 0–5 cm H_2O

(6,7,11,14). Expiratory pressures of at least 4–5 cm H_2O are recommended for "bilevel" ventilators to provide an adequate bias flow to minimize the impact of rebreathing (43). Also, in patients with acute COPD exacerbations, EPAPs of 4–5 cm H_2O are desirable because of the need to counterbalance autoPEEP (see Chap. 12). Higher EPAP levels may sometimes be helpful to enhance patient-ventilator synchrony in patients with high levels of auto-PEEP, to improve oxygenation, or to ventilate patients with obstructive sleep apnea and acute respiratory failure. In general, within these constraints the lowest effective EPAP level is used so that the IPAP level need not be excessive.

The authors' practice is to begin with an IPAP of 8–12 cm H_2O and an EPAP of 4–5 cm H_2O based on the presumption that relatively low initial pressures enhance patient tolerance (Table 4). Inspiratory pressures are then increased gradually as tolerated by the patient. The strategy is to balance the relief of respiratory distress afforded by the greater inspiratory pressure against the increasing discomfort associated with greater pressures applied to the nasal passages, sinuses, and ears. It is acknowledged that other authors have described the use of substantially higher initial pressures (14). If volume-limited ventilation is used, tidal volumes of 10–15 mL/kg are recommended to allow for leak compensation.

When using a mode with a timed back-up, such as assist/control or spontaneous/timed on "bilevel" devices, a back-up rate must be selected. This is useful to prevent apneas and to assure machine triggering when air leaks render the ventilator insensitive to patient triggering. Based on the assumption that most acutely ill patients are more comfortable if allowed to trigger their own breaths, a back-up rate lower than the spontaneous rate (i.e., 12–16 breaths per minute) is usually selected. However, in very fatigued or weak patients, rates exceeding

Table 4 Suggested Ventilator Settings for Pressure-Limited NPPV in the Acute Setting

Inspiratory pressure	Initial	8–10 cmH$_2$O
	Eventual	12–20 cmH$_2$O
Expiratory pressure	Initial	4–5 cmH$_2$O
	Eventual	4–8 cmH$_2$O
	(higher pressures for auto-PEEP, to improve oxygenation, eliminate obstructive apneas, or eliminate rebreathing)	
Back-up rate		12–20/min
Oxygenation	"Bilevel" ventilators	O$_2$ flow of 2–15 L/min via mask or circuit
	"Critical care" ventilators	Titrate F$_{IO_2}$ or flow for O$_2$ sat > 90–92%
Humidification	Heated passover humidifier recommended for >24 h applications	

20 breaths per minute may control breathing and allow for complete respiratory muscle rest.

D. Adjuncts to NPPV

Oxygenation

Several adjuncts to NPPV may be necessary either to enhance gas exchange or to improve patient comfort. Hypoxemic patients require supplemental oxygen adjusted to maintain the oxygen saturation at the desired level, usually greater than 90%. With "critical care" or noninvasive ventilators equipped with oxygen blenders, this is easily achieved by adjusting the fraction of inspired oxygen (FIO_2). However, with bilevel ventilators that lack oxygen blenders, oxygen tubing is connected directly to the mask or to a T-connector in the ventilator tubing near the ventilator. Unless an oxygen blender is used, the precise FIO_2 that the patient receives is difficult to ascertain. Dilution of the delivered oxygen is the result of mixing supplemental oxygen with ambient air delivered by the ventilator. This is especially important in severely hypoxemic patients in whom delivered oxygen concentration may decrease if pressure support is increased. In this situation, use of ventilators equipped with oxygen blenders is advisable.

Successful noninvasive ventilation prevents excessive CO_2 retention that may otherwise occur in COPD patients treated with a high FIO_2 (44). Therefore, clinicians should not hesitate to use sufficient supplemental oxygen to achieve adequate oxygen saturation, provided that $PaCO_2$ is checked periodically. With bilevel ventilators, oxygen saturation in hypoxemic patients may continue to improve even when oxygen supplementation rates are increased as necessary up to 15 L/min (authors' personal observation). However, these rates have not been evaluated with regard to effects on machine triggering or cycling.

Humidification

Humidification of inspired air is potentially useful during NPPV. However, since the normal air-conditioning mechanisms (i.e., nose and upper airway) are left intact, humidification is usually unnecessary for short-term acute applications. On the other hand, patients who have frequent expectoration of secretions, the need for long-term use, or substantial air leaks may benefit from humidification. Richards et al. (45) have observed increases in nasal resistance if large air leaks occur during application of nasal CPAP, presumably because of mucosal cooling and drying. The use of a heated humidifier reverses this effect. If humidification is desired during use of bilevel ventilation, a heated "passover" humidifier should be used. Pass-through humidifiers or heat and moisture exchangers may reduce delivered pressures and alter triggering sensitivities and therefore should be avoided.

Aerosol Treatments

Nebulizer or aerosol treatments may be delivered directly via the ventilator tubing during use of critical care or bilevel ventilators without interruption of noninvasive ventilatory assistance. No studies have evaluated the pulmonary distribution of the aerosol, either in COPD patients or in those with other forms of respiratory failure. However, increases in FEV_1 have been observed after aerosol administration during "bilevel" ventilation (46). Alternatively, if the patient is sufficiently stable, ventilation can be interrupted and the respiratory treatment administered using standard nebulizer or aerosol techniques.

E. Patient Adaptation to NPPV

Once NPPV is initiated, most patients have mask- or air pressure–related discomfort and require a period of adjustment prior to clinical stabilization and improvement. Virtually all patients need coaching and encouragement to leave the mask in place, relax as much as possible, and allow the ventilator to assist breathing. Inspiratory pressure should be adjusted to maximize patient comfort. If a nasal mask is used, oral air leaks can be reduced by simply coaching cooperative patients to close their mouths. Otherwise, placement of a chin strap to enhance mouth closure or switching to an oronasal mask may suffice to reduce persistent air leaks. Within 1–2 hours of NPPV application, successful patients usually appear much more comfortable, with decreased respiratory and heart rates in addition to an obvious reduction or even cessation of accessory muscle use (47,48).

Because of dyspnea-related sleep deprivation, the relief of respiratory distress may induce sleep almost immediately as patients can finally rest. The differentiation between sleep deprivation and somnolence due to CO_2 retention because of worsening ventilatory status is a critical distinction that requires careful observation and examination of patients. Vital signs, pulse oximetry, occasional blood gases and clinical response should be closely monitored. Further ventilator adjustments should be based on arterial blood gas results and patient tolerance. If hypercapnia fails to improve, the level of pressure support should be increased within the limits of patient tolerance. Particularly in chronically hypercapnic COPD patients, initial decreases in $Paco_2$ may be small (7) but this need not be cause for concern as long as other parameters, such as respiratory rate or sternocleidomastoid muscle activity, improve.

Persistent hypoxemia can be treated by increasing either the supplemental oxygen flow or EPAP. Importantly, unless the IPAP is simultaneously increased or patient effort increases, an increase in EPAP decreases the level of pressure support resulting in smaller tidal (V_T) and minute volumes. Any adjustment in pressure settings must be monitored closely, as increased pressure may reduce patient comfort and adversely affect patient tolerance. Fortunately, most appropriately selected patients can be helped to adapt successfully by skilled, experienced, and attentive clinicians.

F. Patient Location and Monitoring

The best location for delivery of NPPV depends on the acuity of the patient's illness and the availability of critical care beds. For patients who are unstable and would be threatened by even brief discontinuation of ventilatory assistance, monitoring in an intensive care unit is advisable. Most studies on acute applications of NPPV have been performed in such settings (Table 5) (6,7). Patients are often initiated in the Emergency Department and transferred to the Critical Care Unit (6). More institutions are adding respiratory care units, which are also suitable for most patients treated noninvasively. Admission of patients with acute respiratory insufficiency to general medical wards has been described, mainly from countries that lack sufficient numbers of intensive care or respiratory care unit beds (49). Such admissions are discouraged in acutely ill patients, and, in

Table 5 Location and Monitoring for Acute Applications of NPPV

Location
    Emergency department (for initiation, then transfer)
    Critical care unit
    Respiratory care unit
    General medical/surgical unit (if stabilized and capable of spontaneous breathing for >20–30 min)
Monitoring
    "Eyeball test"
    Respiratory distress
    Patient discomfort
    Vital signs; respiratory rate, heart rate, blood pressure
    Sternocleidomastoid muscle activity
    Patient-ventilator synchrony
    Gas exchange
      Continuous pulse oximetry
      Occasional blood gases
      End-tidal/transcutaneous CO_2 not recommended
    Ventilation variables
      Pressure
      Flow
      Tidal volume
      Leaks
      F_{IO_2}
    Complications (see Table 6)

the authors' judgment, transfer to general medical wards should be deferred until patients are capable of breathing without ventilatory support for at least 20–30 minutes, depending on the monitoring capabilities of the particular floor.

The most important aspect of monitoring during use of NPPV is direct bedside observation (i.e., the "eyeball" test). The observer can quickly determine the level of patient comfort, alleviation of respiratory distress, reduced sternocleidomastoid muscle activity, the presence of air leaks, appropriateness of mask fit and strap tension, and whether the patient's breathing is well synchronized with the ventilator. Vital signs are also important to monitor. Perhaps the best early indicator of NPPV success is a drop in respiratory rate (48). Heart rate also usually promptly drops, and blood pressure remains steady, although, as discussed below, blood pressure alterations may occur. Continuous pulse oximetry is advisable until the patient stabilizes, and occasional blood gases should be obtained as clinically indicated. In patients with hypercapnic respiratory failure, an initial blood gas within the first hour or two of initiation is mandatory to demonstrate that $Paco_2$ is gradually dropping and not rising. Noninvasive measures of CO_2 tension such as end-tidal or transcutaneous are not sufficiently reliable to supplant occasional blood gases (50).

Monitoring capabilities of ventilators vary greatly, as discussed above, but fortunately, the patient-related monitoring variables are more important than the ventilator ones. At a minimum, ventilators should be capable of monitoring mask pressure and have alarms for disconnection and low pressure. Monitoring of tidal volume and air leak is helpful, but most bilevel ventilators offer only estimates, which can be quite inaccurate. Critical care ventilators are more accurate for monitoring these variables.

G. Weaning from Noninvasive Ventilation

The weaning process should be initiated gradually. As patients stabilize, NPPV can be interrupted for short periods of time to allow for eating, drinking, and conversation. Before even temporary discontinuation of NPPV, patients should have a substantial reduction in respiratory rate and stabilization of oxygen saturation at levels of $\geq 90\%$ with an Fio_2 of $\leq 40\%$ or the equivalent while using the ventilator. Initially, the interruptions in NPPV use are short in duration but are lengthened as the patient improves. Patients often communicate to their caretakers that they no longer require assisted ventilation. During periods of discontinuation, patients should be monitored closely so that NPPV can be resumed if respiratory distress occurs or vital signs or gas exchange deteriorate. If no deterioration occurs, then NPPV need not be resumed. An alternative approach to weaning is to gradually lower the pressure support level, but this is less often used with NPPV. Some patients, such as those with COPD and severe CO_2 retention (≥ 52

Table 6 Frequency of Complications of NPPV with Possible Preventative Therapies

	Occurrence (%)[a]	Possible therapies
Mask-related		
discomfort	30–50	Check fit, adjust strap, apply water-based jelly to mask contact points, try new mask type
Facial skin erythema	20–34	Loosen strap tension, apply artificial skin
Claustrophobia	5–10	Smaller mask, sedation
Nasal bridge ulceration	5–10	Loosen strap tension, apply artificial skin, new mask
Acneiform rash	5–10	Topical steroids or antibiotics
Air pressure– or flow–related		
Nasal congestion	20–50	Nasal steroids, decongestants/antihistamine
Sinus/ear pain	10–30	Reduce pressure if intolerable
Nasal/oral dryness	10–20	Nasal saline, add humidifier, reduce air leak
Eye irritation	10–20	Check mask fit, readjust straps
Gastric insufflation	5–10	Reassure, simethacone, reduce pressure if intolerable
Air leaks	80–100	Encourage mouth closure, try chin straps, oronasal mask if using nasal mask, apply water-based jelly to mask contact points, reduce pressure slightly
Major complications		
Aspiration pneumonia	<2	Careful patient selection
Hypotension	<2	Reduce pressure
Pneumothorax	<2	Reduce pressure

[a] Adapted from Ref. 52.

mmHG) and nocturnal desaturations or sleep apnea that predate the acute exacerbation may be candidates for long-term nocturnal NPPV (51).

H. Complications and Adverse Effects of Noninvasive Ventilation

Most complications associated with NPPV are related to the mask interface. Table 6 lists mask-related complications derived from a number of series using nasal and oronasal masks. Up to 28% of patients fail to tolerate nasal interfaces despite adjustments in strap tension, repositioning, and trials of different sizes and types

(52). Nasal pain, erythema, and skin abrasions account for the majority of complications with both nasal and oronasal masks and occur in up to 34% of patients (52). These can be reduced or prevented by assuring proper mask fit, avoiding excessive strap tension, and applying artificial skin to the bridge of the nose prior to mask application.

Other common adverse effects are related to air pressure or flow (Table 6). During initiation, sinus and/or ear burning and/or pain occur frequently and may be alleviated by lowering inspiratory pressure slightly. Nasal and oral dryness are also common and may be treated with nasal saline or humidification. Nasal congestion and/or discharge are also frequent complaints and can be effectively treated with nasal steroids, antihistamine/decongestant combinations, or decongestant nose drops (52). Conjunctivitis occurs when air leaks underneath the mask seal into the eyes, causing irritation. This is alleviated by readjusting or changing the mask to minimize leak, or if all else fails, eye patches. Gastric insufflation occurs commonly during NPPV, but is rarely uncomfortable enough to render patients intolerant. Patients usually pass gas spontaneously and may occasionally respond to simethacone. The most feared complication of high positive airway pressure, pneumothorax, is virtually unheard of during NPPV in the acute care setting, probably because of the relatively low inflation pressures used compared to invasive ventilation.

Air Leaks

Although air leakage through the mouth (with nasal masks) or around the mask occurs in virtually all patients treated with NPPV, leaks large enough to cause failure can usually be avoided. Air escaping through the mouth is associated with the reappearance of substantial phasic diaphragm electromyographic activity (53), so every attempt should be made to minimize leaks without causing undue patient discomfort. Mask leaks can be reduced by ensuring proper mask fit. Although tightening the head straps to maintain a mask seal is tempting, this may reduce patient comfort and cause skin ulceration; pulling outward on the mask to reseal the silicon gasket may be more effective. Using a thin layer of water-based jelly between the mask and skin may also improve seal and comfort without the need for increased head strap tension. Petroleum jelly should be avoided in light of case reports of lipoid pneumonia associated with aspiration of these products (54). With nasal masks, mouth leaks can be minimized by encouraging patients to keep their mouths closed. Application of chin straps or switching to an oronasal mask may help, but air leaks often persist despite these interventions. Pressure-limited ventilators compensate for these leaks by sustaining high inspiratory flow for a longer duration, thus maintaining the prescribed mask pressure and assisting ventilation even in the face of substantial leaks.

Aspiration

Nasogastric tube insertion has been advocated to prevent one of the most feared complications of oronasal NPPV: gastric distention leading to emesis and aspiration. However, problems with gastric distention or aspiration are infrequent even when nasogastric tubes are not used. In the only report of a patient who aspirated, a nasogastric tube was in place (55). Aspiration can be prevented by giving at-risk patients nothing by mouth until they are more stable and by using NPPV cautiously, if at all, in patients with illnesses that predispose to vomiting. A nasogastric tube can be inserted if patients develop excessive gastric distention. Due to the risk of air insufflation, NPPV should not be applied to patients with recent high esophageal or tracheal surgery or injuries or to patients with basilar skull fractures in whom pneumocephalus has been reported (56).

Rebreathing

Rebreathing may occur with large volume oronasal facemasks, particularly during use of bilevel ventilators. Most bilevel ventilators use a single ventilator circuit, with gases passing through a single tube for both inspiration and expiration. A continuous leak through a small port in the mask or ventilator tubing is used to exhaust exhaled CO_2. Several laboratory reports have demonstrated that substantial rebreathing occurs under certain circumstances during use of these ventilators (43,57), but the problem has never been evaluated in patients undergoing therapy in a critical care setting. In general, this is probably not an important problem as long as adequate expiratory pressures (4–5 cm H_2O) are used during "bilevel" ventilation to flush out CO_2. However, if difficulty is encountered in lowering $Paco_2$, nonrebreathing valves may be added to the circuit (Plateau valve, Respironics) or a lower volume mask may be tried.

Hemodynamic Effects

Positive pressure ventilation, whether administered endotracheally or noninvasively, may have either adverse or beneficial hemodynamic effects depending on fluid volume status and cardiac systolic function. In the normal heart, preload (and thus venous return) is the most important determinant of cardiac output under usual circumstances (58). With the application of CPAP, increased intrathoracic pressure reduces venous return, leading to a fall in preload and cardiac output. Similar findings are seen among congestive heart failure (CHF) patients with pulmonary artery wedge pressures < 12 mmHg. In contrast, CHF patients with pulmonary artery wedge pressures > 12 mmHg show significant increases in cardiac output after the application of CPAP (59). This augmentation is probably related to a CPAP-induced increase in intrathoracic pressure, resulting in decreased LV transmural pressure (LV intramural pressure minus pericardial pressure) and thereby reduced afterload. Also, reduction in left ventricular end diastolic volume by the same mechanism reduces LV transmural tension via the Law of La Place, contributing to reduced afterload (60,61). Thus, although NPPV may have beneficial hemodynamic effects on patients with CHF and impaired left ventricular systolic function, adverse effects may also be encountered. Even though the risk of hypotension during use of NPPV is reduced because of lower inflation pressures when compared to invasive ventilation, it is still important to monitor blood pressures closely, particularly in dehydrated patients who may be starting with low filling pressures.

I. Overview of NPPV Application

The application of NPPV, more than almost any other form of mechanical ventilation, tests the clinical skills of the critical care team. Selection of appropriate recipients is key to success, and physicians who are responsible for making this judgment rely largely on their experience while applying general selection guidelines. Respiratory therapists in the United States and nurses in many other countries are then responsible for initiating NPPV under the direction of physicians, making informed choices about mask and ventilator selection. These personnel must be willing to spend time at the patient's bedside, making initial adjustments and readjustments to optimize patient comfort. They must coach patients to allow the ventilator to assist their breathing, gaining the patient's confidence and reassuring the patient that success will come with cooperation. Heavy sedation and paralysis are not options during NPPV, so communication skills are very helpful in calming patients. In addition, close monitoring of acutely ill patients is necessary so that temporary disconnections, problems expectorating, or abrupt desaturations related to air leaking or mucus plugs can be promptly handled. Despite its challenges, proper application of NPPV is generally safe and rewarding, particularly when one considers that it can usually be administered with greater patient comfort and reduced morbidity compared to invasive mechanical ventilation.

VI. Effects of NPPV on Patient Outcomes

The use of NPPV for acute respiratory failure has been evaluated in numerous clinical trials involving well over 1000 patients. Thus, the effects on numerous patient outcomes have been well studied. The best known effects are on short-term physiological outcomes and the need for intubation, as demonstrated in numerous uncontrolled or historically controlled trials. However, well-designed randomized controlled trials, although not numerous, have also demonstrated effects on global outcomes such as morbidity and mortality rates. The following will briefly review these effects on outcomes, relying heavily on results from the few controlled trials that have been done.

A. Physiological Outcomes

Vital Signs

One of the earliest benefits of noninvasive ventilation is a rapid reduction in respiratory and heart rate. This effect is almost immediate, occurring as soon as the patient is able to synchronize breathing efforts with the ventilator and tolerates sufficient inspiratory pressures. Figure 2 shows the typical time course of respiratory and heart rate over the first 24 hours. The failure to observe a drop in respiratory rate within the first 2 hours of initiation of NPPV is considered an important indicator of impending failure (48). The blood pressure response to NPPV is more variable, but most patients experience either a stable blood pressure response or a slight decrease as respiratory distress and, presumably, catecholamine levels diminish. Increasing blood pressure and persisting hypertension may indicate failure to alleviate respiratory distress.

Work of Breathing and the Sensation of Dyspnea

Studies in subacutely ill patients with severe COPD demonstrate unequivocally that NPPV is capable of reducing breathing effort as determined by the magnitude of esophageal pressure swings and the sum of the diaphragmatic EMG signal (53) (Fig. 3). The precise physiological mechanisms by which this phenomenon occurs are unclear, but it is evident that central drive is suppressed in response to the provision of inspiratory assistance. Outward manifestations of this adaptation include reductions in respiratory rate and sternocleidomastoid muscle activity. The reduction in respiratory effort is associated with a prompt alleviation in the sensation of dyspnea and usually anxiety, as well (Fig. 4).

Gas Exchange

As with vital signs, gas exchange improves rapidly as patients with acute respiratory failure adapt to NPPV (6). As shown in Figure 5, patients with hypercapnic respiratory failure experience 5–10 mmHg decreases in $Paco_2$ and patients with hypoxemic respiratory failure experience dramatic increases in PaO_2, both within the first hour. As with respiratory rate, if no improvement in gas exchange is seen within the first 2 hours, NPPV failure is likely (47,48). It is important to bear in mind, however, that occasional patients with hypercapneic respiratory failure may not manifest large decreases in $Paco_2$ immediately (7). This is acceptable as long as respiratory rate, accessory muscle use, and the sensation of dyspnea are all diminishing.

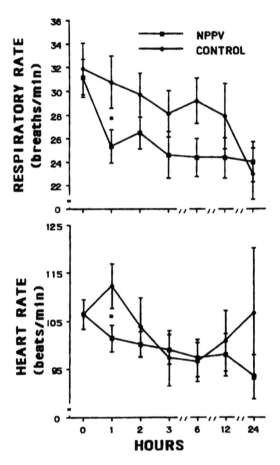

Figure 2 Time course of responses of respiratory and heart rates to noninvasive ventilation in patients treated with NPPV as opposed to controls treated conventionally. Respiratory rate drops promptly whereas the drop in heart rate is more gradual. *$p < 0.05$ compared to control group. (From Ref. 6.)

B.   Intubation, Morbidity, and Mortality

Need for Intubation

Among nonphysiological outcome variables, the reduction in the need for intubation is the best established. A number of randomized, controlled trials have demonstrated marked reductions in the need for intubation, not only in patients with COPD, but more recently in patients with hypoxemic respiratory failure as well as acute community-acquired pneumonia (Table 7). Among these controlled studies,

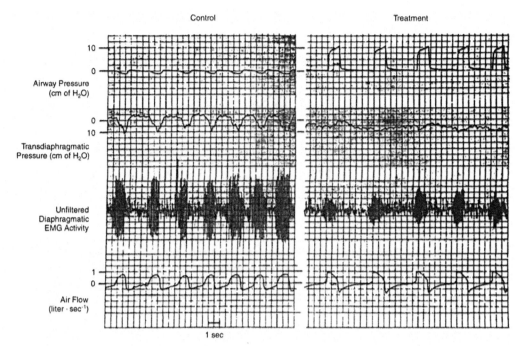

Figure 3 Response to noninvasive pressure support ventilation in COPD patients Breathing spontaneously (on left) and with ventilatory assistance (on right). Note the decline in the amplitude in the EMG signal and reduction in respiratory rate. (From Brochard et al. N Engl J Med 1990; 323:1523–1530.)

average intubation rates declined from approximately 50% in controls to 20% among NPPV-treated patients. In a meta-analysis of controlled trials on NPPV, Keenan et al. (16) also found a strongly significant reduction in the need for intubation. In fact, virtually every controlled trial of NPPV has found a significant reduction in intubations. Exceptions include a trial on patients with non-COPD causes of respiratory failure in which nonhypercapnic patients had high intubation rates despite use of NPPV (27) and a trial on patients with relatively mild COPD exacerbations, none of whom needed intubation (62). As discussed earlier, more recent studies suggest that many non-COPD patients with acute respiratory failure also avoid intubation if treated with NPPV (26,28)

Morbidity and Complication Rates

Most controlled trials have demonstrated decreases in complication rates among patients using NPPV compared to those treated conventionally. Not unexpect-

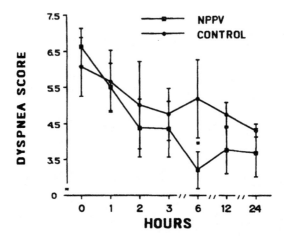

Figure 4 Time course of relief of dyspnea in patients with acute respiratory failure treated with NPPV compared with controls, as determined by a visual analog scale. Dyspnea diminishes gradually over several hours with a significantly greater drop in NPPV patients at 6 hours. *$p < 0.05$ compared with controls. (From Ref. 6.)

edly, this reduction has been in complications attributable to prolonged intubation, such as accidental extubations as well as infection rates. The reduction in nosocomial pneumonias has been quite large but has been inconsistent among studies (Table 7), largely because the definition and reporting of complications has been quite variable between studies. One recent outcome study calculated that the risk of nosocomial pneumonia was reduced by approximately fourfold when patients were treated with NPPV as opposed to endotracheal intubation, even after adjustment for severity of illness (63). Reductions in the incidence of sinusitis and episodes of sepsis have also been reported (26).

Mortality

A number of randomized controlled trials have shown either significant or at least trends toward reductions in mortality rate in patients using NPPV compared to those conventionally treated (Table 7). In their meta-analysis, Keenan et al. (16) calculated that mortality rates were significantly reduced by use of NPPV among patients with COPD exacerbations, although the effect was not as great as that on intubations. Whether NPPV reduces mortality rates in patients with non-COPD forms of respiratory failure has not been established. Recent randomized controlled studies on these patients have shown significant reductions in ICU, but not overall hospital mortality (20,22) (Table 7). Some studies have raised concerns that NPPV, when applied to such patients, may actually be harmful if it is used in patients with excessive secretions or leads to inordinate delays

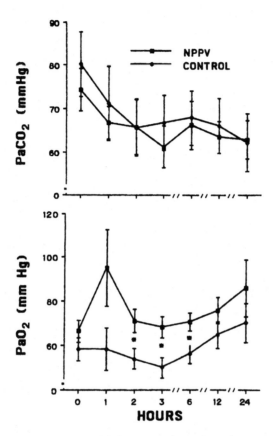

Figure 5   Time course of response of $Paco_2$ and Pao_2 in patients treated with NPPV compared with controls. Oxygenation improves significantly more in NPPV-treated than in controls, accompanied by a gradual drop in $Paco_2$. The control group experienced a similar drop in $Paco_2$, mainly because patients in the control group who failed (of patients at 6 hours) were intubated and were no longer monitored. $*p < 0.05$ compared with controls. (From Ref. 6.)

in needed intubation (64). These latter observations underline the importance of careful patient selection and the advisability of proceeding with intubation if there is no evidence of improvement within the first few hours.

C. Resource Utilization

Hospital and ICU Lengths of Stay

Several controlled trials have demonstrated reductions in ICU and/or hospital lengths of stay in patients treated with NPPV compared to conventional therapy,

Table 7 Effects of NPPV on Intubation, Nosocomial Pneumonia, and Mortality Rates in Randomized Trials on Patients with Acute Respiratory Failure

Author	Ref.	Diagnoses	n	Intubations (%)		Complications		Mortality (%)	
				NPPV	Control	NPPV	Control	NPPV	Control
Bott	5	COPD	60	—	—	—	—	10	30*
Kramer	6	Mainly COPD	31	31	73*	—	—	6	13
Brochard	7	COPD	85	25	74*	16(5)[a]	48(17)*	9	29*
Wysocki	27	Non-COPD Mixed	41	62	70	—	—	33	50
Barbe	63	COPD	24	0	0	—	—	0	0
Celikel	11	COPD	30	7	40*	53	—	0	7
Wood	64	Mixed	27	44	45	10	5	25	0
Antonelli	26	Hypoxia	64	30	100*	38(3)	38(31)	28	47*†
Confalonieri	21	Pneumonia	56	21	50*	4	14	25	21
Antonelli	22	Pneumonia	40	20	70*	20	50*	20	50*†
Martins	28	Mixed	61	28	59*	20	14	16	34†

— = not reported; *p < 0.05 c/w control; † = ICU mortality.
[a] Numbers in parentheses are numbers of pneumonias plus sinusitis.

Table 8 Length of ICU and/or Hospital Stays Among Patients Treated Noninvasively Compared to Controls

Author	Ref.	ICU stay (days)		Hospital stay (days)	
		NPPV	Control	NPPV	Control
Bott	5	—	—	9	9
Kramer	6	—	—	15	17
Brochard	7	—	—	23	35*
Wysocki	27	17	25	—	—
Barbe	63	—	—	10.6	11.3
Celikel	11	—	—	11.7	14.6*
Wood	64	5.8	4.9	17.4	9.1
Antonelli	26	6.6	14*	—	—
Confalonieri	26	1.8	6*	17	18
Antonelli	22	5.5	9**	—	—

* $p < 0.05$ compared with controls.
** $p < 0.05$ compared with controls for survivors.

but other studies have shown no such effect (Table 8). The ability to demonstrate such reductions probably depends to a certain extent on regional practices relating to admission and discharge. For example, in the European multicenter trial by Brochard et al. (7) (Table 8), the average length of hospital stay among controls was 35 days, and this was reduced to 17 days among NPPV-treated patients. In a comparable group of patients who had almost identical initial blood gases treated in the United States, Kramer et al. (6) observed a slight decline in hospital days from 17 days among controls to 15 days among NPPV-treated patients, a nonsignificant difference. The great pressure exerted in the United States by managed care organizations to discharge patients as soon as possible may have been responsible for the substantially shorter hospital stays among controls in the Kramer study, making it more difficult to demonstrate a significant reduction among NPPV-treated patients. Thus, although NPPV appears to improve the efficiency of hospital utilization under some circumstances, this has not been a universally consistent finding. Also, in recent studies on non-COPD patients, patients moved out of the ICU sooner, but total hospital stay was not shortened with noninvasive ventilation (21,22,26).

Some evidence suggests that the use of NPPV during an initial hospitalization may have a lingering benefit. Vitacca et al. (65) demonstrated that the frequency of ICU use during the subsequent year was 0.3 per patient among those treated with invasive mechanical ventilation and only 0.12 per patient among those treated with noninvasive ventilation only during the initial hospitalization, a statistically significant reduction. However, this was not a randomized prospective trial, and it is conceivable that patients treated with NPPV were less severely impaired than recipients of invasive ventilation.

Costs and Reimbursement of NPPV

Few studies have examined the costs of administering NPPV. Kramer et al. (6) observed no significant reduction in hospital charges among patients treated with NPPV (average $40,000 per hospitalization) compared to those treated conventionally ($37,000 per hospitalization). Nava et al. (66) examined costs in terms of personnel time expenditure and utilization of laboratory and radiological services and again found no differences between patients treated with NPPV or invasively. NPPV-treated patients had average costs of $806 per hospital day as opposed to $865 per hospital day for conventionally treated patients, but the difference was not statistically significant. Although it seems quite likely that hospital costs would be reduced if hospital lengths of stay are shortened by NPPV, the studies showing significant reductions in ICU and hospital lengths of stay did not examine costs.

Even if costs are lowered by use of NPPV, however, the benefit for care providers may not be apparent unless they are adequately reimbursed. Criner et al. (67) monitored costs and reimbursement for NPPV in their ventilation weaning unit. They found that the Diagnosis Related Group (DRG) classification system used for Medicare reimbursement in the United States consistently undervalued the cost associated with administering NPPV. On average, there was a deficit of $9,701 per patient because of the shortfall. They recommend modification of the DRG payment scales, but this has not yet been done.

Utilization of Personnel Time

An early study on acute applications of NPPV pointed out that the modality was quite expensive in terms of nursing time consumption (68). In fact, for the three patients with COPD exacerbations in this study, nurses were present at the bedside for 91% of the time that the ventilator was in use. Subsequent studies have found that although NPPV usually does not require quite as much personnel time as this early study suggested, it does require more time for initiation than invasive mechanical ventilation. Kramer et al. (6) found that respiratory therapists tended to spend more time during the first 8 hours on patients receiving NPPV than on those receiving invasive ventilation, and this time consumption fell significantly during the second 8 hours, when time consumption was comparable between the two ventilator modalities (Table 9). In this study, nursing time consumption was not affected by ventilator modality. In addition, the nurses rated NPPV as no more difficult to administer than invasive ventilation. It should be borne in mind when interpreting these studies that Switzerland did not employ respiratory therapists at the time of the early study, so nurses served the respiratory therapy role.

Table 9 Respiratory and Nursing Time at Bedside and Difficulty Scores[a]

	First 8 h		Second 8 h	
	Min/8 h[b]	Difficulty score[c]	Min/8 h[b]	Difficulty score
Respiratory				
NPPV	100 ± 27	3.1 ± 0.4	34 ± 9*	4.0 ± 0.8
Control	44 ± 15	3.0 ± 0.7	59 ± 43	4.8 ± 1.1
Nursing				
NPPV	96 ± 15	2.8 ± 0.8	82 ± 15	2.6 ± 0.8
Control	139 ± 40	3.4 ± 1.2	66 ± 28	4.0 ± 1.8

[a] Data are mean + SEM. Values in parentheses are number of patients.
[b] Mean number of minutes in 8 h spent at the bedside as recorded by nurses and respiratory therapists.
[c] Difficulty score was analog: 1 = least difficult; 10 = most difficult.
* $p < 0.05$ compared with the first 8-h period.
Source: Ref. 6.

A third study from Italy (66) found that although time expenditure by physicians and nurses was similar whether administering NPPV or invasive mechanical ventilation, respiratory therapy time expenditure was greater during the administration of NPPV.

These studies support the contention that NPPV requires more time for initiation than invasive mechanical ventilation, amounting to an additional hour or so. Once patients have successfully adapted, time consumption is no greater. At times when respiratory therapy staffing is light, however, the need to spend additional time on a ventilator modality may affect attitudes toward its implementation and limit the therapist's ability to spend the requisite bedside time to optimize success.

VII. Summary and Conclusions

The greater use of NPPV in the acute care setting during the past decade has stimulated the performance of studies examining effects on outcomes and efficiency of resource utilization. These studies have demonstrated unequivocally that NPPV is highly effective at bringing about rapid improvements in vital signs, dyspnea scores, and gas exchange, particularly in patients with COPD. In so doing, NPPV is also highly effective at reducing the need for intubation. In addition, complications attributable to prolonged intubation are usually reduced, particularly infectious ones. In accordance with the reduction in complications, mortality rates are reduced in patients with COPD, with less consistent reductions in patients with non-COPD causes for acute respiratory failure.

Studies of the effects of NPPV on resource utilization have not provided clear answers yet. A number of studies have demonstrated reductions in the time of ICU and total hospital lengths of stay, but this has not been universal. In addition, although it is reasonable to assume that reductions in lengths of stay should lead to decreased costs, this has not been definitively demonstrated in controlled studies. Furthermore, resource consumption in terms of respiratory therapy time is increased by the use of NPPV, at least during initiation. In addition, some evidence suggests that NPPV utilization, at least in the United States, is not reimbursed at adequate rates to compensate for costs, and until Diagnosis Related Groups are created that adequately compensate for NPPV, its use could conceivably contribute to hospital financial losses.

On the other hand, it should be borne in mind that a lack of evidence is not tantamount to a lack of effect. The likelihood that the optimal use of NPPV will improve the efficiency of resource utilization seems overwhelming when the results of the randomized trials are combined. In addition, none of the studies thus far have examined an extremely important component in the decision to choose one ventilator modality over the other, patient preference. In the authors' experience, patients who have experienced both noninvasive and invasive approaches almost invariably prefer noninvasive ventilation.

References

1. Wilson JL. Acute anterior poliomyelitis. N Engl J Med 1932; 206:887–893.
2. Bach JR, Alba AS. Management of chronic alveolar hypoventilation by nasal ventilation. Chest 1990; 97:52–57.
3. Kerby GR, Mayer LS, Pingleton SK. Nocturnal positive pressure ventilation via nasal mask. Am Rev Respir Dis 1987; 135:738–740.
4. Meduri GU, Conoscenti CC, Menashe P, et al. Noninvasive face mask ventilation in patients with acute respiratory failure. Chest 1989; 95:865–870.
5. Bott J, Carroll MP, Conway JH, et al. Randomized controlled trial of nasal ventilation in acute ventilatory failure due to chronic obstructive airways disease. Lancet 1993; 341:1555–1557.
6. Kramer N, Meyer TJ, Meharg J, et al. Randomized, prospective trial of noninvasive positive pressure ventilation in acute respiratory failure. Am J Respir Crit Care Med 1995; 151:1799–1806.
7. Brochard L, Mancebo J, Wysocki M, et al. Noninvasive ventilation for acute exacerbations of chronic obstructive pulmonary disease. N Engl J Med 1995; 333:817–822.
8. Pingleton SK. Complications of acute respiratory failure. Am Rev Respir Dis 1988; 137:1463–1493.
9. Dreyfuss D, Saumon G. Ventilator-induced lung injury. Lessons from experimental studies. Am J Respir Crit Care Med 1998; 157:294–323.
10. Ambrosino N, Foglio K, Rubini F, et al. Noninvasive mechanical ventilation in acute

respiratory failure due to chronic obstructive pulmonary disease: correlates for success. Thorax 1995; 50:755–757.

11. Celikel T, Sungur M, Ceyhan B, Karakurt S. Comparison of noninvasive positive pressure ventilation with standard medical therapy in hypercapnic acute respiratory failure. Chest 1998; 114:1636–1642.

12. Meduri GU, Cook TR, Turner RE, Cohen M, Leeper KV. Noninvasive positive pressure ventilation in status asthmaticus. Chest 1996; 110:767–774.

13. Hodson ME, Madden BP, Steven MH, et al. Noninvasive mechanical ventilation for cystic fibrosis patients—a potential bridge to transplantation. Eur Respir J 1991; 4: 524–527.

14. Meduri GU, Turner RE, Abou-Shala N, Wunderink R, Tolley E. Noninvasive positive pressure ventilation via face mask. Chest 1996; 109:179–193.

15. Piper AJ, Sullivan CE. Effects of short-term NIPPV in the treatment of patients with severe obstructive sleep apnea and hypercapnia. Chest 1994; 105:434–444.

16. Keenan SP, Kernerman PD, Cook DJ, Martin CM, McCormack D, Sibbald WJ. The effect of noninvasive positive pressure ventilation on mortality in patients admitted with acute respiratory failure: a meta-analysis. Crit Care Med 1997; 25:1685–1692.

17. Rasanen J, Vaisanen IT, Heikkila J, et al. Acute myocardial infarction complicated by left ventricular dysfunction and respiratory failure. Chest 1985; 87:158–162.

18. Lin M, Yang Y, Chiany H, Chang M, Chainy BN, Chitlin MD. Reappraisal of continuous positive airway pressure therapy in acute cardiogenic pulmonary edema: short-term results and long-term follow-up. Chest 1995; 107:1379–1386.

19. Bersten AD, Holt AW, Vedig AE, et al. Treatment of severe cardiogenic pulmonary edema with continuous positive airway pressure delivered by face mask. N Engl J Med 1991; 325:1825–1830.

20. Mehta S, Jay GD, Woolard RH, Hipona RA, et al. Randomized prospective trial of bilevel versus continuous positive airway pressure in acute pulmonary edema. Crit Care Med 1997; 25:620–628.

21. Confalonieri M, Potena A, Carbone G, Della Porta R, Tolley EA, Meduri GU. Acute respiratory failure in patients with severe community-acquired pneumonia. Am J Respir Crit Care Med 1999, 160:1585–1591.

22. Antonelli M, Conti G, Bufi M, Costa MG, Lappa A, Rocco M, Gasparetto A, Meduri GU. Noninvasive ventilation for treatment of acute respiratory failure in patients undergoing solid organ transplantation. JAMA 2000; 283:235–241.

23. Rocker GM, Mackensie M-G, Williams B, Logan PM. Noninvasive positive pressure ventilation. Successful outcome in patients with acute lung injury/ARDS. Chest 1999; 115:173–177.

24. Finlay G, Concannon D, McDonell TJ. Treatment of respiratory failure due to kyphoscoliosis with nasal intermittent positive pressure ventilation (NIPPV). Irish J Med Sci 1995; 164:28–30.

25. Bach JR, Ishikawa Y, Kim H. Prevention of pulmonary morbidity for patients with Duchenne muscular dystrophy. Chest 1997; 112:1024–1028.

26. Antonelli M, Conti G, Rocco M, Bufi M, DeBlasi RA, Vivino G, Gasparetto A, Meduri GU. A comparison of noninvasive positive-pressure ventilation and conventional mechanical ventilation in patients with acute respiratory failure. N Engl J Med 1998; 339:429–435.

27. Wysocki M, Laurent T, Wolff MA, et al. Noninvasive pressure support ventilation in patients with acute respiratory failure. A randomized comparison with conventional therapy. Chest 1995; 107:761–768.

28. Martin TJ, Hovis DK, Constantino JP, et al. A randomized, prospective evaluation of noninvasive ventilation for acute respiratory failure. Am J Respir Crit Care Med 2000, 161:807–813.

29. Pennock BE, Kaplan PD, Carlin BW, et al. Pressure support ventilation with a simplified ventilatory support system administered with a nasal mask in patients with respiratory failure. Chest 1991; 100:1371–1376.

30. Pennock BE, Crawshaw L, Kaplan PD. Noninvasive nasal mask ventilation for acute respiratory failure. Chest 1994; 105:441–444.

31. Aguilo R, Togores B, Pons S, Rubi M, Barbe F, Agusti AGN. Noninvasive ventilation support after lung resectional surgery. Chest 1997; 112:117–121.

32. Joris JL, Sottiaux TM, Chiche JD, Desaive CJ, Lamy ML. Effect of bi-level positive airway pressure (BiPAP) nasal ventilation on the postoperative pulmonary restrictive syndrome in obese patients undergoing gastroplasty. Chest 1997; 111:665–670.

33. Gregoretti C, Burbi L, Berardino M, et al. Noninvasive mask ventilation (NIMV) in trauma and major burn patients. Am Rev Respir Dis 1992; 145:A75.

34. Benhamou D, Girault C, Faure C, et al. Nasal mask ventilation in acute respiratory failure. Experience in elderly patients. Chest 1992; 102:912–917.

35. Meduri GU, Fox RC, Abou-Shala N, et al. Noninvasive mechanical ventilation via face mask in patients with acute respiratory failure who refused endotracheal intubation. Crit Care Med 1994; 22:1584–1590.

36. Nava S, Ambrosino N, Clini E, Prato M, Orlando G, et al. Non-invasive mechanical ventilation in the weaning of patients with respiratory failure due to chronic obstructive pulmonary disease: a randomized study. Ann Intern Med 1998; 128:721–728.

37. Girault C, Daudenthun I, Chevron V, Tamion F, Leroy J, Bonmarchand G. Noninvasive ventilation as a systematic extubation and weaning technique in acute-on-chronic respiratory failure. Am J Resir Crit Care Med 1999, 160:86–92.

38. Hilbert G, Gruson D, Portel L, Gbikpi-Benissan G, Cardinaud JP. Noninvasive pressure support ventilation in COPD patients with post-extubation hypercapnic respiratory insufficiency. Eur Respir J 1998; 11:1349–1353.

39. Patrick W, Webster K, Ludwig L, Roberts D, Weibe P, and Younes M. Noninvasive positive pressure ventilation I acute respiratory distress without prior chronic respiratory failure. Am J Respir Crit Care Med 1996; 153:1005–1011.

40. Mehta S, Hill N. Noninvasive ventilation in acute respiratory failure. Respir Care Clin North Am 1996; 2(2):267–292.

41. Girault C, Richard J-C, Chevron V, Tamion F, Pasquis P, Leroy J, Bonmarchand G. Comparative physiologic effects of noninvasive assist-control and pressure support ventilation in acute hypercapnic respiratory failure. Chest 1997; 111:1639–1648.

42. Vitacca M, Rubini F, Foglio K, Scalvini S, Nava S, Ambrosino N. Noninvasive modalities of positive pressure ventilation improved the outcome of acute exacerbations in COLD patients. Intensive Care Med 1993; 19:450–455.

43. Ferguson GT, Gilmartin M. CO_2 rebreathing during BiPAP ventilatory assistance. Am J Respir Crit Care Med 1995; 151:1126–1135.

44. Aubier M, Murciano D, Milic-Emili J, Touaty E, Daghfous J, Pariente R, Derenne

JP. Effects of the administration of O_2 on ventilation and blood gases in patients with chronic obstructive pulmonary disease during acute respiratory failure. Am Rev Respir Dis 1980; 122(5):747–754.

45. Richards GN, Cistulli PA, Ungar G, Berthon-Jones M, Sullivan CE. Mouth leak with nasal continuous positive airway pressure increases nasal airway resistance. Am J Respir Crit Care Med 1996; 154:182–186.

46. Pollack CJ, Fleisch K, Dowsey K. Treatment of acute bronchospasm with beta-adrenergic agonist aerosols delivered by a nasal bilevel positive airway pressure circuit. Ann Emerg Med 1995; 26(5):552–557.

47. Meduri GU, Abou-Shala N, Fox RC, et al. Noninvasive face mask mechanical ventilation in patients with acute hypercapnic respiratory failure. Chest 1991; 100:445–454.

48. Soo Hoo GW, Santiago S, Williams J. Nasal mechanical ventilation for hypercapnic respiratory failure in chronic obstructive pulmonary disease: determinants of success and failure. Crit Care Med 1994; 27:417–434.

49. Plant PK, Owen JL, Elliott MW. Use of noninvasive ventilation (NIV) in acute exacerbations of COPD-subgroup analysis of multicenter randomized controlled trial. Am J Resp Crit Care Med 1999, 159:A15.

50. Sanders MH, Kern NB, Costantino JP, et al. Accuracy of end-tidal and transcutaneous PCO_2 monitoring during sleep. Chest 1994; 106:472–483.

51. Consensus Conference: Clinical indications for noninvasive positive pressure ventilation in chronic respiratory failure due to restrictive lung disease, COPD, and nocturnal hypoventilation—a consensus conference report. Chest 1999; 116:521–534.

52. Hill NS. Complications of noninvasive positive pressure ventilation. Respir Care 1997; 42:432–442.

53. Carrey Z, Gottfried SB, Levy RD. Ventilatory muscle support in respiratory failure with nasal positive pressure ventilation. Chest 1990; 97:150–158.

54. Brown AC, Slocum PC, Puthoof SL, Wallace WE, Foresman BH. Exogenous lipoid pneumonia due to nasal application of petroleum jelly. Chest 1994; 105:968–969.

55. Meduri GU, Abou-Shala N, Fox RC, et al. Noninvasive face mask mechanical ventilation in patients with acute hypercapnic respiratory failure. Chest 1991; 100:445–454.

56. Klopfenstein CE, Forster A, Suter PM. Pneumocephalus: a complication of continuous positive airway pressure after trauma. Chest 1980; 78:656–657.

57. Lofaso F, Brochard L, Touchard D, Hang T, Harf A, Isabey D. Evaluation of carbon dioxide rebreathing during pressure support ventilation with BiPAP devices. Chest 1995; 108:772–778.

58. Luce JM. The cardiovascular effects of mechanical ventilation and positive end-expiratory pressure. JAMA 1984; 252:807–811.

59. Bradley TD, Holloway RM, McLaughlin PR, et al. Cardiac output response to continuous positive airway pressure in congestive heart failure. Am Rev Respir Dis 1992; 145:377–382.

60. Fewell JE, Abendschein DR, Carslon CJ, et al. Continuous positive-pressure ventilation decreases right and left ventricular end-diastolic volumes in the dog. Circ Res 1980; 46:125–132.

61. Johnston EW, Vinten-Johansen J, Santamore WP, et al. Mechanism of reduced car-

diac output during positive end expiratory pressure in the dog. Am Rev Respir Dis 1989; 140:1257–1264.

62. Barbe F, Togores B, Rubi M, Pons S, Maimo A, Agusti AGN. Noninvasive ventilatory support does not facilitate recovery from acute respiratory failure in chronic obstructive pulmonary disease. Eur Respir 1996; 9:1240–1245.

63. Nourdine K, Combes P, Carton MJ, Beuret P, Cannamela, Ducreux JC. Does noninvasive ventilation reduce the ICU nosocomial infection risk? A prospective clinical survey. Intensive Care Med 1999; 25:567–573.

64. Wood KA, Lewis L, Von Harz B, Kollef MH. The use of noninvasive positive pressure ventilation in the emergency department. Chest 1998; 113:1339–1346.

65. Vitacca M, Clini E, Rubini F, Nava S, Foglio K, Ambrosino N. Non-invasive mechanical ventilation in severe chronic obstructive lung disease and acute respiratory falure: Short and long-term prognosis. Intensive Care Med 1996; 22:94–100.

66. Nava S, Evangesliti I, Rampulla C, Campagnoni ML, et al. Human and financial costs of noninvasive mechanical ventilation in patients affected by COPD and acute respiratory failure. Chest 1997; 111:1631–1638.

67. Criner GJ, Kreimer DT, Tomaselli M, Pierson W, Evans D. Financial implications of noninvasive positive pressure ventilation (NPPV). Chest 1995; 108:475–481.

68. Chevrolet JC, Jolliet P, Abajo B, et al. Nasal positive pressure ventilation in patients with acute respiratory failure. Chest 1991; 100:775–782.

7

New Modes of Ventilation

DEAN HESS

Harvard Medical School
and Massachusetts General Hospital
Boston, Massachusetts

RICHARD D. BRANSON

University of Cincinnati
Cincinnati, Ohio

I. Introduction

Breath delivery during mechanical ventilation is described by the trigger, control, limit, cycle, and conditional variables (1). The trigger initiates a breath. The control variable remains constant throughout inspiration regardless of changes in respiratory system impedance. The limit variable is held constant throughout inspiration and is often the same as the control variable. Inspiration ends when the cycle is reached. The conditional variable results in a change in output by the ventilator such as synchronized intermittent mandatory ventilation (SIMV), in which the ventilator delivers the mandatory breath in synchrony with the patient's inspiratory effort or automatically if the patient is apneic. The relationship between the various possible breath types and conditional variables is the mode of ventilation (2). Practically speaking, ventilator modes are either pressure or volume controlled. A mode can include pressure and volume controlled breaths and even be sophisticated enough to switch from one control variable to the other.

With each generation of ventilators, new modes and variations on previous modes become available. There now exist numerous ventilator modes from a variety of manufacturers. The purpose of this chapter is to describe the technical aspects of new modes of ventilation, most of which have become available within the past 10 years. In addition, relevant studies related to these modes are reviewed. Modes such as assist/control and SIMV will not be discussed since most clinicians are familiar with these.

II. The Ventilator Trigger

A breath is triggered either by the ventilator or by the patient. A breath initiated by the ventilator is time-triggered and based on the set respiratory frequency. A second form of ventilator-triggered breath occurs when the clinician activates a manual breath from the ventilator control panel. Patient triggering of the ventilator is usually pressure- or flow-triggered, but theoretically any signal can be used as a trigger variable.

A. Pressure Triggering

Pressure triggering requires sufficient patient inspiratory effort to cause airway pressure to fall from the set end-expiratory level to a threshold level (sensitivity) set by the clinician (Fig. 1). Sensitivity is expressed in cm H_2O and preceded by

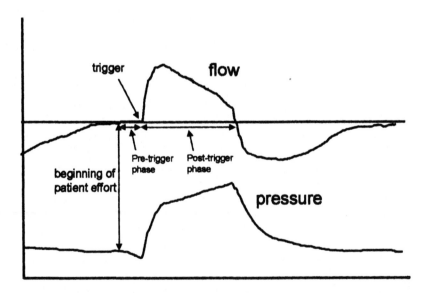

Figure 1 Pressure triggering. Note that there is no flow to the patient during the pretrigger phase. The decrease in pressure below baseline represents the patient's inspiratory effort, which triggers the ventilator when the pressure sensitivity is reached.

a negative sign. The smaller the absolute value, the easier the ventilator is to trigger. Sensitivity settings from -0.5 to -2.0 cm H_2O are used safely and effectively in most situations. More sensitive settings may result in auto-triggering due to signal noise such as leaks, patient movement, and water in the ventilator circuit. The inspiratory and expiratory valves must be closed during pressure-triggering. Closure of the expiratory valve requires patient effort to move it to the closed position. This may explain the effect of expiratory valve resistance on the inspiratory work-of-breathing (3). This may also represent one of the advantages of flow triggering, where both the inspiratory and expiratory valves remain open during triggering.

Sassoon and Gruer (4,5) described pressure triggering in detail. During the pretrigger phase, the patient generates effort prior to ventilator response. If prolonged, this delay may produce patient/ventilator dyssynchrony. Factors responsible for this delay include errors due to the speed of the pressure signal, errors due to the frequency response of the pressure transducer, errors in the pressure transducer, errors due to differences in set and actual positive end-expiratory pressure (PEEP), errors due to circuit noise, and position of the pressure transducer in the ventilator circuit. This initial delay is typically <150 ms and represents only a small amount of the work-of-breathing imposed during triggering.

Once a breath is triggered, the ventilator delivers flow and attempts to maintain pressure (the limit variable) in the ventilator circuit until the breath cycles. This portion of the breath delivery, the posttrigger phase, is more important in determining the work-of-breathing than the pretrigger phase. For volume-controlled, pressure-controlled, or pressure-supported breaths, gas flow in the posttrigger phase is dictated by the ventilator settings for these breath types. The algorithm used by the ventilator during pressure-triggered spontaneous breaths (i.e., CPAP mode without pressure support) can be pressure-limited and pressure or flow cycled. For the Nellcor-Puritan-Bennett 7200, gas delivery is triggered when the patient's inspiratory effort is sufficient to reduce airway pressure to the sensitivity setting, the limit variable (i.e., what the ventilator targets during inspiration) is the end-expiratory pressure level minus the sensitivity setting, and the breath is cycled when airway pressure exceeds the end-expiratory pressure by 1 cm H_2O (6). In contrast, the Hamilton Veolar uses different limit and cycle variables for pressure-triggered spontaneous breaths. After the sensitivity threshold has been exceeded, the limit variable is 1.5 cm H_2O above the end-expiratory pressure and the breath is flow-cycled. In fact, the Veolar treats each spontaneous breath like a pressure-supported breath. Comparing the Nellcor-Puritan-Bennett 7200 and the Hamilton Veolar during pressure triggering with a sensitivity of -2 cm H_2O, one ventilator provides 3.5 cm H_2O more pressure than the other during inspiration. Additionally, the breaths are cycled differently, which may also affect patient/ventilator synchrony.

B. Flow Triggering

With flow triggering, breath initiation is based on a flow change in the ventilator circuit beyond some predetermined threshold (Fig. 2). The operational characteristics of flow-triggering systems differ among ventilators. Additionally, the site of flow measurement and accuracy of the flow transducer are important determinants of successful operation (6).

Ventilators that incorporate flow triggering use one of three methods. The first measures a change in flow caused by the patient's inspiratory effort. The second provides a preset, nonadjustable continuous flow through the circuit, from which a change in flow (the flow sensitivity) is detected. The third allows the clinician to set the continuous flow and the flow sensitivity. In this case, a change in flow through the circuit caused by the patient's inspiratory effort reduces the flow below the flow sensitivity setting and a breath is triggered.

The limit and cycle variables with flow triggering may be different from pressure triggering for a spontaneous breath (i.e., during CPAP without pressure support). Once the flow triggered breath is initiated with the Nellcor-Puritan-Bennett 7200, the ventilator maintains airway pressure 1.0 cm H_2O above the end-expiratory pressure and the breath is cycled when flow through the expiratory

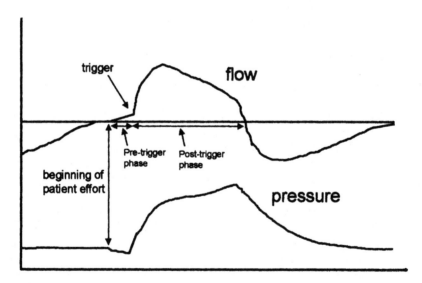

Figure 2 Flow triggering. Note that there is flow to the patient during the pretrigger phase. The increase in flow above baseline represents the patient's inspiratory effort, which triggers the ventilator when the flow sensitivity is reached.

flow transducer is 2 L/min greater than the base flow. With the Hamilton Veolar ventilator, the limit and cycle variables for pressure and flow triggering are identical, but with flow triggering the flow sensor is at the airway whereas the pressure sensor is inside the inspiratory side of the ventilator with pressure triggering (7). The Siemens 300 ventilator uses continuous flows of 2, 1, and 0.5 L/min during flow triggering during adult, pediatric, and neonatal operation, respectively. The sites of pressure and flow measurements are located on the expiratory side of the ventilator. The limit variable in the Siemens 300 with pressure and flow triggering is PEEP + 2 cm H_2O (8).

Potential problems with flow triggering include auto-triggering resulting from system leaks or the presence of water in the ventilator circuit (which can cause auto triggering or failure to trigger). Devices that measure flow at the airway opening eliminate problems associated with circuit condensate. Flow-triggering systems with an adjustable continuous flow can be used to compensate for leaks. In systems with a constant continuous flow, particularly at low levels, leaks may preclude the system from triggering appropriately. Potential advantages of flow triggering include the ability to minimize the effort needed to trigger by leaving both the inspiratory and expiratory valves in the open position during triggering, providing continuous flow to meet the patient's initial demand for flow, and detecting changes in flow more rapidly than changes in pressure can be detected (4).

C. Continuous Flow and Pressure Triggering

Several manufacturers use a continuous flow with pressure triggering. The continuous flow is adjustable from 1 to 30 L/min, and triggering occurs when the pressure sensitivity threshold is reached. The goal of these systems is to provide gas flow for the patient prior to triggering and to compensate for leaks. However, the patient demand for flow must exceed the continuous flow to produce a pressure change in the circuit, close the expiratory valve, and create a negative pressure relative to end-expiratory pressure. In a lung model study, Konyukov et al. (9) compared the effects of increasing continuous flow on the time delay and work to pressure trigger the ventilator in the pressure support mode and found that the work to trigger the ventilator increased as continuous flow was increased. Gurevitch and Gelmont (10) reported patient/ventilator dyssynchrony in an elderly patient with chronic obstructive pulmonary disease (COPD), which was attributed to a continuous flow of 5 L/min in a pressure-triggered ventilator. In a bench model of pressure support ventilation, Holbrook and Guiles (11) compared flow triggering with the Nellcor-Puritan-Bennett 7200ae and Siemens 300 ventilators to a pressure triggered ventilator using a continuous bias flow (Newport E200). They reported no advantage of flow triggering over pressure triggering when the combination of a continuous bias flow, an adjustable sensitivity control, and proximal airway pressure monitoring were used (i.e., with the Newport E200).

D. Pressure Versus Flow Triggering

Sassoon et al. (4,5,12–14) extensively compared pressure and flow triggering with the Nellcor-Puritan-Bennett 7200. In a lung model study, they reported that the response time during flow triggering was shorter than pressure triggering (75 vs. 115 ms), which was attributed to the initial flow meeting patient inspiratory demand and the open position of the expiratory valve (12). However, this does not adequately explain the significant reductions in the work-of-breathing observed in patients during flow versus pressure triggering. This decrease in work-of-breathing can be explained by the differences in limit and cycle variables between pressure and flow triggering with the Nellcor-Puritan-Bennett 7200, producing a small reduction in the response time and several centimeters of pressure support with flow triggering. Sassoon et al. confirmed this by demonstrating that the addition of 5 cm H_2O pressure support during pressure triggering eliminated differences in patient work from flow triggering.

There have been many evaluations of flow-triggered ventilation during spontaneous breathing with continuous positive airway pressure (CPAP). Branson et al. (7) compared pressure and flow triggering with the Nellcor-Puritan-Bennett 7200 and the Hamilton Veolar and found that flow triggering reduced the work-of-breathing during continuous positive airway pressure (CPAP). Saito and colleagues (15) reported similar findings. Compared to pressure triggering, Polese et al. (16) reported a reduction in work-of-breathing when flow triggering was used during spontaneous breathing trials with CPAP. Jager et al. (17), however, found no significant differences in the work-of-breathing or pressure time product between pressure and flow triggering with the Nellcor-Puritan-Bennett 7200.

Heulitt et al. (18) and Carmack et al. (8) compared pressure and flow triggering of the Siemens Servo 300 in a small animal model (e.g., simulating pediatrics) and reported that the flow and pressure triggering capabilities of the Servo 300 were superior to the pressure triggering of the Siemens 900C. They suggested that flow triggering compensates for the work-of-breathing secondary to small endotracheal tubes, which is supported by similar findings of Nishimura et al. (19,20) and El-Khatib et al. (21). The finding of improved triggering with the Servo 300 compared with the Servo 900C is consistent with the findings of others (22).

Giuliani et al. (23) reported improved patient-ventilator synchrony and reduced pressure time product during both spontaneous and mandatory breaths with flow triggering in SIMV mode. In a lung model study using the Servo 300 with pressure support ventilation, Konyukov et al. (24) reported comparable triggering capabilities with pressure and flow triggering. Tutuncu et al. (25) using the Servo 300, and Goulet et al. (26) using the Nellcor-Puritan-Bennett 7200, reported similar patient responses with flow and pressure triggering using pressure support ventilation. Aslanian et al. (27) reported a modest benefit of flow triggering with pressure support ventilation but suggested that this benefit may be too small to affect clinical outcomes. More importantly, they found that the pressure triggers of current generation ventilators are much superior to that available in older ventilators. Although Bunburaphog et al. (28) reported significant differences in the trigger performance of portable pressure ventilators designed for noninvasive ventilation, the clinical implications of this are unclear.

In patients with expiratory airflow obstruction due to dynamic airway closure, the presence of auto-PEEP is a significant impediment to triggering. In order to trigger the ventilator, the patient's effort must first overcome auto-PEEP before a pressure (or flow) change will occur at the proximal airway to trigger the ventilator (Fig. 3). In these patients, the work-of-breathing to overcome auto-PEEP is much greater than the work to trigger the ventilator. The addition of PEEP may counterbalance the auto-PEEP and improve the patient's ability to trigger (29,30). Several studies (23,31,32) reported advantages of flow triggering in patients with auto-PEEP. This is likely due to the effect of the base flow, which causes a small increase in airway pressure due to resistance through the expiratory limb of the ventilation circuit. This increase in expiratory airway pressure counterbalances airway pressure and improves triggering.

From the available evidence, the following recommendations can be made. Flow triggering is superior to pressure triggering during CPAP. Therefore, spon-

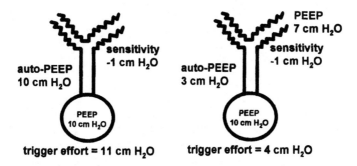

Figure 3 The effect of auto-PEEP on trigger effort. With an auto-PEEP of 10 cm H_2O, the patient must generate an inspiratory effort of 11 cm H_2O to trigger the ventilator. Adding PEEP of 7 cm H_2O counterbalances the auto-PEEP, so only 4 cm H_2O of inspiratory effort is required to trigger. PEEP to counterbalance auto-PEEP may be useful to facilitate triggering in patients with dynamic airway closure (e.g., COPD).

taneous breathing trials with CPAP should be performed using flow triggering. During pressure support, there is not clear superiority of flow triggering and pressure triggering. The choice of trigger type during pressure support should be based on patient response, using the trigger type that produces the best patient comfort. In patients with expiratory flow obstruction and auto-PEEP, flow triggering may partially counterbalance the auto-PEEP and improve triggering. Regardless of whether pressure or flow triggering is chosen, the trigger sensitivity should be set to the most sensitive level that does not produce auto-cycling.

E. Volume Triggering

Volume triggering uses the integral of the flow signal for triggering. Because this is, in essence, an averaging of the flow signal over time, signal noise is reduced. This provides a theoretical advantage of volume triggering over flow triggering. Volume triggering is available on the Respironics Vision, Respironics S/T-D 30, and the Drager Babylog. The Babylog uses an anemometer at the proximal airway and has been shown to provide an adequate trigger response in a lung model (20).

F. Auto-Trak Sensitivity

Auto-Trak is used on the Respironics Vision and S/T-D 30 ventilators. A shape signal is produced by offsetting the actual patient flow signal by 15 L/min and delaying it by 300 ms. This intentional delay causes the ventilator-generated shape signal to be slightly behind the patient's flow rate (Fig. 4). A sudden change

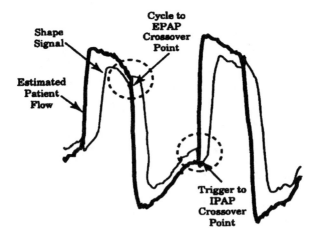

Figure 4 The shape signal used by Respironics Vision for triggering and cycling the ventilator. (Courtesy of Respironics.)

in patient flow will cross the shape signal, causing the ventilator to trigger to the inspiratory phase or cycle to the expiratory phase. No evaluations of this have been reported.

G. Tracheal Pressure Triggering

Tracheal triggering has been explored as a method to bypass the imposed resistance of the endotracheal tube. Banner et al. (33–36) compared pressure triggering, flow triggering, and tracheal pressure triggering in a lung model using a Nellcor-Puritan-Bennett 7200. They disconnected the pressure transducer from the expiratory side of the ventilator and connected it to a catheter with its tip at the distal endotracheal tube. They reported that the imposed work-of-breathing during tracheal pressure triggering was reduced by 300% compared to flow triggering and 382% compared to pressure triggering. A major concern with this work is related to the term pressure triggering. While the system described triggers from a tracheal pressure signal, it also controls the limit and cycle variables from the tracheal pressure signal. The limit variable during pressure triggering is the PEEP minus sensitivity with the Nellcor-Puritan-Bennett 7200. During conventional triggering, the proximal airway pressure will be 3 cm H_2O during the inspiratory phase at a PEEP of 5 cm H_2O and sensitivity of -2 cm H_2O. If the pressure signal is measured on the distal end of the endotracheal tube, a pressure of 3 cm H_2O will be maintained in the trachea during the inspiratory phase. With an 8.0 mm endotracheal tube, this produces a proximal airway pressure of 7–10 cm H_2O (depending on inspiratory flow). The major difference with this method is not the trigger but control of airway pressure at the distal endotracheal tube, resulting in the delivery of pressure support. As such, this technique should be called tracheal pressure control, unless the trigger signal is used solely to activate inspiration (37,38).

Messinger et al. (39) compared tracheal pressure control to pressure and flow triggering in patients with acute respiratory failure and found that tracheal pressure triggering resulted in a significant reduction in the work-of-breathing because it created an effect similar to pressure support ventilation. Bhatt et al. (40) compared tracheal pressure control to an equivalent level of pressure support ventilation in the proximal airway with conventional triggering. They found that tracheal pressure control reduced the initial pressure drop seen at the start of inspiration, but the differences in imposed work-of-breathing between the techniques was very small.

The use of tracheal pressure control has several limitations. The first is related to obtaining the signal. This could be accomplished by use of a special endotracheal tube with a pressure monitoring lumen imbedded in the tube wall. This may require reintubation of patients. Alternatively, a catheter could be inserted into the endotracheal tube. The possibility of catheter kinking or contamination would require a redundant conventional pressure triggering system and alarms. Purging the catheter with a continuous or intermittent flow might be required. The presence of a catheter in the airway would increase flow resistance of the tube and interfere with suctioning. None of these problems is insurmountable, but the cost of tracheal pressure control needs to be balanced carefully against the benefit, particularly in light of alternative methods of overcoming endotracheal tube resistance.

H. Esophageal Pressure Triggering

When lung mechanics are abnormal, transmission of the inspiratory signal to the ventilator may be delayed. This is particularly an issue when auto-PEEP is present. Under such conditions, pleural or esophageal pressure triggering may be advantageous. Using a lung model and PSV, Takahashi et al. (41) reported the value of pleural pressure triggering. Barnard et al. (42) demonstrated the feasibility of esophageal pressure triggering in normal volunteers. However, neither pleural triggering nor esophageal triggering has been reported in mechanically ventilated patients. Despite the attractiveness of this approach, it has several limitations. First, it requires an invasive procedure. Second, esophageal pressure is subject to artifacts, such as cardiac oscillations and peristaltic contractions, which could complicate this approach.

I. Respiratory Impedance Triggering

Because of the difficulties associated with measuring respiratory efforts in neonates and the small endotracheal tubes required, alternative triggers have been explored. With the Sechrist SAVI, the ventilator is triggered by a respiratory impedance signal. Standard ECG electrodes are used and as the chest wall expands, the change in impedance initiates inspiration. Once inspiratory effort is detected, the control of ventilator limit and cycling variable returns to airway pressure. This method of triggering is not commonly used, and its effectiveness is unclear.

J. Motion Triggering

Infrasonics (Nellcor-Puritan-Bennett, Carlsbad, CA) uses a motion sensor for triggering the neonatal ventilator. This device (Star Sync) utilizes an abdominal sensor to detect inspiration. The sensor is a small, air-filled balloon enclosed in a capsule, which is taped to the infant's abdomen midway between the umbilicus and the xiphoid. As the abdomen rises, the change in balloon pressure triggers the ventilator. Pressure in the sensor is sampled 8 times every 5 ms, and the response time from the onset of patient effort to breath delivery is 47 ms. From a technical standpoint, this is pressure-triggered ventilation. Nikischin et al. (43)

also attempted motion triggering from abdominal and chest wall signals in neonates. Chest wall motion was measured using impedance monitoring, and tidal volume was measured using a hot wire anemometer at the endotracheal tube. They found that abdominal inductance monitoring had the shortest signal delay (triggering actually occurred prior to airflow being measured) and shortest trigger delay. Volume triggering was comparable to abdominal triggering, and both were superior to impedance triggering. There were few failed triggers with any of the techniques, but the percentage of auto-triggered breaths was significantly greater with chest wall impedance compared to volume or abdominal inductance. These findings suggest that volume and abdominal movement signals are reliable signals for patient-triggered ventilation in neonates, while chest wall impedance triggering was slower and less reliable.

K. Triggering from Diaphragmatic Electromyographic Activity

Diaphragmatic activation can occur with no change in diaphragm pressure generation (44–46). This has been shown to occur in patients with COPD and those with prior polio infection (46). In this case, inspiratory efforts may not trigger the ventilator using pressure or flow monitoring at the proximal airway. One solution may be to couple the ventilator trigger to diaphragm electromyographic activity. However, this approach is investigational at the present time and its clinical usefulness remains to be determined.

III. Pressure Ventilation

Traditionally, positive pressure ventilation of adults has been volume-controlled. In contrast, positive pressure ventilation of neonates is achieved using pressure-limited ventilation. In recent years, however, there has been increasing interest in the use of pressure-limited ventilation in adults. There are two principal advantages of pressure-limited ventilation over volume-limited ventilation. First, pressure ventilation limits the pressure applied to the airway and thus may prevent overdistension injury in patients with acute lung injury. Second, unlike volume-controlled ventilation, in which inspiratory flow is fixed, inspiratory flow is variable with pressure-controlled ventilation. This variable inspiratory flow may improve patient-ventilatory synchrony for patients assisting the ventilator. The limitation of pressure ventilation is that tidal volume and minute ventilation vary, which may be a problem in patients sensitive to hypercarbia (e.g., head-injured patients).

A. Pressure-Controlled Ventilation

Pressure-controlled ventilation (PCV) is either patient or ventilator triggered and time cycled. During PCV, inspiratory flow is determined by the pressure applied to the airway (i.e., the pressure control setting), airways resistance, and the time constant (Fig. 5) (47,48):

$$\dot{V} = (\Delta P/R) \cdot (e^{-t/\tau})$$

where ΔP is the pressure applied to the airway above PEEP, R is airways resistance, t is the elapsed time after initiation of the inspiratory phase, e is the base of the natural logarithm, and τ is the product of airways resistance and respiratory system compliance (the time constant of the respiratory system). The area of the flow-time curve (Fig. 5) is the delivered tidal volume. Thus, tidal volume during PCV is determined primarily by the pressure control setting, airways resistance, respiratory system compliance, and inspiratory time. Note, however, that the inspiratory time will not affect the delivered tidal volume if the flow has decelerated to zero. The delivered tidal volume will also be affected during PCV by auto-PEEP. An increase in auto-PEEP effectively decreases the driving pressure and thus the tidal volume decreases. Active inspiratory efforts increase ΔP and thus increase tidal volume during pressure-limited ventilation.

With PCV, flow decelerates exponentially during the inspiratory phase. Compared with constant-flow (square wave) volume ventilation, the end-inspiratory flow is lower with PCV. Therefore, the peak inspiratory pressure (PIP)

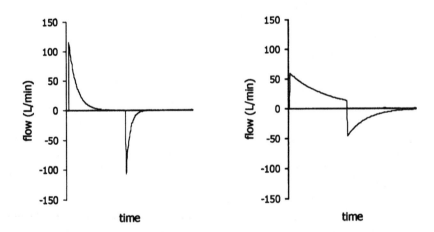

Figure 5 During pressure-controlled ventilation, the inspiratory flow pattern is determined by airways resistance and respiratory system compliance. (Left) Airways resistance of 10 cm $H_2O/L/s$ and respiratory system compliance of 20 mL/cm H_2O. The inspiratory time is 1.5 s and the resulting tidal volume (the area under the flow curve) is 400 mL. (Right) Airways resistance of 20 cm $H_2O/L/s$ and respiratory system compliance of 50 mL/cm H_2O. The inspiratory time is 1.5 s and the resulting tidal volume (the area under the flow curve) is 775 mL.

is lower with PCV. If the flow decelerates to zero during PCV, PIP will equal the peak alveolar pressure. A longer inspiratory time will be required with PCV to deliver the same tidal volume due to the decelerating flow, and thus the mean airway pressure is increased. The increased mean airway pressure and lower end-inspiratory flow may improve arterial oxygenation in some patients. The beneficial effects of PCV on PIP and oxygenation appear to be due to the inspiratory flow pattern rather than PCV per se. In fact, several groups reported similar findings with PCV and volume-controlled ventilation (VCV) with a decelerating flow waveform (49–51). The decelerating flow waveform during VCV is different than that during PCV in several ways. First, the flow decelerates linearly with the VCV decelerating waveform (unlike the exponential flow decrease with PCV). Second, the flow may decelerate to zero with PCV, whereas it decelerates to a ventilator-preset flow with the decelerating waveform and VCV (e.g., 5 L/min end-inspiratory flow with the decelerating waveform during VCV with the Nellcor-Puritan-Bennett 7200).

Unlike VCV with a decelerating flow waveform, peak alveolar pressure is limited with PCV. This may be beneficial as a lung protection strategy to avoid alveolar overdistension. Uncontrolled (52) and controlled (53) studies suggest a mortality benefit when PCV is used to prevent overdistension lung injury in patients with ARDS. With PCV, no alveolus can receive a pressure greater than the pressure set on the ventilator. Rappaport et al. (54) conducted a prospective randomized trial of PCV versus VCV in severe respiratory failure and reported that PCV was well tolerated as an initial mode of ventilation, was associated with a sustained reduction in PIP, and was associated with a more rapid improvement in respiratory system compliance.

That inspiratory workload with assisted VCV can be substantial has long been appreciated (55,56). With VCV, the flow from the ventilator is fixed. However, inspiratory flow with PCV is variable because the ventilator will vary its flow output to maintain a constant airway pressure. Several studies suggest that PCV may be superior to VCV during assisted ventilation (57,58). MacIntyre et al. (58) reported that the variable flow with PCV reduced patient effort and patient-ventilator dyssynchrony during assisted ventilation (Fig. 6).

B. Pressure-Controlled Inverse-Ratio Ventilation

The early reports (59–62) of improved oxygenation with pressure-controlled inverse-ratio ventilation (PCIRV) generated considerable enthusiasm for this method. The basic approach is to use an inspiratory time greater than the expiratory time to increase mean airway pressure and improve arterial oxygenation. PCV is often used with inverse ratio ventilation to limit inspiratory pressure, although VCV with inverse ratio has also been described (63–65). Following the initial enthusiasm for this ventilatory approach, a number of subsequent con-

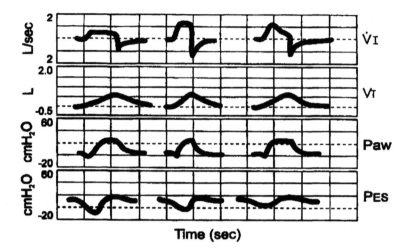

Figure 6 Ventilator flow, tidal volume, airway pressure, and esophageal pressure for a patient receiving constant flow volume ventilation at 30 L/min (left), constant flow volume ventilation at 75 L/min (center), and pressure control at 22 cm H₂O (right). Note the lower patient effort (PES) and improved synchrony with pressure control ventilation. (From Ref. 58.)

trolled studies reported no benefit or marginal benefit of PCIRV over more conventional approaches to ventilatory support of patients with ARDS (66–72). Although PCIRV can be applied without producing auto-PEEP (73), auto-PEEP commonly occurs with PCIRV (74). Due to the heterogeneous nature of the lungs with ARDS, auto-PEEP occurring with PCIRV may be distributed in the lungs in an inhomogeneous manner (75). The elevated mean airway pressure that occurs with PCIRV may also adversely affect hemodynamics.

Based on the available evidence, there seems to be no clear role for PCIRV in the management of patients with ARDS. The oxygenation of some patients may benefit from the use of a longer inspiratory time to increase mean airway pressure. However, the target variable should be the inspiratory time and not the I:E ratio per se. The likelihood of an improvement in oxygenation using inverse ratio ventilation is small, and the risk of auto-PEEP and hemodynamic compromise is great. Lung recruitment maneuvers followed by PEEP sufficient to maintain recruitment might be a better approach to improving mean airway pressure and arterial oxygenation in these patients (76).

C. Pressure Support Ventilation

Pressure support ventilation (PSV) has been shown to effectively assist respiratory muscles during invasive (77,78) and noninvasive ventilation (79). PSV is patient triggered and primarily flow cycled. Secondary cycling mechanisms with PSV are pressure and time. In other words, PSV will cycle to the expiratory phase when the flow decelerates to a ventilator-determined level, when the pressure rises to a ventilator-determined level, or the inspiratory time reaches a ventilator-determined limit. Although PSV is often considered a simple mode of ventilation (80–83), in reality it can be quite complex (Fig. 7). First, the ventilator must recognize the patient's inspiratory effort, which depends on the trigger sensitivity of the ventilator. Second, the ventilator must deliver an appropriate flow at the onset of inspiration. A flow that is too high can produce a pressure overshoot, whereas a flow that is too low can produce patient flow starvation and dyssynchrony. Third, the ventilator must appropriately cycle to the expiratory phase without the need for active exhalation by the patient.

Like PCV, flow deceleration during PSV is largely a function of the resistance and compliance of the respiratory system (Fig. 5). The flow at which the ventilator cycles can be either a fixed absolute flow, a flow based on the peak inspiratory flow, or a flow based on peak inspiratory flow and elapsed inspiratory time (Table 1). In some cases, the cycle is quite sophisticated. With the Respironics Vision ventilator, for example, inspiration cycles to the expiratory phase

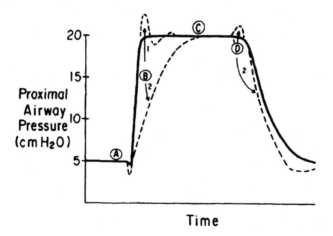

Figure 7 A pressure support breath with 5 cm H_2O PEEP and 15 cm H_2O pressure support. The breath is triggered at A. The rise in pressure (B) may be very rapid (B1), producing a pressure overshoot and ringing in the system, or the rise in pressure may be very slow (B2), which may not satisfy the patient's initial inspiratory flow requirement. There is a pressure plateau (C) at the pressure support plus PEEP level. Termination of the patient's inspiratory effort occurs at D. If termination is delayed, the patient will actively exhale (D1). If termination is premature, the patient will continue to have inspiratory effort. (From Ref. 82.)

Table 1 Cycle Criteria for Commonly Used Critical Care Ventilators

Ventilator	Flow cycle	Pressure cycle	Time cycle
Nellcor-Puritan-Bennett 7200	5 L/min	Set pressure + 1.5 cm H_2O	5 seconds
Nellcor-Puritan-Bennett 840	Variable (1–45% of peak expiratory flow), 10% default setting	Set pressure + 1.5 cm H_2O	Minimum 2 seconds; variable based upon patient size
Nellcor-Puritan-Bennett 740	10 L/min or 25% of peak flow	Set pressure + 3 cm H_2O	3.5 seconds for adults and 2.5 seconds for pediatrics
Servo 900C	25% of peak flow	Set pressure + 3.0 cm H_2O	80% of set cycle time
Servo 300	5% of peak flow	Set pressure + 20 cm H_2O	80% of set cycle time
Drager Evita 4	25% of peak flow in adult mode; 6% of peak flow in pediatric mode		4 seconds in adult mode and 1.5 seconds in pediatric mode
Bear 1000	25% of peak flow	High pressure limit	5 seconds
Hamilton Veolar	25% of peak flow	High pressure limit	3 seconds
Hamilton Galileo	Variable, 10–40% of peak inspiratory flow		3 seconds
Infrasonics Star	4 L/min	Set pressure + 3.0 cm H_2O	3.5 seconds
Bird 8400 and TBird	25% of peak flow		3 seconds
Pulmonetics LTV	Variable, 10–40% of peak inspiratory flow		Variable, 1–3 seconds
Newport Wave	Variable, based on peak flow and elapsed time	Set pressure + 2.0 cm H_2O	3 seconds

either due to the shape signal, due to an expiratory threshold based on inspiratory time and flow, or when an inspiratory time of three seconds is reached.

Several studies have reported dyssynchrony with PSV in subjects having airflow obstruction (e.g., COPD) (84–89). With airflow obstruction, the inspiratory flow decelerates slowly during PSV, the flow necessary to cycle may not be reached, and this stimulates active exhalation to pressure cycle the breath (Fig. 8 and 9). This problem increases with higher levels of PSV and with higher levels of airflow obstruction. Two approaches can be used to solve this problem. PCV can be used, with the inspiratory time set short enough so that the patient does not contract the expiratory muscles to terminate inspiration (e.g., 0.8–1.2 s). The inspiratory time is adjusted by observing patient comfort and avoiding a period of zero flow at the end of inspiration (which can be observed from flow graphics) (Fig. 6). A second approach, available on newer generation ventilators, allows the clinician to adjust the termination flow at which the ventilator cycles (Table 1). Using this approach, the termination flow can be adjusted to a level appropriate for the patient (90,91).

The flow at the onset of the inspiratory phase may also be important during PSV (90,92–94). This is called rise time and refers to the time required for the ventilator to reach the PSV level at the onset of inspiration. Flows that are either

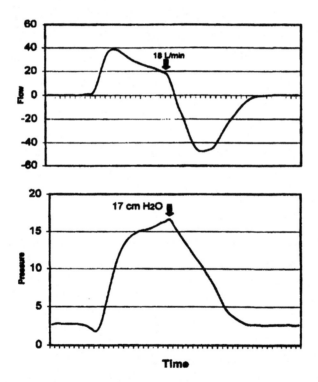

Figure 8 An example of delayed termination of the inspiratory phase with pressure support ventilation and the Puritan-Bennett 7200. Pressure exceeds the preset pressure by >1.5 cm H_2O at a flow of 18 L/min rather than 5 L/min. (From Ref. 83.)

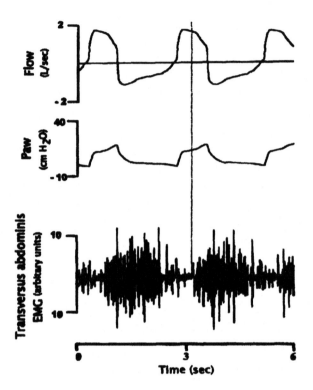

Figure 9 Flow, airway pressure (Paw), and transversus abdominis EMG in a critically ill patient with COPD receiving pressure support ventilation at 20 cm H$_2$O. The onset of expiratory muscle activity (vertical dotted line) occurred when mechanical inflation was only partly completed. (From Ref. 86.)

too high or too low at the onset of inspiration can produce dyssynchrony. Several of the newer generation of ventilators allow adjustment of the rise time during PSV (Table 2). The rise time should be adjusted to patient comfort and ventilator graphics may be useful to guide this setting (Fig. 10). With the Servo 900C ventilator, the rise time is determined by the setting of the working pressure on the ventilation. It has been shown that setting the working pressure too high produces an excessive flow at the onset of inspiration, a pressure overshoot, ringing in the ventilator circuit, and reduced inspiratory time and tidal volume (95).

Bonmarchand et al. (96) compared four rise times during pressure support ventilation (Drager Evita ventilator) in intubated patients with restrictive lung disease. They reported the lowest work of breathing with the fastest rise time (i.e., the one that reached the set level of pressure support in 0.1 s compared to 0.5, 1, and 1.5 s), which was associated with highest flow at the onset of inspiration. A

Table 2 Critical Care Ventilators with Adjustable Rise Time During PSV

Bear 1000 (pressure slope): variable from -9 to $+9$, where -9 produces the slowest rise in pressure and $+9$ produces the fastest rise in pressure
Hamilton Galileo (pressure ramp): pressure rise time adjustable from 50 to 200 ms
Nellcor-Puritan-Bennett 840 (flow acceleration): the greater the flow acceleration setting, the more rapid the rise in inspiratory pressure
Drager Evita 4: pressure rise time is adjustable from 64 ms to 2 s
Pulmonetics LTV: variable on a scale of 1 to 9, where 1 is the fastest and 9 is the slowest

high inspiratory flow at the onset of inspiration, however, may not be beneficial (97). First, if the flow is higher at the onset of inspiration, the inspiratory phase may be prematurely terminated if the ventilator cycles to the expiratory phase at a flow that is a fraction of the peak inspiratory flow. Second, several studies have demonstrated the existence of a powerful, graded, flow-related inspiratory terminating reflex (98–102). The result of activation of this reflex is a shortening of neural inspiration, which could result in brief, shallow inspiratory efforts (particularly at low pressure support settings). The clinical effects of this inspiratory flow-terminating reflex remain to be determined. At the least, it suggests that manipulation of rise time during pressure support may result in a complex interaction between ventilator function and physiology (97).

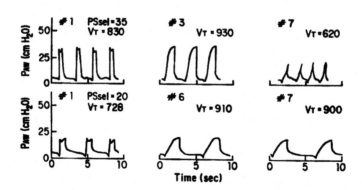

Figure 10 Examples of airway pressure waveforms from two patients with different rise times during pressure support ventilation. The maximal rise time is #1 and the minimal rise time is #7. Note that the optimal rise time for the first patient (top) is at a high setting, whereas the optimal rise time for the second patient (bottom) is at a slow setting. (From Ref. 90.)

Another issue with PSV is the presence of leaks in the system (e.g., bronchopleural fistula, cuffless airway, mask leak with noninvasive ventilation). If the leak exceeds the termination flow at which the ventilator cycles, either active exhalation will occur to terminate inspiration or a prolonged inspiratory time will be applied (Table 1). With a leak, either PCV or a ventilator that allows an adjustable termination flow should be used.

PSV has been used effectively to ventilate many patients. However, the issues related to trigger, rise time, and cycle during PSV should be appreciated. Unfortunately, issues related to patient-ventilator synchrony during PSV are not commonly appreciated.

D. Proportional Assist Ventilation

Proportional assist ventilation (PAV) was designed to increase (or decrease) airway pressure in proportion to patient effort (103,104), which should improve patient-ventilator synchrony. This is accomplished by a positive feedback control that amplifies airway pressure proportionally to instantaneous inspiratory flow and volume. Unlike other modes of ventilatory support, which deliver a preset tidal volume or inspiratory pressure at the airway, with proportional assist ventilation the amount of support changes with patient effort, assisting ventilation with a uniform proportionality between ventilator and patient (Fig. 11). The advantage of a proportional (as opposed to a fixed) ventilatory support lies in its ability to track changes in ventilatory effort that may occur abruptly in patients with respiratory failure. To the extent that inspiratory effort is a reflection of ventilatory demand, this form of support may result in a more physiological breathing pattern. Patient effort determines the ventilating pressure, determined by the central drive and the respiratory mechanics.

Proportional unloading of ventilatory effort (i.e., of inspiratory flow, volume, or both) was proposed many years ago (105–107) but has only recently been used to ventilate patients (106). Proportional unloading that is limited to inspiratory flow (i.e., "resistive unloading") has been used to investigate ventilatory control during sleep (108) and exercise (105–107). Younes et al. (103) developed a prototype ventilator for clinical use that is capable of delivering positive pressure at the airway in proportion to both inspiratory flow and volume and described the effect of this ventilator to deliver PAV. While the theory of PAV has been extensively modeled mathematically (109), few published data exist that test predictions from this theory.

The principles of PAV have been extensively described elsewhere (103,104,109). PAV is a positive feedback controller where respiratory elastance and resistance are the feedback signal gains, defined as K_1 (cm H_2O/L) and K_2 (cm $H_2O/L/s$), respectively. In such a system, the pressure at the airway opening is adjusted according to the equation:

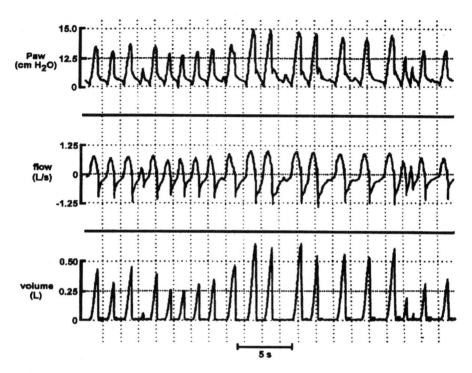

Figure 11 Airway pressure, flow, and volume waveforms for proportional assist ventilation. Note that the airway pressure varies with the inspiratory flow and volume demands of the patient. (From Ref. 117.)

$$P_{APPL} = K_1 \cdot V + K_2 \cdot \dot{V}$$

where P_{APPL} is the total pressure applied at the airway [the sum of the pressure developed by the respiratory muscles (P_{MUS}), and the pressure supplied by the ventilator (P_{AW})], V is inspiratory volume, and V is inspiratory flow. This equation is derived from the Law of Motion of the respiratory system (110):

$$P_{APPL} = P_{MUS} + P_{AW} = P_E + P_R$$

where P_E and P_R are the fractions of P_{APPL} dissipated against respiratory elastance and resistance, respectively. This equation can also be stated as:

$$P_{AW} = \text{elastance} \cdot V + \text{resistance} \cdot \dot{V}$$

where elastance can be substituted by K_1 and resistance by K_2, the volume and flow gains of the proportional assist ventilator. For the airway pressure to be amplified in proportion to the pressure developed by the respiratory muscles, K_1

and K_2 must be set to $<100\%$ of the patient's elastance and resistance. If K_1 and K_2 are $\geq 100\%$ of elastance and resistance, "runaway" occurs where the ventilator no longer tracks inspiratory effort (103,104).

The use of PAV requires knowledge of the patient's inspiratory airways resistance and respiratory system elastance. These can be estimated by use of an end-inspiratory pause method and the calculation of inspiratory resistance (R_I) as:

$$R_I = (PIP - Pplat)/\dot{V}$$

and respiratory system compliance (C) as:

$$C = V_T/(Pplat - PEEP)$$

Elastance (E) is the inverse of compliance ($E = 1/C$). In other words, a compliance of 50 mL/cm H_2O is an elastance of 20 cm H_2O/L. The amount of unloading of resistance and elastance is set on the ventilator. For example, consider a patient who has an inspiratory airways resistance of 20 cm $H_2O/L/s$ and an elastance of 20 cm H_2O/L. To unload 50% of the patient's inspiratory effort, a flow assist of 10 cm $H_2O/L/s$ (half of the resistance) and a volume assist of 10 cm H_2O/L (half of the elastance) is set on the ventilator. At any point during inspiration, the pressure applied to the airway will be flow measured at that time multiplied times the flow assist (10 cm $H_2O/L/s$ in this example) and the inspired volume times the volume assist (10 cm H_2O/L in this example). Because flow decreases and volume increases throughout inspiration, flow assist is greatest at the beginning of inspiration and volume assist is greatest at the end of inspiration. Because flow and volume vary breath by breath, the airway pressure during PAV varies breath by breath. Thus, PAV allows the respiratory rate, inspiratory time, and inspiratory pressure to vary. This is in contrast to PSV, which has a fixed pressure, and PCV, which has a fixed pressure and inspiratory time.

The measurement of elastance and resistance in a spontaneously breathing patient is difficult. The necessity of accurate measurements of these variables represents the Achilles heel of PAV. When PAV performs appropriately, the output of the ventilator (pressure) is less than the pressure required to overcome the impedance of the respiratory system. However, if impedance is overestimated, the ventilator output (pressure) will exceed the pressure required to overcome respiratory system impedance. The result is a "runaway" condition. The difficulty in measuring elastance and resistance is further complicated by the common fluctuations in these values in mechanically ventilated patients. Finally, the algorithm for control of PAV assumes that elastance and resistance characteristics are linear. In patients with respiratory failure, the nonlinearity of these variables may result in inappropriate ventilation. Leaks in the patient/ventilator system can also create problems. However, PAV has been used successfully for noninvasive ventilation (110–113) in which resistance and elastance cannot be easily measured and leaks are common. In this application, the settings of flow assist and volume assist are titrated to patient comfort—much like setting the pressure during PSV.

One method for selecting the correct settings for PAV uses the "runaway" method. The volume assist is set at 2 cm H_2O/L (with a flow assist of 1 cm $H_2O/L/s$) and raised in 2 cm H_2O/L increments until runaway occurs. The patient's elastance is estimated as this level of volume assist minus 1 cm H_2O/L. The flow assist is set at 1 cm $H_2O/L/s$ (with a volume assist of 2 cm H_2O/L) and raised in 1 cm $H_2O/L/s$ increments until runaway occurs. The patient's airways resistance is estimated as the flow assist minus 1 cm $H_2O/L/s$ (111).

In the original piston-driven PAV device described by Younes (103), the forward motion of the piston increases in proportion to the patient demand. With the use of rapidly responding flow sensors and gas-delivery mechanisms, PAV can be provided by solenoid-based, piston-based, and blower-based ventilators. The investigational use of PAV for noninvasive ventilation using a blower device has been reported (112). PAV has been available on the Drager Evita 4 as proportional pressure support (PPS).

Bigatello et al. (114) reported that PAV provided uniform unloading of the work-of-breathing in a lung model where ventilatory drive was varied. Patient studies, mainly from Canada or Europe, have confirmed the feasibility of PAV in a variety of patient conditions (103,111–1113,115–120). Experience with this mode is limited in the United States, where the Food and Drug Administration (FDA) has not yet approved it for commercial use. Although its physiological basis is sound, the clinical role of PAV remains to be established.

E. Automatic Tube Compensation

A properly positioned endotracheal tube effectively bypasses upper airway obstruction. However, the resistance to flow through an endotracheal tube is greater than that of a normal native upper airway (121–124). Lofaso et al. (127) proposed the Blasius Resistance Formula to estimate the effective diameter of endotracheal tubes:

$$\Delta P = K \cdot (L/D^{4.75}) \cdot \mu^{0.25} \cdot \rho^{0.75} \cdot \dot{V}^{1.75}$$

where ΔP is the pressure drop along the length (L) of the endotracheal tube, K depends upon the shape of the tube cross section (K = 0.24 for circular tubes), D is the diameter of the tube, μ is gas viscosity, ρ is gas density, and $\dot{V}$ is flow through the tube. Guttman et al. (122) reported a nonlinear approximation of the pressure drop across the endotracheal tube (ΔP_{ETT}):

$$\Delta P_{ETT} = K1 \cdot \dot{V}^{K2}$$

where K1 and K2 are coefficients, which were determined in the laboratory and validated in intubated patients. For example, K1 and K2 for an uncut 8 mm endotracheal tube are 6.57 and 1.94, respectively. It should also be appreciated that endotracheal tube resistance increases in situ (127,132,133), most likely due to progressive reduction of tube diameter secondary to mucus deposition. Nasal intubation does not produce greater resistance than oral intubation for comparable endotracheal tube sizes (121). Conversion of endotracheal intubation to tracheostomy has been reported to decrease the work-of-breathing (134).

Several investigators have advocated using PSV to overcome the imposed work of the endotracheal tube. Brochard et al. (135) reported that PSV of 3.4–14.4 cm H_2O was sufficient to compensate for the additional work of the endotracheal tube. Fiastro et al. (136) reported that a PSV of 2–20 cm H_2O eliminated the imposed work from the ventilator and endotracheal tube. In both of these studies, there was wide variability among patients in the appropriate level of pressure support needed to overcome the imposed work. Under static conditions, pressure support can effectively eliminate endotracheal tube resistance. However, variable inspiratory flow and changing demands of the patient cannot be met by a single level of pressure support. During periods of tachypnea, the previously chosen level of pressure support will no longer eliminate work imposed by the endotracheal tube. Additionally, the resistance of the endotracheal tube creates a condition where early in the breath when ventilator flow is high, tracheal pressure remains low and undercompensation for imposed work occurs. Late in the breath, pressure support overcompensates, prolongs inspiration, and may exacerbate overinflation.

Guttman et al. (122) described a technique for continuously calculating tracheal pressure in intubated, mechanically ventilated patients. This system uses the known resistive component of the endotracheal tube and the measurement of flow to calculate tracheal pressure. The technique was validated in a group of mechanically ventilated patients, with good correlation between calculated and measured tracheal pressure. This led to the introduction of automatic tube compensation (ATC) on the Drager Evita 4 (137–140). ATC compensates for endotracheal tube resistance via closed loop control of *calculated* tracheal pressure. The proposed advantages of ATC are to overcome the work-of-breathing imposed by artificial airways, to improve patient/ventilator synchrony as a result of variable inspiratory flow commensurate with demand (similar to PAV), and to reduce air trapping as a result of compensation for imposed expiratory resistance. This system uses the known resistive coefficients of the tracheal tube (tracheostomy or endotracheal) and measurement of instantaneous flow to apply pressure proportional to resistance throughout the total respiratory cycle. The equation for calculating tracheal pressure is:

$$\text{Tracheal pressure} = \text{proximal airway pressure} - (\text{tube coefficient} \cdot \text{flow}^2)$$

Most of the interest in ATC revolves around eliminating the imposed work-of-breathing during inspiration. However, during expiration there is also a flow-dependent pressure drop across the tube. ATC compensates for this flow resistive component and may reduce expiratory resistance and unintentional hyperinflation. During expiration, the calculated tracheal pressure is greater than airway pressure. Under these conditions a negative pressure at the airway may reduce expiratory resistance. Since this is not always desirable or possible, ATC can reduce PEEP to no less than 0 cm H_2O during exhalation to facilitate compensation of expiratory resistance posed by the endotracheal tube. Because in vivo tracheal tube resistance tends to be greater than in vitro resistance, incomplete compensation for endotracheal tube resistance may occur. Additionally, kinks or bends in the tube as it traverses the upper airway and accumulation of secretions in the inner lumen will change the tube's resistive coefficient and result in incomplete compensation.

Stocker et al. (141) reported that ATC was superior to pressure support in overcoming endotracheal tube resistance and eliminating dynamic hyperinflation. They demonstrated that PSV, unlike ATC, was associated with an increase in auto-PEEP and ineffective ventilator triggering. Stocker et al. (141) also introduced the term "electronic extubation," which suggests that the patient's breathing pattern during ATC mimics their breathing pattern when extubated (142). In a group of eight postoperative patients, the pressure time product was unchanged between ATC and when the patient was extubated. This is an interesting concept, which deserves further study. A potential pitfall is the incomplete upper airway control in some patients after extubation, which may render this technique a poor predictor of successful extubation.

Investigations by Fabry et al. (139,140) and Guttman et al. (140) demonstrated improved patient comfort during ATC compared to PSV (Fig. 12), much of which was due to prevention of hyperinflation by ATC. Fabry (139) also showed that with changing patient demand, ATC consistently eliminated imposed work, but pressure support was unable to compensate for changes in patient demand. The concept of ATC appears to have advantages compared to pressure support ventilation. Future studies should address the appropriate application of this technique (137).

Whether endotracheal tube resistance poses a clinical concern for increased work-of-breathing in adults is controversial. The imposed work-of-breathing through the endotracheal tube is modest at usual minute ventilations for the tube sizes most commonly used for adults. Several recent studies cast doubt on the importance of endotracheal tube resistance during short trials of spontaneous breathing. Estaban et al. (143) reported similar outcomes when spontaneous breathing trials were conducted with PSV (7 cm H_2O) or with a T-piece. Strauss et al. (144) reported that the work-of-breathing through the endotracheal tube amounted to only about 10% of the total work-of-breathing. That study further

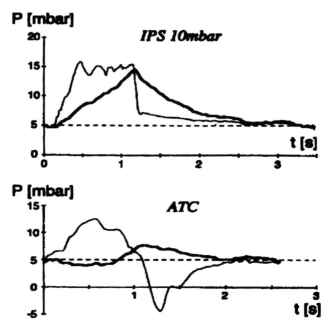

Figure 12 Pressure waveforms from the trachea (heavy lines) and the proximal airway (light lines) during inspiratory pressure support (IPS) and automatic tube compensation (ATC). Note that the tracheal pressure fluctuated very little during ATC. (From Ref. 139.)

reported that the work-for-breathing during a 2-hour spontaneous breathing trial with a T-piece was similar to the work-of-breathing immediately following extubation. Although prolonged spontaneous breathing through an endotracheal tube is not desirable due to the resistance of the tube, this may not be important for short periods of spontaneous breathing to assess extubation readiness.

F. Airway Pressure-Release Ventilation

Airway pressure-release ventilation (APRV) produces alveolar ventilation as an adjunct to CPAP. Airway pressure is transiently released to a lower level, after which it is quickly restored to reinflate the lungs (Fig. 13). For a patient with no spontaneous breathing efforts, APRV is similar to PCIRV. Unlike PCIRV, APRV allows spontaneous breathing at any time during the respiratory cycle. Since PIP during APRV does not exceed the CPAP level, the hazards associated with high airway pressure may be minimized (e.g., alveolar overdistension, hemodynamic compromise). Because the patient is allowed to breathe spontaneously at both

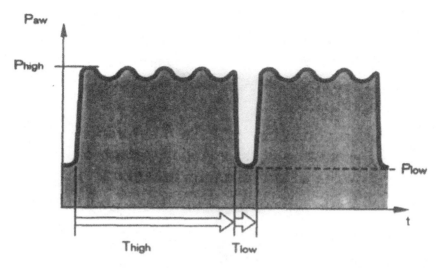

Figure 13 Pressure waveform for APRV. Note that the patient can breathe at both levels of pressure and that the pressure release is brief. (Courtesy of Drager.)

levels of CPAP, the need for sedation may also be decreased. Tidal volume for the APRV breath depends on lung compliance, airways resistance, the magnitude of the pressure release, the duration of the pressure release, and the magnitude of the patient's spontaneous breathing efforts. Of concern is the potential for alveolar derecruitment during the release of pressure with APRV. Clinical reports (145–149), including a prospective multicenter trial (150), suggest that APRV is a feasible alternative to conventional ventilation in patients with acute respiratory failure. However, it has not received widespread application in the United States, and its precise role in the management of acute respiratory failure is unclear. APRV can be provided using a modified CPAP circuit in which the CPAP level is modified by opening or closing a release valve connected to a timer (Fig. 14). APRV is available on the Drager Evita 4 Ventilator.

Biphasic intermittent positive pressure (BIPAP) is a modification of APRV (Fig. 15) (151). Unlike APRV, the I:E ratios used with BIPAP are not reversed. BIPAP is also partially synchronized to the patient's inspiratory efforts, allowing the inspiratory and expiratory times to be reduced by as much as 25% based on the patient's respiratory efforts. Without spontaneous breathing, BIPAP is similar to PCV. There are few clinical reports of BIPAP (152–154), and its role is unclear. One potential advantage of BIPAP is that the exhalation valve is active during both the inspiratory and expiratory phase. Prior to the current generation of ventilators, the exhalation valve was active during the expiratory phase but

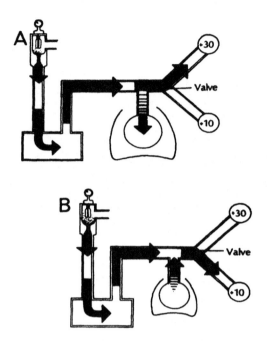

Figure 14 Schematic representation of APRV with an inflation pressure of 30 cm H_2O and a release pressure of 10 cm H_2O. Pressure is determined by the flow through the system and the threshold CPAP valves. A timer determines the time at each level of CPAP. (A) Inflation phase. (B) Release phase. (From Ref. 146.)

closed completely during the inspiratory phase. An active exhalation valve during the inspiratory phase will open as necessary to maintain a constant inspiratory pressure. This may improve patient-ventilator synchrony and prevent inadvertent overpressurization when auxiliary gas flows are added to the system (e.g., nebulizer therapy, tracheal gas insufflation) (155). BIPAP (also called PCV+) is available on the Drager Evita 4. It is also available as BiLevel on the Nellcor–Puritan–Bennett 840. BIPAP should not be confused with BiPAP; BiPAP (Respironics, Inc.) is the brand name of a commercially available portable pressure ventilator for noninvasive ventilation.

Another variation to APRV is intermittent mandatory pressure release ventilation (IMPRV) (156,157). During IMPRV (CESAR ventilator, TAEMA, Air Liquide, France), the pressure release occurs according to the patient's spontaneous breathing efforts. IMPRV also allows PSV to be used with the patient's

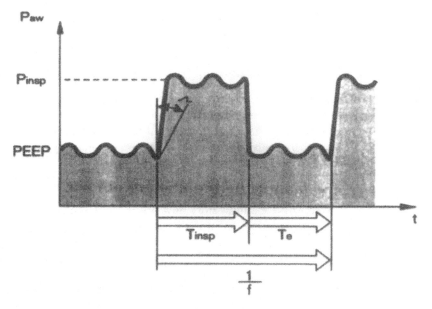

Figure 15 Pressure tracing for BIPAP (PCV+). Note that the patient can breathe at both levels of pressure. Also note that the I:E ratio is relatively normal. (Courtesy of Drager.)

inspiratory efforts. IMPRV is not available on any ventilator used in the United States.

IV. Dual Control Modes

Recently developed modes allow the ventilator to control pressure or volume based on a feedback loop (dual control). However, it is important to remember that the ventilator is controlling only pressure or volume, not both at the same time. These modes are classified as dual control within a breath or dual control breath-to-breath (158). Dual control within a breath describes a mode where the ventilator switches from pressure control to volume control during the breath. These techniques are known as volume assured pressure support (VAPS) and pressure augmentation (158–160). Dual control breath-to-breath is simpler because the ventilator operates in either the pressure support or the pressure control mode. The only difference is that the pressure limit increases or decreases to maintain a clinician selected tidal volume. These modes are analogous to having a respiratory therapist at the bedside who increases or decreases the pressure limit of each breath based on the tidal volume of the previous breath.

A. Dual Control Within a Breath

The proposed advantage of this approach is a reduced work-of-breathing while maintaining constant minute volume and tidal volume. Examples include volume assured pressure support (VAPS) (Bird 8400Sti and Tbird) and pressure augmentation (PA) (Bear 1000). Both approaches operate during mandatory breaths or pressure supported breaths. Conceptually, VAPS and PA are meant to combine the high initial flow of a pressure-limited breath with the constant volume delivery of a volume-limited breath (Fig. 16) (48,101).

During VAPS or PA the inspiratory flow waveform is square (constant). Additionally, the initial pressure target is the pressure support level. Selecting the appropriate pressure support is critical for the successful use of VAPS, yet no studies have reported the best method for choosing this pressure. One approach is to set the pressure support setting at a level equivalent to the plateau pressure obtained during a volume control breath at the desired tidal volume. The peak flow setting is also important and should be adjusted to allow for the appropriate inspiratory time for the patient. A VAPS or PA breath may be patient or ventilator triggered. Once the breath is triggered, the ventilator attempts to reach the pressure support setting as quickly as possible. This portion of the breath is the pressure control portion and is associated with a high variable flow, which may reduce the work-of-breathing. As this pressure level is reached, the ventilator's microprocessor determines the volume which has been delivered from the machine, compares this to the desired tidal volume, and determines if the minimum desired tidal volume will be reached. Note that the ventilator monitors the delivered tidal volume and not the exhaled tidal volume, so as to provide control within the breath rather than on the subsequent breath.

There are several differences in ventilator output based on the relationship between the volume delivered and the minimum set tidal volume (Fig. 17). If the delivered tidal volume and set tidal volume are equal, the breath is a pressure support breath. That is, the breath is pressure limited at the pressure support setting and flow cycled. With the Bear and Bird ventilators, this occurs at 25% of the initial peak flow (Fig. 17A). If the patient's inspiratory effort is diminished, the ventilator delivers a smaller volume at the set pressure level, and when delivered and set volume are compared, the microprocessor will determine that the minimum set tidal volume will not be delivered. As the flow decelerates and reaches the set peak flow, the breath changes from a pressure-limited to a volume-limited breath (Fig. 17B). Flow remains constant, increasing the inspiratory time until the volume has been delivered. It is important to remember that the volume is volume exiting the ventilator, not exhaled tidal volume. During this time the

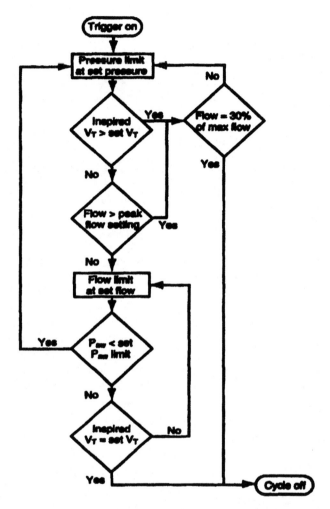

Figure 16 Control logic for the pressure augmentation function of the Bear 1000 ventilator. (From Ref. 161.)

pressure will rise above the set pressure support setting. Setting the high-pressure alarm remains important during VAPS. If pressure increases abruptly, the high-pressure alarm setting will be reached and the breath will be pressure cycled. A similar condition can occur if there is an acute decrease in lung compliance or increase in airway resistance (Fig. 17C). This breath demonstrates the possibility of a prolonged inspiratory time during a VAPS breath. There are secondary cycle characteristics for these breaths and an inspiratory time lasting longer than 3

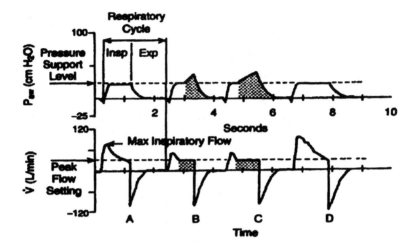

Figure 17 Pressure and flow waveforms illustrating volume-assured pressure-support mode. See text for details. (From Ref. 158.)

seconds will be automatically time cycled. This finding suggests that when used for patients with airflow obstruction, intrusions of the constant flow on the patient's expiratory time should be carefully evaluated. Finally, the VAPS breath can allow the patient a tidal volume larger than the set volume (Fig. 17D). Because the pressure limit remains the same, this breath is also a pressure support breath (i.e., it is pressure limited and flow cycled). This allows for normal variations in patient tidal volume, sighing, and increased volumes during times of hyperpnea.

Choosing the appropriate pressure and flow settings is critical to successfully using VAPS and PA. If the pressure is set too high, all breaths will be pressure support breaths and the volume guarantee will be negated. The same problem applies to selecting a minimum tidal volume that is too low. If the constant flow setting is too high, all the breaths will switch from pressure to volume control. If the peak flow is set too low, the switch from pressure to volume will occur late in the breath and inspiratory time may be unnecessarily prolonged.

Amato et al. (162) described the technique of volume-assisted pressure support as an alternative to VCV. They reported a reduction in work-of-breathing of nearly 50% with VAPS as well as improvements in dynamic compliance, airways resistance, and auto-PEEP. This was attributed to the higher inspiratory flow provided during VAPS. They also suggested that VAPS improved patient/ventilator synchrony by matching ventilator output to patient demand. One criticism of this study (162) is the relatively low peak flow during VCV (46 L/min) and the significantly larger tidal volume delivered during VAPS (0.72 L vs. 0.59 L). This increase in tidal volume may explain the decrease in the work-of-breathing. It could be argued that no differences would have been identified if tidal volume and inspiratory flow during VCV were equivalent to that during VAPS. However, peak inspiratory pressure would increase by increasing tidal volume and flow during VCV. Additionally, regardless of the chosen peak flow during VCV, fluctuating patient demands appear to be better met by VAPS than VCV.

Haas et al. evaluated VAPS as provided by the Bird 8400STi (160). They attempted to replicate the findings of Amato et al. (162) while optimizing tidal volume and inspiratory flow during VCV. This was accomplished by setting the pressure limit during VAPS to produce a tidal volume equivalent to VCV and by setting inspiratory flow to closely approximate patient demand during VCV prior to initiating VAPS. They reported a significant reduction in patient effort with VAPS compared to VCV as well as significant reductions in respiratory drive and esophageal pressure changes. Despite attempts to maintain constant tidal volume over the course of the 40-minute study period, it rose slightly during VAPS. This is an important observation, in that as patients' demands vary, the ability to increase tidal volume may play an important role in the sensation of breathlessness.

MacIntyre et al. (159) evaluated the PA function of the Bear 1000 in a lung model at varying degrees of simulated patient demand and reported that the PA breath allowed for more effective matching of ventilator output to simulated patient demand than traditional volume ventilation. They suggested that this breath type could replace both volume and pressure control breaths on future ventilators. Clinicians could then select the VAPS breath with a high pressure limit to provide enhanced patient/ventilator synchrony or at a lower pressure limit to assure constant tidal volume and inspiratory time.

B. Dual Control Breath to Breath—Pressure-Limited Flow-Cycled Ventilation

Breath-to-breath dual control is available as Volume Support (VS) (Siemens 300, Siemens Medical Systems, Inc., Danvers, MA) and Variable Pressure Support (Venturi, Cardiopulmonary Corporation, New Haven, CT). Its proposed advantages are to provide the positive attributes of pressure support ventilation with constant minute volume and tidal volume and automatic weaning of pressure limit as patient compliance improves and/or patient effort increases.

This technique is a closed-loop control of pressure support ventilation. VS is PSV that uses tidal volume as a feedback control for continuously adjusting the pressure support level. All breaths are patient triggered, pressure limited, and flow cycled (Fig. 18) (48,161). When using the Siemens 300 ventilator, VS is initiated by delivering a "test breath" with a peak pressure of 5 cm H_2O

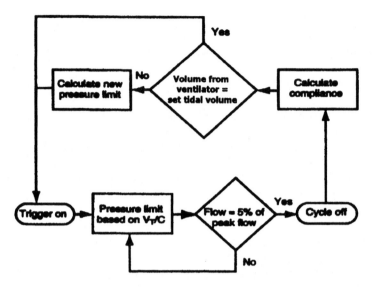

Figure 18 Control logic for the volume support mode of the Servo 300. (From Ref. 161.)

(Fig. 19). The delivered tidal volume (again, this is not exhaled tidal volume, but volume exiting the ventilator) is measured and total system compliance is calculated. The following three breaths are delivered at a pressure support level of 75% of the pressure calculated to deliver the minimum set tidal volume. From breath to breath the maximum pressure change is <3 cm H_2O and can range from 0 cm H_2O above PEEP to 5 cm H_2O below the high-pressure alarm setting.

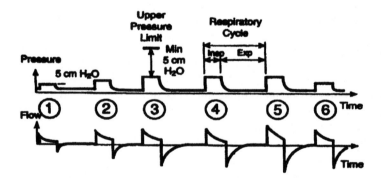

Figure 19 Pressure and flow waveforms for volume support mode. See text for details. (From Ref. 158.)

Since all breaths are pressure-support breaths, cycling normally occurs at 5% of the initial peak flow. A secondary cycling mechanism is activated if inspiratory time exceeds 80% of the set total cycle time. There is also a relationship between the set ventilator frequency and tidal volume. If the desired tidal volume is 500 mL and the respiratory frequency is set at 15 breaths per minute, the minute volume setting will be 7.5 L/min. If the patient's respiratory frequency decreases below 15 breaths per minute, the tidal volume target will be automatically increased by the ventilator up to 150% of the initial value (in this example 750 mL). This is done in an effort to maintain the minute volume constant.

Considerable speculation, but few data, suggests that VS will wean the patient from pressure support as patient effort increases and lung mechanics improve. Unfortunately, patients do not always attempt to take over the work-of-breathing, and weaning may not progress. If the pressure level increases in an attempt to maintain tidal volume in the patient with airflow obstruction, auto-PEEP may result. In cases of hyperpnea, as patient demand increases, ventilator support will decrease. This may be the opposite of the desired response. Additionally, if the minimum tidal volume chosen by the clinician exceeds the patient demand, the patient may remain at that level of support and weaning may be delayed. The issues related to increasing tidal volume during a low spontaneous respiratory frequency should also be considered when using VS.

Keenan and Martin (163) reported their experience with VS in a retrospective case series in which this mode was used in infants and children. They reported a reduction in PIP and set tidal volume when children were switched to VS. They also reported that PIP and tidal volume further decreased over the course of VS ventilation. They reported a failure to wean and extubate from VS of nearly 50% (i.e., patient switched to another mode to complete weaning), much of which was attributed to clinician unfamiliarity with this mode.

C. Dual Control Breath to Breath—Pressure-Limited Time-Cycled Ventilation

This approach is available as Pressure Regulated Volume Control (PRVC) (Siemens 300, Siemens Medical Systems, Danvers, MA), Adaptive Pressure Ventilation (APV) (Hamilton Galileo, Hamilton Medical, Reno, NV), Auto-Flow (Evita 4, Drager Inc., Telford, PA), or Variable Pressure Control (Venturi, Cardiopulmonary Corporation, New Haven, CT). Proposed advantages of this approach are the positive attributes of pressure-control ventilation with a constant assured minute volume and tidal volume, and automatic lowering of the pressure limit as patient compliance improves and/or patient effort increases.

Each of these modes is a form of pressure-limited, time-cycled ventilation that uses tidal volume as a feedback control for continuously adjusting the pressure limit (Fig. 20). The volume signal used for ventilator feedback is not exhaled

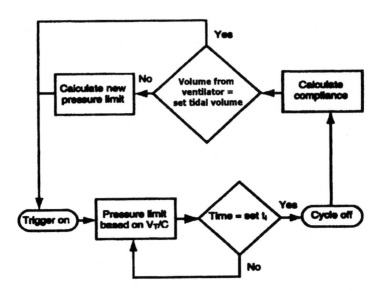

Figure 20 Control logic for pressure-regulated volume control mode of the Servo 300. (From Ref. 161.)

tidal volume, but volume exiting the ventilator. This prevents runaway that could occur if a leak in the circuit interferes with accurate measurement of exhaled tidal volume. Despite the fact that each manufacturer's mode has a different name, operation is fairly consistent between devices. All breaths in these modes are time or patient triggered, pressure limited, and time cycled. One difference between devices is that the Siemens 300 only allows PRVC in the CMV mode, whereas the other ventilators allow dual control breath to breath using CMV or SIMV. During SIMV, the mandatory breaths are the dual control breaths. Volume measurement for the feedback signal is also different between ventilators. The Siemens 300 uses the volume leaving the inspiratory flow sensor. The Hamilton Galileo uses the flow sensor at the airway and the inspiratory flow sensor to determine an average volume. This latter technique eliminates compressible volume and can detect the presence of leaks and may be the preferred method of volume monitoring in dual control. Rather than describe the individual nuances of each version of dual control, the operation of PRVC will be discussed.

As with VS, PRVC delivers a "test breath" and calculates total system compliance (Fig. 21). The next three breaths are delivered with an inspiratory pressure limit that is 75% of that necessary to achieve the desired tidal volume based on the compliance calculation. The ensuing breaths will increase or decrease the pressure by no more than 3 cm H_2O per breath in an attempt to deliver

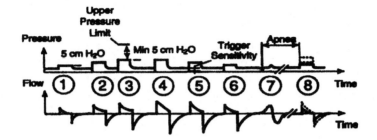

Figure 21 Pressure and flow waveforms illustrating the pressure-regulated volume control mode. See text for details. (From Ref. 158.)

the desired tidal volume. The pressure limit will fluctuate between 0 cm H_2O above the PEEP level to 5 cm H_2O below the upper pressure alarm setting. The ventilator will alarm if the tidal volume and maximum pressure limit settings are incompatible. The proposed advantage of PRVC and other dual control, breath-to-breath modes is, like that of VS, maintaining the minimum peak pressure that provides a constant set tidal volume and automatic weaning of the pressure as the patient improves. Likewise, during periods of limited staffing, these modes will maintain a more consistent tidal volume as compliance decreases or increases. Perhaps the most significant advantage of these modes is the ability of the ventilator to change inspiratory flow to meet patient demand while maintaining a constant minute volume.

Because these modes provide pressure-limited, time-cycled ventilation with a fluctuating pressure limit that depends on a measured tidal volume, any errors in tidal volume measurement will result in decision errors. If the patient's effort increases during assisted breaths because of increased dyspnea, the pressure level may diminish at a time when support is most necessary. Additionally, as the pressure level is reduced, mean airway pressure will fall, potentially resulting in a fall in oxygenation.

Piotrowski et al. (164) compared PRVC to volume-controlled IMV in 60 neonates with respiratory distress syndrome and reported a reduction in the length of mechanical ventilation and the incidence of bronchopulmonary dysplasia without any differences in outcome variables or complications. Alvarez et al. (165) compared volume-controlled ventilation, pressure-limited time-cycled ventilation, and PRVC in 10 adult patients with acute respiratory failure and reported that PRVC resulted in a lower peak airway pressure and a slight improvement in carbon dioxide elimination. Kesecioglu et al. (166,167) compared VCV and PRVC in a pig model of ARDS and reported similar oxygenation with both modes but (not surprisingly) lower peak inspiratory pressure with PRVC.

V. AutoMode

AutoMode is available on the Siemens 300A ventilator (Siemens Medical Systems, Danvers, MA). Its proposed advantages are automatic weaning from pressure control to pressure support and automated escalation of support as patient condition worsens or effort diminishes. AutoMode combines VS and PRVC in a single mode. If the patient is paralyzed, the ventilator will provide PRVC. All breaths are mandatory breaths that are time triggered, pressure limited, and time cycled. The pressure limit increases or decreases to maintain the desired tidal volume set by the clinician. If the patient breathes spontaneously for two consecutive breaths, the ventilator switches to VS. In this case, all breaths are patient triggered, pressure limited, and flow cycled. If the patient becomes apneic for 12 seconds in the adult setting, 8 seconds in the pediatric setting, or 5 seconds in the neonatal setting, the ventilator switches back to the PRVC mode. The change from PRVC to VS is accomplished at equivalent peak pressures. This mode is the combination of two existing modes using the conditional variable of patient effort to decide if the next breath will be time cycled or flow cycled.

AutoMode also switches between pressure control and pressure support or volume control to VS. In the volume control to VS switch, the VS pressure limit will be equivalent to the pause pressure during volume control. If an inspiratory plateau is not available, the pressure level is calculated as:

(Peak pressure − PEEP) · 50% + PEEP

AutoMode has only recently been introduced. One concern is that during the switch from time-cycled to flow-cycled ventilation, mean airway pressure will fall. This may result in hypoxemia in the patient with acute lung injury. The ventilator's algorithm is fairly simple and the patient is either assisting all or none of the breaths. This all-or-none type of decision making may require modification. Perhaps more importantly, no clinical studies have evaluated AutoMode, and no evidence suggests that this type of weaning is either necessary or useful.

VI. Mandatory Minute Ventilation

Mandatory minute ventilation (MMV) was first described in 1977 by Hewlett et al. (168) as a mode that guaranteed minute ventilation during weaning. If the patient's spontaneous ventilation does not match a target minute ventilation set by the clinician, the ventilator supplies the difference between the patient's minute ventilation and the target minute ventilation (169–171). If the patient's spontaneous minute ventilation exceeds the target, no ventilator support is provided. MMV is thus a form of closed-loop ventilation in which the ventilator adjusts its output according to the patient's response. MMV is only available on a few ventilator types used in the United States, and its value to facilitate weaning is unclear.

MMV can be provided by altering the rate or the tidal volume delivered from the ventilator. The Bear 1000 and Drager Evita 4 increase the mandatory breath rate if the minute ventilation falls below the target level. This has the potential to result in excessively rapid rates if the tidal volume (and thus the minute ventilation) falls. In contrast to this approach, the Hamilton Veolar increases the level of pressure support when the minute ventilation falls below the target level.

VII. Adaptive Support Ventilation

Adaptive support ventilation (ASV) is available on the Hamilton Galileo. Its proposed advantages are automated escalation or withdrawal of support based on changes in patient effort and lung mechanics and automated selection of initial ventilatory parameters. ASV is based on the minimal work-of-breathing concept developed by Otis (172). This suggests that the patient will breathe at a tidal volume and respiratory frequency, which minimizes the elastic and resistive loads while maintaining oxygenation and acid base balance. This is described mathematically as:

$$\text{Respiratory rate} = (1 + 4\pi^2 RC \cdot (\dot{V}_A/\dot{V}_D) - 1)/(2\pi^2 RC)$$

RC is the respiratory time constant, $\dot{V}_A$ is alveolar ventilation, and $\dot{V}_D$ is dead space ventilation. The ASV algorithm uses this formula along with patient weight (which determines dead space) to adjust a number of ventilator variables. The clinician inputs the patient's ideal body weight; sets the high-pressure alarm, PEEP, and inspired oxygen concentration; and adjusts the rise time and flow cycle variable for pressure support breaths from 10 to 40% of initial peak flow. The ventilator attempts to deliver 100 mL/min/kg of minute ventilation for an adult and 200 mL/min/kg for children. This can be adjusted by a setting known as the % minute volume control, which can be set from 20 to 200%. With 200%, a minute volume of 200 mL/min/kg would be delivered to an adult patient. This setting allows the clinician to provide full ventilatory support or encourage spontaneous breathing and facilitate weaning.

When connected to the patient, the ventilator delivers a series of test breaths and measures system compliance, airways resistance, and auto-PEEP using a least-squares-fit technique (173). This measurement system is important for accurate measurement of variables used in the minimal work equation. The input of body weight allows the ventilator's algorithm to choose a required minute volume. The ventilator then uses the clinician input and measured respiratory mechanics to select a respiratory frequency, inspiratory time, I:E ratio, and pressure limit for mandatory and spontaneous breaths. These variables are measured on a breath-to-breath basis and altered by the ventilator's algorithm to meet the desired targets. If the patient breathes spontaneously, the ventilator will pressure support breaths and encourage spontaneous breathing. However, spontaneous and mandatory breaths can be combined to meet the minute ventilation target. The pressure limit of both the mandatory and spontaneous breaths are always being adjusted. This means that ASV is continuously employing dual control breath-to-breath of mandatory and spontaneous breaths.

The ventilator adjusts the I:E ratio and inspiratory time of mandatory breaths to prevent air trapping and auto-PEEP. This is done by calculation of the expiratory time constant (compliance × resistance) and maintenance of sufficient expiratory time. If the patient is paralyzed, the ventilator determines the respiratory frequency, tidal volume, pressure limit required to deliver the tidal volume, inspiratory time, and the I:E ratio. As the patient begins to breathe spontaneously, the number of mandatory breaths decreases and the ventilator chooses a pressure support level that maintains a tidal volume sufficient to assure alveolar ventilation based on a dead space calculation of 2.2 mL/kg. ASV can provide pressure-limited, time-cycled ventilation, add dual control of those breaths on a breath-to-breath basis, allow for mandatory breaths and spontaneous breaths (a kind of dual control SIMV + PSV), and eventually switch to pressure support with dual control breath to breath (variable pressure with each pressure-supported breath). During mandatory breath delivery, the ventilator sets inspiratory time and I:E ratio.

This very new technique suffers predominantly from a lack of clinical evaluation or clinician experience. Other problems are those previously described for other dual control, breath-to-breath techniques. These include reductions in mean airway pressure resulting in hypoxemia, reductions in inspiratory pressure when an increase might be more appropriate, and appropriate setting of the percent minute volume control to meet the goals of ventilatory support.

Weiler et al. (174) reported that the ASV algorithm provided adequate ventilation for five patients undergoing abdominal surgery. No instances of auto-PEEP were identified, and delivered and target tidal volumes were different by only 28 mL. In a study during thoracic surgery, Weiler et al. (175) also reported that ALV was able to ventilate patients even under the highly variable conditions of one lung ventilation. Laubscher et al. (176) compared the ability of the ASV algorithm to select initial ventilation parameters to clinician settings in 25 adults and 17 children using a version of ASV, which incorporated carbon dioxide monitoring. They reported that the algorithm provided equivalent gas exchange to clinician set parameters. The ventilator consistently delivered smaller tidal volumes and higher respiratory frequencies than the clinicians. These findings were confirmed in a follow-up study of 30 patients ranging in weight from 15 to 100 kg (177). The results of this study demonstrated that the ventilator algorithm provided a slightly smaller tidal volume, slightly higher respiratory frequency, and slightly lower peak pressure than clinician settings. Blood gases were essentially unchanged between the methods of ventilation. Linton et al. (178) and Weiler et al. (179) performed studies similar to those previously described and reported similar findings. Weiler et al. (179) compared ASV to conventional ventilation during changes in patient position. They found that during extreme changes in position, the ASV algorithm "adapted" to provide more appropriate ventilator settings in response to position induced changes in lung mechanics. Campbell et al. (180) compared ASV to clinician-set parameters in a group of paralyzed postoperative patients and reported that ASV provided similar gas exchange with lower tidal volumes, lower peak pressures, higher respiratory rates, and lower dead space. These studies demonstrate the feasibility of allowing the ventilator to automatically select parameters and to make changes in response to patient efforts and lung mechanics.

VIII. Conclusions

Many new ventilator modes have become available over the past decade that claim to improve the efficiency and safety of mechanical ventilation. Some also claim to facilitate the weaning process while reducing the need for direct clinician input. Clinicians should understand these new ventilator techniques and appreciate the nuances in ventilator algorithms. The decision to apply a particular mode of ventilation, however, should also be based upon an understanding of the underlying physiology. Just because a new mode does what it claims does not mean it will be clinically more useful than existing modes. Unfortunately, there are very few clinical outcome data upon which to base a decision regarding the choice of ventilator mode. The choice of a particular mode is often based on clinician experience and bias, institutional preferences, and the capabilities of the ventilators available at that institution.

References

1. Chatburn RL. A new system for understanding mechanical ventilators. Respir Care 1992; 36:1123–1155.
2. Branson RD, Chatburn RL, East TD, et al. Consensus statement on the essentials of mechanical ventilators—1992. Respir Care 1992; 37:1000–1008.
3. Banner MJ, Downs JB, Kirby RR. Effects of expiratory flow resistance on inspiratory work of breathing. Chest 1988; 93:795–799.
4. Sassoon CSH. Mechanical ventilator design and function: The trigger variable. Respir Care 1992; 37:1056–1069.
5. Sassoon CSH, Gruer SE. Characteristics of the ventilator pressure and flow trigger variables. Intensive Care Med 1995; 21:159–168.

6. Branson RD. Flow triggering systems. Respir Care 1994; 39:892–896.
7. Branson RD, Campbell RS, Davis K, et al. Comparison of pressure and flow triggering systems during continuous positive airway pressure. Chest 1994; 106:540–544.
8. Carmack J, Torres A, Anders M, et al. Comparison of inspiratory work of breathing in young lambs during flow-triggered and pressure triggered ventilation. Respir Care 1995; 40:28–34.
9. Konyukov Y, Takahashi T, Kuwayama N, et al. Estimation of triggering work of breathing. Chest 1994; 105:1836–1841.
10. Gurevitch MJ, Gelmont D. Importance of trigger sensitivity to ventilator response delay in advanced chronic obstructive pulmonary disease with acute respiratory failure. Crit Care Med 1989; 17:354–359.
11. Holbrook PJ, Guiles SP. Response time of four pressure support ventilators: effect of triggering method and bias flow. Respir Care 1997; 42:952–959.
12. Sassoon CSH, Giron, AE, Ely, EA, Light RW. Inspiratory work of breathing on flow-by and demand-flow continuous positive airway pressure. Crit Care Med 1989; 17:1108–1114.
13. Sassoon CSH, Lodia R, Rheeman CH, et al. Inspiratory muscle work of breathing during flow-by, demand-flow, and continuous-flow systems in patients with chronic obstructive pulmonary disease. Am Rev Respir Dis 1992; 145:1219–1222.
14. Sassoon CSH, del Rosario N, Fei R et al. Influence of pressure- and flow-triggered synchronous intermittent mandatory ventilation on inspiratory muscle work. Crit Care Med 1994; 22:1933–1941.
15. Saito S, Tokioka H, Kosaka F. Efficacy of flow-by during continuous positive airway pressure ventilation. Crit Care Med 1990; 18:654–656.
16. Polese G, Massara A, Poggi R, et al. Flow-triggering reduces inspiratory effort during weaning from mechanical ventilation. Intensive Care Med 1995; 21:682–686.
17. Jager K, Tweedale M, Holland T. Flow-triggering does not decrease the work of breathing and pressure time product in COPD patients. Respir Care 1994; 39:892–896.
18. Heulitt MJ, Torres A, Anders M, et al. Comparison of total resistive work of breathing in two generations of ventilators in an animal model. Pediatr Pulmonol 1996; 22:58–66.
19. Nishimura M, Imanka H, Yoshiya I, et al. Comparison of inspiratory work of breathing between flow-triggered and pressure-triggered demand flow systems in rabbits. Crit Care Med 1994; 22:1002–1009.
20. Nishimura M, Hess D, Kacmarek RM. The response of flow-triggered infant ventilators. Am J Respir Crit Care Med 1995; 152:1901–1909.
21. El-Khatib MF, Chatburn RL, Potts DL, et al. Mechanical ventilators optimized for pediatric use decrease work of breathing and oxygen consumption during pressure-support ventilation. Crit Care Med 1994; 22:1942–1948.
22. Tan IK, Bhatt SB, Tam YH, et al. Superimposed inspiratory work of the Siemens Servo 300 ventilator during continuous positive airway pressure. Intensive Care Med 1995; 21:1023–1026.
23. Giuliani R, Mascia L, Recchia F, et al. Patient-ventilator interaction during synchro-

nized intermittent mandatory ventilation. Effects of flow triggering. Am J Respir Crit Care Med 1995; 151:1–9.

24. Konyukov YA, Kuwayama N, Fukuoka T, et al. Effects of different triggering systems and external PEEP on trigger capability of the ventilator. Intensive Care Med 1996; 22:363–368.
25. Tutuncu AS, Cakar N, Camci E, et al. Comparison of pressure- and flow-triggered pressure-support ventilation on weaning parameters in patients recovering from acute respiratory failure. Crit Care Med 1997; 25:756–760.
26. Goulet R, Hess D, Kacmarek RM. Pressure vs. flow triggering during pressure support ventilation. Chest 1997; 111:1649–1653.
27. Aslanian P, el Atrous S, Isabey D, et al. Effects of flow triggering on breathing effort during partial ventilatory support. Am J Respir Crit Care Med 1998; 157:135–143.
28. Bunburaphog T, Imanaka H, Nishimura M, et al. Performance characteristics of bilevel pressure ventilators. A lung model study. Chest 1997; 111:1050–1060.
29. Ranieri VM, Grasso S, Fiore T, et al. Auto-positive end-expiratory pressure and dynamic hyperinflation. Clin Chest Med 1996; 17:379–394.
30. MacIntyre NR, Cheng KC McConnell R. Applied PEEP during pressure support reduces the inspiratory threshold load of intrinsic PEEP. Chest 1997; 111:188–193.
31. Nava S, Ambrosino N, Bruschi C, et al. Physiological effects of flow and pressure triggering during non-invasive mechanical ventilation in patients with chronic obstructive pulmonary disease. Thorax 1997; 52:249–254.
32. Ranieri VM, Mascia L, Petruzzelli V, et al. Inspiratory effort and measurement of dynamic intrinsic PEEP in COPD patients: effects of ventilator triggering systems. Intensive Care Med 1995; 21:896–903.
33. Banner MJ, Blanch PB, Kirby RR. Imposed work of breathing and methods of triggering a demand-flow, continuous positive airway pressure system. Crit Care Med 1993; 21:183–190.
34. Banner MJ, Kirby RR, Blanch PB. Site of pressure measurement during spontaneous breathing with continuous positive airway pressure: effect on calculating imposed work of breathing. Crit Care Med 1992; 20:528–533.
35. Messinger G, Banner MJ, Blanch PB, et al. Using tracheal pressure to trigger the ventilator and control airway pressure during continuous positive airway pressure decreases work of breathing. Chest 1995; 108:509–514.
36. Blanch PB, Banner MJ. Is tracheal pressure ventilator control comparable to an equivalent level of pressure support ventilation. Respir Care 1997; 42:1022–1033.
37. Branson RD. What is tracheal pressure triggering?—and do we need it? No! We don't need it! Respir Care 1996; 41:526–528.
38. MacIntyre NR. What is tracheal pressure triggering?—and do we need it? Yes! We do need it! Respir Care 1996; 41:524–525.
39. Messinger G, Banner MJ. Tracheal pressure triggering a demand-flow continuous positive airway pressure system decreases patient work of breathing. Crit Care Med 1996; 24:1829–1834.
40. Bhatt SB, Patel CB, Tan IKS, et al. Imposed work of breathing during tracheal pressure-triggering using a demand-valve CPAP system. Respir Care 1996; 41:512–518.

41. Takahashi T, Takezawa J, Kimura T, et al. Comparison of inspiratory work of breathing in T-piece breathing, PSV and pleural pressure support ventilation. Chest 1990; 100:1030–1034.
42. Barnhard M, Shukla A, Lovell T, et al. Esophageal-directed pressure support ventilation in normal volunteers. Chest 1999; 115:482–489.
43. Nikischin W, Gerhardt T, Everett R, et al. Patient triggered ventilation: a comparison of tidal volume and chestwall and abdominal motion as trigger signals. Pediatr Pulmonol 1996; 22:28–34.
44. Beck J, Sinderby C, Lindstrom L, et al. Crural diaphragm activation during dynamic contractions at various inspiratory flow rates. J Appl Physiol 1998; 85:451–458.
45. Sinderby C, Nandesi P, Beck J, et al. Neural control of mechanical ventilation in respiratory failure. Nature Med 1999; 5:1433–1436.
46. Sinderby C, Beck J, Spahija J, et al. Voluntary activation of the human diaphragm in health and disease. J Appl Physiol 1998; 85:2146–2158.
47. Marini JJ, Crooke PS. A general mathematical model for respiratory dynamics relevant to the clinical setting. Am Rev Respir Dis 1993; 147:14–24.
48. Chatburn RL. Classification of mechanical ventilators. In: Branson RD, Hess DR, Chatburn RL, eds. Respiratory Care Equipment. Philadelphia: Lippincott Williams and Wilkins, 1999:359–393.
49. Davis K, Branson RD, Campbell RS, Porembka DT. Comparison of volume control and pressure control ventilation: Is flow waveform the difference? J Trauma 1996; 41:808–814.
50. Munoz J, Guerrero JE, Escalante JL, et al. Pressure-controlled ventilation versus controlled mechanical ventilation with decelerating inspiratory flow. Crit Care Med 1993; 21:1143–1148.
51. Ravenscraft SA, Burke WC, Marini JJ. Volume-cycled decelerating flow. An alternative form of mechanical ventilation. Chest 1992; 101:1342–1351.
52. Hickling KG, Walsh J, Henderson S, Jackson R. Low mortality rate in adult respiratory distress syndrome using low-volume, pressure-limited ventilation with permissive hypercapnia: a prospective study. Crit Care Med 1994; 22:1568–1578.
53. Amato MB, Barbas CS, Medeiros DM, et al. Effect of a protective-ventilation strategy on mortality in the acute respiratory distress syndrome. N Engl J Med 1998; 338:347–354.
54. Rappaport SH, Shpiner R, Yoshihara G, et al. Randomized, prospective trial of pressure-limited versus volume-controlled ventilation in severe respiratory failure. Crit Care Med 1994; 22:22–32.
55. Marini JJ, Capps JS, Culver BH. The inspiratory work of breathing during assisted mechanical ventilation. Chest 1985; 87:612–618.
56. Marini JJ, Rodriquez RM, Lamb V. The inspiratory workload of patient-initiated mechanical ventilation. Am Rev Respir Dis 1986; 134:902–909.
57. Cinnella G, Conti G, Lofaso F, et al. Effects of assisted ventilation on the work of breathing: volume-controlled versus pressure-controlled ventilation. Am J Respir Crit Care Med 1996; 153:1025–1033.
58. MacIntyre NR, McConnell R, Cheng KG, Sane A. Patient-ventilator flow dyssynchrony: flow-limited versus pressure-limited breaths. Crit Care Med 1997; 25:1671–1677.

59. Gurevitch MJ, Van Dyke J, Young ES, Jackson K. Improved oxygenation and lower peak airway pressure in severe adult respiratory distress syndrome. Treatment with inverse ratio ventilation. Chest 1986; 89:211–213.

60. Lain DC, DiBenedetto R, Morris SL, Van Nguyen A. Pressure control inverse ratio ventilation as a method to reduce peak inspiratory pressure and provide adequate ventilation and oxygenation. Chest 1989; 95:1081–1088.

61. Tharratt RS, Allen RP, Albertson TE. Pressure controlled inverse ratio ventilation in severe adult respiratory failure. Chest 1988; 94:755–762.

62. Abraham E, Yoshihara G. Cardiorespiratory effects of pressure controlled inverse ratio ventilation in severe respiratory failure. Chest 1989; 96:1356–1359.

63. Mang H, Kacmarek RM, Ritz R, et al. Cardiorespiratory effects of volume and pressure controlled ventilation at various I:E ratios in an acute lung injury model. Am J Respir Crit Care Med 1995; 151:731–736.

64. Ludwigs U, Klingstedt C, Baehrendty S, et al. Volume-controlled inverse ratio ventilation in oleic acid induced lung injury: effects on gas exchange, hemodynamics, and computed tomographic lung density. Chest 1995; 108:804–809.

65. Willms D, Nield M, Gocka I. Adult respiratory distress syndrome: outcome in a community hospital. Am J Crit Care 1994; 3:337–341.

66. Chan C, Abraham E. Effects of inverse ratio ventilation on cardiorespiratory parameters in sever respiratory failure. Chest 1992; 102:1556–1561.

67. Lessard MR, Guerot E, Lorino, et al. Effects of pressure-controlled with different I:E ratios versus volume-controlled ventilation on respiratory mechanics, gas exchange, and hemodynamics in patients with adult respiratory distress syndrome. Anesthesiology 1994; 80:983–991.

68. Mercat A, Titiriga M, Anguel N, et al. Inverse ratio ventilation (I/E = 2/1) in acute respiratory distress syndrome: a six-hour controlled study. Am J Respir Crit Care Med 1997; 155:1637–1642.

69. Mercat A, Graini L, Teboul J, et al. Cardiorespiratory effects of pressure-controlled ventilation with and without inverse ratio in the adult respiratory distress syndrome. Chest 1993; 104:871–875.

70. Zavala E, Ferrer M, Polese G, et al. Effect of inverse I:E ratio ventilation on pulmonary gas exchange in acute respiratory distress syndrome. Anesthesiology 1998; 88:35–42.

71. Yanos J, Watling SM, Verhey J. The physiologic effects of inverse ratio ventilation. Chest 1998; 114:834–838.

72. Gore DC. Hemodynamic and ventilatory effects associated with increasing inverse inspiratory-expiratory ventilation. J Trauma 1998; 45:268–272.

73. Armstrong BW, MacIntyre NR. Pressure-controlled, inverse ratio ventilation that avoids air trapping in the adult respiratory distress syndrome. Crit Care Med 1995; 23:279–285.

74. Kacmarek RM, Hess D. Pressure-controlled inverse-ratio ventilation: panacea or auto-PEEP (editorial). Respir Care 1990; 35:945–948.

75. Kacmarek RM, Kirmse M, Nishimura M, et al. The effects of applied versus auto-PEEP on local lung unit pressure and volume in a four-unit lung model. Chest 1995; 108:1073–1079.

76. Medoff BD, Harris RS, Kesselman H, et al. Use of recruitment maneuvers and

high positive end-expiratory pressure in a patient with acute respiratory distress syndrome. Crit Care Med 2000; 28:1210–1216.

77. Brochard L, Pluskwa F, Lemaire F. Improved efficacy of spontaneous breathing with inspiratory pressure support. Am Rev Respir Dis 1997; 136:411–415.

78. Kreit JW, Capper MW, Eschenbacher WL. Patient work of breathing during pressure support and volume-cycled mechanical ventilation. Am J Respir Crit Care Med 1994; 149:1085–1091.

79. Girault C, Jean-Christophe R, Chevron V, et al. Comparative physiologic effects of noninvasive assist-control and pressure support ventilation in acute hypercapnic respiratory failure. Chest 1997; 111:1639–1648.

80. Brochard L. Pressure-support ventilation: still a simple mode? Intensive Care Med 1996; 22:1137–1138.

81. Campbell RS, Branson RD. Ventilatory support for the 90s: pressure support ventilation. Respir Care 1993; 38:526–537.

82. MacIntyre N, Nishimura M, Usada Y, et al. The Nagoya conference on system design and patient-ventilator interactions during pressure support ventilation. Chest 1990; 97:1463–1466.

83. Branson RD, Campbell RS. Pressure support ventilation, patient-ventilator synchrony, and ventilator algorithms (editorial). Respir Care 1998; 43:1045–1047.

84. Fabry B, Guttmann J, Eberhard L, et al. An analysis of desynchronization between the spontaneously breathing patient and ventilator during inspiratory pressure support. Chest 1995; 107:1387–1394.

85. Jubran A, van de Graff W, Tobin MJ. Variability of patient-ventilator interaction with pressure support ventilation in patients with chronic obstructive pulmonary disease. Am J Respir Crit Care Med 1995; 152:129–136.

86. Parthasarathy S, Jubran A, Tobin MJ. Cycling of inspiratory and expiratory muscle groups with the ventilator in airflow limitation. Am J Respir Crit Care Med 1998; 158:1471–1478.

87. Yamada Y, Du H. Effects of different pressure support termination on patient-ventilator synchrony. Respir Care 1998; 43:1048–1057.

88. Nava S, Bruschi C, Rubini F, et al. Respiratory response and inspiratory effort during pressure support ventilation in COPD patients. Intensive Care Med 1995; 21:871–879.

89. Nava S, Bruschi C, Fracchia C, et al. Patient-ventilator interaction and inspiratory effort during pressure support ventilation in patients with different pathologies. Eur Respir J 1997; 10:177–183.

90. MacIntyre NR, Ho L. Effects of initial flow rate and breath termination criteria on pressure support ventilation. Chest 1991; 99:134–138.

91. Branson RD, Campbell R, Davis K, et al. Comparison of the effects of pressure support ventilation delivered by two ventilators. Respir Care 1990; 35:1049–1055.

92. Branson RD, Campbell RS, Davis K, et al. Altering flowrate during maximum pressure support ventilation (PSVmax): Effects on cardiorespiratory function. Respir Care 1990; 35:1056–1064.

93. Bonmarchand G, Chevron V, Chopin C, et al. Increased initial flow rate reduces inspiratory work of breathing during pressure support ventilation in patients with

exacerbation of chronic obstructive pulmonary disease. Intensive Care Med 1996; 22:1147–1154.

94. Mancebo J, Amaro P, Mollo JL, et al. Comparison of the effects of pressure support ventilation delivered by three different ventilators during weaning from mechanical ventilation. Intensive Care Med 1995; 21:913–919.

95. Cohen IL, Bilen Z, Krishnamurthy S. The effects of ventilator working pressure during pressure support ventilation. Chest 1993; 103:588–592.

96. Bonmarchand G, Chevron V, Menard J, et al. Effects of pressure ramp slope values on the work of breathing during pressure support ventilation in restrictive patients. Crit Care Med 1999; 27:715–722.

97. Jubran A. Inspiratory flow: more may not be better (editorial). Crit Care Med 1999; 27:670–671.

98. Puddy A, Younes M. Effect of inspiratory flow rate on respiratory output in normal subjects. Am Rev Respir Dis 1992; 146:787–789.

99. Georgopoulos D, Mitrouska I, Bshouty Z, et al. Effect of breathing route, temperature and volume of inspired gas and airway anesthesia on the response of respiratory output to varying inspiratory flow. Am J Respir Crit Care Med 1996; 153:168–175.

100. Corne S, Gillespie D, Roberts D, et al. Effect of inspiratory flow rate on respiratory rate in intubated ventilated patients. Am J Respir Crit Care Med 1997; 156:304–308.

101. Manning HL, Molinary EJ, Leiter JC. Effect of inspiratory flow rate on respiratory sensation and pattern of breathing. Am J Respir Crit Care Med 1995; 151:751–757.

102. Fernandez R, Mendez M, Younes M. Effect of ventilator flow rate on respiratory timing in normal subjects. Am J Respir Crit Care Med 1999; 159:710–719.

103. Younes M, Puddy A, Roberts D, et al. Proportional assist ventilation. Results of an initial clinical trial. Am Rev Respir Dis 1992; 145:121–129.

104. Younes M. Proportional assist ventilation, a new approach to ventilatory support. Theory. Am Rev Respir Dis 1992; 145:114–120.

105. Poon CS, Ward SA, Whipp BJ. Influence of inspiratory assistance on ventilatory control during moderate exercise. J Appl Physiol 1987; 62:551–560.

106. Harries JR, Tyler JM. Mechanical assistance to respiration in emphysema. Results of a patient-controlled servo-respirator. Am J Med 1964; 36:68–78.

107. Younes M, Bilan D, Jung D, et al. An apparatus for altering the mechanical load of the respiratory system. J Appl Physiol 1987; 62:2491–2499.

108. Meza S, Younes M. Ventilatory stability during sleep studied with proportional assist ventilation (PAV). Sleep 1996; 19:S164–S166.

109. Younes M. Patient-ventilator interaction with pressure-assisted modalities of ventilatory support. Semin Respir Med 1993; 14:299–322.

110. Mead J, Agostoni E. Dynamics of breathing. In: Fenn WO, Rhan H, eds. Handbook of Physiology. Washington, DC: American Physiologic Society, 1964:411–422.

111. Ambrosino N, Vitacca M, Polese G, et al. Short-term effects of nasal proportional assist ventilation in patients with chronic hypercapnic respiratory insufficiency. Eur Respir J 1997; 10:2829–2834.

112. Gay P, Hess D, Hollets S, et al. A randomized, prospective trial of noninvasive

proportional assist ventilation vs. pressure support ventilation to treat acute respiratory insufficiency (abstr). Am J Respir Crit Care Med 1999; 159:A14.

113. Patrick W, Webster K, Ludwig L, et al. Noninvasive positive-pressure ventilation in acute respiratory distress without prior chronic respiratory failure. Am J Respir Crit Care Med 1996; 153:1005–1111.

114. Bigatello LM, Nishimura M, Imanaka H, et al. Unloading of the work of breathing by proportional assist ventilation in a lung model. Crit Care Med 1997; 25:267–272.

115. Ranieri VM, Grasso S, Mascia L, et al. Effects of proportional assist ventilation on inspiratory muscle effort in patients with chronic obstructive pulmonary disease and acute respiratory failure. Anesthesiology 1997; 86:79–91.

116. Ranieri VM, Giuliani R, Mascia L, et al. Patient-ventilator interaction during acute hypercapnia: pressure support vs. proportional assist ventilation. J Appl Physiol 1996; 81:426–436.

117. Marantz S, Patrick W, Webster K, et al. Response of ventilator-dependent patients to different levels of proportional assist. J Appl Physiol 1996; 80:397–403.

118. Bianchi L, Foglio K, Pagani M, et al. Effects of proportional assist ventilation on exercise tolerance in COPD patients with chronic hypercapnia. Eur Respir J 1998; 11:422–427.

119. Appendini L, Purro A, Gudjonsdottir M, et al. Physiologic response of ventilator-dependent patients with chronic obstructive pulmonary disease to proportional assist ventilation and continuous airway positive pressure. Am J Respir Crit Care Med 1999; 159:1510–1517.

120. Giannouli E, Webster K, Roberts D, et al. Response of ventilator-dependent patients to different levels of pressure support and proportional assist. Am J Respir Crit Care Med 1999; 159:1716–1725.

121. Kil HK, Bishop MJ. Head position and oral vs nasal route as factors determining endotracheal tube resistance. Chest 1994; 105:1794–1797.

122. Guttman J, Eberhard L, Fabry B, et al. Continuous calculation of intratracheal pressure in tracheally intubated patients. Anesthesiology 1993; 79:503–513.

123. Gal TJ. Pulmonary mechanics in normal subjects following endotracheal intubation. Anesthesiology 1980; 52:27–35.

124. Bolder PM, Healey TEJ, Bolder AR, et al. The extra work of breathing through adult endotracheal tubes. Anesth Analg 1986; 65:853–859.

125. Conti G, De Blasi RA, Lappa A, et al. Evaluation of respiratory system resistance in mechanically ventilated patients: the role of the endotracheal tube. Intensive Care Med 1994; 20:421–424.

126. Heyer L, Louis B, Isabey D, et al. Noninvasive estimate of work of breathing due to the endotracheal tube. Anesthesiology 1996; 85:1324–1333.

127. Lofaso F, Louis B, Brochard L, et al. Use of the Blasius resistance formula to estimate the effective diameter of endotracheal tubes. Am Rev Respir Dis 1992; 146:974–979.

128. Sullivan M, Paliotta J, Sakland M. Endotracheal tube as a factor in measurement of respiratory mechanics. J Appl Physiol 1976; 41:590–592.

129. Tipping TR, Sykes MK. Tracheal tube resistance and airway and alveolar pressures during mechanical ventilation in the neonate. Anaesthesia 1991; 46:565–569.

130. Shapiro M, Wilson RK, Casar G, et al. Work of breathing through different sized endotracheal tubes. Crit Care Med 1986; 14:1028–1031.
131. Yung MW, Snowdon SL. Respiratory resistance of tracheostomy tubes. Arch Otolaryngol 1984; 110:591–595.
132. van Surell C, Louis B, Lofaso F, et al. Acoustic method to estimate the longitudinal area profile of endotracheal tubes. Am J Respir Crit Care Med 1994; 149:28–33.
133. Wright PE, Marini JJ, Bernard GR. In-vitro versus in-vivo comparison of endotracheal tube airflow resistance. Am Rev Respir Dis 1989; 140:10–16.
134. Diehl J, el Atrous S, Touchard D, et al. Changes in the work of breathing induced by tracheotomy in ventilator-dependent patients. Am J Respir Crit Care Med 1999; 159:383–388.
135. Brochard L, Rua F, Lorino H, et al. Inspiratory pressure support compensates for the additional work of breathing caused by the endotracheal tube. Anesthesiology 1991; 75:739–745.
136. Fiastro JF, Habib MP, Quan SF. Pressure support compensation for inspiratory work due to endotracheal tubes and demand continuous positive airway pressure. Chest 1988; 93:499–505.
137. Ranieri VM. Optimization of patient-ventilator interactions: closed-loop technology to turn the century. Intensive Care Med 1997; 23:936–939.
138. Fabry B, Guttman J, Eberhard L, et al. Automatic compensation of endotracheal tube resistance in spontaneous breathing patients. Technol Health Care 1994; 1: 281–291.
139. Fabry B, Haberthur C, Zappe D, et al. Breathing pattern and additional work of breathing in spontaneously breathing patients with different ventilatory demands during inspiratory pressure support and automatic tube compensation. Intensive Care Med 1997; 23:545–552.
140. Guttmann J, Bernhard H, Mols G, et al. Respiratory comfort of automatic tube compensation and inspiratory pressure support in conscious humans. Intensive Care Med 1997; 23:1119–1124.
141. Stocker R, Fabry B, Haberthur C. New modes of ventilatory support in spontaneously breathing intubated patients. In: Vincent JL, ed. Yearbook of Intensive Care and Emergency Medicine. 1997:514–533.
142. Kuhlen R, Rossaint R. Electronic extubation—Is it worth trying? (editorial). Intensive Care Med 1997; 23:1105–1107.
143. Esteban A, Alia I, Gordo F, et al. Extubation outcome after spontaneous breathing trials with T-tube or pressure support ventilation. The Spanish Lung Failure Collaborative Group. Am J Respir Crit Care Med 1997; 156:459–465.
144. Straus C, Louis B, Isabey D, et al. Contribution of the endotracheal tube and the upper airway to breathing workload. Am J Respir Crit Care Med 1998; 157:23–30.
145. Bratzke E, Downs JB, Smith RA. Intermittent CPAP: a new mode of ventilation during general anesthesia. Anesthesiology 1998; 89:334–340.
146. Cane RD, Peruzzi WT, Shapiro BA. Airway pressure release ventilation in severe acute respiratory failure. Chest 1991; 100:460–463.
147. Davis K, Johnson DJ, Branson RD, et al. Airway pressure release ventilation. Arch Surg 1993; 128:1348–1352.

148. Falkenhain SK, Reilley TE, Gregory JS. Improvement in cardiac output during airway pressure release ventilation. Crit Care Med 1992; 20:1358–1360.
149. Florete OG, Banner MJ, Banner TE, et al. Airway pressure release ventilation in a patient with acute pulmonary injury. Chest 1989; 96:679–682.
150. Rasanen J, Cane RD, Downs JB, et al. Airway pressure release ventilation during acute lung injury: a prospective multicenter trial. Crit Care Med 1991; 19:1234–1241.
151. Silver MR. BIPAP: Useful new modality or confusing acronym? (editorial). Crit Care Med 1998; 26:1473–1474.
152. Staudinger T, Kordova H, Roggla M, et al. Comparison of oxygen cost of breathing with pressure-support ventilation and biphasic intermittent positive airway pressure ventilation. Crit Care Med 1998; 26:1518–1522.
153. Calzia E, Linder KH, Witt S, et al. Pressure-time product and work of breathing during biphasic continuous positive airway pressure and assisted spontaneous breathing. Am J Respir Crit Care Med 1994; 150:904–910.
154. Kiehl M, Schiele C, Stenzinger W, Kienast J. Volume-controlled versus biphasic positive airway pressure ventilation in leukopenic patients with severe respiratory failure. Crit Care Med 1996; 24:780–784.
155. Kirmse M, Fujino Y, Hromi J, et al. Pressure-release tracheal gas insufflation (TGI) reduces airway pressures in lung injured sheep maintaining eucapnia. Am J Respir Crit Care Med 1999; 160:1462–1467.
156. Rouby JJ, Ameur B, Jawish D, et al. Continuous positive airway pressure (CPAP) vs. intermittent mandatory pressure release ventilation (IMPRV) in patients with acute respiratory failure. Intensive Care Med 1992; 18:69–75.
157. Rasanen J. IMPRV—synchronized APRV, or more? (editorial). Intensive Care Med 1992; 18:65–66.
158. Branson RD, MacIntyre NR. Dual-control modes of mechanical ventilation. Respir Care 1996; 41:294–305.
159. MacIntyre NR, Gropper C, Westfall T. Combining pressure limiting and volume cycling features in a patient-interactive mechanical ventilation. Crit Care Med 1994; 22:353–357.
160. Haas CF, Branson RD, Folk LM, et al. Patient determined inspiratory flow during assisted mechanical ventilation. Respir Care 1995; 40:716–721.
161. Chatburn RL. Reply to Blanch and Desautels (letter). Respir Care 1994; 39:764–772.
162. Amato MBP, Barbos CSV, Bonassa J, et al. Volume assisted pressure support ventilation (VAPSV): a new approach for reducing muscle workload during acute respiratory failure. Chest 1992; 102:1225–1234.
163. Keenan HT, Martin LD. Volume support ventilation in infants and children: analysis of a case series. Respir Care 1997; 42:281–287.
164. Piotrowski A, Sobala W, Kawczynski P. Patient initiated, pressure regulated, volume controlled ventilation compared with intermittent mandatory ventilation in neonates: a prospective, randomised study. Intensive Care Med 1997; 23:975–981.
165. Alvarez A, Subirana M, Benito S. Decelerating flow ventilation effects in acute respiratory failure. J Crit Care 1998; 13:21–25.
166. Kesecioglu J, Telci L, Tutuncu AS, et al. Effects of volume controlled ventilation

with PEEP, pressure regulated volume controlled ventilation and low frequency positive pressure ventilation with extracorporeal carbon dioxide removal on total static lung compliance and oxygenation in pigs with ARDS. Adv Exp Med Biol 1996; 388:629–636.

167. Kesecioglu J, Gultuna I, Pompe JC, et al. Assessment of ventilation inhomogeneity and gas exchange with volume controlled ventilation and pressure regulated volume controlled ventilation on pigs with surfactant depleted lungs. Adv Exp Med Biol 1996; 388:539–544.

168. Hewlett AM, Platt AS, Terry VG. Mandatory minute volume. Anesthesia 1977; 32:163–169.

169. Quan SF, Parides GC, Knoper SR. Mandatory minute volume (MMV) ventilation: an overview. Respir Care 1990; 35:898–905.

170. East TD, Elkhuizen PHM, Pace NL. Pressure support with mandatory minute ventilation supplied by the Ohmeda CPU-1 prevents hypoventilation due to respiratory depression in a canine model. Respir Care 1989; 34:795–800.

171. Quan SF. Mandatory minute ventilation. In: Tobin MJ, ed. Principles and Practice of Mechanical Ventilation. New York: McGraw-Hill, 1994:333–339.

172. Otis AB, Fenn WO, Rahn H. Mechanics of breathing in man. J Appl Physiol 1950; 2:592–607.

173. Iotti GA, Braschi A, Brunner JX, et al. Respiratory mechanics by least squares fitting in mechanically ventilated patients: applications during paralysis and during pressure support ventilation. Intensive Care Med 1995; 21:406–413.

174. Weiler N, Heinrichs W, Kessler W. The AVL-mode: a safe closed loop algorithm for ventilation during total intravenous anesthesia. Int J Clin Monit Comput 1994; 11:85–88.

175. Weiler N, Eberle B, Heinrichs W. Adaptive lung ventilation (AVL) during anesthesia for pulmonary surgery: automatic response to transitions to and from one-lung ventilation. J Clin Monit 1998; 14:245–252.

176. Laubscher TP, Frutiger A, Fanconi S, et al. Automatic selection of tidal volume, respiratory frequency and minute ventilation in intubated ICU patients as start up procedure for closed-loop controlled ventilation. Int J Clin Monit Comput 1994; 11:19–30.

177. Laubscher TP, Frutiger A; Fanconi S; Brunner JX. The automatic selection of ventilation parameters during the initial phase of mechanical ventilation. Intensive Care Med 1996; 22:199–207.

178. Linton DM, Potgieter PD, Davis S, et al. Automatic weaning from mechanical ventilation using an adaptive lung controller. Chest 1994; 106:1843–1850.

179. Weiler N, Eberle B, Latorre F, et al. Adaptive lung ventilation. Anaesthetist 1996; 45:950–956.

180. Campbell RS, Sinamban RP, Johannigman JA, et al. Clinical evaluation of a new closed loop ventilation mode: adaptive support ventilation. Respir Care 1998; 43: 856.

8

Closed Loop Mechanical Ventilation

BRIAN A. KIMBLE and MITCHELL M. LEVY

Brown University School of Medicine
Providence, Rhode Island

I. Introduction

In the 30 years since their introduction, positive pressure mechanical ventilators have become increasingly complex. From the original controlled mechanical ventilation (CMV) mode, the number of ventilatory modes has increased dramatically to include other volume preset modes (assist control, synchronized intermittent mandatory ventilation), pressure preset modes (pressure control ventilation, pressure support ventilation), mixed modes (pressure-regulated volume control), and high-frequency modes (high-frequency jet ventilation). While it is true that some modes may promote better patient-ventilator interaction in a given situation or offer theoretical advantages in gas exchange, there are currently no studies showing that any one mode is "superior" with regard to patient outcomes. Until recently (1) there were insufficient data to conclude that the manner in which clinicians ventilate patients has an impact on survival at all. So while ventilators have become more and more complex, it is unclear whether this increased complexity translates into better patient care and improved clinical outcomes. While still in its infancy, closed loop ventilation (CLV) has the potential to simplify the clinician's task of adjusting the ventilator and to do this in a more timely manner than is possible with current ventilators.

II.   What Is Closed Loop Ventilation?

The goal of CLV is for the ventilator to dynamically adjust itself to the changing ventilatory needs of the patient without clinician intervention. In a manner analogous to the process used by clinicians, the ventilator acquires relevant data inputs, analyzes these data to determine if a problem exists with the current ventilator settings, and then institutes appropriate changes.

A good example of a closed loop system is the household thermostat. The occupants set a desired temperature, the actual temperature is measured by a thermometer, and the two values are compared. If the desired and actual temperatures do not agree, the system makes adjustments to either increase or decrease the temperature as needed. While it would be possible to manually adjust the temperature in the household, the presence of the closed loop system is more convenient and efficient. It continuously monitors and adjusts the temperature in a dynamic manner that minimizes extremes of temperature fluctuation.

Obviously, the management of mechanically ventilated patients is a far more challenging task than regulating household temperature. What input variables are important? Should some be given more weight than others? Is there more than one way to interpret the variables, and, if so, how does one decide on the "correct" interpretation? Finally, what is the optimal change in ventilator settings based on this interpretation? These questions are often difficult for a skilled clinician to answer, and the problem is magnified when trying to develop a computer algorithm to address them.

III.   Computer Decision Support Systems Versus True Closed Loops

There are many different ways to use computers in the care of mechanically ventilated patients. A CLV strategy will adjust ventilator settings based on monitored variables obtained from patient data. Not only does the ventilator acquire and analyze these patient data, it adjusts its own operation to reflect the patient's current ventilatory status. The approach is somewhat different in a computerized decision support process. In a series of papers published between 1989 and 1993, Morris and coworkers (2–9) described their experience with a computer decision support system aimed at assisting clinicians in adjusting ventilator settings. The system described by Morris et al. generated computer-derived recommendations based on data input by physicians, nurses, respiratory therapists, and the laboratory. Implementation of these recommendations was the responsibility of the medical team caring for the patient. Thus, this system is an example of an open loop that requires active intervention by clinicians, rather than a true closed loop.

IV. How Does Closed Loop Ventilation Work?

The traditional interface between clinician and ventilator involves the integration of data pertaining to gas exchange and pulmonary mechanics into a ventilatory strategy. If a ventilator is to qualify as a closed loop system, it must mimic this process of data acquisition and analysis. A true closed loop ventilator must also have the ability to appropriately adjust itself based on this information to optimize ventilatory support and facilitate the weaning process, all under dynamic conditions.

V. Inputs

What possible variables can be incorporated into ventilatory strategies? In order for CLV to function at a high level, the ventilator should incorporate as many patient-derived variables as possible into a presigned ventilatory strategy. Some of the possible inputs to the CLV system include variables relating to gas exchange ($Paco_2$, pH, Pao_2, Sao_2), pulmonary mechanics (compliance, resistance, intrinsic PEEP), and patient respiratory drive ($P_{0.1}$). While other factors, such as hemodynamics, may influence clinical decision making and should ideally be incorporated as inputs into a strategy for CLV, they are not available on the current generation of ventilators.

VI. Gas Exchange

A. Ventilation

In order to accurately determine minute ventilation requirements, it is necessary to have measurements of CO_2 production, $Paco_2$, and pH. Currently available ventilators lack the ability to measure and integrate these variables. Although not commercially available, several systems relying on end-tidal CO_2 as a marker of the adequacy of ventilation have been developed which operate in a closed loop fashion (10–14). One potential problem that arises from utilizing end-tidal CO_2 concentration is that this method fails to differentiate between alveolar hyperventilation and increased physiological dead space. Ohlson and coworkers (10) examined dogs ventilated with this type of closed loop ventilator. When they increased physiological dead space by either blocking one branch of the pulmonary artery or injecting air into the venous system, the $Paco_2$ increased. However, the end-tidal CO_2, as one would expect, fell as a result of the increased dead space. This decrease in end-tidal CO_2 was interpreted by the ventilator as a signal that the experimental animal was being hyperventilated. It thus responded by lowering minute ventilation, which resulted in a further increase in $Paco_2$. While such dramatic alterations in the ventilation/perfusion ratio are not common in clinical practice, they do occur (e.g., massive pulmonary embolus). In such cases the end-tidal CO_2 is not an accurate reflection of the patient's $Paco_2$. For this reason ventilators relying on this parameter may not provide appropriate levels of ventilation.

B. Oxygenation

While several decision support systems incorporate Pao_2 in their algorithms, the current generation of closed loop mechanical ventilators have failed to do so. Likely this is due to the problems and expense associated with in-line blood gas analyzers in clinical practice. As these devices become reliable, cost-effective, and widely available, closed loop ventilators may be able to adjust the Fio_2 and PEEP levels to optimize oxygenation, as well as assess ventilation by means of $Paco_2$ and pH.

VII. Mechanics

Perhaps the most important aspect of the current generation of closed loop ventilators is their ability to measure pulmonary mechanics on a breath-by-breath basis. Pulmonary mechanics play an important role in the clinical assessment of mechanically ventilated patients. For example, compliance can serve as an indicator of disease severity in the acute respiratory distress syndrome (ARDS), and persistently elevated resistance can indicate the need for additional therapy in reactive airways disease. Ventilators capable of accurately assessing pulmonary mechanics on a breath-by-breath basis could not only provide clinicians with information about a patient's compliance (C), resistance (R), and intrinsic positive end expiratory pressure $(PEEP_i)$, but could also potentially incorporate these variables into a closed loop ventilation strategy.

Mathematically, pulmonary mechanics can be expressed by the following equation (15):

$$\Delta P = \frac{1}{C} \cdot V + R \cdot V' + I \cdot V'' \tag{1}$$

where ΔP is transpulmonary pressure, C is compliance, V is lung volume, R is resistance, V' is gas flow (dV/dt), I is inertance, and V'' is gas acceleration (d^2V/dt^2). Equation (1) represents the flow of liquid through a tube or, in the case of respiration, of air through the lungs. This equation assumes a one compartment lung model, meaning that resistance and compliance are equal throughout the lungs, as if there were one conducting airway and one giant alveolus. While many disease states such as COPD and ARDS are characterized by regional differences in compliance and resistance, it is common practice to apply Eq. (1) when describing the behavior of the respiratory system with mathematical modeling.

As shown by Mead (16), inertance accounts for less than 5% of the total pressure change and for this reason is often dropped, yielding the simplified equation:

$$\Delta P = \frac{1}{C} \cdot V + R \cdot V' \tag{2}$$

During passive ventilation of intubated patients, transpulmonary pressure equals airway pressure (P_{aw}) minus total PEEP ($PEEP_{tot}$). With this information in mind, Eq. (2) can be modified to read:

$$(P_{aw} - PEEP_{tot}) = \frac{1}{C} \cdot V + R \cdot V' \tag{3}$$

At the bedside, clinicians routinely calculate values for C, R, and $PEEP_{tot}$ by performing simple maneuvers on standard ventilators. Compliance is calculated after performing an end-inspiratory hold (to measure plateau pressure, P_{plat}) and an end-expiratory hold (to measure $PEEP_{tot}$). Since flow is zero during these maneuvers, the resistance term cancels out of Eq. (3). To obtain the compliance, the tidal volume is divided by the difference in measured pressures, as shown in Eq. (4):

$$C = \frac{V}{(P_{plat} - PEEP_{tot})} \tag{4}$$

In order to calculate resistance, an end-inspiratory hold is applied. The difference between the pressure just prior to the occlusion (P_{peak}) and after occlusion (P_{plat}) represents the ΔP from Eq. (2). Since there is no volume change, the compliance term cancels out. The change in pressure following the hold maneuver is divided by the flow rate, yielding the value for resistance as shown in Eq. (5):

$$R = \frac{(P_{peak} - P_{plat})}{V'} \tag{5}$$

While simple to perform, calculation of pulmonary mechanics in this manner has its drawbacks. A constant flow rate must be maintained throughout the breath in order to obtain an accurate measurement of resistance. It is therefore impossible to measure this variable in decelerating flow modes such as pressure control ventilation (PCV) or pressure support ventilation (PSV). Performance of occlusion maneuvers requires a brief interruption of ventilation and the presence of trained personnel. Additionally, the values of C, R, and $PEEP_{tot}$ reflect a measurement at a single point in time and do not account for the dynamic character of pulmonary mechanics in an acutely ill patient.

A. Least-Squares-Fit Method for Determining Pulmonary Mechanics

Over the past several years, as microprocessor and ventilator function have become more integrated, mathematical models have been borrowed from the field of engineering. This has allowed for the calculation of pulmonary mechanics on a breath-by-breath basis without the need for hold maneuvers or constant flow rates. The most widely employed of these models is the least-squares-fit (LSF) method, first described in 1969 by Wald et al. (17) and soon modified into a more practical form by Uhl and Lewis (15). For continuous data, Eq. (3) can be modified to read:

$$P_{aw}(t) = \frac{1}{C} \cdot V(t) + R \cdot V'(t) + \text{PEEP}_{tot} \tag{6}$$

where $P_{aw}(t)$ is airway pressure at time t, $V(t)$ is volume at time t, and $V'(t)$ is air flow at time t. $P_{aw}(t)$ and $V'(t)$ are measured variables. $V(t)$ is the area under the flow curve or the integral of $V'(t)$. This leaves three unknowns, C, R, and PEEP_{tot}, which are assumed to remain constant throughout each breath. To solve for these three variables, it is necessary to have three equations describing them. Modern closed loop ventilators utilizing an LSF algorithm sample airway pressure and flow data at 60 cycles/s. For a ventilator rate of 20 breaths/min, this means that each breath lasts approximately 3 s, yielding roughly 180 separate equations per breath from which to solve for the three variables. How does the LSF algorithm determine the "true" values of C, R, and PEEP_{tot}. After the initial 0.05 s of a breath, the ventilator has acquired three sets of data and can solve for the three unknowns. With values for C, R, and PEEP_{tot}, the ventilator can then predict based on Eq. (6) subsequent values of $P_{aw}(t)$ for any given $V(t)$ and $V'(t)$. These predicted values are compared to the actual values as they become available throughout the breath. C, R, and PEEP_{tot} are then recalculated as necessary to minimize the sum of the squared differences between the predicted and actual values of $P_{aw}(t)$. Mathematically, C, R, and PEEP_{tot} are solved for values that produce the minimum error, ϵ, where:

$$\varepsilon = \Sigma \, (P_{aw}(t)_{meas} - P_{aw}(t)_{pred})^2 \tag{7}$$

One early challenge facing researchers was noise inherent in the data obtained during inspiration and expiration. This results from numerous factors such as turbulence in the pneumatic system, mechanical movement, mucus in the trachea, and sensor noise. Since measurements are obtained on the order of milliseconds and the model is a recursive one, any random variation in the measured parameters can have profound effects on the computed best fit curve. This is especially true when all the incoming data are similar with a small number of random outliers. In this instance the system may place undue importance on these anomalous data points. This problem may be addressed by filtering the incoming data in an attempt to minimize the effect of outlying signals. The potential drawback to this approach is that rapid changes in respiratory mechanics (i.e., due to bronchoconstriction) may be erroneously filtered out.

Lauzon et al. (18) developed an estimator to test the ability of an LSF model to successfully filter out random noise and at the same time correctly identify rapid changes in pulmonary mechanics. This algorithm performed well when confronted with computer-generated data simulating rapid changes in airways resistance. The algorithm was then applied to experimental animals given a methacholine challenge. Qualitatively appropriate results were observed (i.e., a rise in the calculated resistance following methacholine admininstration), but since resistance and compliance were not measured by traditional methods, this study cannot address the accuracy of the LSF method.

Another potential problem with the LSF method relates to the ability of the system to accurately identify the beginning and end of each breath. Theoretically, since volume is calculated from the flow data, if the initial portion of the breath is not determined accurately, the calculated values for C, R, and $PEEP_i$ may be incorrect. This error could be magnified by modes of ventilation with high initial flow rates, such as pressure control or pressure support ventilation. To investigate this potential concern, Stegmaier and colleagues (19) studied four patients undergoing general anesthesia with muscle relaxation to examine the effect of imprecise breath detection on the calculated values of C, R, and $PEEP_i$. All four patients were ventilated in a volume control mode with a square inspiratory flow pattern. Reference detection of the beginning of inspiration and end of expiration was determined by inline capnography as described by Brunner et al. (20). Using these time points, the data obtained from the patients were divided into discrete breaths, and the values for C, R, and $PEEP_i$ were calculated using the LSF method. The boundaries for the beginning and end of each breath were then shifted back and forth in 16.7 ms intervals to include or exclude the intervening points of data. Values for C, R, and $PEEP_i$ were recalculated based on these "shifted" data windows and compared to the original calculated values. A shift in the initial part of the window corresponding to onset of inspiration by ± 0.5 s did not significantly affect the calculation of C or R. However, a delay in the window start did have a significant effect on the values of $PEEP_i$. The mean error was 20% when the initial portion of the breath was missed by 0.1 s and rose to a mean error of 53% when the initial 0.3 s of data was missed. Shifts in the terminal portion of the data window did not produce significant errors with respect to C or R, while the relative error in $PEEP_i$ remained below 7%. The nonsignificant difference in C and R despite significant errors in $PEEP_i$ can be explained by the observation that values of $PEEP_i$ in these patients was relatively small (4.5 ± 3.4 cm H_2O). Thus the 20% or 53% errors in $PEEP_i$ had minimal effect on C and R as calculated in Eq. (6). While not addressed in this study, imprecise breath detection could significantly affect C and R values in patient populations with higher levels of $PEEP_i$, as in those with obstructive lung disease or high respiratory rates. In these patients, the calculated errors in $PEEP_i$ could have a more profound effect on the calculated values of C and R. Additionally, imprecise breath detection in patients on pressure present modes could significantly impair the ability of the ventilator to accurately calculate C, R, and $PEEP_i$, since the high initial flow rates cause a greater proportion of the tidal volume to be delivered early in the breath. These issues have not been investigated to date and are of potential clinical relevance.

B.   Validation Studies: Least-Squares-Fit Method

Having addressed some of the potential problems with the technical aspects of the LSF method, how well does it compare to standard methods of deriving pulmonary mechanics? Avanzolini and colleagues (21) studied mechanically ventilated human subjects using an estimator similar to that described by Lauzon et al. In this study, respiratory mechanics were monitored using an LSF algorithm in four postoperative cardiac patients. Four different breathing patterns were evaluated: either a high or low respiratory rate (keeping minute ventilation at approximately 10 L/min) in combination with either a square or ascending/descending flow pattern. In most cases, the calculated values of resistance and elastance (the inverse of compliance) were significantly different depending upon which respiratory rate and flow pattern were used. Static measurements were not obtained, making it difficult to assess the accuracy of the derived variables. Of note, for a given rate and flow pattern, the calculated values of resistance and elastance when compared on a breath-by-breath basis were highly reproducible for any given test subject.

In an effort to compare respiratory system mechanics computed by the LSF method to conventional techniques, Guttmann and colleagues (22) studied 17 paralyzed, mechanically ventilated patients. Five were without pulmonary disease following open-heart surgery, and 12 had ARDS. Static compliance and resistance were used as reference values, and $PEEP_i$ was obtained by end-expiratory occlusion. No statistically significant differences between calculated and measured values of C and R were found among the open-heart surgery patients. In the ARDS patients there was no significant difference with respect to compliance, but the calculated resistance was on average 20% higher than the reference value. There was good agreement in $PEEP_i$ between methods.

Iotti et al. (23) compared values of C, R, and $PEEP_i$ obtained by LSF to conventional methods in 11 paralyzed, mechanically ventilated patients studied on CMV. Reference values were obtained by performing traditional hold maneuvers. Calculated and measured values of compliance and resistance were significantly different (ΔC 1.47 $\pm$ 1.52 mL/cm H_2O, p = 0.016, ΔR 3.05 $\pm$ 2.03 cm $H_2O/(L/s)$, p = 0.003), while values of $PEEP_i$ were not ($\Delta PEEP_i$ 0.3 $\pm$ 1.1, p = 0.48). The results of this study suggest that the LSF method can provide reasonably good estimates of pulmonary mechanics in paralyzed patients on a volume preset mode of ventilation.

Larger differences were found in a study by Kimble et al. (24), which compared the values of C and R calculated by the LSF method with those measured using traditional hold maneuvers. Twelve patients with ARDS or COPD ventilated on the Hamilton Galileo ventilator in adaptive support ventilation (ASV) mode were studied. With regard to compliance, there was no difference between the LSF and occlusion methods in patients with measured compliance $\geq$40 (54.4 $\pm$ 13.6 vs. 52.4 $\pm$ 10.9, p = 0.261). A statistically significant difference was found between LSF and occlusion in patients with measured compliance <40 (31.3 $\pm$ 16.6 vs. 24.4 $\pm$ 8.5 mL/cm H_2O, p < 0.001). Calculated and measured values of resistance were different for all patients (18.3 $\pm$ 6.9 vs. 14.2 $\pm$ 7.2 cm $H_2O/(L/s)$, p < 0.001). Values for $PEEP_i$ were not compared in this study.

C. Least-Squares-Fit Method: Summary

As suggested above, the LSF method has several potential benefits over the traditional occlusion method:

1. The simultaneous measurement of C, R, and $PEEP_i$ is possible on a dynamic breath-by-breath basis.
2. Calculation is possible in both volume preset and pressure preset modes of ventilation (22–24).
3. These variables may be measured in spontaneously breathing patients (although the accuracy of the LSF method decreases in the presence of significant patient effort) (23).

It is also important to remember that the LSF method is based on several assumptions:

Intra-alveolar pressure is identical in all alveoli (i.e., one-compartment lung model).
Effects of variations in volume and physical conditions of the gases are insignificant.
The effects of inertia and turbulence can be ignored.

The system is stationary and linear (C and R do not change over the course of the breath).

When evaluating the studies comparing values of compliance and resistance calculated by the LSF method to corresponding measured values, it is important to remember that there are relatively few data available (a total of 40 patients in three studies). While statistically significant differences between the two methods likely exist, the clinical relevance of these differences is unclear at the present time.

D. Intrinsic PEEP

$PEEP_{tot}$ is the pressure that remains in the alveolar space at the end of expiration. It is the sum of applied or extrinsic PEEP ($PEEP_{ext}$) and intrinsic PEEP ($PEEP_i$). $PEEP_i$ represents an additional pressure resulting from incomplete airway emptying, also termed dynamic hyperinflation. In obstructive lung disease, $PEEP_i$ is thought to result from expiratory flow limitation secondary to increased compliance (with a resultant collapse of airways during expiration) and/or increased resistance. In ARDS patients, $PEEP_i$ is more commonly caused by a limited expiratory time related to high respiratory rates. In both cases, PEEP results when the amount of time the patient has to exhale is less than a given multiple of the respiratory system time constant, defined as the product of resistance and compliance.

It has been shown that an exhalation must last three times the time constant for 95% of the maximal volume change to occur and five times the time constant for a 99% volume change (25). The percent of maximal volume change is an exponential function with only 63% of the maximal volume being expelled when the duration of exhalation is limited to the time constant. Insufficient time for exhalation leads to elevated end-expiratory lung volume, manifest as $PEEP_i$.

As previously stated, the standard method of determining $PEEP_{tot}$ (and hence $PEEP_i$) at the bedside is through the use of an end-expiratory hold maneuver. While $PEEP_i$ can be calculated by a closed loop ventilator using the LSF method [Eq. (6)], there have been mixed results when comparisons are made between calculated and measured values (19,22,23). In an additional study, Eberhard and colleagues (26) found in 12 patients with ARDS that calculated values for $PEEP_i$ were universally lower than measured values. This difference increased as expiratory time was shortened. The authors hypothesized that the $PEEP_i$ calculated by the LSF method represents dynamic $PEEP_i$ as opposed to the static $PEEP_i$ measured by the occlusion method. The differences between the two were attributed to inhomogeneity of time constants between different lung units and viscoelastic properties within the lung parenchyma, which resulted in an uneven end-expiratory pressure distribution. This effect was magnified by shorter expiration times. Though this study only examined ARDS patients, the authors conjectured that the differences they found between calculated and measured $PEEP_i$ may be larger in patients with obstructive lung disease.

VIII. Patient Respiratory Drive ($P_{0.1}$)

The final input parameter to be addressed is $P_{0.1}$, an indirect measurement of patient respiratory drive. $P_{0.1}$ is the drop in airway pressure measured 0.1 seconds after an occlusion is performed at end-expiration and reflects the force applied by the inspiratory muscles. Since there is no gas flow and no volume change during the occlusion, $P_{0.1}$ is independent of resistance and compliance. Because the measurement is taken so quickly after the occlusion, it is unaffected by the patient's reaction to the occlusion and probably represents how the following breath was programmed by the respiratory centers. There are numerous caveats to interpreting $P_{0.1}$. It assumes an intact neural circuit from the CNS to the inspiratory muscles. There is large breath-by-breath variability. The measurement is best performed at low lung volumes to achieve maximal muscle stretch and hence maximal force generation. In addition, the ventilator must be set for pressure triggering, since with flow triggering the effective occlusion is delayed and takes place after some inspiration has occurred from the flow-by. This causes both the timing to be off and the volume to be higher than end-expiration.

With these limitations in mind, $P_{0.1}$ can be useful in adjusting the level of pressure support in spontaneously breathing patients. Alberti (et al.) (27) studied 10 patients with acute respiratory failure ventilated in pressure support mode. The level of pressure support was varied and $P_{0.1}$, work of breathing (WOB), and respiratory rate (RR) were measured. Statistically significant correlations between $P_{0.1}$ and WOB ($r = 0.87$) were found, while WOB and RR were less closely associated ($r = 0.53$).

Iotti et al. (28) described a closed loop controller which adjusted the level of pressure support based on the measured $P_{0.1}$. Eight stable patients were ventilated in pressure support mode for 15 minutes at each of four target $P_{0.1}$ levels ranging from 1.5 to 4.5 cm H_2O. The algorithm increased the pressure support level when actual $P_{0.1}$ was higher than the target value and decreased the amount of support when the actual value was lower than the target value. In general, the controller performed well with an average difference between steady-state and target values for $P_{0.1}$ of 0.59 ± 0.27 cm H_2O. However, the controller experienced serious problems in two patients who were coughing and thus had high $P_{0.1}$ levels. The ventilator responded to these patients by continued increases in the level of pressure support, which may have stimulated further coughing. In one instance, the patient had to be removed from the ventilator for a short period of time until the coughing subsided.

IX. Inputs Summary

The discussion thus far has focused on the various inputs available to closed loop ventilators. With regard to gas exchange, there are currently no commercially available ventilators that can acquire information pertaining to oxygenation or ventilation and adjust themselves to optimize these variables. More progress has been made in the area of pulmonary mechanics. Mathematical models have been developed and implemented that can calculate compliance, resistance, and $PEEP_i$ on a breath-by-breath basis without the need for hold maneuvers or a change in the patient's mode of ventilation. While validation studies do not show perfect agreement between the calculated and measured values, the clinical significance of the differences needs to be examined in greater detail. Of the three values, $PEEP_i$ seems to be the most prone to error. Finally, $P_{0.1}$ may be a useful estimate of patient effort and potentially could help ventilators adjust the level of pressure support needed by patients.

X. Outputs

Having addressed the various inputs available to the ventilator, emphasis will now be placed on the uses of these inputs to adjust output variables. Output variables include Fio_2, $PEEP_{ext}$, minute ventilation, optimal tidal volume, and respiratory rate for a given minute ventilation, I:E ratio, and the adjustment of ventilatory support to facilitate liberation of the patient from the ventilator. Most of these outputs are dependent on the availability of appropriate inputs. Without information on oxygenation or ventilation, it would be difficult for a ventilator to change the Fio_2 and PEEP levels or to adjust minute ventilation. Some of the other outputs can be adjusted based on information currently available to ventilators in clinical practice, such as the division of minute ventilation into respiratory rate and tidal volume, choosing an I:E ratio, and exercising the patient's respiratory muscles at an appropriate level.

XI. Respiratory Rate and Tidal Volume

To qualify as a closed loop system, a mechanical ventilator must have a means of assessing the patient's minute ventilation needs and then determining the optimal method of dividing this number into its constituent parts of respiratory rate (RR) and tidal volume (V_t). To assess minute ventilation requirements, a CLV system would need information on CO_2 production, $Paco_2$, and pH. As mentioned previously, current ventilators do not assess these variables. While some experimental systems rely on end-tidal CO_2 (14,29–31), commercially available ventilators rely on estimates of minute ventilation requirements based on ideal body weight.

The clinician then increases or decreases the set minute ventilation based on arterial blood gas values. This method is utilized by the adaptive lung ventilation (ALV) controller currently incorporated into the Hamilton Galileo ventilator (Reno, NV) (13,32–36). The ALV controller is similar in mode to SIMV + pressure support, except that the mandatory breaths are pressure controlled rather than volume controlled.

To determine the optimal breathing frequency, the ALV controller adopts a strategy intended to minimize the work of breathing (WOB) based on equations developed by Otis in 1950 (37). Otis found that in normal subjects for any given minute ventilation there is an optimal respiratory rate that requires the least amount of energy expenditure. The three forces that in combination produce the total WOB are the elastic, viscous, and turbulent forces. The work associated with elastic forces decreases with increasing RR, while that associated with the remaining two forces increases with increasing RR. As shown in Figure 1, when the three forces are combined to yield the total WOB, there is an optimal frequency range where this value is at a minimum. Mathematically, this minimum can be described as follows (13):

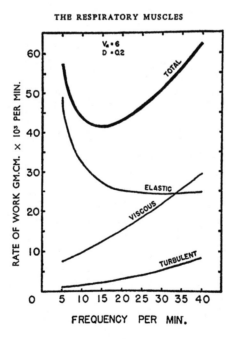

Figure 1   Relationship of elastic, viscous, turbulent, and total work of breathing/min to frequency of breathing. (From Ref. 37.)

$$RR = 30 \frac{\sqrt{1 + \frac{200}{3} \pi RC \frac{(V'_E - V'_D)}{V_D}} - 1}{\pi^2 RC} \tag{8}$$

where RR is respiratory rate, RC is the time constant (the product of resistance and compliance), V'_E is minute ventilation, V'_D is dead space ventilation, and V_D is volume of dead space. The time constant is in both the numerator and the denominator, but in the former case as the square root. Thus, as either R or C increases in magnitude, the denominator grows larger relative to the numerator and the corresponding optimal RR becomes smaller. This is exemplified by the pulmonary mechanics in obstructive lung disease. Conversely, with smaller values of either R or C, as in ARDS, the optimal RR is higher. However, it should be noted that Eq. (8) was derived from healthy humans and animals. The optimal RR is what a normal individual with a given ventilation requirement, resistance, and compliance would adopt to minimize the WOB. It is unknown whether Eq. (8) remains valid in pathological conditions.

In the case of paralyzed or heavily sedated patients who are not assisting the ventilator, the work of breathing for the patient is minimal to nonexistent regardless of the respiratory rate chosen. For spontaneously breathing subjects, the respiratory rate is determined by the patient, not the ventilator. The situation where this optimal RR determination may be useful is in the patient who is in transition from assisted to spontaneous modes. In the ALV controller, as the patient begins to initiate spontaneous breaths, the ventilator decreases the number of delivered mandatory breaths and adjusts the amount of pressure support in an effort to attain the RR and V_t values derived from Eq. (8). In theory this is an attractive strategy, but there are currently no data to validate its use.

Of interest, the ALV controller does not use the calculated values of R and C as derived from the LSF method to determine the optimal respiratory rate. Instead, the time constant is calculated using the slope of the exhalation limb of the flow-volume loop. These two methods of determining the expiratory time constant were shown to be equivalent by Brunner (et al.) (38). The advantage of using the flow-volume loop lies in its ability to account for a two compartment lung model. Figure 2 shows a sample flow-volume loop (25).

Examining the exhalation limb (the portion on the left side of zero-flow) reveals an initial rapid phase of exhalation followed by a slower phase. The slope of this curve is change in volume over change in flow ($\Delta V / \Delta V'$), which has the units of seconds (i.e., this slope is the time constant). This figure has two different slopes on the exhalation limb, meaning that this patient has two different exhalation time constants. It is the second of the two segments with the steeper slope that represents the ''true'' time constant in the sense of temporally limiting the amount of volume change for a given pressure change. The slope of the dotted line drawn from point a to the point of zero flow represents the time constant

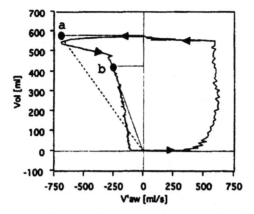

Figure 2 Flow-volume loop in a dynamically hyperinflated patient, paralyzed, in CMV. Point a represents the expiratory tidal volume and expiratory peak flow. Point b represents the 75% of the expiratory tidal volume and the corresponding expiratory flow. (From Ref. 25.)

as it would be calculated assuming a one-compartment lung model. Point b is determined by excluding the initial 25% of exhaled volume (representing the initial rapid exhalation), and the slope of the line connecting this point to the point of zero flow more closely approximates the actual slope of the "slow" portion of the exhalation limb.

XII. I:E Ratio

As discussed above in the section on $PEEP_i$, the major determinant of dynamic hyperinflation is an inadequate exhalation time. In order to minimize $PEEP_i$, the current generation of closed loop ventilators adjusts the I:E ratio in an effort to keep the exhalation time greater than three times the time constant. This allows >95% of the tidal volume to be exhaled.

XIII. Weaning

The goal of mechanical ventilation is to provide ventilatory support and/or airway protection for patients who, because of pulmonary, cardiac, metabolic, or neurological reasons, are in need of external assistance. In an effort to avoid the complications associated with mechanical ventilation, it is the clinician's responsibility to assess the patient's need for ventilatory support and attempt to liberate the patient from the ventilator as quickly as possible. There are numerous approaches to the weaning process as well as multiple indices, which attempt to predict when a patient can be successfully extubated, none of which have been shown to be clearly superior to any other. Closed loop control of the weaning process is a potentially attractive alternative. While it is impractical for clinicians and respiratory therapists to stand by the bedside and continually monitor the progress of the weaning process, this may be possible with closed loop ventilators having an internal weaning algorithm. Three such attempts have been reported to date.

One such system is the adaptive lung ventilation (ALV) controller described above. Linton et al. (36) described their experience with 27 patients having met standard weaning criteria. These patients were placed on ALV, which is designed to prevent excessive dead space ventilation, avoid $PEEP_i$, and discourage rapid shallow breathing by adjusting RR and V_t to minimize the work of breathing. In 22 patients, the ALV controller reduced the level of pressure support to 5 cm H_2O and the number of mandatory breaths to 4/min within 30 minutes of the initiation of weaning. All but one of these patients was successfully extubated within 24 hours. This study did not compare an ALV wean to standard methods of weaning, so the results must be interpreted with caution.

Strickland et al. (39) reported on a different closed loop controller, which adjusted the SIMV rate and pressure support level based on the patient's RR and Vt. Nine patients were weaned by the closed loop system, while six patients were weaned by physicians. They found that seven of the nine CLV patients were successfully weaned compared to two of the six control patients and that the mean duration of weaning was significantly shorter in the CLV group.

In a series of papers published between 1992 and 2000, Dojat and colleagues (14,29–31) have studied a closed loop controller operating in PSV mode, which adjusts the level of pressure support based on RR, V_t, and end-tidal CO_2. With regard to weaning, their system was evaluated for between 2 and 24 hours in 38 patients prior to undergoing a 2-hour T-piece trial (30). Those patients who tolerated the T-piece trial were then extubated. The CLV controller adjusted the level of pressure support and then predicted which patients would tolerate extubation. They found that the positive predictive value of the CLV controller was 89% versus 77% for the successful T-piece trial or 81% for the rapid shallow breathing index.

While the results of weaning with CLV systems are encouraging, further work needs to be done before they can be recommended for routine clinical practice.

XIV. Future Directions

Closed loop ventilation is an exciting field with high aspirations. While still in its infancy, CLV research is making promising strides toward the goal of autonomous ventilators. As more data become available on the optimal strategies for ventilation of patients with diverse pathology, algorithms can be developed to adjust the manner in which ventilators administer supportive care without the need for clinician intervention. The major tasks to be addressed include the identification and incorporation of all appropriate inputs and the translation of these data into rational ventilation strategies that are appropriate in various clinical scenarios. Of particular importance will be the ability of future ventilators to incorporate in a practical manner physiologic data such as CO_2 production, $Paco_2$, pH, and Pao_2 into their operation. Ultimately, outcome studies are needed which show not only that CLV systems are safe, but that they perform as well or better than clinician-driven management.

References

1. Ventilation with lower tidal volumes as compared with traditional tidal volumes for acute lung injury and the acute respiratory distress syndrome. The Acute Respiratory Distress Syndrome Network. N Engl J Med 2000; 342(18):1301–1308.
2. Sittig DF, et al. Clinical evaluation of computer-based respiratory care algorithms. Int J Clin Monit Comput 1990; 7(3):177–185.
3. Sittig DF, et al. Implementation of a computerized patient advice system using the HELP clinical information system. Comput Biomed Res 1989; 22(5):474–487.
4. Sittig DF, et al., Computerized management of patient care in a complex, controlled clinical trial in the intensive care unit. Comput Methods Programs Biomed 1989; 30(2–3):77–84.
5. Thomsen GE, et al. Clinical performance of a rule-based decision support system for mechanical ventilation of ARDS patients. Proc Annu Symp Comput Appl Med Care 1993; 339–343.
6. East TD, et al. A strategy for development of computerized critical care decision support systems. Int J Clin Monit Comput 1991; 8(4):263–269.
7. East TD, et al. A successful computerized protocol for clinical management of pressure control inverse ratio ventilation in ARDS patients. Chest 1992; 101(3):697–710.
8. East TD, et al. Efficacy of computerized decision support for mechanical ventilation: results of a prospective multi-center randomized trial. Proc AMIA Symp 1999; 251–255.
9. Randolph AG, et al. Evaluation of compliance with a computerized protocol: weaning from mechanical ventilator support using pressure support. Comput Methods Programs Biomed 1998; 57(3):201–215.
10. Ohlson KB, Westenskow DR, Jordan WS. A microprocessor based feedback controller for mechanical ventilation. Ann Biomed Eng 1982; 10(1):35–48.
11. Chapman FW, Newell JC, Roy RJ. A feedback controller for ventilatory therapy. Ann Biomed Eng 1985; 13(5):359–372.
12. Schaublin J, et al. Fuzzy logic control of mechanical ventilation during anaesthesia. Br J Anaesth 1996; 77(5):636–641.

13. Laubscher TP, et al. An adaptive lung ventilation controller. IEEE Trans Biomed Eng 1994; 41(1):51–59.
14. Dojat M, et al. Clinical evaluation of a computer-controlled pressure support mode. Am J Respir Crit Care Med 2000; 161(4 Pt 1):1161–1166.
15. Uhl RR, Lewis FJ. Digital computer calculation of human pulmonary mechanics using a least squares fit technique. Comput Biomed Res 1974; 7(5):489–495.
16. Mead J. Measurement of inertia of the lungs at increased ambient pressure. J Appl Physiol 1956; 9:208.
17. Wald A, et al. A computer system for respiratory parameters. Comput Biomed Res 1969; 2(5):411–429.
18. Lauzon AM, Bates JH. Estimation of time-varying respiratory mechanical parameters by recursive least squares. J Appl Physiol 1991; 71(3):1159–1165.
19. Stegmaier PA, et al. Assessment of pulmonary mechanics in mechanical ventilation: effects of imprecise breath detection, phase shift and noise. J Clin Monit Comput 1998; 14(2):127–134.
20. Brunner J, et al. Reliable detection of inspiration and expiration by computer. Int J Clin Monit Comput 1985; 1(4):221–226.
21. Avanzolini G., et al. Influence of flow pattern on the parameter estimates of a simple breathing mechanics model. IEEE Trans Biomed Eng 1995; 42(4):394–402.
22. Guttmann J, et al. Maneuver-free determination of compliance and resistance in ventilated ARDS patients. Chest 1992; 102(4):1235–1242.
23. Iotti GA, et al. Respiratory mechanics by least squares fitting in mechanically ventilated patients: applications during paralysis and during pressure support ventilation. Intensive Care Med 1995; 21(5):406–413.
24. Kimble BA, et al. Measurement of pulmonary mechanics during closed loop ventilation: least squares fit vs. occlusion. Am J Respir Crit Care Med 2000; 161(3):A386.
25. Iotti GA, Braschi A. Measurements of Respiratory Mechanics During Mechanical Ventilation. Rhäzüns, Switzerland: Hamilton Medical Scientific Library, 1999.
26. Eberhard L, et al. Intrinsic PEEP monitored in the ventilated ARDS patient with a mathematical method. J Appl Physiol 1992; 73(2):479–485.
27. Alberti A, et al. P0.1 is a useful parameter in setting the level of pressure support ventilation [see comments]. Intensive Care Med 1995; 21(7):547–553.
28. Iotti GA, et al. Closed-loop control of airway occlusion pressure at 0.1 second (P0.1) applied to pressure-support ventilation: algorithm and application in intubated patients. Crit Care Med 1996; 24(5):771–779.
29. Dojat M, et al. A knowledge-based system for assisted ventilation of patients in intensive care units. Int J Clin Monit Comput 1992; 9(4):239–250.
30. Dojat M, et al. Evaluation of a knowledge-based system providing ventilatory management and decision for extubation. Am J Respir Crit Care Med 1996; 153(3):997–1004.
31. Dojat M, et al. NeoGanesh: a working system for the automated control of assisted ventilation in ICUs. Artif Intell Med 1997; 11(2):97–117.
32. Laubscher TP, et al. Automatic selection of tidal volume, respiratory frequency and minute ventilation in intubated ICU patients as start up procedure for closed-loop controlled ventilation. Int J Clin Monit Comput 1994; 11(1):19–30.

33. Laubscher TP, et al. The automatic selection of ventilation parameters during the initial phase of mechanical ventilation. Intensive Care Med 1996; 22(3):199–207.

34. Weiler N, Heinrichs W, Kessler W. The AVL-mode: a safe closed loop algorithm for ventilation during total intravenous anesthesia. Int J Clin Monit Comput 1994; 11(2):85–88.

35. Weiler N, Eberle B, Heinrichs W. Adaptive lung ventilation (ALV) during anesthesia for pulmonary surgery: automatic response to transitions to and from one-lung ventilation. J Clin Monit Comput 1998; 14(4):245–252.

36. Linton DM, et al. Automatic weaning from mechanical ventilation using an adaptive lung ventilation controller. Chest 1994; 106(6): 1843–1850.

37. Otis AB, Fenn WO, Rahn H. Mechanics of breathing in man. J Appl Physiol 1950; 2:592–607.

38. Brunnel JX, et al. Simple method to measure total expiratory time constant based on the passive expiratory flow-volume curve [see comments]. Crit Care Med 1995; 23(6):1117–1122.

39. Strickland JH, Jr Hasson JH. A computer-controlled ventilator weaning system. A clinical trial. Chest 1993; 103(4):1220–1226.

9

Treatment of Agitation and Its Comorbidities in the Intensive Care Unit

DAVID CRIPPEN

St. Francis Medical Center
Pittsburgh, Pennsylvania

I. Agitation in the ICU

In the critical care setting, we deal with organ system failure by the application of high-technology monitoring and treatment systems. However, our care plan frequently requires that our patients be placed in a very high-stress environment, full of flashing lights, noisome bells, and frenetic activity 24 hours a day (1). We demand that our patients stay very still in uncomfortable positions on uncomfortable bedding for long periods so that our monitoring systems will register truly. This is necessary to accurately identify monitoring points for sophisticated treatment systems. In so doing, we have inadvertently set the stage for the creation of a different kind of organ system failure, exacerbated, if not wholly created, by our care plan. Brain failure is becoming a more common problem in high-technology medicine, and we are learning how to deal with it as effectively as we do heart or renal failure (2).

Brain failure in the critical care setting rarely occurs as an isolated event (3). Generally the stage is set by a predisposing hemodynamic or metabolic decompensation, either intra- or extracranial. Stress such as pain, anxiety, and discomfort may be either accelerate or exacerbate the process (4). The physiological result of brain failure causes dysfunctional processes "downstream" from the failed organ in much the same way as any other kind of organ system failure. With brain failure, the major dysfunction is the phenomenon of delirium. When agitation accompanies delirium in a critical care setting, a severe integrative cerebral failure exists, suggesting a true medical emergency (5).

In part, the central nervous system exists as a processing station for the coordination of incoming stimuli and outgoing responses. Toward this end, alterations in brain metabolism, especially at the levels of neurotransmission, play an important role in modulating practical brain function. When metabolic homeostasis is interrupted or distorted, varying degrees of "brain failure" can occur resulting in distorted and miscoordinated brain functions. Loss of clarity in thinking processes and fragmented cognition due to disordered neurotransmission characterizes the phenomenon of delirium. This process is fueled by metabolic derangement elsewhere in the body.

The typically delirious patient cannot integrate a stream of thoughts and deduce coherent information from them. Interviewing the patient reveals short attention span, short-term memory retention, and disorientation to person, place, and time. The uncomfortable intensive care unit (ICU) environment hastens disrupted sleep patterns resulting in reversed day-night sleep cycles. This eventually causes poorly organized delusions and hallucinations, frequently of a paranoid nature, especially in elderly patients. Unresolved pain may lead to increased catecholamine levels, exacerbating delirium at both the neurohumeral and musculoskeletal level by increasing blood pressure, heart rate, and ventilation rate. Untreated anxiety may rapidly progress to delirium, especially in the elderly patient with decreased coping ability for stress found in the ICU environment. At some point in the brain failure process, delirium, which is primarily a cerebral process, turns to agitation, which opens many somatic complications.

The term "agitation" is different from delirium in that it expresses a syndrome of excessive, nonpurposeful motor activity. Although delirium is a genuine medical emergency and a source of great concern for the intensivist, agitation is a particularly big problem in the ICU because it can alter the diagnosis and course of medical treatment (6). At the least, severe agitation may result in the inability of the patient to cooperate with sensitive monitoring systems that require quiescence for accuracy. A more significant problem is the resulting hemodynamic and respiratory deterioration (7). Musculoskeletal hyperactivity increases oxygen consumption, initiating a reflex in cardiac output. For elderly patients with fixed myocardial blood flow due to coronary artery disease, this increase in myocardial work may result in angina, heart failure, or myocardial infarction. Increased catecholamine activity, a frequent accompaniment of agitation, exacerbates this effect. Hypermetabolism at the muscular level also produces metabolic acidosis with the potential for increased arrhythmias and oxygen delivery imbalances. Disruption and lysis of nonacclimatized muscle tissue increases the potential for rhabdomyolysis, myoglobinuria, and renal failure. Increased musculoskeletal metabolism also increases carbon dioxide production. Chronic lung failure patients and those controlled on mechanical ventilation may manifest sudden increases in pco_2. This results in narcosis and obtundation or further catecholamine release, increasing agitation.

Agitation was a relatively minor issue before the arrival of high-technology monitored areas for critically ill patients. Modern ICUs now have the potential to reverse multiple organ system insufficiency using invasive corrective modalities overseen by close monitoring systems. These monitoring and treatment modalities pin the patient firmly to their bed with tubes, catheters, and appliances, conferring upon the already hemodynamically unstable patient new kinds of stress we never had to deal with before. Crude sedation regimens aimed at suppressing symptomatology are no longer relevant. Agitation episodes that threaten hemodynamic stability are uncommon but are occurring more frequently as ICUs accept wider ranges of critically ill patients for longer periods. Generally, such episodes are signaled by escalating agitation in the face of increasing sedative administration and multiple drugs. Eventually, the underlying causes of agitation combined with pharmacological side effects threaten respiratory and hemodynamic stability (8).

For example, respiratory failure can be exacerbated by the administration of sedation without adequate monitoring has increased the mortality and morbidity of delirium tremens (9). Clearly, escalating magnitudes of antiagitation medications signal a serious problem that must be aggressively evaluated. Initially, a rapid evaluation of emergent medical and surgical disorders should be a priority. The purpose of an ICU is to monitor the patient's ongoing condition so that early, subtle deleterious decompensations can be detected before they bloom into full-blown hemodynamic disasters.

II. Delirium in the ICU

The multifaceted syndrome of clinical delirium can be affected by a wide range of noncerebral metabolic and organic disorders, such as underlying physiological and hemodynamic decompensations and environmental stress factors. Elderly patients manifest a normal loss of cortex neuronal populations and a decrease in acetylcholine activity. This accounts for their increased susceptibility to delirium (11). Drug interactions can cause changes in cerebral function that may enhance susceptibility to delirium, especially multiple, simultaneous drug regimens. The highly stressful environment of the ICU may lead to a loss of orientation to time and place. The onset of delirium is associated with monotonous sensory input, repetitive and noisy monitoring equipment, prolonged immobilization, indwelling life support hardware, interrupted sleep patterns, and social isolation, However, such environmental factors' role is thought to be contributory only and not an initiating event in most patients. Delirium usually results after significant physiological and metabolic insults occur first, resulting in organ system malfunction (12).

The term "ICU stress delirium" would be more applicable for organic brain syndromes occurring in the intensive care unit environment than the often-used term "ICU psychosis" (13). There is a qualitative difference between the psychiatric idea of psychosis and clinical delirium. True delirium as seen in the ICU may exhibit psychotic features such as hallucinations, delusions, and disordered thinking, but "psychosis," as used in the psychiatric literature, is characterized by persistent disorders of brain functioning where no specific organic factors may be causally related. In clinical delirium, organic causation is always present and frequently originates from somatic areas outside the brain. Symptoms of clinical delirium are usually lacking in systematization and are therefore random and purposeless. Psychotic symptoms manifest as bizarre affect but are frequently consistent and well organized.

III. Brain Failure and Delirium

The nervous system is unique in the vast complexity of the control actions that it can perform. The major function of the nervous system is to process incoming information so that coordinated and appropriate motor responses occur as a result. Most sensory information is not used in any coherent form. After the salient sensory stimuli have been selected, they are channeled through many neuronal circuits into proper motor regions of the brain to elicit desired responses. This channeling of stimuli is called the integrative function of the nervous system. The lower control regions are primarily concerned with automatic, instantaneous responses of the body to the sensory stimuli, and the higher regions with deliberate movements controlled by cerebral thought processes. Only a small fraction of selected sensory stimuli elicits an immediate motor response. Most are stored as imprinted memory for nonvolitionally directed control of "learned" motor activities and for cognitive processes. Most of this storage occurs in the cerebral cortex, but spinal cord can also store small amounts of information. Once imprinted memories have been stored in the nervous system, they become part of the processing mechanism and the brain constantly compares new sensory experiences with stored memories, looking for new information that may require variations in action responses. Integrative brain functions help to select the important new sensory information and to channel this into appropriate storage areas for future use or into motor areas to cause somatic responses.

Delirium is a clue that disintegration of normal motor axis integration has occurred and that stimuli are being mischanneled into filogenetically old brain areas such as basal ganglia, reticular formation, vestibular nuclei, and often the red nucleus (extrapyramidal system). Such short-circuiting produces the clinical picture of uncoordinated and nonpurposeful movements. Failure to integrate stimuli effectively results in a continuum of symptoms from confusion to delirium and agitation and ultimately coma. The biochemical and pathophysiological bases of brain failure are characterized by global disorders of cognition and wakefulness and by impairment of psychomotor behavior. Cognitive functions such as perception, deductive reasoning, memory, attention, and orientation are all globally disordered (14). Delirium associated with brain failure is a manifestation of cerebral insufficiency of both a generalized (15) and focal (16) nature, fueled by neurotransmitter system dysregulation (17). These pathophysiological mechanisms are thought to include (1) a cholinergic-dopaminergic imbalance, (2) dopamine and β-endorphin hyperfunction, (3) increased central noradrenergic activity, and (4) damage to intraneuronal enzyme systems (18). Delirium does not have to be associated with an agitational state. When this occurs, the resulting constellation of symptoms is called "agitated delirium." When agitation accompanies brain failure in a critical care setting, there exists a failure to integrate cerebral functioning, and this is a true emergency.

IV. Clinical Presentations of Brain Failure

Brain failure leading to the clinical symptom of delirium is characterized by disorganized thinking and short-term memory deficits resulting in rambling, incoherent thought and speech patterns that may or may not be accompanied by agitation (19). During a delirious state, cognition loses its clarity and goal direction. The delirious patient cannot refit the fragments of miscognition. His perceptions are altered, leading to the development of delusions and hallucinations. In severe delirium, cognition is fragmented and disharmonious and the patient is unable to perceive reality, even with coaching from unaffected onlookers. When they occur, hallucinations are characteristically visual, tactile, or kinesthetic, fleeting and poorly organized. In advanced stages, misperceptions become vivid and frequently threatening. Short-term memory expression and retention are impaired due to short-circuiting and misregistration of neurohumoral stimuli. The delirious patient cannot integrate a stream of incoming stimuli and deduce meaningful information from them, but some random "islands of memory" in a field of amnesia may be preserved. Delirium is usually characterized by fluctuating levels of arousal over the day's course associated with sleep-wake cycle disruption hastened by reversed day-night cycles. Since this psychomotor agitation syndrome usually occurs in the night hours, it has been termed the "sundown syndrome" by intensive care nurses and is virtually diagnostic of stress-induced delirium. The patient tends to sleep fitfully, with frequent interruptions during the day, and then stay awake at night. Although typical delirium is characterized by poorly organized delusions and hallucinations, the presence of "lucid intervals" is very common. This clinical picture differs from agitated dementia, functional psychosis, and psychogenic dissociative states, the symptomatology of which remain constant. When agitation accompanies delirium, however, patients may continually resist restraints and treatment modalities, sometimes to the point of exhaustion.

V. Comorbidities of Brain Failure and Delirium

The probability of developing ICU stress–induced delirium varies with the patient's age, severity of illness, and number of contributing comorbidities. Young people with hemodynamic and metabolic reserve normally do not develop ICU stress–induced delirium following the onset of these comorbidities except after relatively lengthy sojourns in an ICU environment. Older patients with an inability to cope due to advancing age and severity of illness scores develop delirium more quickly in a high-stress environment. The following factors do not necessarily cause delirium but tend to exacerbate it once the stage is set by the placement of patients in a high stress environment.

A. Pain

Pain is the single most common complaint of patients in the ICU (20). Although pain is not necessarily the most commanding etiology of agitation for critical care patients, it is a difficult problem. The severity of pain cannot be measured in strictly objective terms, and its quality frequently varies according to the patient's subjective ability to describe it. The appraisal of pain's qualities is a matter of personal interpretation and is extremely difficult for others to penetrate. An individual's interpretation of pain varies directly with coincident activity such as anxiety, personality type, expectations of treatment outcome, coincident events, and the presence of reassuring support systems (21). It is a truism that pain may hasten agitation in ICU patients, but agitation has many other important etiologies. Most patients who find themselves in ICUs have had an operative or medical procedure that results in pain. Frequently, intubated patients undergoing mechanical ventilation find it almost impossible to express their displeasure, increasing their frustration.

B. Generalized Effect of Pain in the ICU

Pain is a representation of many stress factors resulting in reactionary neuroendocrine changes. Other stress factors include fear, anxiety, apprehension, tissue damage, blood loss, anoxia, effects of anesthetic gases, immobilization, fever, sepsis, and starvation. Pain functions as a beneficial protective mechanism, mandating attention drawn to noxious circumstances even to the point of promoting reflex withdrawal. Pain is a clear warning sign that harm is near and avoidance maneuvers are needed. Nociceptors for the perception of pain reside in the skin and various organs and sense noxious stimuli, transmitting these sensations to the cerebral and limbic cortex via sensory pathways. These specialized receptors encode the location, intensity, and duration of the painful stimuli. Many subjective kinds of pain are perceived, including heat, cold, pressure, and incising, penetrating, and chemical stimuli.

Pain can be mediated and modulated by vasoactive amines and neurotransmitters located in the organs, brain, and spinal column or through the nervous system. Common active mediators include serotonin, bradykinin, histamine, prostaglandins, and potassium ion release from damaged cells. Acute pain sensations are carried by A-delta (larger, thinly myelinated) fibers (22). These afferents carry painful sensations to the dorsal horn cells. Visceral pain is carried by C (unmyelinated, slow conducting) afferent fibers that follow sympathetic afferents to the dorsal root ganglia. C fibers are polymodal in that they can carry more than one kind of pain sensation. On arrival in the horn area, the ganglia from all these cells spread out laterally along the substantia gelatinosa and penetrate deep into this structure. There is no central "pain center" in the brain. Multiple areas are fed by a multiplexity of ganglia. Ultimately, many tracts such as the spinoreticular, spinospinal, and spinothalamic converge to form the reticular formation and feed the thalamus, which in turn fans out fibers to the cortex. Pain perception at the precortex level, especially when influenced by the limbic areas, is perceived only in very crude form.

Stress has two separate components, psychic and somatic, both of which usually combine to stimulate the hypothalamus via a common pathway (23). The more intense the stimuli, the more pronounced the response. Increased catecholamine levels because of the psychic component of pain have been measured in many individuals undergoing stressful situations (24). The levels of norepinephrine generally increase about that of epinephrine and the levels of 11- and 17-hydroxycorticosteroids also increased. Increased catecholamine levels increase heart rate and myocardial contractility to bolster cardiac output for potential trauma. Increases in blood sugar (hyperglycemia of stress), free fatty acids, triglycerides, and cholesterol also occur to fuel possible "fight or flight." Painful stimulation of afferent nerves in a somatic area is a potent activator of neuroendocrine changes. Immediate inhibition of insulin production occurs coincidentally with an increase in glucagon production, resulting in increased blood sugar. Growth hormone and cortisol secretion increase, providing an anti-inflammatory response for potential trauma. Aldosterone production acts to conserve salt and water, bolstering intravascular volume in case of potential blood loss.

The function of the cerebral cortex is to perceive the location, nature, and intensity of the pain sensation. These perceptions are then integrated and relayed via integrated afferent pathways from the hypothalamus to the reticular activating system via the reticular formation, beginning in the medulla and extending to the midbrain. This pathway links the brain with perception of external events. Pain is a very potent activator of this system, and this explains the importance of pain elicitation in the evaluation of consciousness. Modulated signals ultimately reach the medulla oblongata and the sympathetic outflow tracts of the spinal cord leading to the pupils, heart, blood vessels, GI tract, pancreas, and adrenal medulla. Norepinephrine is released from the postganglionic fibers into the target organ, and both epinephrine and norepinephrine are released into the blood stream from the adrenal medulla. The effects of this system are felt in many organ systems.

In the ICU, proper treatment of pain requires accurate assessment of its location, severity, and an assessment of what hemodynamic or ventilatory variables might be affected by effective treatment. The perception of pain is an experience colored by experience and emotion (25). Verbal complaints of pain from patients give very little clue how much therapy might be effective. Although no really objective measurements of what a patient is feeling exist, there are some objective signs that can give clues as to severity of pain. Presence of muscle spasm in areas thought to be painful is a reliable sign. As mentioned elsewhere in this text, the classic triad of systolic hypertension, tachycardia, and tachypnea is a reliable indicator that pain is significant enough to affect hemodynamics. It is unusual for patients exhibiting almost "pure" anxiety to elevate their blood pressure. Hyperventilation and tachycardia are more common in these patients. Patients with severe pain frequently exhibit a mild hyperkinetic musculoskeletal activity. This reaction is commonly seen in renal colic, where the patient is searching for a comfortable position.

However, an elemental "pain avoidance" maneuver is sometimes seen where the patient lies very still and quiet to avoid a pain reflex. This is commonly seen in syndromes like pancreatitis, where undue musculoskeletal movement exacerbates the pain. Physicians are notoriously and inappropriately conservative in their assessment of pain and its treatment (26). Sometimes this results from the clinician's inability to empathize with perceived discomfort, or lack of it. Sometimes it is a result of unwillingness to create drug dependence by long or intense courses of narcotic therapy. The creation of drug addicts in the ICU is extremely rare and should not be a real concern. Non–drug dependent personalities rarely become dependent on pain relief. It makes no sense to allow the vast majority of patients in pain to suffer to avoid an easily treatable, short-term drug reliance in only a few. The presence of pain in the ICU immediately translates into somatic and hemodynamic consequences that increase morbidity and length of stay. There are far more reasons to assume a liberal analgesic stance than not (27).

C. Anxiety

The subjective sensation of anxiety is most prevalent during the first 24 hours of ICU admission. Many factors contribute to the experience of anxiety, including the fear of death or disability, misunderstanding of information provided by staff, discomfort, and restricted ability to do usual activities. These factors may be associated with feelings of helplessness and loss of control. Serotonin has been implicated as a basis for anxiety but the exact role remains undefined (28). Misfunction of GABA-benzodiazepine receptor systems has also been implicated. In the psychiatric practice, anxiety is not usually associated with any organic etiology and affects women more than men (29). A strong quality of anxiety is hyperacute vigilance, improving the ability to avoid a potential threat. However, in the ICU the perceived threats are highly technological and unfamiliar. Anxiety is heightened because there is no clear path of retreat and no obvious defense. Males and females are affected similarly. The most common organ systems involved in anxiety responses are cardiovascular, respiratory, and neurological. Chest pain, tachycardia, and palpitations are frequent. Chest pain is described as "stabbing," is usually unrelated to activity, and can be easily confused with angina. Respiratory complaints include shortness of breath, hyperventilation syndrome, with tetany of the fingers and a choking sensation (30). Complaints of weakness and dizziness are also common. Nausea and vomiting are commonly associated with anxiety.

However described, the perception of anxiety is stressful, painful, and potentially dangerous to ICU patients. Anxiety is a leading cause of sleeplessness, which contributes to the abnormal "sleep-wake cycle" seen in a typical ICU day. Increased heart rate and blood pressure during prolonged anxious periods can speed myocardial decompensation by increasing myocardial oxygen consumption out of proportion to coronary artery flow. In the ICU environment, anxiety may be characterized by hyperactivity or withdrawal and may not necessarily result in a catecholamine response, but may rapidly progress to delirium, especially in elderly patients who have a decreased ability to cope with unusual stress.

D. Environmental Discomfort

Discomfort occurs when environmental situations cause stress. The subjective sensation of discomfort is proportional to the efficiency of coping patterns. In the unique, stressful ICU environment, patients' ability to cope decreases with increasing severity of illness and advancing age. Patients forced to lie still for long periods encumbered by indwelling hardware soon become profoundly uncomfortable and seek more comfortable positions. A particular comfort problem is the patient undergoing mechanical ventilation. Sympathetic stimulation does not necessarily occur during periods of discomfort, but constant musculoskeletal activity may cause physical exhaustion. Restraining patients usually results in attempts to escape confinement, confirming any incipient paranoid ideation and exacerbating agitation. Fighting restraints increases musculoskeletal oxygen demand, promoting a reflex increase in cardiac output that may increase myocardial oxygen consumption above the ability of diseased coronary arteries to supply it, resulting in heart failure or angina. Patients find it particularly difficult to relax and rest while undergoing mechanical ventilation. The need to move about and stretch can become an obsession, especially during sleepless nights, which decreases the patient's ability to cope.

Sedation with benzodiazepines was reported by most patients to decrease the discomforts associated with the ventilator. Most patients treated with morphine sulfate also reported no recollection of the experience (31). Reassurance and comfort measures by the nursing staff were also recollected as an important source of anxiety relief. A national survey showed that most patients received some sort of sedation for mechanical ventilation, but there was not a clear preference for most physicians (32). Most patients vividly recall the discomfort of ventilators, especially musculoskeletal paralysis for facilitation of ventilation function (33). These feelings were described vividly as "agony," "panic," and "insecurity" (32). The discomfort experienced by positive end-expiratory pressure (PEEP) was so profound that student volunteers were unable to tolerate it for more than a few minutes (34). Newer methods of positive pressure mechanical ventilation in patients with high peak airway pressures such as inverse ratio ventilation in the adult respiratory distress syndrome (ARDS) require therapeutic musculoskeletal and potent sedation because the unusual artificial breathing pattern is impossible to tolerate normally (35).

VI. Rational Treatment of Agitation and Its Comorbidities

Intramuscular absorption of drugs is influenced by the ratio of ionized to nonionized drug, site if injection, blood flow to the site region, amount of drug metabolized before entry into the systemic circulation—all variably affected by critical illness (36). In the ICU, medications are generally administered intravenously. Intramuscular injection usually requires musculoskeletal activity and adequate tissue perfusion to enhance absorption into the systemic circulation. Since patients in the ICU generally lie still, they tend to absorb drugs from the muscles erratically. ICU patients also frequently suffer from decreased tissue perfusion because of varying degrees of heart failure and multiorgan insufficiency, also decreasing the reliability of muscular absorption. Intravenous administration of sedatives offers the advantage of close titration, a very big plus in the treatment of unstable patients. Insertion of central venous access is usually indicated to insure that the drug continues access to the central circulation, as peripheral IVs may infiltrate with very little warning, particularly in the middle of the night. Intraarterial catheters are indicated for constant blood pressure monitoring and easy access for blood sampling. Most rapidly acting drugs are very lipid soluble and can only be titrated by intravenous administration. However, the effective titratability of these drugs probably decreases with time as the volume of distribution throughout the body water compartments increases (37). Organ insufficiency, particularly liver failure, also decreases the short-term titratability of most sedatives by prolonging the serum half-life.

Continuous infusions of analgesics and sedatives are a very effective method of avoiding the "valleys" inherent in bolus medication therapies that initiate a "peak" of therapeutic action followed by a variable period of "valley" where the patient has little or no drug effect. Current literature suggests that high-risk cardiac patients are jeopardized by relatively brief periods of analgesia ineffectiveness (38). Intermittent periods of sympathetic stimulation due to ineffective analgesia and sedation can cause relatively profound deleterious effects on compromised myocardium. Continuous intravenous infusions of short-acting agents such as midazolam, propofol, and fentanyl allow titration of plasma level effects to a fluctuating baseline of pain, anxiety, and discomfort. This real-time titration of natural fluctuations may occur with minimum hemodynamic and respiratory suppression. Increased costs of newer short-acting agents are justified if complications are avoided, as patients achieve more effective analgesia and sedation, avoiding blanket effects of less selective regimens. Continuous intravenous administration of short-acting benzodiazepines such as midazolam and propofol are safe and effective in the monitored setting and have been extensively described in the literature (39).

A. Delirium

Major Tranquilizers

It is possible that manipulation of neurotransmitters or their precursors may directly or indirectly improve delirious states. The serotonin precursor L-tryptophan was given to delirious patients in high doses, resulting in significant trends toward improvement in objective clinical assessment scores (40). However, this kind of therapy has not shown consistent results. The phenothiazines are thought to exert a stabilizing effect on cerebral function by antagonizing dopamine-mediated neurotransmission at the synapses. The therapeutic effects also extend to the basal ganglia, potentially enhancing extrapyramidal side effects. Higher intellectual function usually remains intact, but the patient's interest in his environment is diminished, producing a characteristic flat cerebral affect. Abnormal symptomatology such as hallucinations, delusions, and unstructured thought patterns are inhibited. Phenothiazines exert a pronounced anxiolytic and sedative effect, making it useful when sedative qualities are wanted besides the reordering of neurotransmission. Neuroleptics such as haloperidol have the quality of suppressing spontaneous movements and complex behavior patterns that result from disharmonious brain function, with minimal central nervous system (CNS) depressive effect. There is little or no ataxia, incoordination, or dysarthria at ordinary doses.

Chlorpromazine produces an antipsychotic effect and quiescence with less sedation than the CNS-depressing benzodiazepines (41). Chlorpromazine can be useful in stress-induced delirium as it acts as a calming influence beyond resolving disorganized brain chemistry. However, chlorpromazine use in the ICU is limited because of side effects affecting the hemodynamically unstable patient. The therapeutic index of chlorpromazine is narrow, resulting in increased side effects at marginally higher than therapeutic blood levels and inadequate therapeutic function at marginally lower levels. The drug induces a pronounced antihistaminic effect, resulting in dry mucous membranes. Chlorpromazine lowers seizure thresholds and may result in seizures, especially in alcoholics. Electrical conductivity of the heart is altered, resulting in QT and PR interval prolongation, blunting of T waves, and ST segment depression on the electrocardiogram. Therefore, accurate hemodynamic monitoring is necessary during the administration of this drug. Because of the ineffectiveness of the intramuscular mode in most ICU patients, intravenous administration, titrated according to the desired effect, is indicated for delirium when associated with agitation. Other side effects such as tachycardia, vasodilation, and postural hypotension may occur because of blocked α-adrenergic and muscarinic receptors and chlorpromazine's adrenergic agonist activity (42).

Neuroleptics

Haloperidol is thought to exert diffuse depressive effects and a neurotransmitter antagonist action on brain function. Haloperidol may also inhibit catecholamine receptors and block reuptake of neurotransmission in portions of the brain affecting mentation by decreasing the neurotransmitter action of dopamine (43). The neuroleptic haloperidol produces less sedation than phenothiazines and exerts little effect on heart rate, blood pressure, and respiration. A unique effect of haloperidol is suppression of spontaneous musculoskeletal hyperactivity and behavior that results from hyperdopaminergic brain function without pronounced sedation or hypotension. The intravenous administration of haloperidol is not specifically approved by the US. Food and Drug Administration (FDA), but the drug is commonly given by this mode and the current medical literature is replete with examples of efficacy in this mode (44–46).

Continuous infusion of haloperidol has been described to flatten out the peaks and valleys inherent in bolus administrations of the drug (47). Extrapyramidal reactions occur frequently with haloperidol, especially in the first few days of treatment, and usually consist of Parkinson-like symptoms, drowsiness, lethargy, and a fixed stare. These symptoms are usually mild and reverse rapidly on cessation of the drug (48). One study found that dystonia occurred in equal proportions of patients treated with oral or IV doses of haloperidol, but akathisia occurred more in patients given IV doses. Extrapyramidal reactions tended to occur relatively early or late in the treatment course at times when drug concentrations were less than peak values (49). Tardive dystonia, oculogyric crisis, torticollis, and trismis all occur less often and are mostly dose related.

Neuroleptics such as haloperidol have an unpredictable sedative effect, sometimes seen only in high doses. Combined use of benzodiazepines and haloperidol has been reported to be effective in combining antipsychotic effects and sedation with a minimum of side effects (50). Whether these combinations offer any benefit over intravenous chlorpromazine alone is arguable. Patients receiving combination therapy consisting of haloperidol and a benzodiazepine did have significantly less incidence of extrapyramidal reactions that patients on isolated haloperidol therapy alone (51). Haloperidol may be safer to use in alcohol-related delirium than chlorpromazine as it seems to lower seizure thresholds minimally. One study showed that haloperidol did not result in any untoward side effects when used to treat 36 head trauma patients and a series of 90 acutely alcohol intoxicated patients (52). Neuroleptic malignant syndrome rarely occurs with any dose of haloperidol administration, requiring ICU admission and aggressive life support measures.

B.   Pain

General Considerations

There have been major advances in the understanding of pain physiology over the last 10 years. Earlier ideas of a dedicated, simple, spinothalamic pain system are no longer tenable. Much evidence now exists that very complex neural connections involving diverse areas of the nervous system play a part. Pain may be modulated or edited at spinal cord level, in the periaqueductal gray matter and brain stem raphe nuclei before reaching relays and gating mechanisms in the thalamus on the way to the cerebral cortex. The perception of noxious stimuli may depend not only on peripheral stimulation and transmission, but also on modulation occurring in spinal cord and higher structures. Accordingly, the subjective sensation of pain can be effectively blocked at the brain level by narcotic analgesics and at the inflow tract level, explaining the efficacy of spinal or epidural anesthesia.

Normally, agitation caused by pain stimulates humoral catecholamines, resulting in the classic triad of systolic hypertension, tachycardia, and tachypnea, but these symptoms may not occur in elderly patients. The administration of analgesics diminish the stimulus to secrete epinephrine and norepinephrine, and so decreases the end organ response to these catecholamines. Patients who have elevated catecholamine levels because of pain tend to buttress the hemodynamic side effects of the narcotics such as hypotension and respiratory depression. Humoral responses such as hypertension and tachypnea counterbalance the side effects of narcotic analgesics, such as hypotension from histamine release and medullary ventilation center depression (53). Agitation syndromes resulting from pain usually resolve when the primary stimulus and the coincident catecholamine storm diminish.

Morphine Sulfate

The most widely used of all narcotic analgesic/sedatives, morphine may be administered by oral, subcutaneous, intrathecal, epidural, intramuscular, and intravenous routes. The drug is easily titrated in intravenous boluses and continuous infusions and may also be reversible with narcotic antagonists (54). However, morphine has profound effects on ventilation and hemodynamics. Morphine promotes secretion of histamine and decreased cardiac preload capable of producing orthostatic hypotension due to vasodilation in the splanchnic beds (55). The respiratory depressive effect can be profound and unpredictable. A 10 mg dose of morphine sulfate (0.15 mg/kg) has increased pco_2 by 3 torr in normal subjects (6). These side effects, however, are most often seen in patients with unstable hemodynamics initially.

Patients in pain frequently have higher normal blood pressure and respiratory rates that counteract the narcotic's hypotensive and respiratory depressant effects. Intrathecal and epidural morphine provide a more selective effect and do not enter the central circulation, providing safe and effective analgesia in selected patients where respiratory drive inhibitory must be considered (56). Occasionally tabloid newspapers decry the "iatrogenic inducement of addiction" by giving hospitalized patients large doses of morphine for prolonged periods. In fact, this problem is not significant in ICU applications where pathological processes causing pain resolve and the need for analgesia no longer exists. Peridural administration of morphine has been shown to provide excellent analgesia with minimal hemodynamic or ventilatory side effects (57).

Fentanyl

A synthetic opioid with morphine-like activity, fentanyl is approximately 7000 times more lipophilic than morphine, allowing it to penetrate fat-laden brain tissues rapidly. Fentanyl is about 200 times more potent than morphine, and it is used in very small doses. It has a rapid action (1–2 minutes) and short duration (30–40 minutes). Fentanyl promotes less histamine release and significantly less effect on cardiac dynamics than morphine. Like morphine, it is quickly reversible with narcotic antagonists, but its affinity for fat can lead to its accumulation during prolonged use, ultimately "leaching out" after discontinuation of the drug. This effect limits its use in long-term continuous infusion analgesia and sedation in the ICU. Fentanyl combines an analgesic, anxiolytic, and sympatholytic effect and is most effectively used in the continuous infusion mode due to its brief span of action. The administration of fentanyl plus a benzodiazepine has the potential to produce unexpected hypotension and respiratory depression (58). This combination should only be used in monitored settings. Occasionally the rapid administration of high doses of fentanyl has resulted in muscular and glottic rigidity during the induction of anesthesia. This complication is reversible with naloxone or succinyl choline (59,60).

Ketorolac

Ketorolac is the first parenteral nonsteroidal anti-inflammatory agent available for the treatment of acute pain. Ketorolac is most effective for pain of an inflammatory nature such as musculoskeletal trauma and renal colic. It was ineffective in pain with minimal tissue inflammation such as migraine (61) and sickle cell crisis (62). Since its prostaglandin inhibition properties tend to decrease protective barriers to gastric acid, ketorolac is contraindicated in active peptic ulcer disease (63). Like other nonsteroidal anti-inflammatories, ketorolac has also rarely been implicated as a cause of acute renal failure (64) and anaphylactic shock (65). Ketorolac is usually administered by the intramuscular route, but critical care patients generally tolerate intramuscular (IM) injections poorly. Poor peripheral tissue perfusion in patients with cardiac decompensations provides erratic and ineffective absorption of medication deposited outside the intravascular space. There is evidence in the literature that the intravenous administration of ketorolac is safe and effective (66). Intravenous (IV) administration would presumably allow more rapid onset of action, closer titratability, and more predictability of response (67).

Ketorolac is unique in that it has virtually pure analgesic activity with no sedative qualities (68,69). A need for an analgesic with no hemodynamic or respiratory side effects is apparent in hemodynamically unstable ICU patients, where the side effects of narcotic analgesics would be poorly tolerated. Pain prevents postsurgical patients with upper midline abdominal and thoracic incisions from coughing effectively to clear retained secretions resulting from anesthesia and operative endotracheal intubation. If given narcotics, the pain resolves, but respiratory depressive side effects prevent effective coughing, causing difficulty in clearing secretions and an increased incidence of nosocomial pneumonia. A pure analgesic such as ketorolac may facilitate clearing airway secretions effectively with less risk of respiratory depression. ICU patients with unstable hemodynamics who must undergo painful procedures such as invasive vascular catheterization, chest tube thoracostomy, or intra-aortic balloon placement also tolerate narcotic side effects poorly and may benefit from a pure analgesic. Patients treated for painful syndromes in the ICU are also able to give informed consent because there are no CNS depressive actions of ketorolac.

α_6-*Adrenoreceptor Agonists*

These drugs inhibit norepinephrine release from presynaptic junctions by negative feedback mechanisms. As a result, α_2-adrenergic agonists inhibit sympathoadrenal outflow (70). This class of drugs that are normally used as antihypertensives also possess anxiolytic, sedative, and analgesic properties, making them attractive for use in the treatment of agitation and delirium associated with catecholamine storm. α_2-Agonists administered concurrently with benzodiazepines or opiate analgesics provide additive sedation effect while effectively decreasing the effective doses of sedative-narcotics needed to achieve the same therapeutic effect. Among clinically available α_2-agonists, clonidine is the most popular. Clonidine is thought to act by competitively binding opiate catecholaminergic receptors, decreasing the dose of opiates required to get the same sedative effect. Consequently, respiratory depression, hypotension, and other side effects of narcotic sedatives are significantly decreased. Clonidine decreases the amount of anesthesia required to obtain operative analgesia. Ghignone et al. (71) showed a 45% reduction in fentanyl requirements as compared to the control group of patients when clonidine 5.0 µg/kg was administered orally prior anesthesia. Clonidine has been effectively used intrathecally for analgesia in terminal cancer patients who had become tolerant to intrathecal morphine (72). Oral clonidine has also been extensively used on psychiatry wards to attenuate drug withdrawal syndrome after chronic benzodiazepine and alcohol use (73).

Clonidine is quickly absorbed after oral administration, but this route of administration is rarely available in hemodynamically unstable ICU patients. Drug delivery through a transdermal patch takes much longer to reach effective blood levels and a minimum of 2 days to achieve a steady state concentration, making it unattractive for ICU use inpatients with variable blood flow to the skin (74). Intravenous clonidine has been used extensively in Europe but is not yet available in the United States (75). Clinical data are accumulating supporting the use of intravenous clonidine in critical care applications, especially for sedation and analgesia. Postoperative patients after spinal fusion who received 0.3 mg/kg/h continuous intravenous infusion of clonidine required significantly fewer supplementary doses of morphine than those not treated with it (76). Other α_2-agonists are being investigated in Europe. The highly selective α_2-agonist dexmedetomidine also reduces anesthetic requirements and improves recovery from anesthesia, with fewer side effects than clonidine (77). Dexmedetomidine produces anxiolytic effects comparable to benzodiazepines but has fewer negative effects on hemodynamics and ventilation (78). Dexmedetomidine does not significantly affect myocardial contractile force or respiratory depression in the animal model (79,80), and α_2-antagonists such as atipamezole or idazoxan could effectively reverse the hypnotic effect of the drug (81).

C. Regional Anesthesia in the ICU

Epidural analgesia is particularly efficacious for the treatment of pain in the thoracic and abdominal area (82). It reliably produces good long-term analgesia and an alert patient. The selectivity of this route of administration targets the specific area of pain and tends to spare hemodynamics and ventilation from the generalized side effects of system wide analgesics (83). Regional analgesia can be effected with either narcotics or local anesthetics depending on the desirability of sympathetic blockade, muscle relaxation, and affected area. The local anesthetic bipivacaine is the most frequently used agent for initiating pharmacological sympathectomy. Bipivacaine administrated peridurally in low concentrations gives long-acting pain relief with minimal blockade of motor activity. Addition of epinephrine extends the duration of action by limiting spread. Epidural administration of narcotics such as morphine and fentanyl give excellent analgesia through their interactions with opiate receptors on the dorsal horn of the spinal cord. The more lipid-soluble narcotics such as fentanyl produce a more limited spread around the spinal cord because they are rapidly absorbed. More water-soluble narcotics such as morphine (duramorph) remain in the cerebrospinal fluid longer, allowing greater cephalad distribution, widening the analgesia effect, but potentially increasing respiratory depression. The addition of epinephrine to the morphine solution decreases vascular uptake and increases cephalad spread.

Hypotension is a potential complication because of sympathetic blockade and loss of vascular tone. When this occurs, most patients quickly respond to fluid challenge. Respiratory depression can occur as late as 24 hours after epidural administration of morphine, and other side effects such as pruritus, nausea, and urinary retention occur infrequently and are reversible by systemic therapy. If respiratory depression occurs, small doses of naloxone quickly reverse it. Sympathetic blockade also increases bowel motility, promoting nausea and vomiting. These symptoms usually respond to intravenous administration of small doses of prochlorperazine. The possibility of infection as a result of spinal puncture always exists but is minimized by strict aseptic technique during the procedure and the use of inline bacterial filters. Catheters should be pulled as soon as is practical. It is unlikely that an epidural catheter will be in place more than 7 days.

VII. Treatment of Anxiety and Discomfort

A. General Considerations

Patients who find themselves ensconced in a critical care unit are at severe risk for anxiety-related exacerbation of delirium, especially with advancing severity of illnesses (84). The physiological response to postoperative pain, anxiety, and discomfort includes an increase in sympathetic activity and musculoskeletal hyperactivity, which can increase oxygen consumption and myocardial oxygen demand in compromised patients (85). Normally, autonomic hyperarousal and hypervigilance facilitate appropriate rapid behavioral reaction to threat. Stress-induced levels of cortisol may promote metabolic activation necessary for sustained physical demands necessary to avoid further injury. Elevated catecholamine levels increase heart rate and myocardial contractility to bolster cardiac output as potential compensation for injury during "fight or flight." Painful stimulation of somatic afferent nerves is a potent activator of neuroendocrine changes. Immediate inhibition of insulin production occurs coincidentally with an increase in glucagon production, resulting in increased blood sugar (hyperglycemia of stress), free fatty acids, triglycerides, and cholesterol to fuel possible "fight or flight." Growth hormone and cortisol secretion increase, providing an anti-inflammatory response for potential trauma. Aldosterone production acts to conserve salt and water, bolstering intravascular volume in case of potential blood loss (86).

The acute behavioral responses brought about by the activation of these humoral responses by psychological and physical trauma represent evolutionary adaptive responses critical for survival in an uncertain and potentially dangerous environment. These compensatory responses were presumably created at a time in the universe when there were no high-technology surrogates for naturally induced environmental stress. Patients in the hybrid operating room and ICU environment undergo stress but no natural environmental threat. Therefore these maladaptations may translate into deleterious hemodynamic and metabolic function. Agitated patients tend to increase peripheral musculoskeletal metabolism, increasing lactate and carbon dioxide production. Both lactate and increased CO_2 are evolutionary signals that danger is approaching, prompting a responsive response to potential jeopardy. Hypercapnea stimulates the sympathetic centers resulting in tachycardia and mild hypertension and can precipitate panic attacks. During hyperventilation, pco_2 declines causing cerebral vessels to constrict reflexly, further limiting blood flow and oxygen transport to the brain, which can result in cerebral confusion and increased agitation. Musculoskeletal hyperactivity also increases oxygen consumption, initiating a reflex in cardiac output. For elderly patients with fixed myocardial blood flow due to coronary artery disease, this increase in myocardial work may result in angina, heart failure, or myocardial infarction. Increased catecholamine activity exacerbates this effect.

The solution to ameliorating this therapeutic dilemma lies in selecting effective pharmacological regimens, administrating optimal doses of medication, and utilizing the most effective routes of administration for individualized dilemmas rather than a ''shotgun'' approach. Benzodiazepines are the most commonly used sedatives in critical care. This class of drugs attenuate stress-induced increases in norepinephrine release in the hippocampus, cortex amygdaloid, and locus coeruleus region, effectively reducing conditioned fear and generalized anxiety. Variable magnitudes of anterograde amnesia occur as well.

Administering sedative and analgesic medication by the intravenous bolus method can be a problem for this set of patients because the effect cannot be titrated in real time (87,88). Boluses of medication enter the blood stream, accumulate serum concentration quickly, then decay with variable and sometimes unpredictable consequences. A good analogy is a home furnace thermostat. The house heats up quickly, then cools through a ''comfort zone'' until it gets cold again. Just before the thermostat turns on again to repeat the next cycle is a problematic time for patients with unstable or rapidly fluctuating hemodynamics and ventilation. This is when ''breakthrough'' occurs and the patient is unprotected from the effects of pain and agitation that may precipitate complications.

B. Anxiety and Discomfort

Lorazepam

Lorazepam is an intermediate length-of-action benzodiazepine with anxiolytic and sedative qualities. The drug has a mild amnesic effect as well: 4 mg of lorazepam is about equivalent to 10 mg of diazepam, and 1 mg lorazepam approximately equals 4–6 mg of midazolam (89). The drug does not accumulate toxic intermediary products and does not require hepatic oxidative metabolism–only glucuronidation, which makes it attractive in liver insufficiency. Lorazepam has been approved for oral, intramuscular, and intravenous use, and the traditional dose for patients in the intensive care unit has been 1–2 mg every 3–4 hours. Lorazepam has been described as having a synergistic action when used in combination with haloperidol for delirious patients in the ICU setting (90). The effective duration of action of lorazepam has been the subject of some speculation, although no published reports exist as yet, and some interest has been generated in using the drug in a constant infusion for selected applications.

Short-acting benzodiazepines such as midazolam have little indication for long-term sedation of patients expected to be on mechanical ventilation in the ICU for extended periods recovering from prolonged disorders such as the adult respiratory syndrome. For such patients, the benefit of short-term titratability is lost and the expense of using short-duration medication for long-term use can be substantial. A starting dose of 1 mg/h continuous drip has been used, titrating the dose up to as much as 10 mg/h for severe agitation in ventilator patients with no significant hemodynamic effects. Continuous infusion of lorazepam can be problematic because it is a relatively long-acting sedative. It generally requires more concentration per hour to equal a bolus dose, and so several days of continuous infusion may result in prolonged somnolence.

Midazolam

A relatively new short-acting CNS depressant, midazolam is relatively water-soluble compared to other benzodiazepines, increasing the rapidity of its action. The potency of midazolam is about three to four times that of diazepam, and it has a shorter elimination half-life of 1.5–3.5 hours. Sedation after IV injection is achieved within 1–5 minutes, with a duration of action of less than 2 hours. The time of onset is dependent on the total dose administered and the concurrent administration of narcotic premedication. The effect on respiratory pattern has been found to be about the same as diazepam in healthy subjects (110,111). Continuous administration of a sedative/anxiolytic is often indicated for titrated sedation, anxiolysis, and anterograde amnesia in the conscious, restless patient (112). Midazolam is uniquely practical in the ICU environment because its rapid-acting, short-duration properties allow its use as a continuous titrated infusion. In addition, anterograde amnesia occurs almost immediately after IV administration and usually persists for 20–40 minutes after a single dose. Prior studies have shown midazolam to be safe and effective compared to intermittent boluses of diazepam (91) for postoperative cardiac surgery patients. After discontinuation of the drugs, recovery was seen to be faster in the continuous infusion midazolam group than in the untitrated group.

All of the benzodiazepines, including midazolam, have similar side effects and complications. Midazolam potentiates the analgesic effect of opiates and increases the incidence of sudden, unexpected hypotension. The concurrent administration of opiates and midazolam potentiates the respiratory depressive effects of the benzodiazepine. All benzodiazepines reduce the ventilatory response to hypoxia. However, relatively large doses on the order of 100–150 µg/kg are required to produce clinically important respiratory depression (92). In the past, when relatively large doses of midazolam were given for endoscopy procedures in unmonitored settings, unexpected respiratory failure was a noted complication. However, the recommendation for lower initial doses, especially in elderly patients, has resulted in a dramatic decrease in these problems. There is a relatively wide margin of safety when midazolam is administered by continuous infusion in the ICU setting where facilities are available for appropriate monitoring (93). It is of the utmost importance that respiratory and hemodynamic function is monitored during infusion of any benzodiazepine that the proper technology is readily available to treat sudden, unexpected decompensations.

Propofol

Propofol is a new intravenous anesthetic agent chemically unrelated to barbiturate or benzodiazepines. Propofol has been compared to midazolam with regard to its effectiveness as a sedative agent (94), and it was found to be remarkable because of a significantly shorter recovery time, more rapid titration efficacy, reduced post-hypnotic obtundation, and faster weaning from mechanical ventilation. The most desirable features of propofol are its rapid onset of action, rapid titration of effects with rapid and clear emergence from anesthesia or sedation. Propofol produces a rapidly progressive continuum from anxiolysis and hypnosis in low doses to sedation in moderate doses to general anesthesia in high doses, all of which can be effectively maintained by continuous infusion. This unique spectrum of sedative activity may avoid the necessity of titrating one of several sedative, analgesic, or musculoskeletal paralytic agents all simultaneously. Since propofol's rapid response and short duration is a result of its enhanced fat solubility, its use as a long-term intravenous sedative is as questionable as that of fentanyl. Few studies have been done examining this aspect of its use in the ICU setting, but no accumulation of propofol was detected in a patient with severe tetanus when it was being administered in very high dose (20–80 mg/h) for 8 days (95).

The potential complications of propofol are mostly hemodynamic (96–98). Unexpected systemic hypotension resulting from a reduction in systemic vascular resistance has been reported, especially in hypovolemic and low cardiac output patients (99). Anaphylactic reactions have also been reported (100). However, cardiac index has not consistently been shown to be affected when the patient is normovolemic. Minimal ventilatory depression has been observed in patients with chronic lung disease resulting from a decrease in central inspiratory drive. Sympathetic stimulation during intubation usually reverses these declines with the net effect being a rapid return to preinduction hemodynamic status. In patients without intracranial pathology, propofol decreases cerebral blood flow and cerebral metabolic requirements for oxygen to a significant degree. This makes the application of propofol very effective in neurological critical care for the control of elevated intracranial pressure (101).

VIII. Selecting the Most Efficacious Drug Therapy

The selection of medications for use in treating delirium, agitation, pain, discomfort, and anxiety in the critical care setting must be made with surgical accuracy (102). The use of inappropriate drug regimens toward sedation or analgesia problems may result in more complications than simply ineffective resolution of the clinical scenario. The side effects generated by inappropriate drug therapy may interfere with intended treatment, cloud further clinical signs and symptoms, increase length of stay in the ICU, the number of lab tests ordered, consultants contacted, and money spent on the care plan. Treating true delirium with analgesics is ineffective and fraught with hazard. Delirious patients are not necessarily in pain and may not manifest the end organ manifestations of circulating catecholamines. Since there is no pain stimulus, the analgesic effect of morphine is lost and the predominating effect is hemodynamic and ventilatory suppression. The treatment of delirium with CNS depressants such as benzodiazepines confuses the border between psychosis and organic brain dysfunction. Benzodiazepines have no ability to revitalize aberrant cerebral neurotransmission, therefore psychotic patients treated with sedatives become more obtunded and confused simultaneously, further obfuscating the treatment plan.

For patients in pain, attempts to avoid the hemodynamic side effects of morphine by using benzodiazepines as analgesics are also fraught with hazard. The hemodynamic effects of benzodiazepines are less than those of narcotics, but benzodiazepines do not have an analgesic effect and they do not diminish humoral responses to pain. Benzodiazepines have more potential to produce a cloud of CNS depression over pain stimuli, producing the appearance of comfort, but the patient continues to exhibit hypermetabolic humoral responses such as catecholamine storm with the potential for end organ dysfunction. Furthermore, neuroleptics such as haloperidol also have no analgesic effect and an unpredictable sedative effect, sometimes evidenced only in large doses where side effects may predominate. The issue may then be confused by bizarre CNS symptoms additive to the normal humoral response of catecholamines. Attempts to diminish environmental discomfort with narcotic analgesics can be effective, but at the added peril of adverse hemodynamic side effects.

The patient who is uncomfortable may not necessarily be in pain and may have no catecholamine effect. In such situations, the side effects of narcotics such as hypotension and respiratory depression may predominate over the sedative effects. Patients with compromised cardiorespiratory organs tolerate these adverse side effects poorly, even in low doses. The patient may then require more monitoring hardware to gauge hemodynamic side effects, increasing discomfort and leading to more agitation. Patients who are uncomfortable are not necessarily psychotic. Treatment of discomfort-related agitation with antipsychotic neuroleptics is quirky and unpredictable. Haloperidol does not have any musculoskeletal relaxation properties and no antegrade amnesic effect. The sedative properties of haloperidol are undependable and sometimes occur only in large doses, at which exaggerated CNS side effects may materialize. Since sedation is achieved only with large doses, extrapyramidal side effects may also be expressed.

IX. Continuous Infusions in the ICU: Current Experience

Continuous infusions of short-acting sedatives allow the clinician to stand at the bedside and titrate sedative effect to individual patients rather than isolated standards. Small serial boluses of short-acting drugs may achieve an appropriate level of conscious sedation, followed by a variable period of real time maintenance within a comfort band. The literature is replete with examples of the safety and effectiveness of such regimens.

Following cardiac surgery, a period of controlled mechanical ventilation is usually necessary to optimize the patient's hemodynamics and to maintain airway control in the event that emergent operative intervention is needed to control complications such as mediastinal bleeding. In the early hours after open heart surgery, the patient may awaken with discomfort and agitation, still intubated and partially paralyzed due to the remaining effects of neuromuscular blockade (103). Intravenous sedation is usually needed to ameliorate this rather sudden and unexpected discomfort and blunt the sympathetic responses thereof that increase myocardial oxygen demand. Sedation also facilitates mechanical ventilation and airway management and reduces the risk of dislodging catheters and chest tubes. There is evidence that continuous infusions of titratable sedatives are beneficial to this patient population.

Numerous investigators have examined the role of continuous intravenous midazolam in the postoperative sedation of patients after coronary artery bypass graft (CABG) surgery. Westphal and colleagues evaluated the pharmacokinetics of a continuous infusion of midazolam when used for sedation after CABG surgery. Twenty-seven adult patients were randomly assigned to one of the following groups: (1) normal saline placebo, (2) midazolam 1 mg/mL, and (3) midazolam 2 mg/mL. Each patient received a 2 mL loading dose followed by 1 mL/h for 8 hours. Blood levels and vital signs were monitored at predetermined intervals. The two midazolam-treated groups required significantly less morphine than the control group, and the high-dose midazolam group required significantly less vasodilator than the low-dose group. The investigators noted that the hepatic clearance of midazolam was not significantly different from that observed in healthy volunteers. Midazolam worked well for postoperative sedation in open heart surgery patients because of its titratability, it did not adversely affect cardiovascular recovery, and it reduced narcotic requirements (104).

Sedation and recovery were studied in 14 patients requiring overnight mechanical ventilation after CABG surgery. All patients had received high-dose fentanyl during surgery, had an ejection fraction of >50%, and had no hepatic or renal dysfunction. The loading dose of midazolam was 2 mg, followed by 2 mg/h. Patients treated with diazepam received 2 mg as needed for sedation. Compared to the diazepam-treated patients, patients treated with continuous infusion midazolam had fewer episodes of awakening during sedation (3 vs. 12) and had a significantly shorter recovery time after cessation of sedation (310 vs. 471 minutes) (105).

Higgins and colleagues compared the relative safety and efficacy of propofol and midazolam for sedation in 84 mechanically ventilated, post-CABG patients with normal to moderately impaired left ventricular function. Patients were randomized to receive propofol (mean loading dose of 0.24 mg/kg, mean maintenance dose of 0.76 mg/kg/h) or midazolam (mean loading dose of 0.012 mg/kg, mean maintenance dose of 0.018 mg/kg/h) for 8–12 hours. Infusions were titrated to keep patients drowsy, comfortable, and responsive to verbal stimulation. Both regimens lowered blood pressure and heart rate. However, propofol produced significant reductions in heart rate and blood pressure compared with midazolam. Sedation scores were not significantly different between the two groups. The propofol group required less sodium nitroprusside and less opiate. Midazolam and propofol did not differ significantly in time to extubation or ICU length of stay (106).

Propofol is a hemodynamically active sedative. Roekaerts et al. (107) compared continuous infusions of propofol and midazolam in 30 postoperative ventilated patients in an open randomized study. The duration of infusion was approximately 570 minutes in both groups. After a loading dose of propofol (1 mg/kg) or midazolam (0.07 mg/kg), the infusion rates were 2.71 ± 1.13 mg/kg/h and 0.092 ± 0.028 mg/kg/h, respectively. An analgesic infusion of sufentanil was also given in both groups. The time from stopping sedation to patient responsiveness was 118 minutes in the propofol group and 72 ± 70 minutes in the midazolam group, and the time from stopping sedation to extubation was 250 ± 135 minutes and 391 ± 128 minutes, respectively. Following the loading dose of propofol, there was a fall in blood pressure (BP) (mean from 80 ± 11 mmHg to 67.5 ± 10 mmHg). After approximately 15 minutes, BP started to rise but remained below pretreatment level throughout sedation (107).

The sedative and cardiovascular effects of propofol and midazolam were compared in 40 patients who required vasodilators for control of arterial hypertension following CABG surgery. Patients were randomly assigned to receive either midazolam (1–4 mg loading dose followed by 0.1–0.2 mg/kg/h) or propofol (10–40 mg loading dose, followed by 0.5–2.0 mg/kg/h) for 8 hours. A six-point scale was used to assess sedation: 1 = sedated, no response; 2 = responds only to painful stimuli; 3 = responds to verbal commands; 4 = able to be roused, comfortable, and responds to commands; 5 = moderately agitated; 6 = distressed and very restless. The midazolam group required a fourfold greater amount of fentanyl compared with the propofol group. Both agents afforded cardiovascular stability, but propofol produced a higher incidence of hypotension compared with midazolam. Both drugs provided quality sedation, and there was no significant between-group difference in percentage of time spent at each level of sedation. The time to spontaneous ventilation and tracheal extubation was insignificantly shorter in the propofol group (108).

Midazolam was compared with propofol for sedation following prolonged neurosurgery in 20 adults with a mean age of 48.9 years. Nine patients received propofol (mean infusion rate of 2.67 mg/kg/h; range: 0.56–5.15 mg/kg/h) and 11 patients received midazolam (mean infusion rate of 0.075 mg/kg/h; range:

0.026–0.176 mg/kg/h). Propofol-treated patients had a significantly faster recovery time compared with the midazolam group. Time to extubation was shorter with propofol (6.25 h; range: 1.5–8.5 h) compared with midazolam (9.79 h; range: 6–57.5 h). No adverse effects were noted in either group. The author concluded that no major difference in outcome could be observed between propofol and midazolam in this study (109).

Henderson and colleagues performed a study of opiate sedation compared to opiate sedation plus low-dose midazolam (1 mg/h) to assess the effects of each regimen on recall and duration of ventilation. One hundred consecutive postoperative neurosurgery patients were studied. Mean patient age in the midazolam group was 56 ± 18 years and mean age in the placebo group was 63 ± 11.5 years. Midazolam did not affect recall and did not prolong ventilator time (25 ± 20 h) compared to placebo (26 ± 24 h) (110).

Bruder et al. (111) looked at outcome of oxygen consumption (Vo_2) and energy expenditure after cessation of sedation in severe head-injured patients and to assess its usefulness as a predictor of neurological severity in a prospective, descriptive study. Fifteen severe head-injured patients with tracheostomies were mechanically ventilated and sedated at the time of the study. Vo_2 and energy expenditure were measured using indirect calorimetry during and after discontinuation of sedation with continuous infusions of midazolam (2.5–5 mg/h) and fentanyl (250–500 µg/h). After the measurement period the patients were divided into two groups. Group 1 included patients who were completely weaned from sedation; group 2 included patients who had to be sedated again. In both groups energy expenditure was close to basal energy expenditure during sedation and increased to 150% of basal energy expenditure during the recovery period, with maximum hourly values 80% above basal energy expenditure. In group 1, Vo_2 and energy expenditure changed from 284 ± 44 mu/min and 1833 ± 261 kcal/day during sedation to 390 ± 85 mu/min and 2512 ± 486 kcal/day for the period without sedation. During this period, there was a significant correlation between Vo_2 and mean arterial pressure. For the recovery period, there was no difference in mean or maximum Vo_2 between the two groups of patients. At 24 and 48 hours after cessation of sedation, Vo_2 and energy expenditure decrease to 30% above basal energy expenditure. They came to the conclusion that severe head-injured patients during the first 12 hours after the discontinuation of sedation experienced a large increase in Vo_2, energy expenditure, and mean arterial pressure. Methods that blunt these changes which have proven efficacious in anesthesia may be effective for intensive care patients (111).

Nakahashi et al. (112) administered midazolam (0.2 mg/kg) to 10 patients undergoing neurosurgical operation, and its influence on cerebral blood flow was studied under modified neuroleptic anesthesia. Simultaneously, the plasma concentration of midazolam was measured. Heart rate and mean arterial blood pressure showed no significant changes after injection in comparison with the control.

Cerebral blood flow (CBF) decreased for about 15–20% after 5, 10, and 15 minutes in comparison with the control. However, 30 minutes later CBF showed a trend to return to the control. This change in CBF is related to the changes of cerebrovascular resistance. Cerebral metabolism remained constant. They concluded that the sedative dose of midazolam significantly reduced CBF and OMR02 in patients with intracranial hypertension (112).

Hundt et al. (113) studied a continuous intravenous application of alfentanil and midazolam compared to an application of continuously given alfentanil with intermittent midazolam. A sufficient sedation with good neurological judgment was more frequently achieved in 8 out of 15 patients by continuous application of both substances (alfentanil 0.023 mg/kg of body weight (bw)/h, midazolam 0.10 mg/kg bw/h), compared to discontinuous application of midazolam (4.5/ 15 patients; alfentanil 0.028 mg/kg bw/h, midazolam 0.13 mg/kg bw/h). Their results suggested that a continuous application of both agents was superior to an intermittent application of midazolam with continuously given alfentanil. A lower dosage of each substance was necessary to maintain a better state of analgesia and sedation (113).

X. Analgesia and Sedation Combinations: Role of Fentanyl

Fentanyl, a synthetic opioid with morphine-like activity has a rapid analgesic and often underappreciated sedative action (4–5 min) and short duration (30–40 min). Fentanyl promotes less histamine release and significantly less effect on cardiac dynamics than morphine. Fentanyl adds an accurately titratable analgesic and sympatholytic effect to the anxiolytic effects of benzodiazepines and is most effectively used in the continuous infusion mode due to its brief span of action. The administration of fentanyl plus a benzodiazepine has the potential to produce unexpected hypotension and respiratory depression (114). This combination should only be used in monitored settings. Occasionally the rapid administration of high doses of fentanyl has resulted in muscular and glottic rigidity during the induction of anesthesia. This complication is reversible with naloxone or succinylcholine (115).

Newman et al. (110) reviewed the options for adjuvant drug use during cardiac anesthesia and suggested that midazolam supplementation with an opioid is an ideal adjuvant. Given as a continuous infusion or a bolus, potent opioids such as alfentanil, fentanyl, or sufentanil enhance the amnestic and hypnotic effect of midazolam, decreasing the required dose. In addition, the combination of midazolam and narcotics decreases the catecholamine response that either one alone would produce (116). Shapiro et al. (117) reviewed the current sedation literature and developed suggested practice parameters for numerous sedative and analgesic drugs used in critical care. A consensus of experts provided six recommendations with supporting data for intravenous analgesia and sedation in the ICU setting: fentanyl is the preferred analgesic agent for critically ill patients with hemodynamic instability (117).

Chuang et al. (118) assessed the safety and efficacy of intravenous sedation in pediatric upper endoscopy, all elective outpatient procedures performed during a 2-year period. Of 614 children, 553 received intravenous meperidine and midazolam; 61 received fentanyl and midazolam. The mean dose of meperidine was 1.5 ± 0.7 mg/kg and of fentanyl 0.0031 ± 0.0014 mg/kg. Less midazolam was needed for children receiving fentanyl than for those receiving meperidine (0.05 ± 0.03 mg/kg vs. 0.08 ± 0.05 mg/kg. Recovery time (minutes) was shorter for those receiving fentanyl (74.7 ± 22.8 vs. 95.1 ± 23.0; $p < 0.003$). Side effects occurred in 117 patients (19.1%), of which the majority were mild (83%); all were transient with no residual sequelae. Inability to complete the procedure occurred in fewer than 1%. They concluded that the use of fentanyl/midazolam results in a shorter recovery time and a lower dose of midazolam (118).

Hiew et al. (119) reviewed the use of intravenous analgesia and anxiolytics in interventional radiological procedures. They found that fentanyl and midazolam is an effective combination, exhibiting little cardiovascular depression and being easily reversible (with naloxone and flumazenil). They found it to be a better alternative to pethidine and diazepam because of enhanced titratability and control (119)

Milgrom et al. (120) examined four drug combinations (midazolam, midazolam-midazolam, fentanyl-midazolam, and fentanyl-midazolam-methohexital) in a placebo-controlled double-blind clinical trial of intravenous sedation. Subjects were 207 mildly anxious young adults having their third molars removed. Cognitive measures of anxiety increased from preoperative levels in the placebo and both midazolam groups. The anxiety response remained the same in the fentanyl-midazolam and fentanyl-midazolam-methohexital groups. Using the log likelihood method, the fentanyl-midazolam group was 8.1 and the methohexital group 9.0 times more likely to have had a favorable outcome than the placebo group (120).

The same author also studied midazolam and midazolam plus fentanyl in a placebo-controlled, double-blind clinical trial, testing the hypothesis that combined drug therapy results in significantly poorer safety but no difference in efficacy compared to the single-drug approach in 207 mildly anxious young adults having their third molars removed. Fentanyl had a significant depressant effect on respiration. Fifty of 79 (63%) subjects who received a midazolam-fentanyl combination became apneic, while only 2 of 78 (3%) who received midazolam alone were apneic. Subjects in the combination group were more than four times more likely to have excellent versus good, fair, or poor sedation at a given level of intraoperative pain, and behavioral (movement and verbalization) but not cognitive measures of anxiety were attenuated (121).

Lau et al. (122) found that midazolam and fentanyl together produce better sedation, analgesia, and amnesia than does either drug alone, but the electrophysiological effects of the combination are unknown. Twenty patients undergoing electrophysiological studies for clinical reasons were studied. Blood pressure, heart rate, respiratory rate, oxygen saturation, and standard variables related to atrioventricular and ventriculoatrial conduction, dual pathways, accessory pathway conduction, sinus node function, and the inducibility of tachycardia were examined before and after intravenous injections of midazolam (0.07 ± 0.03 mg/kg) combined with fentanyl (0.8 ± 0.4 µg/kg). There were no significant changes in the electrophysiological variables or ease of inducibility of tachycardia. The drugs were well tolerated; they produced minor and clinically unimportant reductions in mean blood pressure (99 ± 13 to 89 ± 16 mmHg and respiratory rate (18 ± 4 to 16 ± 3 breaths/min). Excellent sedation was achieved. Major amnesia was reported by 95% of the patients. In conclusion, midazolam combined with fentanyl provides safe and effective sedation for electrophysiological studies without significantly affecting electrophysiological variables or the inducibility of tachyarrhythmias (122).

XI. Management of Agitation in Organ System Failure

Patients in varying degrees of organ system failure often present problems in pain management because of a fear that blood levels of analgesics or sedatives will pile up, creating unpredictable side effects. In fact, patients with multiple organ system insufficiency frequently need highly titrated analgesia and sedation. The problem is determining dosages that will accomplish a desired effect without precipitating unacceptable hemodynamic reactions. Liver insufficiency is a significant cause of delirium and other problems in the use of analgesic and sedative medications. The initial symptoms of brain failure result from an interference with cerebral neurotransmission caused by the introduction of false neurotransmitter toxins backed up into the blood stream after loss of liver detoxification functions. The first symptom is cerebral confusion, followed by progressive drowsiness, stupor, and eventually coma. The principal site of amino acid interconversion is the liver. The bulk of amino acids entering the liver via the portal vein (with the exception of the branch chain amino acids) are catabolized to urea and then transported to the kidney for excretion. Approximately 25% of blood urea is excreted into the intestine, where ammonia (NH_3) is produced. However, most ammonia and other amines are formed in the bowel by the metabolic action of urease containing bacteria and normally carried into the liver for conversion to nontoxic urea via the portal vein. In the presence of gastrointestinal bleeding, even more nitrogenous compounds may be formed by the action of gut bacteria.

The liver has a great deal of reserve, and severe damage is required to demonstrate significant loss of functions. When severe damage occurs, the liver pulp pressure gradient increases, backing up blood flow from the portal vein. As a result, potentially toxic compounds with neurotransmission capabilities "overflow" into the systemic circulation where they may circulate freely through the brain. Since the pK of ammonia is relatively high at 8.9, the presence of alkalemia and hypokalemia favors the entry of ammonia into the brain by shifting the equilibrium between NH_3 and NH_{4+}. This facilitates the more toxic, nonionized NH_3 transmission through active membranes. Here they may competitively or noncompetitively inhibit the action of normal neurotransmitters causing altered consciousness. Abnormal glucose metabolism may also participate in hepatic encephalopathy. Glucose is normally transported to the liver via the portal vein for metabolism. In obstructive liver disease, this glucose load is diverted to the systemic circulation where it may promote increased secretion of insulin. Since circulating insulin is inefficiently cleared by the liver, it accumulates in the systemic circulation, resulting in chronic hypoglycemia, which in turn stimulates release of branch chain amino acids as fodder for gluconeogenesis. This increase in branched-chain amino acids promotes uptake of amino acids, especially the aromatic variety, into the brain, where they tend to alter neurotransmitters (precursors of tryptophan), increasing serotonin levels and promoting cerebral function changes.

Major organ system failure is usually associated with alterations in distributive volume and clearance of drugs. Most analgesics and sedatives are eliminated by both hepatic and renal routes, following some sort of biotransformation. Hepatic clearance is usually dependent on the drug's plasma binding ability, blood perfusion through the liver, and hepatocellular uptake of the drug. Changes of blood flow to the liver in diseases such as cirrhosis and congestive heart failure tend to decrease the amount of the drug presented to the organ. In addition, passive liver congestion resulting from congestive heart failure can limit the ability of individual hepatocytes to assess the drug. Drugs such as meperidine are highly dependent on hepatic flow. Drugs such as diazepam bypassing the liver may actually increase extraction elsewhere since the drug is not taken up much in the liver. Hepatic enzymes such as the P450 system and glucuronidases act to transform lipophilic drugs into bipolar, water-soluble molecules that can be excreted through the kidneys and bile. These systems are important in the breakdown of morphine and meperidine. Hepatocyte degeneration from cirrhosis or other degenerative liver disorders interferes with this biotransformation. Significant alterations in biotransformation also occur when the serum albumin decreases significantly, limiting the binding of analgesics and subsequent delivery to the liver. Reductions in plasma protein concentration results in increased volumes of distribution, delivery of larger amounts of drug, and a greater potential for accentuated drug action on target organs.

In situations such as these, simply decreasing dosage acts to decrease plasma concentrations, avoiding toxic effect. This can be accomplished by either reducing dose size or frequency, depending on individual properties of the drug. Either method will reduce the effective plasma level. Decreasing an individual dose tends to lower peak plasma level proportionally with the trough. Decreasing distance between administrations tends to do the reverse. Renal dysfunction limits the amount of the active or deactivated drug that can be eliminated, tending to keep it active in the body longer. Dosage of highly excreted drugs is very important when renal function has decreased to 50% or more of normal. By determining an accurate creatinine clearance, appropriate dose-adjustment factors can be utilized to determine adjustment of dosages.

XII. Clearance of Commonly Used ICU Sedatives and Analgesics

A. Morphine

Because it is not very lipophilic and highly ionized (water soluble), less than 0.1% of a dose of morphine administered intravenously actually enters the brain. Most administered morphine undergoes glucuronidation, and the morphine-glucuronide is excreted through the kidneys. Only 10% is excreted unchanged. Morphine-glucuronide normally exerts only minimal analgesic activity and does not cross into CNS membranes. In hepatic dysfunction, morphine-glucuronide tends to accumulate and can cause respiratory depression in patients with altered blood-brain permeability. Intravenous morphine should be restricted or attenuated in the presence of active renal or hepatic disease and infections of the CNS (123).

B. Fentanyl

Because it is a very lipophilic drug, fentanyl absorbs into the CNS very rapidly but also quickly binds to plasma proteins and is rapidly cleared by the liver. Fentanyl undergoes extensive metabolism in the liver, producing intermediaries such as norfentanyl which are not active and are usually excreted into both the bile and urine. Since the drug can be excreted by the kidneys as well as cleared by the liver and has no significant active intermediates to accumulate, it is a relatively good drug to use for analgesia in hepatorenal dysfunction. However, since the drug is quickly accumulated into body fat stores, long-term administration of fentanyl may be associated with delayed clearance and prolonged sedative effect (124).

C. Midazolam

Midazolam is a rapid-acting, water-soluble CNS depressant with a pharmacodynamic profile similar to its older relative, diazepam. Midazolam is highly protein bound and has a large volume of distribution but is extensively cleared in the liver by glucuronidation and hydroxylation subsequent to being eliminated in the bile and urine. Therefore, dosage should be attenuated in extensive liver disease. The excretion of midazolam is relatively unaffected by renal disease (125).

D. Ketorolac

Ketorolac trimethamine is a parenteral nonsteroidal anti-inflammatory drug, comparable to morphine in analgesic activity. Following administration, ketorolac is almost completely bound to plasma protein, with a small volume of distribution and limited hepatic clearance. Ketorolac is mainly glucuronidated, and 90% of the conjugate is excreted in the urine. At least half of the free drug is also excreted through the kidneys. In renal insufficiency, the elimination of the drug is prolonged and the effects of active drug protracted. Ketorolac is a good drug for use in hepatic insufficiency. However, since it is a potent prostaglandin inhibitor, patients with active gastrointestinal bleeding should avoid it, and patients with less risk should be started on prophylactic H_2-antagonist therapy if there are no other contraindications (126).

E. Propofol

Propofol is completely glucuronized in the liver, and the conjugated products are excreted in the urine. The drug has a small initial volume of distribution, short half-life in both the distribution and elimination phase, a high plasma clearance, and mostly inactive intermediate metabolites. Steady-state blood concentrations of propofol do not seem to be affected by moderate degrees of renal or hepatic insufficiency. However, it has been recommended that infusions of propofol be reduced in elderly patient populations because of its tendency to cause hypotension, especially in the presence of intravascular depletion and heart failure (127).

XIII. Role of Sedative-Reversal Agents in the ICU

Naloxone is a narcotic antagonist commonly used in emergency departments for reversing the effects of narcotic overdoses. In the absence of opoid drugs, the drug has virtually no effect, making it safe for a wide range of usage in unconscious patients. However, its usage in the ICU is fraught with more hazard. Narcotic reversal with naloxone in post–cardiac surgery patients has been met with unexpected, precipitous ventricular tachycardia and fibrillation (128). Attempts to uncover possible narcotic-induced stupor versus obtundation as a result of intracranial catastrophe by the administration of naloxone is fraught with hazard. If the patient with increased intracranial pressure is suddenly awakened from a narcotic-induced sleep and becomes agitated, intracranial pressure can rise precipitously, causing intracranial bleeding or other disasters. Naloxone is very effective in the reversal of respiratory depression caused by narcotics. However, with a half-life of 20 minutes, it is rather short acting and requires continuous infusion for the most effective result. Rate of infusion can be easily titrated to the patient's clinical condition.

Flumazenil is a new benzodiazepine antagonist that acts as a competitive inhibitor at the GABA-benzodiazepine receptor site (129). Flumazenil has a 1- to 2-minute onset after intravenous administration and a 30-minute duration or more. A dose of 0.2 mg can be given IV initially and every minute thereafter, titrated to the desired effect. Titrated continuous IV infusions beginning at 0.5 mg/h are effective in maintaining benzodiazepine reversal. A maximum dose of 3 mg/h is recommended. Flumazenil has not yet been associated with severe side effects, but tonic-clonic seizures have been reported. Flumazenil is indicated in the event of accidental overdose of benzodiazepines during procedures such as endoscopy, colonoscopy, or bronchoscopy. Its main use in the emergency department is benzodiazepine overdose combined with alcohol toxicity, where respiratory depression is additive. In the ICU, flumazenil may be useful in a continuous infusion as an aid in weaning from mechanical ventilation by hastening recovery from long-term administration of benzodiazepines (130–132).

XIV. Life-Threatening Agitation in the ICU

Agitation episodes that threaten hemodynamic stability are becoming more common as critical care units accept broader populations of critically ill patients for longer periods of time. Episodes of life-threatening delirium and agitation are signaled by escalating agitation in the face of increasing sedative administration and the addition of multiple drugs. Eventually a point is reached where the deleterious side effects of pharmacological agents threaten respiratory and hemodynamic stability. Escalating dosages of sedatives in the face of increasing agitation is a genuine medical emergency that must be dealt with aggressively. Hemodynamic deterioration from the effects of agitation can precipitate angina, heart failure, and cardiac arrhythmias by increasing myocardial work and oxygen consumption in the face of a fixed coronary artery output. Increased muscular activity and hypermetabolism increases CO_2 production. Patients controlled on mechanical ventilation and chronic lung failure patients may manifest sudden increases in pCO_2, resulting in narcosis and obtundation or further catecholamine release, increasing agitation.

Hypermetabolism at the muscular level also produces metabolic acidosis and the potential for rhabdomyolysis, myoglobinuria, and renal failure. Prolonged agitation episodes can precipitate physical injury to the patient or attending staff. It is extremely important to search until the exact etiology of any agitation episode is identified and treated precisely. Effective prioritization hallmarks the initial appraisal of a severely agitated patient in the acute care setting. Initially, a rapid evaluation of emergent medical and surgical disorders can be quickly performed by inventorying monitoring devices ubiquitous to the ICU setting. Emergent airway decompensations resulting in elevated end-tidal carbon dioxide can be rapidly ruled out by capnography. Acute cardiac decompensations can be rapidly detected by continuous mixed venous oximetry. Acute hypoxia can be quickly detected by continuous pulse oximetry. Most of these devices come equipped with alarms, which signal exceeded parameters before actual hemodynamic decompensation occurs.

Following the ruling out of acutely reversible metabolic or respiratory decompensations, the somatic effects of unrelenting agitation should be ameliorated as quickly as possible while the search continues for the etiology of the agitation episode. End organ damage from catecholamine storm and musculoskeletal hyperactivity happens in real time and while sedation regimens are instituted and titrated. Getting control of hemodynamics and ventilation will facilitate the search for the underlying etiology without concurrent end organ impairment. The effects of hypertension with concomitant tachycardia can be safely resolved using titrated intravenous infusions of β-adrenergic antagonists. Labetalol, a drug manifesting both α-adrenergic agonist and β-adrenergic antagonistic properties, effectively decreases blood pressure and controls reflex tachycardia when administered in continuous infusions, atenolol, a relatively water-soluble β-adrenergic antagonist is cleared by the renal route or metoprolol, a highly lipid-soluble short-acting β-antagonist cleared by the hepatic route. Esmolol, a short-acting, rapidly titratable β-adrenergic blocking agent, has been demonstrated to manifest a negative chronotropic effect and can be titrated by continuous infusions.

For severe, life-threatening agitation, more potent sedation than benzodiazepines alone may be necessary. For this population of patients with life-threatening agitation syndromes, time spent loading sedatives with variable onsets of action make hypnotic effects erratic and unpredictable. The ideal sedative agent for severe, life-threatening agitation should combine properties of decreasing unrestrained brain activity, the effects of catecholamine storm on end organs, and hyperkinetic musculoskeletal activity. The short-acting anesthetic drug propofol used as a sedative has many of these ideal characteristics because it is potent and titratable.

XV. Anxiolysis During Withdrawal of Life Support

Few patients or families are willing to continue the discomfort of life support systems after a reasonable trial has demonstrated their benefit has come to the point of diminishing returns. Typically one of the most vivid concerns of families is that death, once accepted as inevitable, will progress painlessly. Weaning alert patients off futile life support systems is a vastly different proposition than terminal weaning of moribund, unconscious patients. Patients who opt for death rather than continuance of fruitless life support systems are alert enough to feel discomfort when these devices are discontinued. The principle of autonomy affords patients and their families the right to discontinue ineffectual life support systems, but they also demand the right to die in a "comfortable" fashion once removed. This puts the physician in the difficult position of having to diminish pain and discomfort during the dying process without facilitating death as a result (133–135).

The "principle of double effect," which mandates physicians to administer analgesia or sedation to the dying patient knowing that the dying process may be hastened as a result, has been well established in the medical ethics literature (136,137). For example, the administration of morphine decreases discomfort in greater proportion than it hastens an already established respiratory failure. However, societal proscriptions against euthanasia or assisted suicide mandate that the patient must still ultimately die as a consequence of the natural dying process, not a therapeutic maneuver on the part of a physician. Therefore, the administration of narcotics must not act in such a fashion that the patient succumbs from the effects of morphine rather than the underlying disease. This is a very fine line to tread.

XVI. Palliating the Dying Process During Respiratory Failure

For the most part, moribund patients undergoing withdrawal of life support die of respiratory failure. Since the patient is awake during the wean from mechanical ventilator support, the chief problem to be overcome in maintaining comfort is dyspnea, the sensation of breathlessness. Dyspnea is qualitatively different from simple tachypnea, which may be present without discomfort. In the setting of terminal weaning from mechanical ventilation, dyspnea occurs when the metabolic demand for ventilation exceeds the patient's ability to respond. As respiratory failure proceeds, increased pco_2 and resultant respiratory acidosis stimulate central chemoreceptors in the medulla, instantly inducing increased ventilation and a strong sensation of dyspnea (138). Sudden increases of pco_2 as small as 3 mmHg cause intense stimulation of ventilation. Tissue hypoxia increases ventilatory drive by stimulating peripheral chemoreceptors located in the carotid body and the aortic arch. However, hypoxia is not as potent a stimulus for dyspnea as it is an inducer of hyperventilation, and its onset is much slower than increases in pco_2. Hypoxia in the face of respiratory failure and resultant hypercarbia usually precipitates catecholamine release, systolic hypertension, tachypnea, tachycardia, and agitation. However, hypoxia in the face of normocarbia usually results in initial hyperventilation as chemoreceptors sense low po_2, followed by somnolence without agitation.

Patients experiencing the subjective sensation of dyspnea frequently exhibit tachypnea with shallow respirations. Maintenance of effective tidal volumes with mechanical ventilation may lessen the sensation of dyspnea resulting from hypoxia as long as tidal volumes are adequate. If the airway is maintained patent by endotracheal intubation, apnea, with its resultant pco_2 increase, is avoided by continuing ventilator support. Hypoxemia without concomitant hypercarbia results in somnolence without agitation, especially when combined with coincident sedation. The phenothiazine methotrimeprazine has sedative qualities resembling chlorpromazine,but tachycardia and dry mouth is less frequent. It also has effective analgesic qualities. The sedative and analgesic action of this drug has been specifically recommended in the psychiatry literature for restless patients dying of terminal cancer (139).

Benzodiazepines have actions that promote anxiolysis, hypnosis, anticonvulsion, and skeletal muscle relaxation. The opiate analgesics tend to lessen the subjective sensation of dyspnea. In normo- or hypocapnic patients with severe COPD, a single dose of 1 mg/kg dihydrocodeine reduced breathlessness by 20% and improved exercise tolerance by 18%. Postulated mechanisms of action include altered central perception of breathlessness, reduction of ventilatory drive, and reduction in oxygen consumption (140,141). Fentanyl is a very effective adjunct to life support withdrawal during the dyspnea stage. It combines effective sedation, analgesia, anxiolysis, and sympatholysis in a rapid-acting and titratable manner. Sedation can be initiated by an initial bolus followed by a continuous infusion. Any resulting agitation or discomfort from the weaning process can be effectively ameliorated by increasing fentanyl infusion as needed (142). The use of barbiturates has been advocated, rendering the patient unconscious in general anesthesia during the weaning process (143), but the administration of general anesthesia in terminal weaning is not yet completely accepted.

References

1. Crippen DW, Ermakov S. Stress, Agitation and brain failure in critical care medicine. Crit Care N Q 1992; 15(2):52–74.
2. Lipowski ZJ. Delirium: acute brain failure in man. Springfield, IL: Charles C Thomas Publishers, 1980:152–197.
3. Blachly PH, Kloster FF. Relation of cardiac output to postcardiotomy delirium. J Thorac Cardiovasc Surg 1966; 52:423.
4. Layne OL, Yudofsky SC. Postoperative psychosis in cardiotomy patients; the role of organic and psychiatric factors. N Engl J Med 1971; 284:518.
5. Clinton JE, et al. Haloperidol for sedation of disruptive emergency patients. Ann Emerg Med 1987; 16:319–322.

6. Wise NH, Cassem NH. Confusion in critically ill patients. In: Psychiatric aspects of critical care medicine. Probl Critical Care 1988; 2(1):146–167.

7. Romano J, Engel GL. Physiologic and psychologic considerations of delirium. Med Clin North Am 1944; 28:629–638.

8. Crippen DW. The role of sedation in the ICU patient with pain and agitation. Crit Care Clin 1990; 6(2):369–392.

9. Wedington WW. The mortality of delirium: an underappreciated problem? Psychosomatics 1982; 23:1232.

10. Wright SW. Conscious sedation in the emergency department: the value of capnography and pulse oximetry. Ann Emerg Med 1992; 21:551–55.

11. Francis J, Martin D, Kapoor WN. A prospective study of delirium in hospitalized elderly. JAMA 1990; 263(8):1097–1101.

12. Diagnostic and Statistical Manual of Mental Disorders (DSM-III-R), 3rd ed. Washington, DC: American Psychiatric Association, 1987:97–103.

13. Layne OL, Yudofsky SO. Postoperative psychosis in cardiotomy patients; the role of organic and psychiatric factors. N Engl J Med 1971; 284:518.

14. Hales RE, Yudofsky SO. Textbook of Neuropsychiatry. Washington, DC: American Psychiatric Press, 1987:89–103.

15. Lipowski ZJ. Delirium (acute confusional states). JAMA 1987; 258:1789–1792.

16. Mesulam MM, Waxman SG, Geschwind N, et al. Acute confusional states with right middle cerebral artery infarction. J Neurol Neurosurg Psychiatry 1977; 49: 861–864.

17. Medina JL, Chokroverty S, Rubino FA. Syndrome of agitated delirium and visual impairment: a manifestation of medial temporo-occipital infarction. J Neurol Neurosurg Psychiatry 1977; 49:861–864.

18. Lipowski ZJ. Delirium: transient cognitive disorders (delirium, acute confusional state) in the elderly. Am J Psychiatry 1983; 140:1426–1436.

19. Diagnostic and Statistical Manual of Mental Disorders (DSM-III-R), Washington, DC: American Psychiatric Association, 1987:97–103.

20. Greer KA, Hoyt JW. Pain: theory, anatomy, and physiology. Crit Care Clin 1990; 6(2):227–233.

21. Craven JL. Postoperative organic mental syndromes in lung transplant recipients. J Heart Transplant 1990; 9(2):129–132.

22. Kehlet H. Pain relief and modification of the stress response. In: Cousins MJ, Phillips GD, eds. Acute Pain Management. New York: Churchill Livingstone, 1986:46.

23. Basbaum EI, Fields HL. Endogenous pain control systems: brainstem spinal pathways and endorphin circuitry. Ann Rev Neurosci 1984; 7:309–338.

24. Barinaga-M. Playing 'telephone' with the body's message of pain. Science 1992; 258(5085):1085.

25. Li J, Ji YP, Qiao JT, et al. Suppression of nociceptive responses in parafascicular neurons by stimulation of substantia nigra: an analysis of related inhibitor pathways. Brain Res 1992; 591(1):109–115.

26. Berre J. Relief of pain in intensive care unit patients. Resuscitation 1984; 11:157–164.

27. Perry S, et al. Management of pain during debridement: a survey of US burn centers. Pain 1982; 13:275.

28. Barlow DH. Anxiety and Its Disorders. New York: The Gail Ford Press, 1988.
29. Kercher EE. Anxiety. Emerg Med Clin North Am 1991; 9(1):161–187.
30. Bell JA, Weissberg MP. Recognizing anxiety disorders and facilitating early, specific care. Emerg Med Rep 1986; 7(12):145–152.
31. Hallenberg B, Bergbom EI, Haljamae H. Patients' experiences of postoperative respiratory treatment—influence of anaesthetic and pain treatment regimens. Acta Anaesthesiol Scand 1990; 34(7):557–562.
32. Hansen-Flaschen JH, Brazinsky S, Basile C, et al. Use of sedating drugs and neuromuscular blocking agents in patients requiring mechanical ventilation for respiratory failure. A national survey. JAMA 1991; 266(20):2870–2875.
33. Parker MO. Perceptions of a critically ill patient experiencing therapeutic paralysis. Crit Care Med 1984; 12(1):69–71.
34. Bergbom EI, Haljamae H. Assessment of patients' experience of discomforts during respirator therapy. Crit Care Med 1989; 17(10):1068–1072.
35. Reisner L, Hohr J, Dunnington G, et al. Teaching mechanical ventilation. Surg Gynecol Obstet 1991; 173(3):227–228.
36. Granneman GR, Sennello LT, Steinberg FJ, Sonders RC. Intramuscular and intravenous pharmacokinetics of cefmenoxime, a new broad-spectrum cephalosporin, in healthy subjects. Antimicrob Agents Chemother 1982; 21(1):141–145.
37. Malacrida R, Fritz ME, Suter PM, et al. Pharmacokinetics of midazolam administered by continuous intravenous infusion to intensive care patients. Crit Care Med 1991; 20(8):1123–1126.
38. Mangano DT, Siliciano D, Hollerberg M, et al. Postoperative myocardial ischemia: therapeutic trials using intensive analgesia following surgery. Anesthesiology 1992; 76:342–353.
39. Sanchez-Izquierdo-Riera JA, Caballero-Cubedo RE, Perez-Vela JL, Ambrose-Checa A, Cantalapiedra-Santiago JA, Alted-Lopez E. Propofol versus midazolam: safety and efficacy for sedating the severe trauma patient. Anesth Analg 1998; 86: 1219–1224.
40. Hebenstreit GF, Fellerer K, Twerdy B, et al. L-tryptophan in pre-delirium and delirium conditions. Infusionstherapie 1989; 16(2):92–96.
41. Fielding S, Lal H. Behavioral actions of neuroleptics. In: Iversen SD, Snyder SH, eds. Handbook of Psychopharmacology. 2d ed. New York: Plenum Press, 1978: 91–128.
42. Baldessarini RJ. Drugs and the treatment of psychiatric disorders. In: Goodman A, Rall TW, Nies AS, et al., eds. The Pharmacological Basis of Therapeutics. 8th ed. New York: Pergamon Press, 1990:396.
43. Settle EC, Ayd FJ. Haloperidol: a quarter century of experience. J Clin Psychiatry 1983; 44:440–448.
44. Ayd FJ. Intravenous haloperidol therapy. Int Drug Ther Newslett 1978; 13:2330.
45. Settle EC, Ayd FJ. Haloperidol: a quarter century of experience. J Clin Psychiatry 1983; 44:440–448.
46. Tesar GE, Murray GB, Cassem NH. Use of haloperidol for acute delirium in intensive care setting. J Clin Psychopharmcol 1985; 5:344–347.
47. Riker RR, Fraser GL, Cox PM. Continuous infusion of haloperidol controls agitation in critically ill patients. Crit Care Med 1994; 22:433–440.

48. Chernow B, ed. The Pharmacologic Approach the the Critically Ill Patient. 2d ed. New York: Williams & Wilkins, 1988.
49. Geringer ES, Stern TA. Anxiety and depression in critically ill patients. In: Wise MG, ed. Psychiatric Aspects of Critical Care Medicine. Problems in Critical Care. Philadelphia: J.B. Lippincott Company, 1988:35–46.
50. Adams F. Emergency intravenous sedation of delirious, medically ill patient. J Clin Psychiatry 1988; 49(suppl):22–27.
51. Menza MA, Murray GB, Homes VF, et al. Controlled study of extrapyramidal reactions in the management of delirious, medically ill patients: intravenous haloperidol versus intravenous haloperidol plus benzodiazepines. Heart Lung 1988; 17(3):238–241.
52. Clinton JE, et al. Haloperidol for sedation of disruptive emergency patients. Ann Emerg Med 1987; 16:19–322.
53. Kehlet H. Pain relief and modification of the stress response. In: Cousins MJ, Phillips GD, eds. Acute Pain Management. New York: Churchill Livingstone, 1986:46.
54. Veselis RA. Intravenous narcotics in the ICU. Crit Care Clin 1990; 6(2):295–313.
55. Hare BD. The opioid analgesics: rational selection of agents for acute and chronic pain. Hosp Formul 1987; 22:64–83.
56. Rawal N, Tandon B. Epidural and intrathecal morphine in intensive care units. Intensive Care Med 1985; 11:129–133.
57. Jorgenson BC, Anderson HB, Engquist A. Influence of epidural morphine on postoperative pain, endocrine, metabolic and renal responses to surgery: a controlled study. Acta Anaesthesiol Scand 1982; 26:63–68.
58. Coombs DW, Saunders RL, Lachance D. Intrathecal morphine tolerance: use of intrathecal clonidine, DAADLE, and intraventricular morphine. Anesthesiology 1985; 62:358–363.
59. Klausner JM, Caspi J, Lelcuk S, et al. Delayed muscular rigidity and respiratory depression following fentanyl anesthesia. Arch Surg 1988; 123:66–67.
60. Svamman FL. Fentanyl-O_2-NO_2 rigidity and pulmonary compliance. Anesth Analg 1983; 62:332–334.
61. Larkin GL, Prescott JE. A randomized, double blind, comparative study of the efficacy of ketorolac tromethamine versus meperidine in the treatment of severe migraine. Ann Emerg Med 1992; 21:919–924.
62. Wright SW, Norris RL, Mitchell TR. Ketorolac for sickle cell vaso-occlusive crisis pain in the emergency department: Lack of a narcotic-sparing effect. Ann Emerg Med 1992; 21:925–928.
63. Estes LL, Fuhs DW, Heaton AH, et al. Gastric ulcer perforation associated with the use of injectable ketorolac. Ann Pharmacother 1993; 27:42–43.
64. Boras-Uber LA, Brackett-Newton C. Brief clinical observations: Ketorolac-induced acute renal failure. Am J Med 1992; 92(4):450–452.
65. Goetz CM, Sterchele JA, Harchelroad FP. Anaphylactiod reaction following ketorolac tromethamine administration. Ann Pharmacother 1992; 26:1237–1238.
66. Brown CR, Wild VM, Bynaum L. Comparison of intravenous ketolorac tromethamine and morphine sulfate in postoperative pain (abstr). Clin Pharmacol Ther 1988; 43:142.
67. Camu F, Van Overberge L, Bullingham R, et al. Hemodynamic effect of intrave-

nous doses of ketorolac tromethamine compared with morphine. Pharmacotherapy 1990; 10(2):122S–126S.

68. Jung D, Mroszczak E, Bynum L. Pharmacokinetics of ketorolac in humans after intravenous, intramuscular and oral administration. Eur J Clin Pharmacol 1988; 35(4):423–425.

69. Buckley MM, Brogden RN. Ketorolac. A review of its pharmacodynamic and pharmacokinetic properties, and therapeutic potential. Drugs 1990; 89:86–109.

70. Hokfelt B, Hedeland H, Hasson BG. The effect of clonidine and penbutol, respectively on catecholamines in blood and urine, plasma renin activity ad urinary aldosterone in hypertensive patients. Arch Int Pharmacodyn 1975; 213:307–321.

71. Ghignone M, Quintin L, Kehler CH, et al. Effects of clonidine on narcotic requirements and hemodynamic response during induction of fentanyl anesthesia and endotracheal intubation. Anesthesiology 1986; 64:36–42.

72. Coombs DW, Saunders RL, Fratkin JD, et al. Continuous intrathecal hydromorphone and clonidine for tractable cancer pain. J Neurosurg 1986; 64:890–894.

73. Cushman PJ, Sowers JR. Alcohol withdrawal syndrome: clinical and hormonal responses to α-2 adrenergic treatment. Alcoholism 1989; 13:361–364.

74. Toon S, Hopkins KJ, Aarons L, Rowland M. Rate and extent of absorption of clonidine from a transdermal therapeutic system. J Pharm Pharmacol 1989; 41:17–21.

75. Zochowski RJ, Lada W. Intravenous clonidine treatment in acute myocardial infarction (with comparison to a nitroglycerin-treated and control group). J Cardiovasc Pharmacol 1986; 8(S3):S41–45.

76. Wing LM, Reid JL, Hamilton CA, et al. Effects of clonidine on biochemical indices of sympathetic function in normotensive man. Clin Sci Mol Med 1977; 53:45–53.

77. Aantaa RE, Kanto JH, Scheinin M. Dexmedetomidine premedication for minor gynecologic surgery. Anesth Analg 1990; 4:407–413.

78. Aantaa RE, Kanto JH. Dexmedotomidine, an alpha 2-adrenoceptor agonist, reduces anesthetic requirements for patients undergoing minor gynecologic surgery. Anesthesiology 1990; 73:230–235.

79. Scheinin H, Virtanen R, MacDonald E, et al. Medetomidine—a novel α_2-adrenoceptor agonist: a review of its pharmacodynamic effects. Prog Neuropsychopharmacol Biol Psychiatry 1989; 13:635–651.

80. Weitz JD, Foster SD, Waugaman WR, et al. Anesthetic and hemodynamic effects of dexmedetomidine during isoflurane anesthesia in a canine model. Nurse Anesth 1991; 2:19–27.

81. Savola JM. Cardiovascular actions of medetomidine and their reversal by atipamezole. Acta Vet Scand Suppl 1989; 85:39–47.

82. Ibanez J, et al. Thoracic epidural analgesia and chest trauma. Intensive Care Med 1987; 13:297.

83. Shulman M, et al. Post thoracotomy pain and pulmonary function following epidural and systemic morphine. Anesthesiology 1984; 61(5):569–575.

84. Stern TA, Caplan RA, Cassem NH. Use of benzodiazepines in a coronary care unit. Psychosomatics 1987; 28:163.

85. Mangano DT, Siliciano D, Hollenberg M, et al. Postoperative myocardial ischemia. Anesthesiology 1992; 76:342–353.

86. Crippen D. Understanding neurohumoral causes of anxiety in the ICU. J Crit Illness 1995; 10(8):550–560.
87. Crippen DW. Pharmacologic treatment of brain failure and delirium. Crit Care Clin 1994; 10:7.
88. Ronan KP, Gallagher TJ, George B, et al. Comparison of propofol and midazolam for sedation of intensive care patients. Crit Care Med 1995; 23(2):286–293.
89. Greenblatt DJ, et al. Kinetic and dynamic study of intravenous lorazepam: comparison with intravenous diazepam. J Pharmacol Exp Ther 1989; 250(1):134–140.
90. Salzman C. Anxiety in the elderly: treatment strategies. J Clin Psychiatry 1990; 51(S):18–21.
91. Berggren L, Erikson I, Mollenholt P, et al. Changes in respiratory pattern after repeated doses of diazepam and midazolam in healthy subjects. Acta Anaesthesiol Scand 1987; 31:667–672.
92. Behne M, et al. Continuous midazolam infusion for sedation of respirator patients. Anesthetist 1987; 36:228–232.
93. Reves JG, Fragen RJ, Vinik HR, et al. Midazolam: pharmacology and uses. Anesthesiology 1985; 62:310–324.
94. Barvais L, Dejonckheere M, Dernovoi B, et al. Continuous infusion of midazolam or bolus of diazepam for postoperative sedation cardiac surgical patients. Acta Anaesthesiol Belgica 1988; 39:239–245.
95. Vinik HP. Midazolam infusion: Introduction and overview. In: Vinik HR, ed. Midazolam Infusion for Anesthesia and Intensive Care. Princeton: Excerpta Medica, 1989:1–9.
96. Fish DN. Treatment of delirium in the critically ill patient. Clin Pharm 1991; 10(6): 456–466.
97. Aitkenhead AR, Willatts SM, Collins CH, et al. Comparison of propofol and midazolam for sedation in critically ill patients. Lancet; 1989; 23:704–708.
98. Albanese J, Martin C, Lacarelle B. Pharmacokinetics of long-term propofol infusion used ation in ICU patients. Anesthesiology 1990; 73:214–217.
99. Skues MA. The pharmacology of propofol. J Clin Anesth 1989; 1:387–400.
100. Sebel PS, Lowdon JD. Propofol: a new intravenous anesthetic. Anesthesiology 1989; 71:260–277.
101. White PF. Propofol: pharmacokinetics and pharmacodynamics. Semin Anesthesia 1988; (suppl 1):4–20.
102. Clayes MA, Gepts E, Camu F. Haemodynamic changes during anaesthesia induced and maintained with propofol. Br J Anaesth 1988; 60:3–9.
103. Easton C, et al. Sensory-perceptual alterations in the intensive care unit. Heart-Lung 1988; 17:229–235.
104. Westphal LM, Cheng EY, White PF, et al. Use of midazolam infusion for sedation following cardiac surgery. Anesthesiology 1987; 67:257–262.
105. Barvais L, Dejonckheere M, Dernovoi B, et al. Continuous infusion of midazolam or bolus of diazepam for postoperative sedation in cardiac surgical patients. Acta Anaesthesiol Belg 1988; 39(4):239–245.
106. Higgins TL, Yared JP, Estafanous FG, et al. Propofol versus midazolam for intensive care.

107. Roekaerts PM, Huygen FJ, de-Lange S. Infusion of propofol versus midazolam for sedation in the intensive care unit following cardiac surgery. J Cardiothorac Vasc Anesth 1993; 7(2):142–147.

108. Chaudhri S, Kenny GNC. Sedation after cardiac bypass surgery: comparison of propofol and midazolam in the presence of a computerized closed loop arterial pressure controller. Br J Anaesth 1992; 68:98–99.

109. Clarke TNS. Propofol compared with midazolam for sedation following prolonged neurosurgery. J Drug Dev 1991; 4:108–109.

110. Henderson A, Dipplesman J, Miller J. Failure of intravenous low dose midazolam to influence memory recall in drug paralyzed postoperative patients sedated with papaveretum. Aust Crit Care 1994; 7:22–24.

111. Bruder N, Lassegue D, Pelissier D, et al. Energy expenditure and withdrawal of sedation in severe head-injured patients. Crit Care Med 1994; 22(7):1114–1119.

112. Nakahashi K, Yomosa H, Matsuzawa N, et al. Effect on cerebral blood flow of midazolam during modified neuroleptic-anesthesia. Masui Jpn J Anesthesiol 1991; 40(12):1787–1792.

113. Hundt F, el Gindi M, Brandt L. Analgesia and sedation in neurosurgical intensive care patients. Anasthesie Intensivther Notfallmed 1990; 25(4):281–286.

114. Crippen DW, Ermakov S. Stress, agitation and brain failure in critical care medicine. Crit Care N Q 1992; 15(2):52–74.

115. Klausner JM, Caspi J, Lelcuk S, et al. Delayed muscular rigidity and respiratory depression following fentanyl anesthesia. Arch Surg 1988; 123:66–67.

116. Newman M, Reves JG. Midazolam is the sedative of choice to supplement narcotic anesthesia. J Cardiothor Vasc Anesth 1993; 7(5):615–619.

117. Shapiro BA, Warren J, Egol AB, et al. Practice parameters for intravenous analgesia and sedation for adult patients in the intensive care unit: an executive summary. Crit Care Med 1995; 23(9):1458–1459.

118. Chuang E, Wenner WJ, Piccoli DA, et al. Intravenous sedation in pediatric upper gastrointestinal endoscopy. Gastrointest Endosc 1995; 42(2):156–160.

119. Hiew CY, Hart GK, Thomson KR, et al. Analgesia and sedation in interventional radiological procedures. Austral Radiol 1995; 39(2):128–134.

120. Milgrom P, Weinstein P, Fiset L, et al. The anxiolytic effects of intravenous sedation using midazolam alone or in multiple drug techniques. J Oral Maxillofacial Surg 1994; 52(3):219–224, 225.

121. Milgrom P, Beirne OR, Fiset L, et al. The safety and efficacy of outpatient midazolam intravenous sedation for oral surgery with and without fentanyl. Anesthesia Prog 1993; 40(3):57–62.

122. Lau W, Kovoor P, Ross DL. Cardiac electrophysiologic effects of midazolam combined with fentanyl. Am J Cardiol 1993; 72(2):177–182.

123. Aitkinhead AR, Vater M, Acholas K, et al. Pharmacokinetics of single dose IV morphine in normal volunteers and patients with end stage renal failure. Br J Anaesth 1984; 56:813–818.

124. Haberer JP, Schoeffler P, Couderc E, et al. Fentanyl pharmacokinetics in anaesthetized patients with cirrhosis. Br J Anaesth 1982; 54:1267–1270.

125. Greenblatt DJ, Arendt RM, Abernathy DR, et al. In vivo quantitation of benzo-

diazepine lipophilicity: relation to in vivo distribution. Br J Anaesth 1983; 55:985–989.

126. Micaela M, Buckley T, Brogden RN. Ketorolac: a review of its pharmacodynamic properties, and therapeutic potential. Drugs 1990; 39:86–109.

127. Cockshott ID. The pharmacokinetics of propofol in the ICU patient. J Drug Dev 1991; 4(suppl 3):29–36.

128. Michaelis LL, Hickey PR, Clark TA. Ventricular irritability associated with the use of naloxone hydrochloride. Ann Thor Surg 1974; 18:608–614.

129. Dunton AW, Schwam E, Pitman V, et al. Flumazenil: US clinical pharmacology studies. Eur J Anesthesiol Suppl 1988; 2:81–95.

130. Hojer J, Baehrendtz S, Magnusson A, et al. A placebo controlled trial of flumazenil given by continuous infusion in severe benzodiazepine overdosage. Acta Anaesthesiol Scand 1991; 35(7):584–590.

131. Hojer J, Baehrendtz S, Forsstrom A, et al. The stability of flumazenil in infusion solution. Acta Pharma Nord 1990; 2(2):101.

132. Osnes J, Hermanson L. Acid-base balance after maximal exercise of short duration. J Appl Physiol 1972; 32:59–63.

133. Wanzer SH, Federman DD, Adelstein SA, et al: The physician's responsibility toward hopelessly ill patients. N Engl J Med 1989; 320(13):844–849.

134. Schneiderman LJ, Spragg RG. Ethical decisions in discontinuing mechanical ventilation. N Engl J Med 1988; 818:984–988.

135. Guidelines on the termination of life-sustaining treatment and the care of the dying. A report by the Hasting Center. Briarcliff Manor, New York: The Hasting Center, 1987.

136. Wanzer SH, Adelstein SJ, Cranford RE. The physician's responsibility toward hopelessly ill patients. N Engl J Med 1984; 310:955–959.

137. Crippen D. Practical aspects of life support withdrawal: a critical care physician's opinion. Clin Intensive Care 1991; 2:260–265.

138. Hoyt JW, ed. Critical Care Practice. Philadelphia: W.B. Saunders, 1991:49–80.

139. Oliver DJ. The use of methotrimeprazine in terminal care. Br J Clin Pract 1985; 339–340.

140. Woodcock AA, Gross EA, Gellert A, et al. Effects of dihydrocodeine, alcohol, and caffeine on breathlessness and exercise tolerance in patients with chronic obstructive lung disease and normal blood gases. N Engl J Med 1982; 305:1611–1216.

141. Robin ED, Burke CM. Single-patient randomized trial: opiates for intractable dyspnea. Chest 1986; 90:888–892.

142. Crippen DW. Terminally weaning awake patients from life sustaining mechanical ventilation: the critical care physicians role in comfort measures during the dying process. Clin Intensive Care 1992; 3:206–212.

143. Garber AM. Barbiturates in the care of the terminally ill. N Engl J Med 1992; 1678.

10

Optimal Airway Management in Ventilated Patients

GEORGE B. BUCZKO

Brown University School of Medicine
Providence, Rhode Island

I. Introduction

Mechanical ventilation in the critical care setting can be invasive or noninvasive (1). This chapter focuses on the management of the artificial airway in adult patients requiring invasive mechanical ventilatory support. Airway management in this situation consists of artificial airway placement, maintenance, and discontinuation. In most cases, placement refers to trans-laryngeal intubation (endotracheal intubation) or to tracheostomy. Airway placement requires skill and an understanding of indications, equipment, medications, physiological disturbances, routes, complications, and special circumstances related to securing the airway. Optimal maintenance includes avoidance of complications of prolonged trans-laryngeal intubation as well as a reasonable sense of timing of tracheostomy. In addition, endotracheal tube exchange may become necessary during the course of airway maintenance. The artificial airway may be discontinued when the patient is successfully weaned from mechanical ventilation. It must be clear, however, that there is minimal risk of postextubation airway obstruction and that the patient can protect his or her airway from pulmonary aspiration.

Information presented in this chapter has been obtained from original investigations, review articles, textbooks, practice guidelines of the American Society of Anesthesiologists, and from personal experience. This paragraph summarizes the value of management recommendations made in this chapter. *Standards* represent recommendations that reflect a high degree of clinical certainty. Evidence for standards comes from methodologically sound prospective randomized controlled trials (class 1 evidence). *Guidelines* represent recommendations that reflect a moderate degree of clinical certainty. Evidence for guidelines comes from prospectively collected data and includes observational studies, cohort studies, prevalence studies, and case-control series (class 2 evidence). *Options* represent all other recommendations. Evidence for options comes from retrospectively collected data and includes clinical series, case reviews, case reports, and expert opinion (class 3 evidence). Assessment of medical devices may fall outside of these definitions (2,3). Most of the recommendations in this chapter fall under the category of options.

II.   Artificial Airway Placement

Artificial airway placement has been reviewed extensively (4–7). An artificial airway can be placed after induction of general anesthesia, after topical or local anesthesia with intravenous sedation, or without any anesthesia if the patient's level of consciousness is sufficiently depressed. Routes include naso-tracheal, oro-tracheal, and via tracheostomy or cricothyroidotomy. In mechanically ventilated patients, trans-laryngeal airway placement may be necessary after a planned but failed extubation and may also be required after unplanned extubation, which is reported to occur in 3–13% of mechanically ventilated patients (8).

A.   Indications

The indications for endotracheal intubation are summarized in Table 1 and include new or ongoing requirement for mechanical ventilatory support in patients who are poor candidates for noninvasive ventilation, relief of acute upper airway obstruction, and requirement for airway protection from pulmonary aspiration (6).

   The indications for mechanical ventilation include cardiopulmonary arrest, ventilatory insufficiency, and the need for hyperventilation for the treatment of acutely increased intracranial pressure. The presence of ventilatory insufficiency should be detected by clinical examination, which contributes significantly to the decision to reinsert an artificial airway in the setting of unplanned extubation (8). Signs of impending ventilatory failure in patients include elevated respiratory rate, (9), suprasternal and intercostal indrawing (10), and paradoxical breathing (loss of thoraco-abdominal coordination) (11).

   In complete acute upper airway obstruction, the patient may manifest distress, failure of phonation, paradoxical breathing, intercostal indrawing, cyanosis, and lack of air movement. With incomplete acute upper airway obstruction, inspi-

Table 1 Indications for Endotracheal Intubation

I. Requirement for mechanical ventilation
  A. Cardiopulmonary arrest
  B. Impending ventilatory failure
    1. Patient complains of severe shortness of breath
    2. Respiratory rate greater than 30 breaths per minute
    3. Paradoxical breathing (loss of thoraco-abdominal coordination)
    4. Intercostal indrawing
    5. Other evidence of distress (systemic hypertension, tachycardia)
    6. Cyanosis or saturation by pulse oximetry $< 90\%$ with $Fio_2 > 0.6$)
    7. Behavioral changes (lack of cooperation, agitation)
  C. Treatment of increased intracranial pressure
    1. Hyperventilation
II. Symptoms and signs of upper airway obstruction
  A. Incomplete
    1. The signs and symptoms of impending ventilatory failure
    2. Inspiratory stridor
  B. Complete
    1. The signs and symptoms of impending ventilatory failure
    2. Failure of phonation
    3. Lack of air movement (by auscultation or palpation)
III. Airway protection against aspiration pneumonitis
  A. Deep coma

---

ratory stridor can be present in addition to these signs (12). Whether or not there is clinical evidence of ventilatory failure, patients in deep coma require endotracheal intubation for airway protection against aspiration pneumonitis (13).

B. Equipment

Equipment for endotracheal intubation should be immediately available in the critical care setting and checked on a regular basis. At a minimum, the patient should be monitored with continuous EKG, pulse oximetry, and frequent blood pressure measurements (14). Recommended mandatory equipment is listed in Table 2 and includes all of the following: suction apparatus, an oxygen source, a self-inflating bag and mask for delivery of positive pressure ventilation, oral and nasal airways, a layngoscope handle and various blades, endotracheal tubes of various adult sizes, a 10 cc syringe for cuff inflation, an intubating stylet, and a stethoscope (5). In addition, a device that confirms endotracheal tube placement (described below) must be available.

Recommendations for appropriate oral endotracheal tube size must take into account several considerations, which are reviewed in subsequent parts of

Table 2 Equipment for Endotracheal Intubation

I. Mandatory equipment
  A. Source of oxygen
    1. Wall or tank
  B. Suction apparatus
    1. Tube for oropharyngeal suction
    2. Catheter for tracheal suction
  C. Equipment for application of manual positive pressure ventilation
    1. Anesthesia facemasks of various sizes
    2. Oropharyngeal and nasopharyngeal airways of various adult sizes
    3. Self-inflating bag (e.g., Ambu or Laerdal)
  D. Equipment for laryngoscopy
    1. Laryngoscope handle
    2. Curved blades with functioning light source (e.g., #3 and #4 Macintosh)
    3. Straight blades with functioning light source (e.g., #2 and #3 Miller)
    4. Magill forceps to retrieve foreign objects
  E. Equipment for intubation
    1. Endotracheal tubes sizes 6.0–8.5 mm ID
    2. Intubating stylet
    3. 10 cc syringe for cuff inflation
  F. Equipment for confirmation of tube placement
    1. Quantitative carbon dioxide analyzer (capnometer)
    2. Qualitative carbon dioxide detection device (e.g., Easy Cap)
    3. Air aspiration device (e.g., TubeChek)
II. Monitors (minimum requirements) for endotracheal intubation
  A. Pulse oximetry
  B. Electrocardiogram
  C. Frequent blood pressure measurements
  D. Stethoscope

---

this chapter. Smaller tube sizes are thought to limit pressure on the posterior laryngeal structures and may cause less injury to those areas than larger tubes. On the other hand, smaller tubes may require high cuff pressures to achieve an airway seal sufficient for leak-free positive pressure ventilation, and these high cuff pressures may increase the risk of tracheal injury. Larger tubes, while applying greater pressure to the posterior larynx, do facilitate both clearance of tracheal secretions and performance of fiberoptic bronchoscopy. The endotracheal tube sizes that appear to balance these considerations are 8.0–8.5 mm internal diameter (ID) for men and 7.0–7.5 mm ID for women (15,16). In the case of difficult intubation or if there is airway obstruction, it may be necessary to insert a smaller tube. Intubating techniques are described in several sources (4,5,15). Endotracheal tubes should be inspected for defects, the inflated cuff should be checked for leaks (17,18), and the cuff should then be deflated prior to insertion.

C. Medications

Anesthesia Induction Agents

Anesthesia induction agents can be used to facilitate endotracheal intubation in awake patients or in uncooperative patients who require artificial airway placement (19,20). Available choices and usual doses are listed in Table 3 and include thiopental, propofol, etomidate, and ketamine. All are rapid-onset anesthetic induction agents of relatively short duration. Short-acting benzodiazepines and narcotics may also be used.

Thiopental

Thiopental is an ultra-short-acting thiobarbiturate (21). Nervous system effects include loss of consciousness, ventilatory depression, and obliteration of protective airway reflexes, especially with high dosage. Cardiovascular effects include myocardial depression and venodilatation leading to systemic hypotension and reflex tachycardia. Therefore, use of thiopental is undesirable in patients with circulatory shock of any etiology, uncontrolled congestive heart failure, critical coronary artery stenosis, severe cardiac valvular stenosis, and hemodynamically significant pericardial disease. Intravenous dosage is 2.5–4.5 mg/kg in healthy patients and should be reduced in geriatric and in critically ill patients. Onset of action is under one minute, and duration of action is 5–8 minutes after a single bolus injection. This short duration is due to redistribution to fat. Because it decreases cerebral blood flow and cerebral metabolic rate, thiopental may be useful in artificial airway insertion in patients with raised intracranial pressure.

Propofol

Propofol is a phenol (22) with central nervous, cardiovascular, and respiratory system effects that are similar to those of thiopental. Consequently, the use of propofol is also undesirable in patients with circulatory shock of any etiology, uncontrolled congestive heart failure, critical coronary artery stenosis, severe cardiac valvular stenosis, and hemodynamically significant pericardial disease. Preservation of airway reflexes at low anesthetic doses is markedly blunted with the concomitant use of narcotics (23). Propofol does limit neurally mediated bronchoconstriction in response to endotracheal intubation in animal experiments (24) and may be a useful induction agent in patients with asthma. Intravenous dosage is 2–2.5 mg/kg in healthy patients and should be reduced in geriatric and in critically ill patients. Onset of action is under one minute, and duration of action is 3–8 minutes after a single bolus injection. Its short duration is due to redistribu-

Table 3 Anesthesia Induction Agents and Neuromuscular Blocking Agents

Drug	Class	Dose (mg/kg)	Onset (min)	Duration (min)	Effects	
Induction agents:						
Thiopental	Thiobarbiturate	2.5–4.5	<1	5–8	CNS:	Loss of consciousness, decreased cerebral blood flow, ventilatory depression, loss of protective airway reflexes
					CVS:	Myocardial depression, venodilatation, hypotension, reflex tachycardia
Propofol	Alkylphenol	2–2.5	<1	3–8	CNS:	Loss of consciousness, ventilatory depression
					CVS:	Myocardial depression, hypotension
					Resp:	? Bronchodilatation
Etomidate	Imidazole	0.3	<1	5–15	CNS:	Loss of consciousness, decreased cerebral blood flow
					CVS:	Minimal effects
					Endo:	Adrenal suppression
Ketamine	Phencyclidine	1–2	1	15–30	CNS:	Neuroleptic state, increased cerebral blood flow, emergence reactions
					CVS:	Hypertension, tachycardia
					Resp:	Bronchodilatation
Neuromuscular blocking agents:						
Succinylcholine	Depolarizing blocker	1–1.5	0.5	<10		Neuromuscular blockade, dysrhythmias, increased intracranial pressure, increased intraocular pressure, hyperkalemia, malignant hyperthermia trigger, allergic reactions
Rocuronium	Nondepolarizing blocker	0.4–0.6	1	30		Neuromuscular blockade, slight tachycardia

tion, rapid hepatic metabolism, and extrahepatic metabolism. Propofol may cause pain at the injection site.

Etomidate

Etomidate is an imidazole derivative (22). Its chief advantage lies in its minimal effect on cardiovascular function. Because it lowers intracranial pressure while maintaining cerebral perfusion pressure, it is also a desirable induction agent in patients with increased intracranial pressure. Drawbacks include adrenal suppression, pain at the injection site, and a high rate of nausea and vomiting. Intravenous dosage is 0.3 mg/kg with an onset of action less than one minute and duration of action 5–15 minutes.

Ketamine

Ketamine is a phencyclidine (22). Nervous system effects include loss of consciousness although recipient patients may keep their eyes open (the neuroleptic state) and retain some protective airway reflexes. Ketamine also increases intracranial pressure, and some patients experience emergence reactions such as excitement, confusion, euphoria, and fear. Cardiovascular effects include systemic hypertension and tachycardia associated with norepinephrine release. Respiratory effects include bronchodilatation and minimal respiratory depression. Ketamine may be used to facilitate endotracheal intubation in hemodynamically unstable patients. The usual dosage of a single bolus injection is 1–2 mg/kg. The onset of action is one minute and duration of action is 15–30 minutes.

Other Agents

Benzodiazepines and opioids have been used to facilitate intubation (25), but because of a longer duration of action than the usual induction agents, they are used primarily in small doses as adjuncts to hypnosis.

Neuromuscular Blocking Agents

Neuromuscular blocking agents are administered in conjunction with anesthetic induction agents to further facilitate trans-laryngeal artificial airway placement in emergency situations (19,20). They are frequently used during routine induction of general anesthesia in the operating room for the same reason (26,27). For urgent situations, agents with a rapid onset of action, namely succinylcholine and rocuronium, are the most desirable (28).

Succinylcholine

Succinylcholine (29) is a rapid-onset depolarizing neuromuscular blocking agent that is composed of two acetylcholine molecules that stimulate the acetylcholine receptor at the myoneural junction. Intravenous dosage is 1–1.5 mg/kg and onset of action is about one minute, with initial acetylcholine-receptor stimulation resulting in muscle fasciculations. Complete recovery of neuromuscular function occurs in less than 10 minutes, due to rapid metabolism of succinylcholine by plasma pseudocholinesterase. Succinylcholine has many potential complications and side effects that include allergic reactions, cardiac dysrhythmias, increased intracranial pressure, increased intraocular pressure, and a modest rise in serum potassium levels. Exaggerated increases in serum potassium occur if succinylcholine is administered to patients with spinal cord injury or with significant burns. Succinylcholine is also a trigger for malignant hyperthermia. The drug continues to be used despite these drawbacks because its combination of rapid onset and short duration remains unique among neuromuscular blocking agents (30). Of note, duration of action is significantly prolonged in patients with pseudocholinesterase deficiency, a rare condition.

Contraindications to succinylcholine include the following: lack of resuscitative equipment, allergy to the drug, severe burns, spinal cord injury, malignant hyperthermia, myotonic dystrophy, and pseudocholinesterase deficiency. Succinylcholine should not be used in the case of anticipated difficult airway (see below).

Rocuronium

Rocuronium (31) is a quaternary aminosteroid. Its onset of action is 1.5–2 minutes with an intravenous dose of 0.6 mg/kg, and its duration of action is about 30 minutes. It can be used to facilitate artificial airway placement in an emergency situation, especially if there is a contraindication to succinylcholine. Rocuronium has minimal cardiovascular effects but has a tendency to increase heart rate.

Summary

No single agent is ideal for trans-laryngeal airway placement in critically ill patients, and each has advantages and disadvantages. The clinician must weigh these to decide which agent to use when anesthetic induction agent is deemed necessary in the intensive care setting. In my experience, the most commonly used anesthetic induction agent and neuromuscular blocking agent are thiopental and succinylcholine, respectively.

Awake Intubation

There are instances when the use of anesthetic induction agents and neuromuscular blocking agents is undesirable (32). Intravenous injection of these agents may cause hemodynamic disturbances that are dangerous in many critically ill patients. The agents also render the patient apneic. If trans-laryngeal intubation cannot be accomplished quickly and if the patient is difficult to ventilate manually, cardiac arrest and anoxic brain damage may result. When hemodynamic instability or anticipated difficult intubation preclude use of induction agents, intubation should be attempted after adequate topical local anesthesia and intravenous sedation with benzodiazepines, with maintenance of spontaneous ventilation. Intravenous benzodiazepines must be used with caution since, at high doses, they contribute to systemic hypotension and respiratory depression (33).

D. Physiological Disturbances

The physiological disturbances (4) induced by anesthetic induction agents and neuromuscular blocking agents were described above. Laryngoscopy and intubation can stimulate the sympathetic nervous system and cause tachycardia and systemic hypertension, which may be poorly tolerated in patients with critical coronary artery stenosis or with ruptured cerebral arterial aneurysms. Beta-adrenergic blocking agents and narcotics have been used to attenuate the sympathetic manifestations of laryngoscopy and intubation (34,35).

E. Routes

Artificial airway placement may be surgical or nonsurgical (6). Surgical airway placement is achieved with tracheostomy or cricothyroidotomy. Cricothyroidotomy is useful when nonsurgical attempts have failed to establish an airway in an emergency situation, while tracheostomy usually requires more time and is best employed electively (7). Nonsurgical airway placement is achieved via the oral or nasal route. Both require laryngoscopy, although the blind nasal route can be used if the patient is ventilating spontaneously. The blind nasal intubation route is ill-advised in patients with maxillofacial trauma or basal skull fractures since the endotracheal tube may be introduced via a mucosal tear into a surrounding tissue space. Nonetheless, naso-tracheal intubation has been successfully accomplished in this circumstance with the aid of a fiberoptic laryngoscope (36). The nasal route necessitates a smaller endotracheal tube than the oral route (37) and is associated with nosebleeds (38–40), which can obscure the laryngoscopist's view. The oral route is the one most commonly used by most practitioners (6).

F. Complications: Confirmation of Endotracheal Tube Placement

Complications of trans-laryngeal intubation are listed in Table 4 and include failure to intubate, misplacement of the endotracheal tube, and traumatic injury to various structures in and around the upper airway. These include the teeth, the pharynx, larynx, trachea, and spinal cord if the cervical spine is unstable. The most immediately devastating complication is unrecognized misplacement of the endotracheal tube (38). Tube position can be checked clinically by auscultation of the chest, with a chest radiograph and by detection of exhaled CO_2. A fiberoptic

Table 4 Early Complications of Translaryngeal Intubation

I. Complications of medications
   A. Hypoventilation or apnea with resulting hypoxemia
   B. Systemic hypotension
   C. Cardiac dysrhythmias
   D. Aspiration pneumonitis
II. Complications of laryngoscopy
   A. Sympathetic stimulation with resulting systemic hypertension and tachycardia
   B. Trauma
      1. Lips, tongue, epiglottis, glottis
      2. Teeth
      3. Cervical spinal cord if cervical spine unstable
   C. Retching, coughing, vomiting
III. Complications of endotracheal tube insertion
   A. Trauma
      1. Supraglottic structures
      2. Vocal cords
      3. Trachea
      4. Esophagus
   B. Malposition or migration
      1. Esophagus
      2. Right mainstem bronchus
      3. Oropharynx
   C. Tube problems
      1. Kink
      2. Obstruction with blood or mucus
      3. Cuff failure
   D. Failure to intubate

---

bronchoscope may also be used to verify tracheal placement of the endotracheal tube.

Clinical verification of tube position includes observation of entry via the larynx and auscultation of breath sounds, although auscultation of bilateral breath sounds does not exclude endobronchial intubation (41,42). Clinical verification of correct tube position also includes observation of depth of insertion of the tube. In the case of oro-tracheal intubation, the tip of the endotracheal tube should be 23 cm from the incisors in men and 21 cm in women (43). In the case of naso-tracheal intubation, the tip of the endotracheal tube should be 25 and 23 cm in men and women, respectively, from the opening of the naris. Chest radiography reliably detects endobronchial intubation (44), but the chest x-ray is usually obtained too slowly to be of value in the rapid detection of esophageal intubation. Fiberoptic bronchoscopy also reliably confirms accurate endotracheal tube placement (45), but the equipment is not always readily available.

Since the lungs are the only source of CO_2, the American Society of Anesthesiologists mandates exhaled CO_2 detection for confirmation of proper endotracheal tube placement (14). CO_2 detection devices include capnometers and portable devices that change color when exposed to CO_2 (e.g., Easy Cap). Portable CO_2-detecting devices function well except in the case of cardiac arrest, when CO_2 elimination ceases. Devices that check aspiration of air also function well, even during cardiac arrest. These include the TubeChek (46), a 60 cc syringe with an adapter that attaches to an endotracheal tube connector. Aspiration of air into the syringe after intubation confirms endotracheal positioning, whereas failure to aspirate air indicates esophageal intubation (46). The TubeChek-B is a self-inflating bulb that is compressed and then attached to the endotracheal tube connector. If the bulb fills with air when released, then the tube has entered the trachea (32). Although false-negative and false-positive findings occur with any of the devices, one review favors use of the TubeChek (46). The author's preference is to use the Easy Cap, a reliable device in most clinical situations. Regardless of the CO_2-detection device used, a pulse oximeter should also be used to verify adequate oxygenation after intubation (14).

Emergency endotracheal intubation in critically ill patients is associated with increased risk compared to elective intubation. One prospective observational study of emergency intubations noted an 8% rate of difficult intubation, a 4% rate of pulmonary aspiration, and 3% mortality within 30 minutes of the procedure (47).

G. Avoiding Complications of Intubation

Identifying Patients at Increased Risk of Aspiration Pneumonitis

Most intravenous anesthetic agents blunt airway reflexes that protect against pulmonary aspiration (48). When these agents are administered to a patient with increased gastric contents, aspiration pneumonitis can occur if the gastric contents are regurgitated during the intubation procedure (49). Conditions that predispose to increased gastric contents include recent food intake (49) and conditions that delay gastric emptying. Conditions that delay gastric emptying include active peptic ulcer disease, gastritis, pregnancy, obesity, stress, pain, narcotic use, elevated intracranial pressure (50), and diabetes with autonomic neuropathy (51,52). Aspiration risk is also higher in patients with nasogastric tubes (50) and in those patients with acute abdominal pathology (especially bowel obstruction) (53).

Reducing the Risk of Aspiration in Patients Receiving Enteral Feeds

Controversy exists regarding the need to discontinue enteral feeds prior to elective reintubation. While one study suggests that patients fed by jejunostomy are at low risk of developing aspiration pneumonitis (54), another has noted the aspiration risk to be equal to that of patients fed by gastrostomy (55). Based on

available data, temporary discontinuation of enteral feeds prior to elective intubation (e.g., planned reintubation) is an option. However, current preoperative fasting guidelines of the American Society of Anesthesiologists recommend a 6-hour
fast prior to induction of anesthesia to avoid aspiration (56).

Reducing the Risk of Aspiration During Intubation

An endotracheal tube placed in the trachea with its cuff inflated provides significant (though not complete) protection against aspiration of gastric contents (57).
If gastric contents are increased when artificial airway placement is required and
the patient is not comatose, then either rapid sequence induction with intravenous
anesthetic agents or topical anesthesia and sedation should be used to facilitate
intubation to minimize the risk of aspiration (5). Rapid sequence induction was
devised to prevent aspiration during endotracheal intubation by making the interval between anesthesia and endotracheal intubation as brief as possible and by
minimizing passive regurgitation of stomach contents into the oropharynx. The
interval between anesthesia and intubation is decreased by rapid intravenous injection at predetermined dosages of an induction agent and rapid-onset neuromuscular blocking agent, followed in 45–60 seconds by endotracheal intubation and
rapid cuff inflation. Passive regurgitation is minimized by cricoid pressure (58)
and by limiting gastric insufflation of air (4). Application of cricoid pressure is
a skill that requires instruction and practice to be performed correctly (59). Since
the cricoid cartilage is the only complete cartilaginous ring in the upper airway,
digital pressure applied to the cricoid cartilage compresses the esophagus against
the cervical spine, physically blocking the passage of gastric contents. Cricoid
pressure should be maintained by an assistant from the time of injection of anesthetic agents until confirmation of endotracheal tube position in the trachea. Gastric insufflation of air is minimized by cricoid pressure and by avoiding positive
pressure ventilation. However, avoiding positive pressure ventilation may result
in hypoxemia. This is attenuated by administration of 100% oxygen prior to induction of anesthesia (preoxygenation) (60), although effective preoxygenation
may be difficult to achieve in critically ill patients requiring urgent trans-laryngeal
airway placement.

Difficult Intubation

Definition of Difficult Intubation

Difficult intubation (32,61) is defined by the American Society of Anesthesiologists as the proper insertion of an endotracheal tube requiring more than three
attempts or more than 10 minutes in experienced hands (62). For general anesthesia, intubations are difficult in 1.5–13% of cases (61) and fail entirely in 0.13–
0.3% of cases (61). Difficulty in applying effective mask ventilation occurs in

about 0.07% of patients at induction of anesthesia (63). It is estimated that the catastrophe of inability to intubate and to ventilate the patient occurs about 1 in 10,000 cases (64).

Predicting Difficult Intubation

Accurate prediction of a difficult intubation would permit choosing between anesthetic induction and awake intubation to secure the airway, thereby minimizing risk and maximizing patient comfort. Patients at high risk for difficult intubation could be identified and potential pitfalls avoided. Awake endotracheal intubation is less comfortable for the patient and therefore less desirable in a patient with a normal airway (personal opinion). Predictors of difficult intubation are listed in Table 5 and include a history of previous difficult intubation and physical

Table 5 Factors That Identify Patients at Risk of Difficult Intubation

I. History
    A. Acute
        1. Severe trauma to mouth or neck
    B. Chronic
        1. History of previous difficult intubation
        2. Symptoms of chronic and progressive upper airway obstruction
II. Physical examination
    A. Signs of upper airway obstruction
        1. Respiratory distress with difficulty phonating
        2. Inspiratory stridor
        3. Thoraco-abdominal dyscoordination
    B. Conditions that may predict upper airway obstruction after anesthesia
        1. Large airway tumor
        2. Large airway abscess
        3. Large neck mass
        4. Significant neck swelling
    C. Physical characteristics that may be associated with difficult intubation
        1. Poor mouth opening
        2. Large protuberant teeth
        3. Micrognathia
        4. Noncompliant mandibular soft tissue
        5. Large neck (muscular or obese)
        6. Limited neck movement
III. Laboratory
    A. Radiology
        1. Soft tissue lateral radiograph of neck demonstrating airway narrowing
IV. Mallampati classification
    A. (see Fig. 1)

characteristics including a small mouth, limitation of head extension, pharyngeal restriction, and noncompliance of submandibular soft tissue (65). Other physical characteristics predictive of difficult intubation include significant obesity, a receding mandible, and protuberant teeth (66). Mallampati has proposed a classification of the airway (Fig. 1) based on the view of the uvula and tonsillar pillars through a wide-open mouth (67). A revised form of this classification (68) is widely used in anesthetic practice (4,5). In a Class 1 airway, the soft palate, the fauces, the uvula, and the tonsillar pillars are all visible. In a Class 2 airway, the soft palate, the fauces, and part of the uvula are visible. In a Class 3 airway, only the soft palate and the base of the uvula are visible. In a Class 4 airway, even the soft palate is not visible. The classes predict intubation difficulty, with Class 1 being the easiest and Class 4 the most difficult. Sensitivity of this technique ranges from 42 to 81% and the specificity from 66 to 84%. (69). Although the above predictors are not completely reliable (70), observation for the above physi-

Figure 1   Mallampati classification for prediction of difficult intubation: findings in the seated patient with the head in neutral position and the mouth fully open (stylized illustrations).

cal characteristics and use of the classification scheme can help to predict difficulty with trans-laryngeal airway insertion (69).

Approach to the Anticipated Difficult Intubation

Steps to be taken for managing a difficult airway are listed in Table 6. When a difficult intubation is anticipated, the airway should be secured while the patient is awake and breathing spontaneously (32,61). There is a low risk of aspiration of gastric contents in the awake patient. If the oral route is chosen, topical anesthesia should be applied to the oropharynx. This can be supplemented by lingual and glossopharyngeal nerve blocks to abolish the gag reflex. If the nasal route is chosen, a vasoconstricting agent should be applied to the nasal mucosa in addition to topical anesthesia. Sedation should be administered in appropriate dosage. Options for viewing the larynx include fiberoptic bronchoscopy, fiberoptic laryngoscopy, illuminating stylets (light wands) and direct laryngoscopy.

Approach to the Unanticipated Difficult Intubation

If laryngeal intubation proves impossible after injection of anesthesia induction agents and neuromuscular blocking agents, then 100% oxygen should be adminis-

Table 6 Approach to the Difficult Intubation

I. Anticipated difficult intubation
   A. Have help available
   B. Preserve spontaneous ventilation
   C. Awake intubation with sedation and topical anesthesia
      1. Direct laryngoscopy
      2. Fiberoptic laryngoscopy/bronchoscopy
      3. Illuminating fiberoptic stylet (light wand)
   D. Consider tracheostomy under local anesthesia
II. Unanticipated difficult intubation after induction of anesthesia
   A. Call for help
   B. Reposition and reattempt intubation with a smaller endotracheal tube
   C. Establish mask ventilation
      1. Mask ventilation successful
         a. Reattempt intubation (maximum three laryngoscopic attempts)
         b. If still unsuccessful, insert laryngeal mask airway and use as conduit for endotracheal tube
         c. If still unsuccessful, allow patient to awaken and proceed as anticipated difficult intubation
      2. Mask ventilation unsuccessful
         a. Insert laryngeal mask airway or esophageal tracheal combitube
         b. If still unsuccessful, establish transtracheal jet ventilation
         c. Emergency tracheostomy

tered with manual positive pressure ventilation by mask and self-inflating bag. If mask ventilation is successful in providing adequate ventilation and oxygenation, then the patient can be awakened and the approach to the anticipated difficult intubation followed. If mask ventilation is unsuccessful, then a critical situation exists, which may lead to cardiac arrest. Ventilation must be established immediately. Available devices for assisted ventilation in this situation are described below and include the laryngeal mask airway (LMA) and the esophageal tracheal combitube (ETC) as well as trans-tracheal jet ventilation (TTJV) via cricothyroidotomy (32).

Laryngeal Mask Airway. The laryngeal mask airway (LMA) was first described in 1983 (71,72), and its usefulness in difficult airway management was suggested in 1984 (73). The LMA consists of a large-bore curved tube with a connector compatible with respiratory circuits at one end and an inflatable mask made of silicone, which "cups" against the larynx at the other end. There are two flexible bars at the entry of the tube into the mask to prevent obstruction by the epiglottis (74). The LMA is available in many sizes; #3 is usually appropriate for small adults, #4 for normal adults, and #5 for large adults (74). It is easy to insert (75) and is effective as a ventilatory assist device if ventilation difficulty is due to unfavorable anatomy but not if it is due to glottic pathology (32). It does not protect the lungs from aspiration of gastric contents if a predisposing cause exists, but the reported incidence of aspiration pneumonitis is low (76). The LMA can serve as a conduit for the passage of an endotracheal tube, although a standard #4 LMA will only allow passage of a 6.0 mm ID endotracheal tube (77). An intubating LMA has been devised that allows passage of larger endotracheal tubes (78). Use of an LMA is the preferred back-up strategy for the cannot intubate, cannot ventilate circumstance (77).

Esophageal Tracheal Combitube. The esophageal tracheal combitube (ETC) is a double lumen tube, which is inserted blindly. A large proximal balloon is inflated to isolate the mouth from the nose. Two circumferential stripes are depth guides and should be at the teeth or gums. One lumen resembles a cuffed endotracheal tube and is shorter proximally. This lumen usually ends up in the esophagus. The other lumen is longer proximally and has a blind end. This lumen has several perforations along its length. The patient is usually ventilated via the perforations, which should be above the glottis (32). Pulmonary ventilation is confirmed if breath sounds are heard in the chest but not over the stomach. If this is not the case, the shorter lumen is probably in the trachea, and this lumen can then be used to apply positive pressure ventilation (79). The ETC is easy to use but can cause esophageal perforation (75,80) and the upper cuff can obstruct the trachea if it is advanced too far (79). The ETC cannot be used as a conduit for endotracheal intubation.

Transtracheal Jet Ventilation. This is a last resort in the cannot intubate, cannot ventilate situation. Not only is some skill required to insert the ventilation needle through the cricothyroid membrane, but also the equipment must adhere to strict specifications and needs to be preassembled. Risk of barotrauma is substantial. A definitive airway (e.g., tracheostomy) must be established as soon as possible after transtracheal jet ventilation (TTJV) is initiated. Two extensive reviews discuss this topic in detail (64,75).

Intubation of the Patient with an Unstable Cervical Spine

Endotracheal intubation in patients with cervical spine instability appears to be safe. The likelihood of further neurological injury is low and similar to that of hospitalized patients with unstable cervical spines, who do not require intubation. Options for securing the airway include awake intubation and intubation after induction of anesthesia as long as the neck remains immobile (81). To assure safety, patients with cervical spine instability should be intubated only by skilled personnel and an assistant should be present to maintain neck stabilization. One source has suggested that credentialing be introduced as a requirement for allowing personnel to intubate such patients (82). Individuals who provide medical coverage should be proficient with intubation so that expert service can be provided nor only to patients with unstable necks but also to all critically ill patients on a 24-hour basis.

III. Artificial Airway Maintenance

A. Endotracheal Tubes

Description

Standard endotracheal tubes are latex-free and made of polyvinylchloride (PVC), which is stiff at room temperature and softens at body temperature (79). The stiffness facilitates intubation and the subsequent softness allows the tube to conform to the shape of the upper airway. PVC is also nonirritating to mucosa and smooth, which allows easy passage of the tube into the larynx and of suction catheters and bronchoscopes into the tracheobronchial tree via the lumen of the tube. The proximal end has a detachable connector, which allows attachment of the tube to an external breathing system. The distal end is beveled to facilitate introduction past the vocal cords. Near the distal tip, opposite the bevel, is a circular opening, known as the Murphy eye, that allows gas flow if the end of the tube abuts a mucosal surface. Bronchoscopes should not be passed through the Murphy eye because they may be impossible to withdraw afterward. A radio-opaque stripe is imbedded along the length of the endotracheal tube to allow assessment of tube position on a chest radiograph. The tube also has markings that indicate distance in centimeters from the distal end.

Reinforced tubes have a metal spiral reinforcing wire throughout most of the length of the tube. Because this design resists kinking, the tube may be used during anesthesia for head and neck surgery or tracheal surgery where bending or compression of the tube may occur. Case reports have documented airway obstruction due to permanent deformation from patients' biting these tubes. Therefore, if a patient with a reinforced tube requires continued intubation into the postoperative period, the reinforced tube should be changed to a regular PVC endotracheal tube (79).

Cuffs

Adult-sized endotracheal tubes have a cuff located near the distal end that is connected via a small lumen in the tube wall and an external inflation catheter to a pilot balloon with an inflation valve. The inflation valve allows controlled inflation and deflation of the cuff with a syringe. Inflated cuffs serve not only to provide a seal for effective positive pressure ventilation, but also to provide protection against pulmonary aspiration (57) although the protection is not complete (83–85). In addition, an inflated cuff minimizes contact of the tube itself with the tracheal mucosa. High-volume, low-pressure cuffs create an effective seal due to the large area of contact with the tracheal wall. Low pressure reduces the risk of tracheal wall pressure necrosis during prolonged intubations (86). Provided that the cuff is not overstretched, cuff pressure measured at the inflation valve can be used to estimate pressure exerted against the tracheal wall (87), although this has been disputed (88). Overstretching is caused by excessive inflation with the syringe and by high-pressure positive pressure ventilation, which presses on the cuff from below during inspiration (89).

Acceptable cuff pressure is the pressure that creates an effective seal but does not compress the tracheal mucosa enough to interrupt capillary perfusion. Since tracheal capillary pressure is approximately 25 cm H_2O (18 mmHg), pressures above 18 mmHg theoretically interfere with perfusion of the tracheal mucosa. One study in dogs has suggested that maximum cuff pressures exceeding 20 mmHg interfere with tracheal blood flow (90), and a study in patients undergoing surgery has suggested that maximum cuff pressure should be 22 mmHg or 30 cm H_2O (91). On the other hand, cuff pressures below 18 mmHg may not generate an effective cuff seal (79). There is no Class 1 or 2 evidence to recommend either maximum pressure or frequency of cuff pressure checks. Periodic cuff deflation has been ineffective, at least in one animal model, in preventing tracheal injury (92). A survey of cuff management practices published in 1996 found that in two thirds of critical care units that responded, cuff pressures were measured one to three times daily and that maximum allowable cuff pressures ranged from 15 to 30 mmHg (93).

Manometers are commercially available that are specifically designed to measure cuff pressure (79), but measurements are prone to error unless impeccable technique is used (94). Techniques for cuff inflation include the minimal occlusive volume and minimal leak techniques (93). The minimal occlusive volume is the smallest volume added to a cuff to prevent an air leak during a positive pressure inspiration. The minimal leak technique allows for a small leak on inspiration. While there is no demonstrated superiority of one technique over the other, the minimal occlusive volume technique appears to be the most commonly used.

Endotracheal Tube Position

The tip of the tube needs to be situated above the carina to avoid the ventilation perfusion mismatch caused by endobronchial intubation. As already stated, tube position can be evaluated clinically, with a chest radiograph or with fiberoptic bronchoscopy (41,45). Clinical evaluation consists of auscultation for bilateral breath sounds and inspection of the endotracheal tube for depth of insertion from the teeth or gums. These indicators can detect gross malposition but not as reliably as a chest radiograph (41). Fiberoptic bronchoscopy is an excellent tool for determining endotracheal tube position (45) but requires cleaning and sterilization and increases costs.

Routine chest radiography also adds to workload and costs but has the advantage of simultaneous assessment of cardiopulmonary structures, as well as position of monitors and therapeutic devices. One cost analysis of daily chest films in a medical intensive care unit reported that 6% of routine chest films demonstrated a finding that prompted an action that shortened patient length of stay (95). The proportion of abnormal findings related to endotracheal tube malposition varies (42,96). Because of this, one review recommends daily chest radiographs in mechanically ventilated patients (44). The endotracheal tube can move up to 2 cm from the neutral position with flexion or extension of the head. On the chest radiograph, the tip of the tube should be more than 2 cm above the carina with the head in the neutral position (44). One source suggests positioning the tube tip 3–4 cm above the carina to avoid laryngeal impingement as well as endobronchial misplacement (89).

Work of Breathing Related to the Endotracheal Tube

Resistive work of breathing imposed by the breathing apparatus can be significant and increases not only with decreasing internal diameter of the endotracheal tube but also with increasing minute ventilation (97,98). Shapiro et al. (98) calculated that the work of breathing through a 6.0 mm ID tube was almost double the work of breathing through an 8.0 mm ID tube at a minute ventilation of 10 L. The tension-time index, an indirect measure of oxygen consumption by the diaphragm, did not approach fatigue levels in either case.

The respiratory apparatus can impose a workload sufficient to interfere with weaning from mechanical ventilation (99), but this can be overcome by inspiratory pressure support (100,101). There is insufficient information to recommend changing a 6.0 mm ID tube to a wider internal diameter tube in every adult. This decision should be made on an individual basis, taking into account ease of intubation and the level of extra pressure support required to achieve satisfactory patient weaning performance.

Dead Space

The volume of an endotracheal tube is generally less than that of the oro-pharyngeal and supra-laryngeal spaces in adults. Therefore, dead space is usually less in intubated than in unintubated patients (79).

Nasal Versus Oral Route

Key differences between the nasal and oral routes for intubation are listed in Table 7. The nasal route is said to be better tolerated by awake patients than the oral route for prolonged trans-laryngeal intubation (5,79). However, no controlled studies have provided evidence for this, and reviewers who state this offer no supportive references. Moreover, one study found no difference in comfort in the short term between oral and nasal endotracheal tube placement (39).

Naso-tracheal tubes are said to be more stable and less likely to dislodge than oro-tracheal tubes, while oral tubes may be more likely to dislocate spontaneously (102). However, a prospective observational study of self-extubations over one year did not confirm this (103). On the other hand, naso-tracheal intubation has been implicated as a significant risk factor in the development of paranasal sinusitis. Whereas one randomized study found no difference in the incidence of sinusitis between patients with oro- or naso-tracheal tubes (104), another ran-

Table 7 Oral Versus Nasal Intubation

	Oral	Nasal
Method of visualizing larynx	Direct laryngoscopy or fiberoptic laryngoscopy	Direct laryngoscopy or fiberoptic laryngoscopy or "blind" intubation
Tube size	8.0–8.5 mm ID (men) 7.0–7.5 mm ID (women)	6.5–7.0 mm ID (men) 6.0–6.5 mm ID (women)
Preparation	Induction of anesthesia or topical anesthesia and sedation	Same as for oral plus topical vasoconstricting agent
Early complications	Failure to intubate, trauma to structures in and around the airway, tube misplacement	Same as for oral plus epistaxis, difficulty suctioning via smaller tube
Delayed complications	Laryngeal injury, tracheal injury	Same as for oral plus paranasal sinusitis

domized prospective study found a marked increase in the development of paranasal sinusitis related to naso-tracheal intubation (105). Several observational studies have also found a relationship between naso-tracheal intubation and sinusitis (106–108). The incidence of sinusitis increases with duration of intubation (106), and, according to one study, the condition abates after changing to an oro-tracheal tube (109). Nasogastric intubation may also play a role in the pathogenesis of sinus inflammation (105). While one review suggests that laryngeal damage may be less with naso-tracheal intubation (37), a prospective observational study of prolonged naso-tracheal intubations found a significant number of laryngeal lesions (110). Smaller tubes are usually required in naso-tracheal versus oro-tracheal intubation (37). This increases airway resistance and may interfere with effective suctioning. Finally, naso-tracheal intubation may be associated with a higher rate of ventilator-associated pneumonia (111). Based on these observations, the author recommends the oro-tracheal route for prolonged intubations.

Complications of Prolonged Trans-Laryngeal Intubation

One source defines prolonged trans-laryngeal intubation as greater than 24 hours (112); another, as greater than 96 hours (113); a third, as 5–7 days (114). Complications of prolonged intubation are listed in Table 8. Sinusitis, the complication associated with prolonged nasal intubation has been discussed above. It is important because of its association with sepsis (109) and orbital as well as intracranial extension of infection (115). Other complications of prolonged trans-laryngeal intubation include laryngeal and tracheal damage, pulmonary infection, upper airway obstruction that results from accumulation of dried secretions in the lumen, and inability to provide a seal for mechanical ventilation.

Laryngeal and Tracheal Damage

Damage to the upper airway from prolonged trans-laryngeal intubation may be due to the tube (38,114) or to the cuff (86,89)

Damage Due to the Endotracheal Tube. Because of their conformation, endotracheal tubes exert pressure on the posterior larynx at the posterior portion of the vocal cords, the medial surfaces of the arytenoid cartilages, the interarytenoid region posteriorly (114,116), and the posterior lamina of the cricoid cartilage in the subglottic region (89,117). This pressure is sufficient to cause mucosal erosions that often heal without sequelae after extubation but may progress in a variety of ways during prolonged intubation. Mucosal ulcers can create deep troughs, which may leave furrows in the upper airway structures after healing. Furrows may cause moderate dysphonia (14), which has been described as a "leaky voice" (89). Alternatively, healing may take place with significant fibrosis leading to a stenotic airway. Symptoms can range from hoarseness to shortness of breath accompanied by stridor. Stenosis can be subglottic or posterior glottic.

Table 8 Complications of Prolonged Intubation

I. Endotracheal tube
  A. Oral
    1. Pressure injury to the posterior larynx by the tube
      a. Ulceration and dysphonia
      b. Fibrosis and stenosis
      c. Granuloma formation and voice changes
      d. Granulation tissue and glottic incompetence
    2. Pressure injury to the trachea by the cuff
      a. Tracheal stenosis
      b. Tracheomalacia
    3. Abnormal swallowing reflexes
    4. Accidental extubation
    5. Dysfunction
      a. Obstruction with secretions
      b. Kinking
      c. Defective cuff system
  B. Nasal (all of oral plus)
    1. Paranasal sinusitis
      a. Local infection with pain
      b. Local extension to orbit or central nervous system
      c. Sepsis
II. Tracheostomy
  A. Airway injury
    1. Tracheal stenosis
    2. Tracheomalacia
    3. Tracheoesophageal fistula
    4. Tracheoinnominate fistula
    5. Exacerbation of laryngeal injury
  B. Ventilator-associated pneumonia
  C. Dysfunction
    1. Defective cuff system

Subglottic stenosis is more common in the pediatric population, while posterior glottic stenosis occurs more often in adults. Granuloma formation may also occur and may cause a husky voice that appears weeks after extubation (114). Prominent posterior laryngeal granulation can interfere with glottic competency and predispose to aspiration pneumonia (118).

Upper airway damage from endotracheal tubes has been studied in a canine model (119,120). Mucosal ulceration is more pronounced with tube motion and less pronounced if tube motion is minimized. Mucosal damage is also worse with larger endotracheal tubes than with smaller ones (119). Mucosal inflammation is evident after 24 hours, and severe mucosal ulceration occurs within one week.

Arytenoid cartilage inflammation is seen after one week of intubation as well. Between one and 12 weeks of trans-laryngeal intubation in the canine model, no correlation was found between length of intubation and the severity of laryngeal injury (120).

Laryngeal sequelae of trans-laryngeal intubation have also been examined in humans (40,112,113,118). Some degree of mucosal damage is visualized in 54 to 94% of patients endotracheally intubated for more than 24 hours. Two studies have found a correlation between the severity of upper airway mucosal damage and the length of time of trans-laryngeal intubation (113,118), while two others have failed to demonstrate any relation between these variables (40,112). Long-term sequelae have been noted in 7–12% of surviving patients in the above studies with about two thirds of these healing without sequelae by 4 weeks and over three quarters healing by 8 weeks postextubation (121).

One animal model (122) and two human studies (123,124) suggested that altering endotracheal tube design to conform more closely to the shape of the airway might attenuate laryngeal injury caused by excessive pressure, although tubes of such design appear to be unavailable.

Because of the many studies described above, the type, severity, and outcome of laryngeal injuries caused by prolonged endotracheal intubation are well understood. The only factor that can easily be controlled to minimize airway injury in the course of prolonged intubation appears to be tube size. Tube diameter should be as small as possible while permitting an airway seal at the level of the cuff with cuff pressures lower than 25–30 cm H_2O (89). On the other hand, tube size should be large enough to allow effective sectioning of bronchial secretions and not contribute significantly to excessive airway resistance. As already stated, optimal tube sizes which take the above considerations into account are 7.0–7.5 mm ID for women and 8.0–8.5 mm ID for men. Smaller tubes may be necessary for difficult intubations or if significant upper airway obstruction is present.

Damage Due to the Cuff. Microscopic tracheal mucosal erosion has been demonstrated in dogs as early as 5–7 hours after initiation of mechanical ventilation via endotracheal tubes with low-pressure–high-volume cuffs (125). In a canine model, cuff-related tracheal injury was more severe with high-pressure cuffs than low-pressure cuffs (86). Hedden et al. (126) examined the trachea of patients who died after intubation with red rubber tubes and high-pressure cuffs. Two of 19 patients intubated for less than 72 hours had significant tracheal damage, while 6 of 7 patients intubated for greater than 72 hours showed significant tracheal injury at autopsy. Over half of all these patients had hypotensive episodes prior to their demise (126). Laryngeal tomography performed in survivors of prolonged endotracheal intubation has revealed at least 10% narrowing of tracheal diameter at the cuff site in 3 of 27 patients who presented for follow up, but only one of these patients was symptomatic (40). Beyond these studies, there is little information on the incidence of symptomatic tracheal stenosis arising from cuff damage, its outcome, or on the preventable pathogenic factors. This contributes to the difficulty in making precise recommendations about the timing of tracheostomy (see below).

Swallowing Difficulty

Patients intubated via the trans-laryngeal route for more than 24 hours exhibit delayed swallowing reflexes after extubation for 2–7 days (127). The effect of this on aspiration risk is unknown.

Endotracheal Tube Exchange

Endotracheal tube exchange is required when there is inability to provide leak-free positive pressure ventilation. This may result from leak around an intact cuff or loss of air from a defective cuff system (37). Leak around the cuff is most often due to incorrect positioning of the endotracheal tube. Another reason for tube exchange is the perceived need for a larger diameter tube that may be requested in order to facilitate weaning from the mechanical ventilator or to permit fiberoptic bronchoscopy.

If an adequate minute volume cannot be provided because of a cuff leak, then direct laryngoscopy should be performed. If the leak is the result of incorrect positioning, then the tube should be repositioned. Usually this requires advancement of the tube so that the cuff is below the vocal cords. If the leak is due to a defective cuff system, the endotracheal tube must be replaced. Fio_2 should be increased to 1.0 for preoxygenation in preparation for tube exchange. The simplest way to exchange the tube is to maintain the laryngoscopic view of the airway, have an assistant withdraw the defective tube, and then immediately place the new tube. This minimizes the time without supplemental oxygen. If a difficult airway limits the laryngoscopic view, a tube exchanger may be used (128). A rigid long tube with a lumen for insufflation of oxygen is passed into the trachea via the existing endotracheal tube. It serves as a guide over which the existing tube can be withdrawn and the new tube can be inserted. The lumen for insufflation of oxygen provides a margin of safety in case insertion of the new tube proves to be difficult. Endobronchial rupture from the use of a tube exchanger has been reported (129), and this procedure should be limited to practitioners experienced in airway management.

Fiberoptic bronchoscopes vary in diameter with the largest being approximately 6 mm. If fiberoptic bronchoscopy is indicated and the existing endotracheal tube has an internal diameter of 7 mm or less, ventilation during the procedure may be difficult and positive end-expiratory pressure may be excessive (130). Anecdotally, placement of a larger diameter endotracheal tube may be impossible if intubation is known to be difficult and if the laryngoscopic view is limited. Tube exchange may also be hazardous if there is upper airway edema that might impede introduction of a larger tube even over a tube exchanger. In this situation, use of a smaller diameter bronchoscope should be considered. Recommendations that fiberoptic bronchoscopy be performed via a tube no smaller than 8.0 mm ID fail to take into account the potential hazard of tube exchange.

Changing an endotracheal tube to one with a larger internal diameter for facilitation of weaning from mechanical ventilation should be considered if the initial intubation was easy. If the initial intubation was difficult or if significant upper airway edema is present, the patient should be weaned with the existing tube in place, using a higher level of pressure support to compensate for the smaller tube diameter (100).

B. Tracheostomy

The most frequent indication for tracheostomy is prolonged trans-laryngeal intubation. Tracheostomy can be performed using a standard surgical approach (7,131) or percutaneous catheterization (131,132). Arguments can be made for or against either approach. Standard surgical tracheostomy is usually performed in the operating theater. This requires not only availability of a surgeon and of operating room staff, but also patient transport from the critical care area. Percutaneous catheterization is usually performed at the bedside in the critical care area. This obviates the need to coordinate the procedure with a surgical schedule and avoids the risk incurred by transport to and from the operating theater.

Standard surgical tracheostomy provides better surgical exposure. This allows both direct control of unexpected bleeding and placement of a larger tracheostomy tube if necessary. One randomized prospective study could not demonstrate a significant difference in complication rates between the standard and percutaneous approaches (133), although in the small study population, complications tended to be slightly higher with the percutaneous approach. Currently data do not conclusively support the superiority of either approach. Whereas a variety of tracheostomy tubes is available, the usual type inserted in the mechanically ventilated patient is a cuffed, nonfenestrated PVC tube with an inner and an outer cannula. The advantage of the double cannula lies in the ability to easily change the inner cannula if it is obstructed with tenacious secretions, obviating the need to change the entire tracheostomy. The tracheostomy cuff is similar in design to that of translaryngeal endotracheal tubes.

Tracheostomy Care

The tracheal stoma is collapsible for the first 5–7 days after tracheostomy. The tracheostomy tube is difficult to reinsert after removal during this time and should be secured with sutures (7). After about a week, healing at the stomal edges helps maintain stomal patency and makes tube exchange safer. For suctioning, multiple-eyed catheters are preferred because they may cause less tracheal mucosal damage than suction with single-eyed catheters. Closed suctioning systems may reduce the risk of infection (134).

Disadvantages and Complications of Tracheostomy

Tracheostomy is an operative procedure with surgical risks, which include bleeding, infection, pneumothorax, and subcutaneous emphysema. Stauffer and colleagues have reported early complications in up to 36% of tracheostomies (40), an extraordinarily high complication rate. Other sources report early complication rates of 4–8% (135–137). The reason for the lower rates in these sources may be due to greater surgical expertise than in the Stauffer study (138). Late complications of tracheostomy tubes include tracheal stenosis, tracheomalacia, tracheoesophageal fistula, and tracheoinnominate fistula (7). Stenosis can occur at the cuff site or at the site of the stoma (139). Up to 10% of patients who present for follow-up have symptomatic tracheal stenosis (40,140) that develops between 2 and 6 weeks after decannulation (7). Significant tracheal stenosis is treated with segmental tracheal resection, which has a very high success rate (139).

The exact time course of the development of tracheomalacia is unclear, but a study by Law and colleagues found a lesion near the stoma in 29% of patients with long-term tracheostomy (mean duration 4.9 months) (141). Tracheoesophageal fistula has been reported in 0.5% of patients. Risk factors include high cuff pressures, long duration of intubation, use of nasogastric tubes, presence of respiratory infections, and insulin-dependent diabetes (142). The diagnosis of tracheomalacia is suggested by an air leak and loss of delivered tidal volume despite high cuff volumes. Significant gastric insufflation with ventilator breaths may also occur. High-frequency jet ventilation may be useful to maintain ventilation at lower airway pressures (142). The best definitive therapeutic option is esophageal diversion with delay of primary repair until the patient is weaned from mechanical ventilation (143).

Tracheoinnominate fistula occurs in less than 1% of tracheostomies and is related to high cuff pressure and a low site of tracheostomy in the neck. It should be suspected if significant bleeding occurs more than 48 hours after tracheostomy. Any suspected case should be taken promptly to the operating theater for bronchoscopy with preparation for surgical repair (144). The problem is best avoided by controlling high cuff pressures and proper placement of the tracheostomy tube (7).

Laryngeal Injury

A theoretical benefit of tracheostomy for prolonged intubation is to decrease laryngeal injury since the tracheostomy tube bypasses the laryngeal structures. Animal data and human studies, however, suggest that laryngeal injury may be more severe after tracheostomy (113,118,145). Sasaki et al. proposed that this may be due to introduction of bacteria via the tracheostomy stoma into the area of the larynx (145). The laryngeal injuries observed in the above-quoted studies, however, cannot be attributed entirely to tracheostomy because all of the patients had been intubated previously and could have sustained laryngeal injury from the endotracheal tube prior to insertion of the tracheostomy.

Ventilator-Associated Pneumonia

The presence of a tracheostomy is associated with aspiration in about 50% of ventilator-dependent patients (146). Tracheostomy may predispose to bacterial colonization of the lower respiratory tract (147,148) and possibly to pneumonia (149,150). However, endotracheal tubes may have similar effects (151). Heffner points out that the true infection rates in patients with tracheostomy versus endotracheal tubes have not been determined and that any airway predisposes to bacterial entry into the lower respiratory tract. Furthermore, it is difficult to separate artificial airways as factors predisposing to pneumonia independently of other patient variables (138).

Advantages of Tracheostomy

A tracheostomy is a more stable airway than a trans-laryngeal tube and has a significantly lower rate of accidental extubation (40). A retrospective analysis of early (within the first 6 days) versus late (after 7 days) tracheostomy in blunt trauma patients found a marked reduction in both hospital length of stay and ICU length of stay in patients with early tracheostomy. This was associated with a significant reduction in hospital costs (152). A prospective observational study also noted a significant reduction in ICU length of stay and in the number of days of ventilator dependence in critically ill surgical patients who underwent early tracheostomy (153). Another retrospective review found a much lower complication rate with tracheostomy (14%) than with endotracheal intubation (57%) (135). In the same study, 60 critical care nurses responded to a survey of their attitudes toward prolonged airway management. Over 90% of these nurses preferred caring for patients with a tracheostomy versus an endotracheal tube for prolonged ventilation. Reasons given included perceived patient comfort, ease of suctioning, better handling of secretions, ease of mouth care, and ease of communication with the patient. Seventy-five percent of the nurses felt that the patient was "better psychologically" after tracheostomy insertion (135). Another survey of 72 ICU nurses found that 94% thought that patients with tracheostomies were more comfortable, and 72% would prefer a tracheostomy for themselves if they were patients in this situation (154). It was unclear what percentage of the total ICU nursing population was represented by the responders to the survey.

An observational prospective study found that tracheostomy tubes imposed slightly less work of breathing than endotracheal tubes with an equivalent inside diameter. The difference in work of breathing, measured in intubated patients before and after tracheostomy, did not reach statistical significance when expressed in J/L. However, the difference was statistically significant when work was expressed in J/min. Calculated resistance was also less with tracheostomy tubes (155). These observations support the widely held impression that weaning from mechanical ventilation is facilitated after tracheostomy, but no Class 1 or 2 evidence supports this notion.

Timing of Tracheostomy

There is controversy regarding the appropriate timing of tracheostomy because of conflicting information about the advantages and disadvantages of tracheostomy versus endotracheal intubation. Some studies have noted a relationship between duration of endotracheal intubation and laryngeal injury (113,118) while others have not (40,112). Likewise, some studies have described benefit from early tracheostomy (152,153), while one has not (156). Some sources describe a greater complication rate from tracheostomy than from endotracheal intubation (40,157). However, complications from tracheostomy are significantly lower with greater surgical expertise (138). One review advocates individualization of the timing by not relying solely on number of days intubated when weighing risks and benefits (82); another review suggests a timetable as a guideline (7).

It appears that the later a tracheostomy is performed after endotracheal intubation, the higher the risk of worsening of laryngeal injury (113,145). Therefore, even authors who stress individualization of timing of tracheostomy suggest that if it is clear that a patient will require long-term mechanical ventilation, a tracheostomy should be performed sooner rather than later (82). Heffner advocated an approach to timing of tracheostomy in the intensive care unit that serves as a pragmatic model (138). Tracheostomy is usually not considered until the patient requires endotracheal intubation for more than 7 days. At that time, a determination is made by the attending intensivist, based on the severity of the respiratory failure, as to the anticipated duration of intubation. If it is thought that the patient might meet criteria for extubation within the next week, then the decision to perform a tracheostomy is postponed and the patient is evaluated for extubation on a daily basis. If it appears that intubation will be significantly prolonged, then tracheostomy is performed during the second week. Unless there is a clear contraindication to anesthesia and surgery, patients should be converted from trans-laryngeal to tracheostomy tubes within 3 weeks of intubation.

C. Nasogastric Tubes

Prolonged nasogastric intubation is associated with a higher rate of sinusitis in critically ill patients (105). Also, nasogastric tubes are listed as contributory factors in the development of tracheo-esophageal fistulae, especially in patients with indwelling tracheostomy tubes (142). Bilateral vocal cord paralysis and severe throat pain has been described in diabetic patients with indwelling nasogastric tubes. The presumed mechanism is pressure necrosis and ulceration of the esophagus and the postcricoid area with paresis of the crico-arytenoid muscles (158).

D. Summary

Appropriately sized (7.0–7.5 ID in women and 8.0–8.5 ID in men), well-secured oral endotracheal tubes appear to be the most reasonable choice for early artificial airway maintenance in adults requiring invasive mechanical ventilation. Tracheostomy placement should be considered after about 7 days and performed soon afterwards if it appears that the patient will require mechanical ventilation beyond an additional week. There is a divergence of opinion about timing of tracheostomy, however, arising from confusing and contradictory data. Prolonged nasogastric intubation is also associated with significant complications. Although a safe interval has not been defined, alternative methods of gastric drainage should be considered at the time of tracheostomy placement. Since simultaneous nasogastric intubation and tracheostomy predispose to the development of acquired tracheoesophageal fistula, this combination should be avoided if possible.

IV. Artificial Airway Discontinuation

When the patient is weaned from mechanical ventilatory support and is awake enough to protect his or her airway, the artificial airway should be removed.

A. Extubation Techniques

Extubation techniques must aim to minimize aspiration of material that accumulates above the cuff of the endotracheal tube. Most reports describe techniques for extubation after anesthesia and surgery rather than after prolonged intubation for respiratory failure. One technique involves a 10-degree head-down position and a trailing suction catheter introduced via the endotracheal tube in order to clear secretions as the tube is being removed (159). Another includes delivery of a positive pressure breath just prior to cuff deflation in order to promote a vigorous cough (160). This subject has been reviewed, but there is insufficient evidence to support any specific recommendation (161). Most practitioners, however, thoroughly suction the oropharynx prior to extubation.

B. Difficult Extubation

For the most part, difficult extubation is due either to a persistently inflated cuff and/or to the inadvertent surgical fixation of the tube to surrounding tissue (162). A crimped, ruptured, or defective cuff system may result in failure of cuff deflation. The cuff must then be punctured after visualization using direct laryngoscopy or fiberoptic bronchoscopy. Puncture with a needle passed through the cricothyroid membrane has also been suggested (163). Surgical fixation of the endotracheal tube has been described in association with oral, facial, and thoracic surgery (162). If the patient requires postoperative mechanical ventilation, then this problem will become apparent in the intensive care unit. Fiberoptic bronchoscopy via the endotracheal tube may assist in making the diagnosis by identifying the responsible wire or suture (164). Reoperation may be required to release the tube.

C. Physiological Disturbances

Hypertension and tachycardia frequently result from the extubation process. In those few patients for whom this might cause harm, short-acting β blockers and calcium channel blockers have successfully attenuated the sympathetic response (165,166).

D. Predicting Postextubation Airway Obstruction

Postextubation airway obstruction is relatively common in children younger than 5 years of age who are intubated and mechanically ventilated for longer than 48 hours. One report found that dexamethasone significantly reduced the incidence of this complication (167). Among 700 adults, a French group found an incidence of postextubation airway obstruction of approximately 4%, which increased to 7% if the duration of intubation was greater than 36 hours. Women experienced postextubation airway obstruction more than three times as often as men. Only 1% of patients required reintubation, and, in contrast to the response among children, dexamethasone had no influence on outcome among adults (168).

Some authors have attempted to identify patients at risk for airway obstruction after extubation by determining whether air leaks around a deflated tube cuff (cuff leak test). One group studied 88 nonsurgical patients intubated for more than 24 hours. Six patients had postextubation stridor, and three of these required reintubation. Cuff leak was assessed by measuring cuff leak volume per breath prior to extubation during assist-control ventilation. Cuff leak volume was defined as the difference between delivered and exhaled volume averaged over six breaths. If leak was large, the risk of postextubation stridor was low. Patients with and without postextubation stridor had mean cuff leak volumes of 180 cc and 360 cc, respectively. The authors estimated that a cuff leak volume of less than 110 cc was associated with a high risk of postextubation stridor (169).

Another group assessed 62 patients intubated because of upper airway obstruction. They allowed patients to breathe spontaneously, deflated the cuff, occluded the tube, and found a peritubular leak in 55 patients, all of whom were extubated uneventfully. Of seven patients with no cuff leak, two required reintubation after attempted extubation and five underwent tracheostomy because of repeated failure of the test. Subsequently, 10 additional patients without cuff leak were extubated, 3 of whom required reintubation and 7 of whom did not. The authors concluded that the presence of a cuff leak successfully predicted postextubation upper airway patency, but the absence of a leak did not necessarily predict postextubation upper airway obstruction (170).

There is, unfortunately, no standard cuff leak test. Because secretions can accumulate above the cuff, deflation must be performed with caution after thorough suctioning. Cuff leak volume is a reasonable test to perform because most mechanical ventilators provide a measurement of both delivered and exhaled tidal volume. If the leak is large, the likelihood of postextubation airway obstruction is very small. If the leak is small, the risk of postextubation airway obstruction increases. Possible approaches to extubation in the absence of a cuff leak include postponement of extubation until a leak develops, extubation over an endotracheal tube exchanger, extubation over a fiberoptic bronchoscope, or simple extubation in the presence of a team prepared to secure the airway with reintubation or emergency tracheostomy. Some practitioners proceed directly to tracheostomy (170). Since all of the above are options, the approach must be individualized depending on local expertise and experience.

E. Extubation of Patients with a Known Difficult Airway

Emergency reintubation in a patient with a known difficult airway is potentially hazardous. It may be prudent to extubate in the presence of personnel skilled in airway management and equipped to deal with an airway emergency. In some cases, exubation over an endotracheal tube exchanger inserted into the trachea through the endotracheal tube lumen has been used in order to facilitate reintubation if respiratory failure occurs soon after extubation (161). Proceeding directly to tracheostomy is advisable for a patient who was difficult to intubate when there is no detectable cuff leak. Otherwise, extubation can be performed safely as long as the patient clearly exceeds minimal criteria for extubation.

F. Summary

Artificial airway discontinuation requires more than recognition that the patient no longer requires mechanical ventilatory assistance. Some assessment of the risk of postextubation airway obstruction should be made, and if the risk is high precautions should be taken to avoid catastrophes and to appropriately manage the problem if it occurs.

V. Overall Summary

Despite the large body of data on the subject of airway management in the critical care setting, most has been gathered and presented in a way that does not allow the development of standard specific therapeutic recommendations. In some cases, such as design of endotracheal tubes to minimize laryngeal damage, options are limited by the available tubes. In other cases, such as timing of tracheostomy, there is a great need for a large-scale methodologically sound and practical study examining the factors that could assist in this very important decision.

The requirement for urgent endotracheal intubation should be recognized clinically. If significant respiratory distress is accompanied by the clinical signs of upper airway obstruction and/or respiratory muscle fatigue, then the trachea should be intubated immediately. The equipment for intubation should be readily available, preferably in a prepackaged kit that is regularly inspected. With few exceptions, emergency intubation is safest when performed while the patient is breathing spontaneously. Judiciously administered intravenous sedation along with topical airway anesthesia should be used to facilitate intubation in the conscious patient who requires immediate intubation.

When lack of patient cooperation makes laryngoscopy impossible, intravenous anesthetic induction agents and neuromuscular blockers should be considered. However, these drugs can be associated with life-threatening complications if the patient is difficult to intubate or if the patient has a full stomach. Therefore, they should only be administered by personnel experienced in their use.

Clinicians should be able to identify both patients with a potentially difficult airway and patients at risk for aspiration of stomach contents since both circumstances alter the approach to intubation. A difficult airway can be anticipated if there is a history of difficult intubation or if the patient exhibits certain physical characteristics. Specialized techniques, such as fiberoptic bronchoscopy, improve the chances of visualization of the larynx in the spontaneously breathing patient. The likelihood of successful artificial airway placement is also improved significantly by effective topical airway anesthesia.

If intubation proves to be impossible after intravenous induction of anesthesia, then manual ventilation by mask and self-inflating bag of 100% oxygen should be attempted. The most useful tool in this situation is the laryngeal mask airway (LMA), which not only facilitates ventilation but also serves as a conduit for endotracheal intubation. If the patient cannot be intubated and cannot be ventilated even with an LMA in place, then life-threatening hypoxia may ensue. Transtracheal jet ventilation via crico-thyroid puncture may be the only remaining way to prevent the neural and cardiac sequelae of severe hypoxia while preparing for emergency tracheostomy. After emergency intubation, tracheal placement should be confirmed either with a device that detects exhaled CO_2 or a TubeChek.

The oral route is superior to the nasal route for airway maintenance and is, therefore, the preferred route for endotracheal intubation. Tracheostomy is an alternative choice if there is supra-glottic upper airway obstruction. Ideal endotracheal tube sizes are 8.0–8.5 mm ID for men and 7.0–7.5 mm ID for women. These sizes are large enough for effective suctioning and for leak-free positive pressure ventilation at reasonable cuff pressures. Larger tubes apply excessive pressure on laryngeal structures.

Consideration of converting an artificial airway to a tracheostomy should be given after one week of endotracheal intubation. The decision to proceed to tracheostomy must be individualized but should be made within the succeeding week or two if the chance of weaning the patient from mechanical ventilation appears unlikely.

When the patient no longer requires mechanical ventilatory assistance, the trachea should be extubated. Prior to extubation, however, a cuff leak test should be performed if risk factors for postextubation airway obstruction are identified. Absence of a cuff leak suggests a cautious approach to extubation of the trachea, which may include delay of extubation, extubation in the presence of an experienced airway management team, or conversion to tracheostomy.

The various strategies reviewed in this chapter are supported by a massive body of clinical experience but the quality of the evidence is limited by a dearth of Class 1 evidence. Until the principles of clinical epidemiology are universally and rigorously applied in future studies, the practice of airway management will remain an art rather than a science.

References

1. Meyer TJ, Hill NS. Noninvasive positive pressure ventilation to treat respiratory failure. Ann Intern Med 1994; 120:760–770.
2. Walters BC. Clinical practice parameter development in neurosurgery. In: Bean JR, ed. Concepts in Neurosurgery: Neurosurgery in Transition: The Socioeconomic Transformation of Neurological Surgery. Baltimore: Williams & Wilkins, 1998: 99–111.
3. Eddy DM. Clinical decision making: from theory to practice. Designing a practice policy. Standards, guidelines, and options. JAMA 1990; 263:3077.
4. Stehling LC. Management of the airway. In: Barash PG, Cullen BF, Stoelting RK, eds. Clinical Anesthesia. Philadelphia: J.B. Lippincott, 1989:543–561.
5. Castello DA, Smith HS, Lumb PD. Conventional airway access. In: Ayres SM, Grenvik A, Holbrook PR, Shoemaker WC, eds. Textbook of Critical Care. 3rd ed. Philadelphia: W.B. Saunders Company, 1995:698–712.
6. Vender JS, Shapiro BA. Essentials of artificial airway management in critical care. Acute Care 1987; 13:97–124.
7. Wood DE. Tracheostomy. Chest Surg Clin North Am 1996; 6:749–764.
8. Mort TC. Unplanned tracheal extubation outside the operating room: a quality improvement audit of hemodynamic and tracheal airway complications associated with emergency tracheal reintubation. Anesth Analg 1998; 86:1171–1176.
9. Browning IB, D'Alonzo GE, Tobin MJ. Importance of respiratory rate as an indicator of respiratory dysfunction in patients with cystic fibrosis. Chest 1990; 97:1317–1321.

10. Tobin MJ, Jenouri GA, Watson H, Sackner MA. Noninvasive measurement of pleural pressure by surface inductive plethysmography. J Appl Physiol Respir Environ Exercise Physiol 1983; 55:267–275.

11. Tobin MJ. Respiratory monitoring in the intensive care unit. Am Rev Respir Dis 1988; 138:1625–1642.

12. Dailey RH. Acute upper airway obstruction. Emerg Med Clin North Am 1983; 1: 261–277.

13. Root JD, Plum F. Evaluation of the comatose patient. In: Ayres SM, Grenvik A, Holbrook PR, Shoemaker WC, eds. Textbook of Critical Care. 3rd ed. Philadelphia: W.B. Saunders Company, 1995:1562–1571.

14. American Society of Anesthesiologists. Standards for Basic Anesthetic Monitoring, 1998.

15. Stone DJ, Gal TJ. Airway management. In: Miller RM, ed. Anesthesia. 3rd ed. New York: Churchill Livingstone Inc., 1990:1265–1292.

16. Chandler M, Crawley BE. Rationalization of the selection of tracheal tubes. Br J Anaesth 1986; 58:111–116.

17. Bromley HR, Tuorinsky S. An uncommon leak in the anesthesia breathing circuit. Anesth Analg 1997; 85:707.

18. Lewer BM, Karim Z, Henderson RS. Large air leak from an endotracheal tube due to a manufacturing defect. Anesth Analg 1997; 85:944–945.

19. Sakles JC, Laurin EG, Rantapaa AA, Panacek EA. Airway management in the emergency department: a one-year study of 610 tracheal intubations. Ann Emerg Med 1998; 31:325–332.

20. Knopp RK. Rapid sequence intubation revisited. Ann Emerg Med 1998; 31:398–400.

21. Fragen RJ, Avram MJ. Barbiturates. In: Miller RD, ed. Anesthesia. 3rd ed. New York: Churchill Livingstone Inc., 1990:225–242.

22. Reves JG, Glass PS. Nonbarbiturate intravenous anesthetics. In: Miller RD, ed. Anesthesia. 3rd ed. New York: Churchill Livingstone Inc., 1990:243–279.

23. Tagaito Y, Isono S, Nishino T. Upper airway reflexes during a combination of propofol and fentanyl anesthesia. Anesthesiology 1998; 88:1459–1466.

24. Brown RH, Wagner EM. Mechanisms of bronchoprotection by anesthetic agents. Anesthesiology 1999; 90:822–828.

25. Sivilotti ML, Ducharme J. Randomized, double-blind study on sedatives and hemodynamics during rapid-sequence intubation in the emergency department: The SHRED Study. Ann Emerg Med 1998; 31:313–324.

26. Wiklund RA, Rosenbaum SH. Medical progress: anesthesiology: first of two parts. N Engl J Med 1997; 337:1132–1141.

27. Sparr HJ, Leo C, Ladner E, Deusch E, Baumgartner H. Influence of anaesthesia and muscle relaxation on intubating conditions and sympathoadrenal response to tracheal intubation. Acta Anaesthesiol Scand 1997; 41:1300–1307.

28. Magorian T, Flannery KB, Miller RD. Comparison of rocuronium, succinylcholine, and vecuronium for rapid-sequence induction of anesthesia in adult patients. Anesthesiology 1993; 79:913–918.

29. Miller RD, Savarese JJ. Pharmacology of muscle relaxants and their antagonists.

In: Miller RD, ed. Anesthesia. 3rd ed. New York: Churchill Livingstone Inc., 1990: 389–435.

30. Bevan DR. Succinylcholine. Can J Anaesth 1994; 41:465–568.
31. Hunter JM. Rocuronium: the newest aminosteroid neuromuscular blocking drug. Br J Anaesth 1996; 76:481–483.
32. Cooper SD, Benumof JL. Airway algorithm: safety considerations. In: Morell RC, Eichhorn JH, ed. Patient Safety in Anesthetic Practice. New York: Churchill Livingstone Inc., 1997:221–262.
33. Lowenstein DH, Alldredge BK. Status epilepticus. N Engl J Med 1998; 338:970–976.
34. Kovac AL. Controlling the hemodynamic response to laryngoscopy and endotracheal intubation. J Clin Anesth 1996; 8:63–79.
35. Wang SC, Wu CC, Lin MS, Chang CF. Use of esmolol to prevent hemodynamic changes during intubation in general anesthesia. Acta Anaesthesiol Sin 1994; 32: 141–146.
36. Arrowsmith JE, Robertshaw HJ, Boyd JD. Nasotracheal intubation in the presence of frontobasal skull fracture. Can J Anaesth 1998; 45:71–75.
37. Stone DJ, Bogdonoff D. Airway considerations in the management of patients requiring long-term endotracheal intubation. Anesth Analg 1992; 74:276–287.
38. McCulloch TM, Bishop M. Complications of translaryngeal intubation. Clin Chest Med 1991; 12:507–521.
39. Depoix JP, Malbezin S, Videcoq M, Hazebroucq J, Barbier-Bohm G, Gauzit R, Desmonts JM. Oral intubation v. nasal intubation in adult cardiac surgery. Br J Anaesth 1987; 59:167–169.
40. Stauffer JL, Olson DE, Petty TL. Complications and consequences of endotracheal intubation and tracheotomy. A prospective study of 150 critically ill adult patients. Am J Med 1981; 70:65–76.
41. Schwartz DE, Lieberman JA, Cohen NH. Women are at greater risk than men for malpositioning of the endotracheal tube after emergent intubation. Crit Care Med 1994; 22:1127–1131.
42. Brunel W, Coleman DL, Schwartz DE, Peper E, Cohen NH. Assessment of routine chest roentgenograms and the physical examination to confirm endotracheal tube position. Chest 1989; 96:1043–1045.
43. Owen RL, Cheney FW. Endobronchial intubation: a preventable complication. Anesthesiology 1987; 67:255–257.
44. Henschke CI, Yankelevitz DF, Wand A, Davis SD, Shiau M. Accuracy and efficacy of chest radiography in the intensive care unit. Radiol Clin North Am 1996; 34: 21–31.
45. O'Brien D, Curran J, Conroy J, Bouchier-Hayes D. Fibre-optic assessment of tracheal tube position. A comparison of tracheal tube position as estimated by fibreoptic bronchoscopy and by chest X-ray. Anaesthesia 1985; 40:73–76.
46. Cardoso MM, Banner MJ, Melker RJ, Bjoraker DG. Portable devices used to detect endotracheal intubation during emergency situations: a review. Crit Care Med 1998; 26:957–964.
47. Schwartz DE, Matthay MA, Cohen NH. Death and other complications of emer-

gency airway management in critically ill adults. A prospective investigation of 297 tracheal intubations. Anesthesiology 1995; 82:367–376.

48. Wood M. Intravenous anesthetic agents. In: Wood M, Wood AJ, eds. Drugs and Anesthesia. Pharmacology for Anesthesiologists. 2nd ed. Baltimore: Williams and Wilkins, 1990:179–223.

49. Kallar SK, Everett LL. Potential risks and preventive measures for pulmonary aspiration: new concepts in preoperative fasting guidelines. Anesth Analg 1993; 77: 171–182.

50. Olsson GL, Hallen B, Hambraeus-Jonzon K. Aspiration during anaesthesia: a computer-aided study of 185,358 anaesthetics. Acta Anaesthesiol Scand 1986; 30: 84–92.

51. Ishihara H, Singh H, Giesecke AH. Relationship between diabetic autonomic neuropathy and gastric contents. Anesth Analg 1994; 78:943–947.

52. Reissell E, Taskinen MR, Orko R, Lindgren L. Increased volume of gastric contents in diabetic patients undergoing renal transplantation: lack of effect with cisapride. Acta Anaesthesiol Scand 1992; 36:736–740.

53. Mellin-Olsen J, Fasting S, Gisvold SE. Routine preoperative gastric emptying is seldom indicated. A study of 85,594 anaesthetics with special focus on aspiration pneumonia. Acta Anaesthesiol Scand 1996; 40:1184–1188.

54. Weltz CR, Morris JB, Mullen JL. Surgical jejunostomy in aspiration risk patients. Ann Surg 1992; 215:140–145.

55. Fox KA, Mularski RA, Sarfati MR, Brooks ME, Warneke JA, Hunter GC, Rappaport WD. Aspiration pneumonia following surgically placed feeding tubes. Am J Surg 1995; 170:564–566.

56. American Society of Anesthesiologists. Practice guidelines for preoperative fasting and the use of pharmacologic agents to reduce the risk of pulmonary aspiration: application to healthy patients undergoing elective procedures. A report by the American Society of Anesthesiologists Task Force on Preoperative Testing. Anesthesiology 1999; 90:896–905.

57. Petring OU, Adelhoj B, Jensen BN, Pedersen NO, Lomholt N. Prevention of silent aspiration due to leaks around cuffs of endotracheal tubes. Anesth Analg 1986; 65: 777–780.

58. Fanning GL. The efficacy of cricoid pressure in preventing regurgitation of gastric contents. Anesthesiology 1970; 32:553–555.

59. Herman NL, Carter B, Van Decar TK. Cricoid pressure: teaching the recommended level. Anesth Analg 1996; 83:859–863.

60. Kung MC, Hung CT, Ng KP, Au TK, Lo R, Lam A. Arterial desaturation during induction in healthy adults: Should preoxygenation be a routine? Anaesth Intensive Care 1991; 19:192–196.

61. Crosby ET, Cooper RM, Douglas MJ, Doyle DJ, Hung OR, Labrecque P, et al. The unanticipated difficult airway with recommendations for management. Can J Anaesth 1998; 45:757–776.

62. American Society of Anesthesiologists. Practice guidelines for management of the difficult airway. A report by the American Society of Anesthesiologists Task Force on Management of the Difficult Airway. Anesthesiology 1993; 78:597–602.

63. el-Ganzouri AR, McCarthy RJ, Tuman KJ, Tanck EN, Ivankovich AD. Preopera-

tive airway assessment: predictive value of a multivariate risk index. Anesth Analg 1996; 82:1197–1204.

64. Benumof JL, Scheller MS. The importance of transtracheal jet ventilation in the management of the difficult airway. Anesthesiology 1989; 71:769–778.
65. Bainton CR. Difficult intubation—What's the best test? Can J Anaesth 1996; 43: 541–543.
66. Wilson ME, Spiegelhalter D, Robertson JA, Lesser P. Predicting difficult intubation. Br J Anaesth 1988; 61:211–216.
67. Mallampati SR, Gatt SP, Gugino LD, Desai SP, Waraksa B, Freiberger D, et al. A clinical sign to predict difficult tracheal intubation: a prospective study. Can Anaesth Soc J 1985; 32:429–434.
68. Samsoon GL, Young JR. Difficult tracheal intubation: a retrospective study. Anaesthesia 1987; 42:487–490.
69. Randell T. Prediction of difficult intubation. Acta Anaesthesiol Scand 1996; 40: 1016–1023.
70. Jacobsen J, Jensen E, Waldau T, Poulsen TD. Preoperative evaluation of intubation conditions in patients scheduled for elective surgery. Acta Anaesthesiol Scand 1996; 40:421–424.
71. Asai T, Morris S. The laryngeal mask airway: its features, effects and role. Can J Anaesth 1994; 41:930–960.
72. Brain AI. The laryngeal mask—a new concept in airway management. B J Anaesth 1983; 55:801–805.
73. Brain AI. The laryngeal mask airway—a possible new solution to airway problems in the emergency situation. Arch Emerg Med 1984; 1:229–232.
74. Dorsch JA, Dorsch SE. Laryngeal mask airways. In: Dorsch JA, Dorsch SE, eds. Understanding Anesthesia Equipment. 4th ed. Baltimore: Williams & Wilkins, 1998:463–504.
75. Reed AP. Current concepts in airway management for cardiopulmonary resuscitation. Mayo Clin Proc 1995; 70:1172–1184.
76. Brimacombe JR, Berry A. The incidence of aspiration associated with the laryngeal mask airway: a meta-analysis of published literature. J Clin Anesth 1995; 7:297–305.
77. Benumof JL. Laryngeal mask airway and the ASA difficult airway algorithm. Anesthesiology 1996; 84:686–699.
78. Ferson DZ, Brimacombe J, Brain AI, Verghese C. The intubating laryngeal mask airway. Int Anesthesiol Clin 1998; 36:183–209.
79. Dorsch JA, Dorsch SE. Tracheal Tubes. In: Dorsch JA, Dorsch SE, eds. Understanding Anesthesia Equipment. 4th ed. Baltimore: Williams & Wilkins, 1998:557–675.
80. Vezina D, Lessard MR, Bussieres J, Topping C, Trepanier, CA. Complications associated with the use of the esophageal-tracheal combitube. Can J Anaesth 1998; 45:76–80.
81. Meschino A, Devitt JH, Koch JP, Szalai JP, Schwartz ML. The safety of awake tracheal intubation in cervical spine injury. Can J Anaesth 1992; 39:114–117.
82. Blosser SA, Stauffer JL. Intubation of critically ill patients. Clin Chest Med 1996; 17:355–378.

83. Pavlin EG, VanNimwegan D, Hornbein TF. Failure of a high-compliance low-pressure cuff to prevent aspiration. Anesthesiology 1975; 42:216–219.

84. Seegobin RD, van Hasselt GL. Aspiration beyond endotracheal cuffs. Can Anaesth Soc J 1986; 33:273–279.

85. Badenhorst CH. Changes in tracheal cuff pressure during respiratory support. Crit Care Med 1987; 15:300–302.

86. Cooper JD, Grillo H. Experimental production and prevention of injury due to cuffed tracheal tubes. Surg Gynecol Obstet 1969; 129:1235–1241.

87. Wilder NA, Orr J, Westenskow D. Clinical evaluation of tracheal pressure estimation from the endotracheal tube cuff pressure. J Clin Monitoring Computing 1998; 14:29–34.

88. Black AM, Seegobin RD. Pressures on endotracheal tube cuffs. Anaesthesia 1981; 36:498–511.

89. Vukmir RB, Grenvik A, Lindholm C-E. Laryngotracheal injury from prolonged tracheal intubation. In: Ayres SM, Grenvik A, Holbrook PR, Shoemaker WC, eds. Textbook of Critical Care. 3rd ed. Philadelphia: W.B. Saunders Company, 1995: 712–723.

90. Joh S, Matsuura H, Kotani Y, Sugiyama K, Hirota Y, Kiyomitsu Y, Kubota Y. Change in tracheal blood flow during endotracheal intubation. Acta Anaesthesiol Scand 1987; 31:300–304.

91. Seegobin RD, van Hasselt GL. Endotracheal cuff pressure and tracheal mucosal blood flow: endoscopic study of effects of four large volume cuffs. Br Med J Clin Res Ed 1984; 288:965–968.

92. Powaser MM, Brown MC, Chezem J, Woodburne CR, Rogenes P, Hanson B. The effectiveness of hourly cuff deflation in minimizing tracheal damage. Heart Lung 1976; 5:734–741.

93. Crimlisk JT, Horn MH, Wilson DJ, Marino B. Artificial airways: a survey of cuff management practices. Heart Lung J Acute Crit Care 1996; 25:225–235.

94. Bouvier JR. Measuring tracheal tube cuff pressures—tool and technique. Heart Lung 1981; 10:686–690.

95. Brainsky A, Fletcher RH, Glick HA, Lanken PN, Williams SV, Kundel HL. Routine portable chest radiographs in the medical intensive care unit: effects and costs. Crit Care Med 1997; 25:801–805.

96. Greenbaum DM, Marschall KE. The value of routine daily chest x-rays in intubated patients in the medical intensive care unit. Crit Care Med 1982; 10:29–30.

97. Bolder PM, Healy TE, Bolder AR, Beatty PC, Kay B. The extra work of breathing through adult endotracheal tubes. Anesth Analg 1986; 65:853–859.

98. Shapiro M, Wilson RK, Casar G, Bloom K, Teague RB. Work of breathing through different sized endotracheal tubes. Crit Care Med 1986; 14:1028–1031.

99. Kirton OC, DeHaven CB, Morgan JP, Windsor J, Civetta JM. Elevated imposed work of breathing masquerading as ventilator weaning intolerance. Chest 1995; 108:1021–1025.

100. Brochard L, Rua F, Lorino H, Lemaire F, Harf A. Inspiratory pressure support compensates for the additional work of breathing caused by the endotracheal tube. Anesthesiology 1991; 75:739–745.

101. Banner MJ, Kirby RR, Blanch PB, Layon AJ. Decreasing imposed work of the

breathing apparatus to zero using pressure-support ventilation. Crit Care Med 1993; 21:1333–1338.

102. Ripoll I, Lindholm CE, Carroll R, Grenvik A. Spontaneous dislocation of endotracheal tubes. Anesthesiology 1978; 49:50–52.

103. Coppolo DP, May JJ. Self-extubations. A 12-month experience. Chest 1990; 98: 165–169.

104. Holzapfel L, Chevret S, Madinier G, Ohen F, Demingeon G, Coupry A, Chaudet M. Influence of long-term oro- or nasotracheal intubation on nosocomial maxillary sinusitis and pneumonia: results of a prospective, randomized, clinical trial. Crit Care Med 1993; 21:1132–1138.

105. Salord F, Gaussorgues P, Marti-Flich J, Sirodot M, Allimant C, Lyonnet D, Robert D. Nosocomial maxillary sinusitis during mechanical ventilation: a prospective comparison of orotracheal versus the nasotracheal route for intubation. Intensive Care Med 1990; 16:390–393.

106. Fassoulaki A, Pamouktsoglou P. Prolonged nasotracheal intubation and its association with inflammation of paranasal sinuses. Anesth Analg 1989; 69:50–52.

107. Grindlinger GA, Niehoff J, Hughes SL, Humphrey MA, Simpson G. Acute paranasal sinusitis related to nasotracheal intubation of head-injured patients. Crit Care Med 1987; 15:214–217.

108. O'Reilly MJ, Reddick EJ, Black W, Carter PL, Erhardt J, Fill W, Maughn D, Sadd A, Kratt GR. Sepsis from sinusitis in nasotracheally intubated patients. A diagnostic dilemma. Am J Surg 1984; 147:601–604.

109. Deutschman CS, Wilton P, Sinow J, Dibbell D, Jr., Konstantinides FN, Cerra FB. Paranasal sinusitis associated with nasotracheal intubation: a frequently unrecognized and treatable source of sepsis. Crit Care Med 1986; 14:111–114.

110. Holdgaard HO, Pedersen J, Schurizek BA, Melsen NC, Juhl B. Complications and late sequelae following nasotracheal intubation. Acta Anaesthesiol Scand 1993; 37: 475–480.

111. Cook D, De Jonge B, Brochard L, Brun-Buisson C. Influence of airway management on ventilator-associated pneumonia: evidence from randomized trials. JAMA 1998; 279:781–787.

112. Thomas R, Kumar V, Kameswaran M, Shamim A, Al Ghamdi, Mummigaty AP, et al. Post intubation laryngeal sequelae in an intensive care unit. J Laryngol Otol 1995; 109:313–316.

113. Colice GL, Stukel TA, Dain B. Laryngeal complications of prolonged intubation. Chest 1989; 96:877–884.

114. Benjamin B. Prolonged intubation injuries of the larynx: endoscopic diagnosis, classification and treatment. Ann Otol Rhinol Laryngol 1993; 160(suppl):1–15.

115. Seiden AM. Sinusitis in the critical care patient. New Horizons 1993; 1:261–270.

116. Burns HP, Dayal VS, Scott A, van Nostrand AW, Bryce DP. Laryngotracheal trauma: observations on its pathogenesis and its prevention following prolonged orotracheal intubation in the adult. Laryngoscope 1979; 89:1316–1325.

117. Whited RE. A study of post-intubation laryngeal dysfunction. Laryngoscope 1985; 95:727–729.

118. Whited RE. A prospective study of laryngotracheal sequelae in long-term intubation. Laryngoscope 1984; 94:367–377.

119. Whited RE. A study of endotracheal tube injury to the subglottis. Laryngoscope 1985; 95:1216–1219.

120. Bishop MJ, Hibbard AJ, Fink BR, Vogel AM, Weymuller EA, Jr. Laryngeal injury in a dog model of prolonged endotracheal intubation. Anesthesiology 1985; 62: 770–773.

121. Colice GL. Resolution of laryngeal injury following translaryngeal intubation. Am Rev Respir Dis 1992; 145:361–364.

122. Whited RE. Posterior commissure stenosis post long-term intubation. Laryngoscope 1983; 93:1314–1318.

123. Santos PM, Afrassiabi A, Weymuller EA, Jr. Prospective studies evaluating the standard endotracheal tube and a prototype endotracheal tube. Ann Otol Rhinol Laryngol 1989; 98:935–940.

124. Alexopoulos C, Lindholm CE. Airway complaints and laryngeal pathology after intubation with an anatomically shaped endotracheal tube. Acta Anaesthesiol Scand 1983; 27:339–344.

125. Loeser EA, Hodges M, Gliedman J, Stanley TH, Johansen RK, Yonetani D. Tracheal pathology following short-term intubation with low- and high-pressure endotracheal tube cuffs. Anesth Analg 1978; 57:577–579.

126. Hedden M, Ersoz CJ, Donnelly WH, Safar P. Laryngotracheal damage after prolonged use of orotracheal tubes in adults. JAMA 1969; 207:703–708.

127. de Larminat V, Montravers P, Dureil B, Desmonts JM. Alteration in swallowing reflex after extubation in intensive care unit patients. Crit Care Med 1995; 23:486–490.

128. Cooper RM. Clinical use of an endotracheal ventilation catheter for airway management: 202 consecutive cases. Can J Anaesth 1996; 43:90–93.

129. Seitz PA, Gravenstein N. Endobronchial rupture from endotracheal reintubation with an endotracheal tube guide. J Clin Anesth 1989; 1:214–217.

130. Lindholm CE, Ollman B, Snyder JV, Millen EG, Grenvik A. Cardiorespiratory effects of flexible fiberoptic bronchoscopy in critically ill patients. Chest 1978; 74: 362–368.

131. Vukmir RB, Grenvik A, Lindholm C-E. Surgical airway, cricothyroidotomy, and tracheotomy: procedures, complications and outcome. In: Ayres SM, Grenvik A, Holbrook PR, Shoemaker WC, eds. Textbook of Critical Care. 3rd ed. Philadelphia: W.B. Saunders Company, 1995:724–734.

132. Deblieux P, Wadell C, McClarity Z, deBoisblanc BP. Facilitation of percutaneous dilatational tracheostomy by use of a perforated endotracheal tube exchanger. Chest 1995; 108:572–574.

133. Porter JM, Ivatury RR. Preferred route of tracheostomy—percutaneous versus open at the bedside: a randomized, prospective study in the surgical intensive care unit. Am Surg 1999; 65:142–146.

134. Griggs A. Tracheostomy: suctioning and humidification. Nurs Stand 1998; 13:49–53.

135. Astrachan DI, Kirchner JC, Goodwin WJ Jr. Prolonged intubation vs tracheostomy: complications, practical and psychological considerations. Laryngoscope 1988; 98: 1165–1169.

136. Goldstein SI, Breda SD, Schneider KL. Surgical complications of bedside tracheotomy in an otolaryngology residency program. Laryngoscope 1987; 97:1407–1409.
137. Stock MC, Woodward CG, Shapiro BA, Cane RD, Lewis V, Pecaro B. Perioperative complications of elective tracheostomy in critically ill patients. Crit Care Med 1986; 14:861–863.
138. Heffner JE. Timing of tracheostomy in mechanically ventilated patients. Am Rev Respir Dis 1993; 147:768–771.
139. Grillo HC, Donahue DM, Mathisen DJ, Wain JC, Wright CD. Postintubation tracheal stenosis. Treatment and results. J Thoracic Cardiovascular Surg 1995; 109: 486–492.
140. Friman L, Hedenstierna G, Schildt B. Stenosis following tracheostomy. A quantitative study of long term results. Anaesthesia 1976; 31:479–493.
141. Law JH, Barnhart K, Rowlett W, de la Rocha O, Lowenberg S. Increased frequency of obstructive airway abnormalities with long-term tracheostomy. Chest 1993; 104: 136–138.
142. Payne DK, Anderson WM, Romero MD, Wissing DR, Fowler M. Tracheoesophageal fistula formation in intubated patients. Risk factors and treatment with high-frequency jet ventilation. Chest 1990; 98:161–164.
143. Hilgenberg AD, Grill HC. Acquired nonmalignant tracheoesophageal fistula. J Thoracic Cardiovascular Surg 1983; 85:492–498.
144. Wright CD. Management of tracheoinnominate artery fistula. Chest Surg Clin North Am 1996; 6:865–873.
145. Sasaki CT, Horiuchi M, Koss N. Tracheostomy-related subglottic stenosis: bacteriologic pathogenesis. Laryngoscope 1979; 89:857–865.
146. Elpern EH, Scott MG, Petro L, Ries MH. Pulmonary aspiration in mechanically ventilated patients with tracheostomies. Chest 1994; 105:563–566.
147. Niederman MS, Ferranti RD, Zeigler A, Merrill WW, Reynolds HY. Respiratory infection complicating long-term tracheostomy. The implication of persistent gram-negative tracheobronchial colonization. Chest 1984; 85:39–44.
148. Bryant LR, Trinkle JK, Mobin-Uddin K, Baker J, Griffen, Jr WO. Bacterial colonization profile with tracheal intubation and mechanical ventilation. Arch Surg 1972; 104:647–651.
149. Gunawardana RH. Experience with tracheostomy in medical intensive care patients. Postgrad Med J 1992; 68:338–341.
150. Cross AS, Roup B. Role of respiratory assistance devices in endemic nosocomial pneumonia. Am J Med 1981; 70:681–685.
151. Koerner RJ. Contribution of endotracheal tubes to the pathogenesis of ventilator-associated pneumonia. J Hospital Infect 1997; 35:83–89.
152. Armstrong PA, McCarthy MC, Peoples JB. Reduced use of resources by early tracheostomy in ventilator-dependent patients with blunt trauma. Surgery 1998; 124:763–766.
153. Rodriguez JL, Steinberg SM, Luchetti FA, Gibbons KJ, Taheri PA, Flint LM. Early tracheostomy for primary airway management in the surgical critical care setting. Surgery 1990; 108:655–659.
154. McGeehin WH, Scoma R, Igidbashian L, Smink Jr. RD. Tracheostomy versus en-

dotracheal intubation: the ICU nurse's perspective(abstr). Crit Care Med 1990; 18: S224.

155. Davis KJ, Campbell RS, Johannigman JA, Valente JF, Branson RD. Changes in respiratory mechanics after tracheostomy. Arch Surg 1999; 134:59–62.

156. Sugerman HJ, Wolfe L, Pasquale M, Rogers FB, O'Malley MD, Knudson M, DiNardo L, Gordon M, Schaffer S. Multicenter, randomized, prospective trial of early tracheostomy. J Trauma Injury Infection Critical Care 1997; 43:741–747.

157. Berlauk JF. Prolonged endotracheal intubation vs. tracheostomy. Crit Care Med 1986; 14:742–745.

158. Sofferman RA, Haisch CE, Kirchner JA, Hardin NJ. The nasogastric tube syndrome. Laryngoscope 1990; 100:962–968.

159. Mehta S. The risk of aspiration in presence of cuffed endotracheal tubes. Br J Anaesth 1972; 44:601–605.

160. Jamil AK. Letter: laryngotracheal toilet before extubation. Anaesthesia 1974; 29: 630–631.

161. Miller KA, Harkin CP, Bailey PL. Postoperative tracheal extubation. Anesth Analg 1995; 80:149–172.

162. Hartley M, Vaughan RS. Problems associated with tracheal extubation. Br J Anaesth 1993; 71:561–568.

163. Tavakoli M, Corssen G. An unusual case of difficult extubation. Anesthesiology 1976; 45:552–553.

164. Lang S, Johnson DH, Lanigan DT, Ha H. Difficult tracheal extubation. Can J Anaesth 1989; 36:340–342.

165. Fujii Y, Kihara S, Takahashi S, Tanaka H, Toyooka H. Calcium channel blockers attenuate cardiovascular responses to tracheal extubation in hypertensive patients. Can J Anaesth 1998; 45:655–659.

166. Duane DT, Redwood SR, Grounds RM. Esmolol aids extubation in intensive care patient with ischaemic pulmonary oedema. Anaesthesia 1996; 51:474–477.

167. Anene O, Meert KL, Uy H, Simpson P, Sarnaik AP. Dexamethasone for the prevention of postextubation airway obstruction: a prospective, randomized, double-blind, placebo-controlled trial [see comments]. Crit Care Med 1996; 24:1666–1669.

168. Darmon J-Y, Rauss A, Dreyfuss D, Bleichner G, Elkharrat D, Schlemmer B, Tenaillon A, Brun-Buisson C, Huet Y. Evaluation of risk factors for laryngeal edema after tracheal extubation in adults and its prevention by dexamethasone. Anesthesiology 1992; 77:245–251.

169. Miller RL, Cole RP. Association between reduced cuff leak volume and postextubation stridor. Chest 1996; 110:1035–1040.

170. Fisher MM, Raper RF. The 'cuff leak' test for extubation. Anaesthesia 1992; 47: 10–12.

11

Ventilator Management Strategies for Acute Asthma

THOMAS CORBRIDGE

Northwestern University Medical School
Chicago, Illinois

JESSE B. HALL

University of Chicago
Chicago, Illinois

I. Introduction

The goal of management of patients with acute severe asthma, or status asthmaticus, is to restore, without complications, the state of unlabored breathing. Fortunately, this goal is commonly achieved by pharmacotherapy alone, even in the subgroup of patients with hypercapnic respiratory failure (1). Intubation and mechanical ventilation are important in severe cases and can be life saving. They can also contribute to morbidity and mortality. Fortunately, accumulating data and experience have demonstrated good outcomes in the majority of patients ventilated with a strategy of hypoventilation—unless prior respiratory arrest has resulted in anoxic brain injury (2).

In this paper we will begin with a review of the pathophysiology of acute asthma insofar as it clarifies ventilator management and medication choices. We will review two treatment strategies to help prevent intubation (namely, heliox and noninvasive positive pressure ventilation), indications for intubation, and provide recommendations for safely securing the endotracheal tube. We will examine the mechanism and management of postintubation hypotension and provide recommendations for initial ventilator settings. Next we will review techniques for assessing the degree of lung hyperinflation during mechanical ventilation and, based in large part on this assessment, provide an approach to ongoing ventilator management. Finally, we will discuss pharmacotherapeutic considerations, including recommendations for optimal delivery of bronchodilators and rational use of sedatives and paralytics.

II. Pathophysiology

The pathophysiology of acute asthma consists of variable amounts of bronchospasm, airway wall inflammation, and mucus plugging that worsen over variable periods of time. In slow-onset attacks there is progressive airway wall inflammation, accumulation of intraluminal mucus, airway wall edema, and smooth muscle–mediated bronchospasm. Mucus plugs consist of sloughed epithelial cells, eosinophils, fibrin, and other serum components that leak readily through the denuded airway epithelium. They fill large and small airways and are a striking finding at autopsy (3). Slow-onset attacks are triggered by a variety of infectious, allergic, and nonspecific irritant exposures. They evolve over hours to days and resolve slowly because of the presence of airway inflammation and airway architectural distortion. During this process, most patients escalate their use of β-agonist medications; many miss the opportunity to intervene early with anti-inflammatory therapy (4).

The speed at which acute asthma develops varies among patients (5). In some patients, exacerbations occur suddenly and unexpectedly and resolve quickly. Typically developing in less than 3 hours, this syndrome is called "sudden asphyxic asthma." It represents a purer form of smooth muscle–mediated bronchospasm. Compared with slow-onset attacks, there are fewer airway secretions and more neutrophils than eosinophils in the airway (6–9). Sudden attacks occur as sporadic cases or in outbreaks and may result from use of nonsteroidal anti-inflammatory agents or β-blockers in patients with intolerance to these products, allergen exposure, ingestion of foods containing sulfites, or as a consequence of "crack" cocaine or heroin inhalation. Heroin inhalation may cause sudden yet protracted attacks that are unresponsive to β-agonists, suggesting that there is a significant component of airway wall inflammation (10).

Whether of sudden or slow onset, increased expiratory airway obstruction interferes with alveolar gas emptying. In severe cases it may take as long as 60 seconds for expiratory airflow to stop. Because expiratory time is shorter than this during spontaneous or assisted breathing, there is incomplete emptying of the tidal breath and development of positive end-expiratory alveolar pressure (termed auto-PEEP or intrinsic-PEEP) (11). In this situation, the next breath further elevates lung volume (a state referred to as dynamic lung hyperinflation, or DHI). Fortunately, DHI is self-limiting in mild disease because as lung volume increases so does the elastic recoil pressure of the lung and airway diameter—factors favoring expiratory airflow. These factors are represented by the equation:

$$\dot{V} = \frac{\text{Pel}}{\text{Rus}}$$

where $\dot{V}$ is maximum expiratory airflow, Pel is the lung elastic recoil pressure (inversely related to compliance), and Rus is airway resistance upstream from the equal pressure point.

Thus, at a sufficiently large lung volume, airflow may be adequate to exhale the inspired breath and a new steady state is achieved. End-expired lung volume (auto-PEEP) and functional residual capacity (FRC) are elevated and tidal breathing occurs just below total lung capacity (TLC). During spontaneous breathing, DHI is limited by the inability of the patient to inspire much beyond TLC. This physical limitation to minute ventilation (Ve) contributes (along with elevated dead space and fatigue) to hypercapnia (12). On the other hand, it also protects against further lung hyperinflation. During positive pressure ventilation, inspiration may be pushed beyond TLC, increasing the risk of barotrauma (12–15). If TLC is not surpassed during mechanical ventilation, complications may be avoided (13,16).

Wide variations in lung compliance occur, so that in some cases lung compliance is normal despite severe lung inflation—an observation suggesting a possible stretch-relaxation response of lung parenchymal tissue (17). This state is not favorable to expiratory flow but may protect against complications of lung hyperinflation.

Inspiratory work of breathing is increased by airway narrowing and auto-PEEP, a threshold pressure that must be overcome to establish the pressure gradient necessary for inspiratory flow. In addition, decreased lung compliance requires generation of greater transpulmonary pressure during inspiration. Each of these mechanical loads is imposed on a diaphragm that is placed in a mechanically disadvantageous position by DHI at a time when circulatory abnormalities may result in diaphragm hypoperfusion and respiratory acidosis may decrease diaphragm force generation (18). Ventilatory failure may follow, even in robust and otherwise healthy patients.

Dead space increases in acute asthma, presumably due to hypoperfusion of areas of hyperinflated lung. An increase in the dead space to tidal volume ratio (Vd/Vt) favors hypercapnia, as demonstrated by the following equation:

$$\text{Paco}_2 = \dot{V}\text{co}_2 \times 0.863/\text{Va}$$
$$= \dot{V}\text{co}_2 \times 0.863/[\text{Ve} \times (1 - \text{Vd/Vt})]$$

where $\dot{V}\text{co}_2$ is carbon dioxide production, Va is alveolar ventilation, Ve is minute ventilation, and Vd/Vt is the ratio of dead space to tidal volume.

Despite an increase in dead space, the majority of patients with mild acute asthma develop acute respiratory alkalosis because of increased Ve. If respiratory alkalosis persists for 2–3 days, compensatory wasting of bicarbonate occurs through renal mechanisms resulting in a nonanion gap metabolic acidosis. As the severity of airflow obstruction increases (particularly when FEV_1 is 25% of predicted), $Paco_2$ may increase because of inadequate Va (reflecting an increase in Vd/Vt, and a decrease in Ve as the patient nears respiratory arrest) and possibly an increase in CO_2 production.

Because airway obstruction results in maldistribution of alveolar ventilation relative to perfusion (low V/Q), and not true shunt (19), minimal enrichment of inspired oxygen (1–3 L/min by nasal cannula) corrects hypoxemia. Even patients requiring mechanical ventilation achieve adequate arterial oxygen saturation with Fio_2 of 0.3–0.5; if not, the clinician should consider concurrent pneumonia, aspiration, acute lobar atelectasis, pulmonary embolism, or pneumothorax. There is a correlation between severity of airflow obstruction as measured by the FEV_1 or the peak expiratory flow rate (PEFR) and hypoxemia (20,21). However, no threshold value exists for either measurement that accurately predicts hypoxemia. Hypoxemia resulting from peripheral airway obstruction may occur sooner and/ or resolve later than airflow rates that predominantly reflect large airway function (22,23).

Circulatory abnormalities result from a state of cardiac temponade caused by DHI and large pleural pressure excursions associated with breathing against obstructed airways. Blood return to the right heart decreases during expiration because of positive intrathoracic pressure, but during vigorous inspiration intrathoracic pressure falls and blood flow increases. As the right ventricle fills, the intraventricular septum shifts toward the left ventricle (LV), resulting in a conformational change, diastolic dysfunction, and incomplete filling of the LV. Large negative pleural pressures may also directly impair LV emptying by increasing LV afterload (24,25). This plus LV diastolic dysfunction may rarely cause pulmonary edema (26). Finally, lung hyperinflation increases total pulmonary vascular resistance (27) and may cause transient acute pulmonary hypertension (28).

The net effect of these cyclical respiratory events is to accentuate the normal inspiratory reduction in stroke volume, a phenomenon termed "pulsus paradoxus." The pulsus paradoxus can be a valuable sign indicating asthma severity (29); however, the absence of a widened pulsus paradoxus does not ensure a mild attack because pulsus paradoxus falls in the fatiguing asthmatic unable to generate large swings in pleural pressure (2).

III. Preventing Intubation

Because intubation and mechanical ventilation provide no inherent therapeutic benefit to airflow obstruction in asthma and may be associated with significant morbidity and mortality, it is desirable to avoid intubation whenever possible. Fortunately, this goal is achieved in most cases by pharmacotherapy. A detailed discussion of the pharmacotherapy of acute asthma is beyond the scope of this chapter. However, we would like to comment briefly on two strategies (namely heliox and noninvasive positive pressure ventilation) that may be useful in refractory patients.

Heliox is a gas consisting of 80% helium and 20% oxygen (70:30% and 60:40% mixtures are also available). As the concentration of helium decreases, so does the therapeutic benefit. Concentrations of helium less than 60% are ineffective, precluding its use in severely hypoxemic patients. Heliox is slightly more viscous than air, but significantly less dense, resulting in a more than threefold increase in kinematic viscosity (the ratio of gas viscosity to gas density) compared to air. Theoretically, this property decreases the driving pressure required for gas flow by two mechanisms. First, for any level of turbulent flow, breathing low-density gas decreases the pressure gradient required for flow. Second, heliox decreases the Reynold's number (Re = pdV/u, where p is gas density, d is airway diameter, V is the mean linear velocity, and u is gas viscosity), favoring conversion of turbulent flow to laminar flow (30). Heliox does not treat bronchospasm or airway inflammation.

Heliox promptly improves dyspnea, work of breathing, and arterial blood gas abnormalities in patients with upper airway obstruction (31). Benefits have also been reported in acute asthma in children and adults (32–34). In adult asthmatics treated in the emergency room, an 80:20 mix delivered by tight-fitting face mask increases PEFR and decreases pulsus paradoxus, suggesting improved airway resistance and decreased work of breathing (33). A more recent randomized controlled trial of 23 adults with acute severe asthma similarly demonstrated improved dyspnea and PEFR in heliox-treated patients (34). Eighty-two percent of patients receiving a 70:30 blend of heliox had >25% improvement in PEFR at 20 minutes compared to 17% in the placebo group. However, in another study of 13 acutely ill asthmatics, the authors were unable to demonstrate a benefit with a 70:30 blend of heliox (35). When heliox is effective, it may buy time for concurrent therapies to work and thereby avert the need for intubation. Whether heliox augments the bronchodilator effect of inhaled β-agonists compared to delivery in air is unclear. Data are available demonstrating a benefit to heliox as a driving gas (36), but there are also data to the contrary (36).

Noninvasive positive pressure ventilation (NPPV) by face mask is potentially useful for patients with hypercapnic acute respiratory failure who are not in need of immediate control of the airway. Advantages of NPPV over intubation and mechanical ventilation include decreased need for sedation and paralysis, decreased incidence of nosocomial pneumonia, decreased incidence of otitis and sinusitis, and improved patient comfort (38). Disadvantages include a small increased risk of aspiration of gastric contents when there is gastric insufflation, skin necrosis, and diminished control of the ventilatory status compared with invasive ventilation.

The rationale for providing NPPV is to provide partial ventilatory assistance and reduce work of breathing in order to buy time for medical therapy to work. In this way, intubation and the attendant risks are averted. In this context, noninvasive positive pressure can be administered continuously (continuous positive airway pressure, or CPAP) or each breath can be assisted using pressure support or volume-control ventilation. CPAP alone may reduce work of breathing by counterbalancing auto-PEEP or by stenting airways open during expiration, decreasing resistance at low lung volume (39). By adding inspiratory assistance to CPAP (or extrinsic PEEP), work of breathing may be maximally reduced by reducing the inspiratory load both to initiate and then sustain a breath. In one study of 21 acute asthmatics with a mean PEFR of 144 L/min, nasal CPAP of 5 or 7.5 cmH$_2$O decreased RR and dyspnea compared to placebo (40). In the largest study published to date (39), Meduri and colleagues reported their observational experience with NPPV during 17 episodes of acute severe asthma. NPPV was achieved using a loose-fitting full-face mask with initial settings of 0 cmH$_2$O CPAP and 10 cmH$_2$O pressure support ventilation. CPAP was increased by 3– 5 cmH$_2$O and pressure support ventilation was increased to achieve an exhaled tidal volume of 7 mL/kg or more and a respiratory rate (RR) of < 25/min. In general, NPPV improved dyspnea, arterial blood gases, HR, and RR. Two NPPV-treated patients were intubated for worsening Paco$_2$. There were no complications related to NPPV use. These results are promising but in need of confirmation by randomized trials.

IV. Intubation

The primary goals of intubation and mechanical ventilation are to maintain oxygenation and prevent respiratory arrest. Patients who are intubated before they arrest generally do well (if ventilated appropriately); patients who are intubated after respiratory arrest and the development of anoxic brain injury do not. Approximately 40% of deaths in patients who have received mechanical ventilation for severe asthma are due to cerebral anoxia resulting from respiratory arrest prior to mechanical ventilation (12).

Intubation is indicated for cardiorespiratory arrest, altered mental status, or rapid deterioration in respiratory function despite maximal therapy. Patients who are severely affected, but not in extremis, require careful consideration of all the factors influencing the decision to intubate. Most important in this regard is the general appearance of the patient. Changes in posture, speech, alertness, extent of accessory muscle use, diaphoresis, and RR can all indicate worsening respiratory failure that does not need confirmation by measurement of PEFR or arterial blood gases (2). Patients deteriorating on these grounds should be intubated whether or not $Paco_2$ is climbing; conversely, patients who are more comfortable, more polysyllabic, and less attentive to the task of breathing should not be intubated despite an elevated $Paco_2$. Ultimately, the decision rests on a seasoned clinician's estimate of the ability of a patient to maintain spontaneous respiration.

Patients receiving heliox or noninvasive positive pressure by face mask are at particular risk if it appears they are failing and require intubation. Theoretically, removal of these supportive therapies for the purpose of airway inspection and intubation may hasten the decline in respiratory function. Clinicians must take this into consideration and act quickly, or they may be facing an unexpected cardiorespiratory arrest.

Once the decision to intubate has been made, the goal is to take rapid and complete control of the patient's cardiorespiratory status. Whenever possible, intubation should be performed by a clinician experienced in airway procedures and ventilation. Unskilled airway manipulation in these patients may produce laryngospasm or exacerbate bronchospasm. The approach to intubation should follow standard and accepted clinical guidelines for the intubation of any seriously ill patient (see Chapter 10). Initial preparation includes ensuring the appropriate equipment and drugs, the availability of suction, and proper selection of an endotracheal tube. A preintubation inspection of the patient for potential difficulties with airway intubation is vital to avoid the catastrophic situation of a failed or unnecessarily prolonged intubation. Rapid sequence induction using an intravenous sedative/anesthetic agent in combination with succinylcholine is the preferred choice to secure the airway while protecting against gastric aspiration (12). The addition, intravenous lidocaine, may attenuate reflex bronchospasm associated with tracheal manipulation. Ketamine has sedative, analgesic, and bronchodilating properties that may allow for successful emergency intubation in asthma, but it must be used cautiously because of its sympathomimetic effects and its potential to cause delirium and increased laryngeal secretions (40). Bolus administration of morphine sulfate should be avoided because of its potential to drop systemic blood pressure (BP) through a combination of direct vasodilation, histamine release, and vagally mediated bradycardia (41). Morphine-induced vomiting is also undesirable in the peri-intubation period.

Whenever possible, patients should be intubated via the oral route using a large-sized endotracheal tube (e.g., 8.0 mm ID for adult women, 8.0–9.0 mm ID for adult men). Large tubes facilitate clearance of airway secretions and decrease airway resistance. This is particularly important at high airflow rates. When inspiratory flow is 120 L/min, endotracheal tube airflow resistance is more than twice as much with a 6.0 mm tube than with a 7.0 mm tube in vitro, a difference that may be even greater in vivo (42). Nasal intubation may be better tolerated in an awake patient, but it requires a smaller endotracheal tube and may be complicated by bleeding, nasal polyps, and sinusitis. In selected cases, fiberoptic guidance may help facilitate nasal cannulation.

V. Postintubation Hypotension

The time immediately following intubation can be extremely difficult for the patient with severe airflow obstruction, particularly since airflow obstruction may continue to deteriorate during the first 24 hours of mechanical ventilation (13–16). Considerable care must be taken to stabilize the patient during this period, including the thoughtful use of sedatives, paralytics, bronchodilators, intravenous fluids, and careful delivery of positive pressure ventilation.

The immediate concerns are hypotension and pneumothorax. Hypotension has been reported in 25–35% of patients following intubation (12). It occurs for several reasons. First, there is loss of vascular tone due to a direct effect of sedation and loss of sympathetic activity. Second, many patients are hypovolemic because of high insensible losses and decreased oral fluid intake during their exacerbation. Third, overzealous AMBU bag ventilation can result in dangerous levels of DHI because adequate time is not provided for exhalation of the inspired breath. When this occurs, the patient becomes difficult to ventilate, breath sounds diminish, BP falls, and HR rises. This pathophysiology can be demonstrated by a trial of hypopnea (2–3 breaths/min) or apnea in a preoxygenated patient. As the lung deflates, intrathoracic pressure falls, allowing for greater blood return to the right atrium. Within 30–60 seconds, BP rises and HR falls, and the inspired breath becomes easier to deliver.

Thus, a trial of hypopnea or apnea is diagnostic and therapeutic for DHI. If such a trial does not quickly restore cardiopulmonary stability, consideration should be given to tension pneumothorax. Tension pneumothoraces may have been responsible for >6% of deaths of patients who required mechanical ventilation for severe asthma (12). Hemodynamic improvement during a trial of apnea suggests DHI but does not completely exclude tension pneumothorax. Careful inspection of a chest radiograph is mandatory because there may not be significant lung collapse in the setting of DHI. When pneumothorax is present, the contralateral lung deserves close attention because unilateral pneumothorax causes preferential ventilation of the contralateral lung, increasing the risk of bilateral pneumothoraces. Management of this situation consists of intentional hypoventilation, rapid volume resuscitation, and chest tubes placed bilaterally.

VI. Initial Ventilator Settings

There is no consensus as to which ventilator mode should be used in asthmatics. In paralyzed patients synchronized intermittent mandatory ventilation (SIMV) and assist-controlled ventilation (AC) are equivalent. In patients triggering the ventilator, SIMV is generally preferred because of the unproven concern that Ve will be higher during AC since each triggered breath receives a guaranteed tidal volume. Significant pressure support should not be used because this may enable a patient to elevate his Ve beyond a safe limit. Volume-controlled ventilation (VC) is generally chosen over pressure-controlled ventilation (PC) to allow delivery of a constant inspiratory flow and because there is more familiarity with its use. Pressure-controlled ventilation is being increasingly used and has the theoretical advantages of maintaining dynamic hyperinflation within a safe limit (e.g., 30 cmH$_2$O) when airflow obstruction is severe and automatically increasing Ve as airflow obstruction improves.

Ventilator settings must allow for an adequate expiratory time (Te), which is determined by RR, Vt, and inspiratory flow rate (see Fig. 1). Each of these variables may be set and adjusted during mechanical ventilation to allow for sufficiently long Te and avoidance of excessive DHI. The general strategy com-

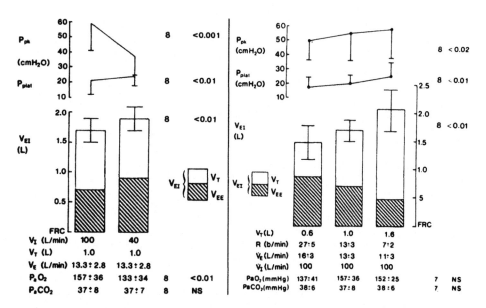

Figure 1 Effects of ventilator settings on airway pressures and lung volumes during normocapneic ventilation of eight paralyzed asthmatics. V_{EE} = lung volume at end expiration; V_{EI} = lung volume at end inspiration; P_{pk} = peak airway pressure; P_{plat} = end inspiratory plateau pressure; V_E = minute ventilation; V_T = tidal volume; V_I = inspiratory flow rate. (left) As inspiratory flow is decreased from 100 L/m to 40 L/m at the same V_E, P_{pk} falls but hyperinflation increases due to dynamic gas trapping. (right) Dynamic hyperinflation is reduced by lowering V_E, but high V_T results in high P_{plat}. (From Ref. 14.)

bines a relatively low Ve (RR × Vt) with a high inspiratory flow rate. To illustrate this strategy, consider the following ventilator settings (43): Vt, 1000 mL; RR, 15 breaths/min; and inspiratory flow rate, 60 L/min. These settings result in a respiratory cycle time (the amount of time required to complete one inhalation/ exhalation cycle) of 4 seconds. Inspiratory time (Ti) is 1 second and Te is 3 seconds, resulting in an I:E ratio of 1:3. Decreasing RR to 12 breaths/min prolongs Te to 4 seconds (i.e., an additional 1 second to exhale the 1000 mL inspired breath) and results in an I:E ratio of 1:4. Doubling inspiratory flow with RR of 15 breaths/min also prolongs Te. Here Ti falls to 0.5 seconds and Te increases to 3.5 s, resulting in an I:E of 1:7. Note that decreasing RR to 12 breaths/min prolongs Te more than doubling inspiratory flow and thereby likely results in less DHI, even though the I:E ratio looks more favorable with the high-flow strategy. Indeed, Ve is a more important determinant of Te than inspiratory flow (14).

Tuxen has recommended that mechanical ventilation be initiated with a Vt of 8 mL/kg and a RR of 10–12 breaths/min resulting in a Ve <115 mL/kg/min (16). He and others have recommended that the Vt be delivered at a high inspiratory flow rate (80 L/min by constant flow) to ensure a short Ti (<0.5 s) and a long Te (>4.0 s) (2,15). These settings for Ve and inspiratory flow have been shown by Williams and coworkers to suit 80% of patients who require mechanical ventilation for severe asthma and result in only mildly excessive DHI in the remainder (16). Rare patients, with exceptionally severe airflow obstruction, may develop a dangerous level of DHI despite this low initial Ve (44–49). Hypotensive patients deserve a trial of apnea; if BP improves they should receive a low Vt and even lower RR (4–6 breaths/min) (46). The use of low Vt helps to prolong Te, but it is also crucial to avoid excessive peak lung inflation, which may occur even when there is an acceptably low Ve (see Fig. 1) (14).

Use of a hypoventilatory strategy helps avoid severe DHI. When patients are ventilated to eucapnia, end-inspiratory lung volume above apneic FRC (termed Vei) can be as large as 3–4 L (see Fig. 2). Hypoventilation invariably causes hypercapnia, although the rise in $Paco_2$ for each decrement in Ve may be less than expected since reduction in hyperinflation may also reduce dead space (see above). When hypercapnia does occur it is generally well tolerated as long as $Paco_2$ is not allowed to rise quickly or to exceed 90 mmHg (50,51).

Associated acidemia is similarly well tolerated, raising the unanswered question of whether buffer therapy should be considered in severe cases. Slow infusions of sodium bicarbonate appear to be safe in patients with severe acidemia, but it is also possible that patients could tolerate several days of acidemia until asthma improves or renal compensation occurs. In animal models, bicarbonate correction of acidemia induced by permissive hypercapnia attenuates hemodynamic and bloods flow changes (52), and it may improve tolerance of hypercapnia

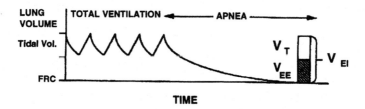

Figure 2 The volume of gas at end-inspiration above apeic FRC (V_{EI}) is determined by collecting the total exhaled volume in a paralyzed patient over 60 seconds of apnea. This volume is the sum of the tidal volume (V_T) and volume at end exhalation above FRC (V_{EE}). A value of V_{EI} greater than 20 mL/kg has been shown to predict complications of hypotension and barotrauma. (From Ref. 15.)

by reducing the acidemic drive to ventilation. Still, bicarbonate has not been shown to be of benefit in patients with moderate hypercapnic acidosis (53). Hypercapneic acidosis does cause cerebral vasodilation, cerebral edema, decreased myocardial contractility, and systemic vasodilation. Accordingly, permissive hypercapnia should be avoided in patients with raised intracranial pressure (as may occur after cardiorespiratory arrest with anoxic brain injury) and in patients with severe myocardial dysfunction.

The use of a high inspiratory flow rate increases peak airway pressure (Ppk) by elevating airway resistive pressure. Theoretically, high inspiratory flow and high airway pressure may redistribute ventilation to low resistance lung units risking barotrauma. These concerns are based largely on mechanical and mathematical lung models (55,56) but have no supporting clinical data. The only clinical data comparing different flow rates suggest that high inspiratory flow rates decrease DHI and improve gas exchange (14,57). There are also preliminary data that use of high inspiratory flow rates in the assist-control mode increases RR in spontaneously breathing patients and thereby decrease Te (58). Note that when Ppk is high, the high-pressure alarm limit must be set sufficiently high to avoid premature termination of the tidal breath.

Peak airway pressures per se do not correlate with morbidity or mortality. Rather it is the state of lung hyperinflation that predicts outcome (see below) (16). It is important to note that ventilator strategies that lower Ppk such as use of a lower constant flow rate or a decelerating flow pattern will shorten Te and worsen DHI.

Ventilator-applied PEEP is not recommended in sedated and paralyzed patients because it may increase lung volume if used excessively (59). In spontaneously breathing patients, we recommend small amounts of ventilator-applied

PEEP (e.g., 5 cmH$_2$O) to help overcome the effects of auto-PEEP and thereby decrease inspiratory work of breathing. We avoid higher levels of ventilator-applied PEEP because the degree of auto-PEEP is difficult to assess in spontaneously breathing patients, and if ventilator-applied PEEP nears or exceeds auto-PEEP it may contribute to lung hyperinflation.

In the peri-intubation period, the fraction of inspired oxygen (Fio$_2$) should be 1.0, although it should be decreased to a nontoxic level once the patient has been stabilized on the ventilator. As stated above, uncomplicated asthma requires minimal enrichment of inspired oxygen (Fio$_2$ 0.3–0.5) to achieve adequate arterial oxygenation. Correction of hypoxemia results in several beneficial effects, including improved oxygen delivery to peripheral tissues (including the respiratory muscles), reversal of hypoxic pulmonary vasoconstriction, and possible airway bronchodilation. Oxygen also protects against the fall in Pao$_2$ resulting from β-agonist–induced pulmonary vasodilation and increased blood flow to low V/Q lung units (60,61).

VII. Assessing Dynamic Hyperinflation

Because the severity of airflow obstruction varies considerably between patients with acute asthma and in the same patient over time, a fixed ventilatory pattern will result in a wide range of DHI that may not ensure ventilation below the safe limit of TLC. An initial ventilatory pattern may be chosen that suites the majority of patients with severe asthma (see above). Thereafter it is essential that the level of DHI be assessed so that Ve can be adjusted either upward or downward to suit the situation. Thus, determination of the severity of dynamic hyperinflation is central to risk management and ongoing ventilator adjustment.

Numerous methods have been proposed to measure dynamic hyperinflation. The volume at end-inspiration, termed Vei, is determined by collecting all expired gas from TLC to FRC during 40–60 seconds of apnea (see Fig. 2) (61). A Vei greater than 20 mL/kg (1.4 L in an average-sized adult) has been shown to predict complications of hypotension and barotrauma (16). Indeed, this is the only measure of dynamic hyperinflation that has been shown to predict barotrauma, even though it may underestimate the degree of air trapping in the presence of noncommunicating (or very slowly communicating) air spaces. Unfortunately, several factors limit the use of Vei at the bedside, including the need for paralysis and the fact that most physicians and respiratory therapists are unfamiliar with expiratory gas collection.

Vei can be calculated if one assumes linear compliance of the respiratory system (which has not been established in clinical studies):

$$Crs = Vt/(Pplat - PEEPi) = Vei/Pplat$$

and

$$Vei = (Vt \times Pplat)/(Pplat - PEEPi)$$

where Crs is static compliance of the respiratory system, Pplat is end-inspiratory plateau pressure, and PEEPi is intrinsic-PEEP or auto-PEEP. (Here we assume no machine-set PEEP.) Validation of calculated Vei is required before it can be recommended for routine assessment of dynamic hyperinflation.

Reasonable, but as yet unproved, surrogate measures of lung hyperinflation are end-inspiratory plateau pressure (Pplat) and auto-PEEP. Unfortunately, both measures are problematic and neither has been shown to predict complications of barotrauma.

The plateau pressure is an estimate of average end-inspiratory alveolar pressures. It reflects the respiratory system pressure change resulting from the delivery of Vt to any level of auto-PEEP. Under conditions of constant flow and patient relaxation, this pressure is easily determined by stopping flow (usually for 0.5 seconds) at end-inspiration (see Fig. 3). Since Pplat is affected by the entire respiratory system including lung tissue and chest wall, significant variations in dy-

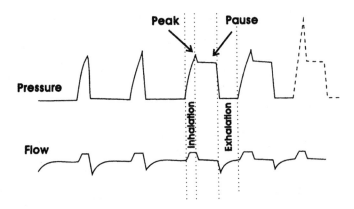

Figure 3 Simultaneous plots of airway pressure and flow in a mechanically ventilated patient. The peak-to-pause or peak-to-plateau gradient is determined by temporarily occluding inspiratory flow (usually for 0.5 s). End-inspiratory occlusions should be measured following a single breath only. An end-inspiratory pause left in place for a series of breaths will shorten Te, worsen DHI, and elevate P_{plat}. Under conditions of constant inspiratory flow and absence of patient effort, the peak-to-plateau gradient can be used as a measure of the severity of inspiratory airway resistance and of the efficacy of bronchodilator therapy. The dotted line indicates a high peak-to-plateau gradient like one would see in acute asthma. The P_{plat} is a reflection of the respiratory system pressure change resulting from the delivery of V_T to any level of auto-PEEP. It is a useful marker for the degree of lung hyperinflation and should be maintained at less than 30 cmH_2O.

namic hyperinflation occur from patient to patient at the same pressure. For example, an obese patient has a higher Pplat than a thin patient for the same degree of dynamic hyperinflation. Williams and colleagues have speculated that the reduced predictive value of Pplat for complications when compared with Vei is due to the variation in chest wall compliance between patients with asthma (16). It is thus possible that trans-pulmonary pressure, enabled by the measurement of esophageal pressure, would be better indicator of the safe level of dynamic hyperinflation than Pplat, but this remains purely speculative (12). Despite these limitations, extensive experience suggests that when Pplat is less than 30 cmH$_2$O, outcome is generally good. It is important to remember that Pplat should be measured following a single breath only. An end-inspiratory pause left in place for a series of breaths will shorten Te and worsen dynamic hyperinflation during that period. This elevates Pplat and is unsafe.

Auto-PEEP is the lowest average alveolar pressure achieved during the respiratory cycle. It is determined during an end-expiratory hold maneuver (see Fig. 4). This maneuver generally allows for equilibration of the airway opening pressure with alveolar pressure, permitting measurement of auto-PEEP. The pres-

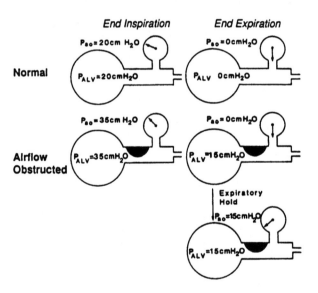

Figure 4 Measurement of auto-PEEP. Under normal conditions, alveolar pressure (P$_{ALV}$) closely tracks the pressure at the airway opening (P$_{ao}$), which is measured by the ventilator manometer. At end-expiration, P$_{ALV}$ and P$_{ao}$ fall to atmospheric pressure (0 cmH$_2$O). In severe asthma, P$_{ALV}$ increases because of gas trapping. At end-expiration P$_{ALV}$ does not fall to atmospheric pressure and does not equal P$_{ao}$. During an expiratory hold maneuver, P$_{ao}$ will rise, reflecting the degree of gas trapping.

ence of expiratory gas flow at the beginning of inspiration also establishes the presence of auto-PEEP. Accurate measurement of auto-PEEP requires patient relaxation, but not necessarily paralysis. One concern with regard to auto-PEEP is that it may underestimate the severity of dynamic hyperinflation. Leatherman and coworkers (62) have reported low levels of auto-PEEP (despite marked increases in Pplat) in four mechanically ventilated asthmatics. They speculated that this occurred because of severe airway narrowing, limiting the communication between the alveolus and mouth so that during an end-exhalation hold maneuver airway, opening pressure did not rise. Still, in the absence of other indicators of severe dynamic hyperinflation, an auto-PEEP of 15 cmH_2O is acceptable.

Keeping Ppk below an arbitrary limit (usually 50–60 cm H_2O) has been suggested by a number of authors. Tuxen and Lane have shown this practice to be unfounded and potentially dangerous because of the opposite effects of inspiratory flow on Ppk and dynamic hyperinflation (see Fig. 1) (14).

VIII. Ventilator Adjustments

With the above considerations in mind, the following initial ventilator settings are recommended: SIMV; RR, 12 breaths/min; Vt, 8 mL/kg; a constant inspiratory flow rate of 80 L/min; PEEP 0 cmH_2O (5 cmH_2O in a spontaneously breathing patient); and Fio_2, 1.0. Subsequent adjustment of these settings is based in large part on the arterial blood gas and airway pressure measurements. The latter requires adequate patient relaxation (with absence of forced inspiration and expiration) and good patient-ventilator synchrony. For these measurements, a constant inspiratory flow rate of 60 L/min to achieve a Vt of 8 mL/k is provided with an inspiratory pause of 0.5 seconds and Ppk and Pplat are recorded on the first interrupted breath. The peak-to-plateau difference represents the pressure to overcome airway resistance (Raw). An inspiratory flow rate of 60 L/min yields Raw in units of $cmH_2O/L/s$. Raw of 15 $cmH_2O/L/s$ is accepted as normal during mechanical ventilation. Elevated Raw is consistent with airflow obstruction as may occur with a narrow or kinked endotracheal tube, a mucus plug, or bronchospasm. Next, an end-exhalation hold maneuver is performed to measure auto-PEEP. This allows calculation of the static compliance of the respiratory system (Crs) (here we assume no machine-set PEEP):

$$Crs = Vt/(Pplat - PEEPi)$$

Normal values for Crs in an intubated patient range from 60 to 80 mL/cmH_2O. Low values demonstrate a stiff respiratory system, which in asthma suggests dynamic hyperinflation and ventilation on the flat portion of the pressure-volume relationship.

Whether RR can be safely increased for the purpose of lowering $Paco_2$ and elevating arterial pH depends in large part on the degree of dynamic hyperinflation. If Pplat is < 30 cmH$_2$O, RR may be increased until Pplat nears that threshold pressure. If the Pplat is > 30 cmH$_2$O, a further decrease in Ve is indicated until this goal is achieved, even if $Paco_2$ continues to rise. If pH is < 7.10 and Ve cannot be increased because of the Pplat limit, sodium bicarbonate may be administered.

As airflow obstruction improves, Raw and dynamic hyperinflation diminish and Ve can be safely increased. This may occur quickly in patients with sudden asphyxic asthma, but more often typically 24–72 hours of aggressive bronchodilator and anti-inflammatory therapy are required before there is convincing patient improvement. When a safe level of Ve (as determined by Pplat) results in eucapnia and Raw falls to < 20 cmH$_2$O/L/s, patients should be considered for extubation (13,16). Judicious use of paralytics and sedatives allows for a quick return to spontaneous breathing and timely extubation. To screen for readiness for extubation, we favor a spontaneous breathing trial using a T-piece or 5–7 cmH$_2$O of pressure support ventilation to overcome endotracheal tube resistance. If the spontaneous breathing is tolerated, we move quickly to extubation if mental status allows. This tempo minimizes endotracheal tube–induced bronchospasm and other risks of prolonged intubation and mechanical ventilation. Close observation in the ICU is recommended for an additional 24 hours, during which time the focus can switch to safe transfer to the medical ward and optimizing the home program.

IX. Sedation and Paralysis

Sedation is indicated to improve comfort, safety, and patient-ventilator synchrony. This is particularly true when hypercapnia serves as a potent stimulus to respiratory drive. Sedation should be used aggressively in an attempt to avoid paralytic agents and the potential for postparalytic myopathy (see below). This is commonly achieved by combining a benzodiazepine or propofol with an opioid. Propofol is particularly attractive when rapid improvement is anticipated (e.g., patients with sudden asphyxic disease) because it can be rapidly titrated to a deep level of sedation and still allow prompt reversal of sedation after discontinuation (63). Benzodiazepines, such as lorazepam and midazolam, are cheaper alternatives and also good choices for sedation of the intubated asthmatic patient (64). Time to awakening after discontinuation of these drugs is longer and less predictable than with propofol (65). Concerns regarding an association between prolonged propofol infusion and seizures, hypertriglyceridemia, and increased CO$_2$ production and the need for frequent changing of the intravenous tubing should not preclude its use in most cases (66).

The addition of an opioid by low-dose continuous infusion provides analgesia and augments the sedating effects of benzodiazepines or propofol without causing the adverse effects associated with bolus administration (67). Morphine and fentanyl are the two most commonly used narcotics. Fentanyl has a quicker onset of action and is slightly more expensive than morphine, although the magnitude of this difference is not large. Morphine has the theoretical disadvantage of histamine release and the potential to worsen bronchospasm.

Ketamine, an IV anesthetic with sedative, analgesic, and bronchodilating properties, is generally reserved for use in intubated patients with severe bronchospasm that precludes safe mechanical ventilation (68,69). Ketamine must be used with caution because of its sympathomimetic effects and ability to cause delirium (70).

When safe and effective mechanical ventilation cannot be achieved by sedation alone, consideration should be given to short-term muscle paralysis. Paralysis augments the beneficial effects of sedation to reduce O_2 consumption, CO_2 production, and lactic acid generation. Eliminating respiratory efforts may also decrease expiratory airway collapse (71). The preferred agents are *cis*-atracurium, atracurium, and vecuronium, all short- to intermediate-acting agents. We prefer *cis*-atracurium because it is essentially free of cardiovascular effects and does not release histamine. It is also eliminated (as is atracurium) by esterase degradation in the serum, whereas both vecuronium and pancuronium rely on intact hepatic and renal function for adequate elimination. Pancuronium is an acceptable alternative in most cases and is the least expensive of the paralytics. However, it is longer acting and has vagolytic effects that may cause unwanted tachycardia. Both pancuronium and atracurium release histamine, but the clinical significance of this property is doubtful. In a study comparing atracurium to vecuronium in acute asthma, there was a greater incidence of hypotension and tachycardia with atracurium, but neither drug affected airway pressures (72).

Paralytics may be given intermittently by bolus or continuous intravenous infusion. Continuous infusions warrant use of a nerve stimulator. Alternatively, the drug should be withheld every 4–6 hours to avoid drug accumulation and prolonged paralysis. Paralytic agents should be discontinued as soon as possible to decrease the risk of postparalytic myopathy. This complication of acute asthma may be mild and of no clinical significance or severe enough to interfere with limb movement and successful extubation. Most patients recover completely, although some require prolonged rehabilitation.

The primary risk factors for development of myopathy are the concurrent use of corticosteroids and a paralytic and the duration of paralysis. Acute myopathy is rare when paralytics are used for less than 24 hours. In one study of 25 ventilated asthmatics, 19 (76%) patients demonstrated an increase in serum creatine kinase; 9 (36%) had clinically detectable myopathy (73). Mechanical ventilation was prolonged in patients with elevated creatine kinase whether or not there was clinically detectable myopathy. In a second retrospective cohort study of 107 episodes of asthma requiring mechanical ventilation, the concurrent use of corticosteroids and a paralytic was associated with muscle weakness in 29% of episodes; corticosteroid treatment alone was not associated with weakness (74). Importantly, this study demonstrated that the duration of paralysis correlated with the incidence of myopathy. Findings of a more recent study confirm this correlation (75).

X. Bronchodilator Delivery During Mechanical Ventilation

Successful treatment of expiratory airflow obstruction further decreases dynamic hyperinflation and improves the chance of timely extubation. With this in mind, inhaled bronchodilators and systemic corticosteroids should be continued during the mechanical ventilation. However, the efficacy of these drugs has not been well established in the intubated patient. Not surprisingly, hospitalized asthmatics have a fairly flat dose-response relationship to β-agonists (76), and there are significant challenges to optimal delivery of bronchodilators to intubated patients. In one study (77), only 2.9% of a radioactive aerosol delivered by nebulizer was deposited in the lungs of mechanically ventilated patients. Other data demonstrate no therapeutic benefit from administration of 100 puffs (9.0 mg) of albuterol without a spacer, stressing the importance of a spacing device on the inspiratory limb of the ventilator to improve drug delivery. In this same study there was an 18% drop in inspiratory flow resistive pressure (as measured by the peak-to-plateau pressure gradient) after 2.5 mg of albuterol delivered by nebulizer (78). Increasing the nebulized albuterol dose to a total of 7.5 mg led to further reductions in airway resistance in 8 of 10 patients but to the development of toxic side effects in half of patients.

Thus, β-agonists may be delivered by MDI with spacer or nebulizer. In either case higher β-agonist doses are required during mechanical ventilation because of poor drug delivery and the flat dose-response relationship to albuterol. When nebulizers are used, they should be placed close to the ventilator, and in-line humidifiers should be stopped during treatments. Inspiratory flow should be reduced to approximately 40 L/min during treatments to minimize turbulence, although this strategy has the potential to worsen lung hyperinflation (see above) and must be time-limited. Patient-ventilator synchrony is crucial to optimize drug delivery (79).

We believe drug dosage should be titrated to a fall in the peak-to-plateau airway pressure gradient or to the development of toxic effects. When no measurable drop in airway resistance occurs, it is important to exclude other causes of elevated airway resistance such as a kinked or plugged endotracheal tube. Bronchodilator nonresponders should also be considered for a drug holiday.

XI. Adjunctive Therapies During Mechanical Ventilation

Rarely, the above strategies are not sufficient to stabilize the patient on the ventilator. In this situation consideration should be given to the use of additional therapies. Halothane and enflurane are general anesthetics with bronchodilating properties that can reduce Ppk and $Paco_2$ (80,81). However, they are associated with myocardial depression, arterial vasodilation, and arrhythmias, and their benefit does not last long after discontinuation of the drug. Heliox delivered through the ventilator circuit may also decrease Ppk and $Paco_2$ (82), but safe use of this gas requires institutional expertise and careful planning, including a trial of heliox use in a lung model prior to patient use. Ventilator flow meters (which measure tidal volume) must be recalibrated for low-density gas flow (83), and a spirometer should be placed on the expiratory port of the ventilator during heliox administration to confirm tidal volume.

The role of magnesium sulfate has yet to be firmly established in acute asthma. Studies have shown no difference in FEV_1 or hospital admission rates in unselected (nonintubated) patients receiving intravenous magnesium sulfate in the ER (84,85). In asthmatics with an FEV_1 <25% of predicted, however, magnesium may improve airflow and decrease hospitalization rates (86). Additional evidence supporting benefit in severe disease comes from an uncontrolled study of five mechanically ventilated asthmatics given magnesium (87). In this study, Ppk fell from 43 to 32 cmH_2O in patients receiving high doses of magnesium sulfate (10–20 g) over one hour. Side effects from the use of magnesium include flushing of skin and hypotension. Its use should be restricted to patients with good renal function.

Strategies to mobilize mucus such as chest physiotherapy or treatment with mucolytics or expectorants have not proved efficacious (2). Bronchoalveolar lavage (BAL) with saline or acetylcysteine may help nonintubated patients clear mucus and improve airflow (88–90). In intubated asthmatics, BAL is theoretically more risky because the bronchoscope increases expiratory airway resistance and may lead to dangerous levels of lung hyperinflation if Ve is not decreased during the procedure. If Ve is reduced, acute hypercapnia may occur during the procedure. For these reasons, BAL cannot be recommended as a part of routine clinical practice.

In extremely rare situations, hypotension may persist despite profound hypoventilation, fluid resuscitation, and isotropic support. Under these conditions, extracorporeal membrane oxygenation may be considered (48–51).

XII. Summary and Conclusions

In the past, the ventilator management of patients with acute respiratory failure was associated with a high risk of morbidity and a substantial potential for mortality. However, advances in the understanding of pathophysiological disturbances associated with mechanical ventilation in patients with obstructive lung diseases have led to changes in ventilator management that have rendered the use of mechanical ventilation much safer. By gaining an appreciation for the factors that predispose to dynamic lung hyperinflation and the potential for barotrauma, ventilator strategies now aim to minimize these adverse consequences. In addition, techniques such as heliox and/or noninvasive positive pressure ventilation are now being widely applied to avoid the need for invasive ventilation and its attendant risks entirely. Although controlled trials are lacking to guide the application of these interventions, the evidence suggests that they are effective in averting intubation.

If invasive mechanical ventilation is unavoidable, then management strategies focus on minimizing dynamic hyperinflation. Adequate inspiratory flow rates (>60 L/min) and lower initial ventilator rates are selected to maximize expiratory time. Smaller tidal volumes than have been recommended in the past are used so that less air must be exhaled, and plateau pressures are kept below 30 cmH_2O. Auto-PEEP levels are monitored as a reflection of dynamic hyperinflation, and marked hypercapnia is tolerated, if necessary, to maintain lower levels of auto-PEEP. Also, if necessary, paralytic agents are used to gain control of the patient's breathing pattern and to minimize energy consumption, but they are discontinued as soon as possible to avoid paralytic-induced myopathy. In the meantime, bronchodilator and anti-inflammatory therapy is optimized to expedite recovery and minimize the duration of airway invasion. Using these strategies, the vast majority of patients with acute respiratory failure due to asthma can be managed safely, with minimal morbidity and virtual elimination of mortality—at least that attributable to ventilator support.

References

1. Mountain RD, Sahn S. Clinical features and outcome in patients with acute asthma presenting with hypercapnia. Am Rev Respir Dis 1988; 138:535.
2. Corbridge T, Hall JB. State-of-the-art: The assessment and management of adults with status asthmaticus. Am J Respir Crit Care Med 1995; 151:1296.
3. Hogg JC. The pathology of asthma. Clin Chest Med 1984; 5:567.
4. Petty TL. Treat status asthmaticus three days before it occurs. J Intensive Care Med 1989; 4:135.
5. Picado C. Classification of severe asthma exacerbations: a proposal. Eur Respir J 1996; 9(9):1775–1778.

6. Arnold AG, Lane DJ, Zapata E. The speed of onset and severity of acute severe asthma. Br J Dis Chest 1982; 76:157.

7. Wasserfallen JB, Schaller MD, Feihl F, Perret CH. Sudden asphyxic asthma: A distinct entity? Am Rev Respir Dis 1990; 142:108.

8. Ried LM. The presence or absence of bronchial mucus in fatal asthma. J Allergy Clin Immunol 1987; 80:415.

9. Sur S, Crotty TB, Kephart GM, Hyma BA, Colby TV, Reed CE, Hunt LW, Gleich GJ. Sudden-onset fatal asthma: a distinct clinical entity with few eosinophils and relatively more neutrophils in the airway submucosa. Am Rev Respir Dis 1993; 148: 713.

10. Cygan J, Trunsky M, Corbridge T. Inhaled heroin-induced status asthmaticus. Chest 2000; 117:272–275.

11. Pepe PE, Marini JJ. Occult positive end-expiratory pressure in mechanically ventilated patients with airflow obstruction: the auto-PEEP effect. Am Rev Respir Dis 1982; 124(2):166–170.

12. Tuxen, D. Mechanical ventilation in asthma. In: Evans T, Hinds C, eds. Recent Advances in Critical Care Medicine, London. Churchill Livingstone, 1996:165–189.

13. Tuxen, D, Williams T, Scheinkestel C, Czarny D, Bowes G. Limiting dynamic hyperinflation in mechanically ventilated patients with severe asthma reduces complications (abstr). Anaesth Intens Care 1993; 21(5):718.

14. Tuxen D, Lane S. The effects of ventilatory pattern on hyperinflation, airway pressures, and circulation in mechanical ventilation of patients with severe airflow obstruction. Am Rev Respir Dis 1987; 136:872–879.

15. Tuxen, D, Williams T, Scheinkestel C, Czarny D, Bowes G. Use of a measurement of pulmonary hyperinflation to control the level of mechanical ventilation in patients with severe asthma. Am Rev Respir Dis 1992; 146(5):1136–1142.

16. Williams T, Tuxen D, Scheinkestel C, Czarny D, Bowes G. Risk factors for morbidity in mechanically ventilated patients with acute severe asthma. Am Rev Respir Dis 1992; 146(3):607–615.

17. Van der Touw T, Mudaliar Y, Nayyar V. Static pressure-volume relationship of the respiratory system and pulmonary hyperinflation in mechanically ventilated patients with acute severe asthma. Am J Respir Crit Care Med 1996; 153:A370.

18. Yanos J, Wood LD, Davis K, Keamy M. The effect of respiratory and lactic acidosis on diaphragm function. Am Rev Respir Dis 1993; 147:616.

19. Rodriguez-Roisin R, Ballester E, Roca J, Torres A, Wagner PD. Mechanisms of hypoxemia in patients with status asthmaticus requiring mechanical ventilation. Am Rev Respir Dis 1989; 139:732.

20. Nowak RM, Tomlanovich MC, Sarker DD, Kvale PA, Anderson JA. Arterial blood gases and pulmonary function testing in acute bronchial asthma: predicting patient outcomes. JAMA 1983; 249:2043.

21. McFadden ER Jr, Lyons HA. Arterial-blood gas tension in asthma. N Engl J Med 1968; 278:1027.

22. Ferrer A, Roca J, Wagner PD, Lopez FA, Rodriguez-Roisin R. Airway obstruction and ventilation-perfusion relationships in acute severe asthma. Am Rev Respir Dis 1993; 147:579.

23. Roca J, Ramis L, Rodriguez-Roisin R, Ballester E, Montserrat JM, Wagner PD.

Serial relationships between ventilation perfusion inequality and spirometry in acute severe asthma requiring hospitalization. Am Rev Respir Dis 1988; 137:1055.

24. Scharf S, Brown R, Saunders N, Green LA. Effects of normal and loaded spontaneous inspiration on cardiovascular function. J Appl Physiol 1979; 47:582.

25. Scharf S, Brown R, Tow D, Parisi AF. Cardiac effects of increased lung volume and decreased pleural pressure. J Appl Physiol 1979; 47:257.

26. Stalcup SA, Mellins RB. Mechanical forces producing pulmonary edema in acute asthma. N Engl J Med 1977; 297(11):592–596.

27. Permutt S, Wise RA. Mechanical interaction of respiration and circulation. In: Fishman A, ed. Handbook of Physiology, Vol 3. Baltimore: Williams and Wilkins, 1986: 647.

28. Corbridge T, Hall JB. Pulmonary hypertension in status asthmaticus. In: Cosentino AM, Martin RJ, eds. Cardiothoracic Interrelationships in Clinical Practice. Armonk, NY: Futura Publishing Co., Inc., 1997:137–156.

29. Knowles G, Clark TJ. Pulsus paradoxus as a valuable sign indicating severity of asthma. Lancet 1973; 2:1356.

30. Madison JM, Irwin RS. Heliox for asthma: a trial balloon. Chest 1995; 107:597–598.

31. Curtis JL, Mahlmeister M, Fink JB, Lampe G, Matthay MA, Stulbarg MS. Helium oxygen gas therapy: use and availability for the emergency treatment of inoperable airway obstruction. Chest 1986; 90:455.

32. Kudukis TM, Manthous CA, Schmidt GA, Hall JB, Wylam ME. Inhaled helium-oxygen revisited: effect of inhaled helium-oxygen during the treatment of status asthmaticus in children. J Pediatrics 1997; 130(2):217–224.

33. Manthous CA, Hall JB, Caputo ME, Walter J, Klocksieben JM, Schmidt GA, Wood LOH. The effect of heliox on pulsus paradoxus and peak flow in non-intubated patients with severe asthma. Am J Respir Crit Care Med 1995; 151:310.

34. Kass JE, Terregino CA. The effect of heliox in acute severe asthma: a randomized controlled trial. Chest 1999; 116:296–300.

35. Verbeek PR, Chopra A. Heliox does not improve FEV1 in acute asthma patients. J Emerg Med 1998; 16:545–548.

36. Melmed A, Hebb DB, Pohlman A, et al. The use of heliox as a vehicle for beta-agonist nebulization in patients with severe asthma. Am J Respir Crit Care Med 1995; 151:A269.

37. Henderson SO, Acharya P, Kilaghbian T, Perez J, Korn CS, Chan LS. Use of heliox-driven nebulizer therapy in the treatment of acute asthma. Ann Emerg Med 1999; 33:141.

38. Meduri GU, Abou-Shala N, Fox RC, Jones CB, Leeper KV, Wunderink RG. Noninvasive face mask mechanical ventilation in patients with acute hypercapnic respiratory failure. Chest 1991; 100:445.

39. Meduri GU, Cook TR, Turner RE, Cohen M, Leeper KV. Noninvasive positive pressure ventilation in status asthmaticus. Chest 1996; 110:767.

40. Corseen G, Gutierrez J, Reves JG, Huber FC. Ketamine in the anesthetic management of asthmatic patients. Anesth Analg 1972; 51:588–596.

41. Wheeler AP. Sedation, analgesia, and paralysis in the intensive care unit. Chest 1993; 104:566–577.

42. Wright PE, Marini JJ, Bernard G. In vitro versus in vivo comparison of endotracheal tube airflow resistance. Am Rev Respir Dis 1989; 140:10–16.
43. Leatherman J. Life-threatening asthma. Clin Chest Med 1994; 15:453–479.
44. Rosengarten, P, Tuxen D, Dziukas L, Scheinkestel C, Merrett K, Bowes G. Circulatory arrest induced by intermittent positive pressure ventilation in a patient with severe asthma. Anaesth Intens Care 1990; 19:118–121.
45. Kollef, M. Lung hyperinflation caused by inappropriate ventilation resulting in electromechanical dissociation: a case report. Heart Lung 1992; 21:74–77.
46. Shapiro M, Kleaveland A, Bartlett R. Extracorporeal life support for status asthmaticus. Chest 1993; 103:1651–1654.
47. King, D, C Smales C, Arnold A, Jones O. Extracorporeal membrane oxygenation as emergency treatment for life threatening acute severe asthma. Postgrad Med J 1986; 62:555–557.
48. Mabuchi N, Takasu H, Ito S, Yamada T, Arakawa M, Hatta M, Katsuya H. Successful extracorporeal lung assist (ECLA) for a patient with severe asthma and cardiac arrest. Clin Intens Med 1991; 2:292–294.
49. Tajimi K, Kasai T, Nakatani T, Kobayashi K. Extracorporeal lung asist (ECLA) for a patient with hypercapnia due to status asthmaticus. Intens Care Med 1988; 14: 588–589.
50. Feihl F, Perret C. State-of-the-art: permissive hypercapnia: how permissive should we be? Am J Resp Crit Care Med 1994; 150:1722.
51. Darioli R, Perret C. Mechanical controlled hypoventilation in status asthmaticus. Am Rev Respir Dis 1984; 129:385.
52. Cardenas VJ Jr, Zwischenberger JB, Tao W, Nguyen PD, Schroeder T, Traber LD, Traber DL, Bidaru A. Correction of blood pH attenuates changes in hemodynamics and organ blood flow during permissive hypercapnia. Crit Care Med 1996; 24(5): 827–834.
53. Cooper D, Cailes J, Scheinkestel C, Tuxen D. Acute severe asthma and acidosis— effect of bicarbonate on cardiac and respiratory function. Anaesth Int Care 1993; 22(2):212–213.
54. Tuxen DV. Permissive hypercapnic ventilation. Am J Respir Crit Care Med 1994; 150:870.
55. Otis A, McKerrow C, Bartlett R, Mead J, McIlroy M, Selverstone N, Radford E. Mechanical factors in distribution of pulmonary ventilation. J Appl Physiol 1956; 8:427–443.
56. Bates J, Rossi A, Milic-Emili J. Analysis of the behavior of the respiratory system with constant inspiratory flow. J Appl Physiol 1985; 58(6):1840–1848.
57. Connors A, McCafree D, Gray B. Effect of inspiratory flow rate on gas exchange during mechanical ventilation. Am Rev Respir Dis 1981; 124:537–543.
58. Corne S, Gillespie D, Roberts D, et al. Effect of inspiratory flow rate on respiratory rate in intubated patients. Am J Respir Crit Care Med 1996; 153:A375.
59. Tuxen DV. Detrimental effects of positive end-expiratory pressure during controlled mechanical ventilation of patients with severe airflow obstruction. Am Rev Respir Dis 1989; 140:5.
60. West JP. State of the art: ventilation-perfusion relationships. Am Rev Respir Dis 1977; 116:919.

61. Ballester E, Reyes A, Roca J, Guitart R, Wagner PD, Rodriguez-Roisin R. Ventilation-perfusion mismatching in acute severe asthma: effects of salbutamol and 100% oxygen. Thorax 1989; 44:258.

62. Leatherman JW, Ravenscraft SA. Low measured auto-positive end-expiratory pressure during mechanical ventilation of patients with severe asthma: hidden auto-positive end-expiratory pressure. Crit Care Med 1996; 24:541.

63. Barrientos-Vega R, MarSanchez-Soria M, Morales-Garcia G, Robas-Gomez A, Cuena-Boy R, Ayensa-Rincon A. Prolonged sedation of critically ill patients with midazolam or propofol: impact on weaning and costs [see comments]. Crit Care Med 1997; 25(1):33–40.

64. Pohlman A, Simpson K, Hall J. Continuous intravenous infusions of lorazepam vs. midazolam for sedation during mechanical ventilatory support: a prospective, randomized study. Crit Care Med 1994; 22:1241.

65. Kress JP, O'Connor MF, Pohlman AS, Olson D, Lavoie A, Toledano A, Hall JB. Sedation of critically ill patients during mechanical ventilation: a comparison of propofol and midazolam. Am J Respir Crit Care Med 1996; 153:1012.

66. Valente JF, Anderson GL, Branson RD, Johnson DJ, Davis K, Porembka DT. Disadvantages of prolonged propofol sedation in the critical care unit. Crit Care Med 1994; 22:710.

67. Murray MJ, DeRuyter ML, Harrison BA. Opioids and benzodiazepines. Crit Care Clin 1995; 4:849.

68. Sarma VJ. Use of ketamine in acute severe asthma. Acta Anaesthesiol Scand 1992; 36:106.

69. Rock MJ, Reyes de la Rocha S, L'Hommedieu E. Use of ketamine in asthmatic children to treat respiratory failure refractory to conventional therapy. Crit Care Med 1986; 14:514.

70. White PF, Way WI, Trevor AJ. Ketamine—its pharmacology and therapeutic uses. Anesthesiology 1982; 56:119.

71. Slutsky AS. Mechanical ventilation. Chest 1993; 104:1833.

72. Caldwell JE, Lau M, Fisher DM. Atracurium versus vecuronium in asthmatic patients. A blinded, randomized comparison of adverse events. Anesthesiology 1995; 83:986.

73. Douglass JA, Tuxen D, Horne M, Scheinkestel CD, Weinmann M, Czarny D, Bowes G. Myopathy in severe asthma. Am Rev Respir Dis 1992; 146:517.

74. Leatherman JW, Fluegel WL, David WS, Davies SF, Iber C. Muscle weakness in mechanically ventilated patients with severe asthma. Am J Respir Crit Care Med 1996; 153:1686.

75. Behbehani NA, Al-Mane F, D'yachkova Y, Pare P, FitzGerald JM. Myopathy following mechanical ventilation for acute severe asthma: the role of muscle relaxants and corticosteroids. Chest 1999; 115:1627.

76. Rodrigo G, Rodrigo C. Early prediction of poor response in acute asthma patients in the emergency department. Chest 1998; 114:1016–1021.

77. MacIntyre NR, Silver RM, Miller CW, et al. Aerosol delivery in intubated, mechanically ventilated patients. Crit Care Med 1985; 13:81.

78. Manthous CA, Hall JB, Schmidt GA, Wood LDH. Metered-dose inhaler versus nebulized albuterol in mechanically ventilated patients. Am Rev Respir Dis 1993; 148:1567.

79. Manthous CA, Hall JB. Update on using therapeutic aerosols in mechanically ventilated patients. J Crit Illness 1996; 11:457.
80. Saulnier FF, Durocher AV, Deturck RA, et al. Respiratory and hemodynamic effects of halothane in status asthmaticus. Intens Care Med 1990; 16:104.
81. Echeverria M, Gelb AW, Wexler HR, Ahmad D, Kenefick P. Enflurane and halothane in status asthmaticus. Chest 1986; 89:153.
82. Gluck EH, Onorato DJ, Castriotta R. Helium-oxygen mixtures in intubated patients with status asthmaticus and respiratory acidosis. Chest 1990; 98:693.
83. Tassaux D, Jolliet P, Thouret JM, Roeseler J, Dorne R, Chevrolet JC. Calibration of seven ICU ventilators for mechanical ventilation with helium-oxygen mixtures. Am J Respir Crit Care Med 1999; 160:22–32.
84. Green SM, Rothrock SG. Intravenous magnesium for acute asthma: failure to decrease emergency treatment duration or need for hospitalization. Ann Emerg Med 1992; 21:260.
85. Tiffany BR, Berk W, Todd IK, White SR. Magnesium bolus or infusion fails to improve expiratory flow in acute asthma exacerbations. Chest 1993; 104:831.
86. Bloch H, Silverman R, Mancherje N, Grant S, Jagminas L, Scharf SM. Intravenous magnesium sulfate as an adjunct in the treatment of acute asthma. Chest 1995; 107: 1576.
87. Sydow M, Crozier TA, Zielmann S, Radke J, Burchardi H. High-dose intravenous magnesium sulfate in the management of life-threatening status asthmaticus. Intens Care Med 1993; 19:467.
88. Smith DL, Deshazo RD. Bronchoalveolar lavage in asthma. State-of-the-art. Am Rev Respir Dis 1993; 148:523–532.
89. Millman M, Millman FM, Goldstein IM, Mercandetti AJ. Use of acetylcysteine in bronchial asthma—another look. Ann Allergy 1985; 54:294.
90. Lang DM, Simon RA, Mathison DA, Timms RM, Stevenson DD. Safety and possible efficacy of fiberoptic bronchoscopy with lavage in the management of refractory asthma with mucous impaction. Ann Allergy 1991; 67:324.

12

Ventilator Management Strategies for COPD Patients

DENIS LIN

Brown University School of Medicine
Providence, Rhode Island

NICHOLAS S. HILL

Miriam Hospital
Rhode Island Hospital
Brown University School of Medicine
Providence, Rhode Island

I. Introduction

Chronic obstructive pulmonary disease (COPD) is the most frequent cause of chronic respiratory insufficiency in the developed world today and is a common underlying etiology for acute ventilatory failure (1). Until recently, invasive positive pressure ventilation was the most commonly used mode of ventilatory assistance in patients with respiratory failure caused by COPD. Complications of barotrauma and respiratory infection occur frequently with invasive ventilation leading to increased patient morbidity and high health care costs. In recent years, newer pathophysiological insights and the increasing use of noninvasive positive pressure ventilation (NPPV) have changed the ventilatory management of COPD (2). The following reviews the respiratory pathophysiology of COPD that is relevant to mechanical ventilation, discusses the evidence supporting use of noninvasive ventilation for acute exacerbations of COPD, makes recommendations for the selection and optimal management of patients receiving invasive mechanical ventilation, and examines evidence on outcomes.

II. Pathophysiology of Ventilatory Impairment in COPD

A. Increased Airway Resistance

Increased airway resistance is the *sine qua non* of COPD, and virtually all other pathophysiological abnormalities derive from it. In contrast to normals who have relatively equal inspiratory and expiratory airway resistance at all but the lowest lung volumes, COPD patients have greatly increased expiratory resistance. Ratios of expiratory to inspiratory resistance in COPD patients are 2:1 near total lung capacity and climb to 10:1 at low lung volumes (3). This marked increase in airway resistance at low lung volumes is related to collapse of smaller airways during expiration. This phenomenon is thought to be caused by destruction of alveoli and supporting connective tissue structures that help to tether airways and prevent collapse when surrounding pressures exceed intraluminal pressures during exhalation. Lacking these structures, the airways in COPD patients collapse during exhalation, even at relatively high lung volumes, creating what is referred to as "flow limitation" and contributing to air trapping (Fig. 1). Since

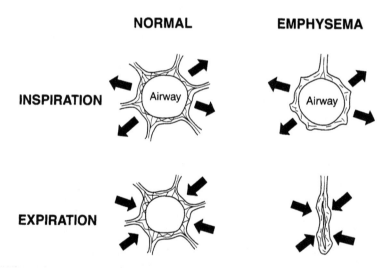

Figure 1 Diagram shows how alveolar walls tether normal small airways but not emphysematous small airways. During inspiration (top diagrams), the pressure gradient favors airway patency (outward pointing arrows) in both normal patients (top left) and patients with emphysema (top right). During expiration (bottom diagrams), the pressure gradient is reversed, favoring airway collapse (inward pointing arrows). In normal patients (bottom left), the alveolar walls contain connective tissue fibers that work like radiating spokes, tethering the airways open. In emphysema (bottom right), tethering alveolar walls have been destroyed, allowing airways to collapse. (From Ref. 2.)

more forceful expiratory efforts serve only to further compress collapsed airways, this phenomenon is sometimes referred to as a flow-limiting "choke point" (4). As will be seen, many of the ventilatory abnormalities in COPD patients result from this expiratory flow limitation, and the strategies of mechanical ventilation have been devised to address this defect.

B. Respiratory Muscle Dysfunction in Acute Exacerbations of COPD

Respiratory muscle dysfunction contributes significantly to the development of respiratory failure in patients with COPD. The factors that predispose to respiratory muscle dysfunction include mechanical and physiological abnormalities related specifically to obstructive airway disease. In addition, the adverse consequences of therapeutic interventions such as steroids or paralytic agents may cause myopathy, which in turn contributes to respiratory pump failure and retards the recovery of the ability to breathe spontaneously.

Hyperinflation, associated with severe expiratory flow limitation, is a major factor in the respiratory muscle dysfunction of COPD. The hyperinflation arises partly due to reduced lung elastance and partly due to the need to breathe at higher lung volumes to maintain airway patency. Greater lung volumes permit generation of high alveolar pressures during exhalation, thereby maintaining a driving pressure sufficient to overcome "choke points" caused by collapsed airways that obstruct expiratory flow (5). With hyperinflation, inspiratory muscles become mechanically disadvantaged, as depicted in Figure 2. The flattened diaphragm occupies a disadvantageous position on the length-tension curve, and the overall sarcomere length shortens, diminishing the diaphragm's capacity to generate maximal force (6). According to the law of La Place, the greater radius of diaphragmatic curvature increases muscle tension, which consequently impedes blood flow, further compromising muscle function. In addition, the zone of apposition between the diaphragm and chest wall is reduced, limiting the bucket-handle action on the ribs that augments chest wall expansion during inspiration. The recruitment of accessory inspiratory muscles necessitated by the hyperinflation greatly increases the oxygen cost of breathing. This high oxygen demand, combined with increased impedance to blood flow, predisposes to the development of an energy supply/demand imbalance and respiratory muscle fatigue (7).

During an exacerbation, usually caused by a viral or bacterial infection, airway resistance increases and airflow at a given lung volume decreases (Fig. 3). Because expiratory flow in a patient with severe airway obstruction is already maximal at resting lung volume, the patient's only recourse is to breathe at an even higher lung volume if airflow is to be maintained. The patient becomes tachypneic, resulting in shorter expiratory times that aggravate hyperinflation.

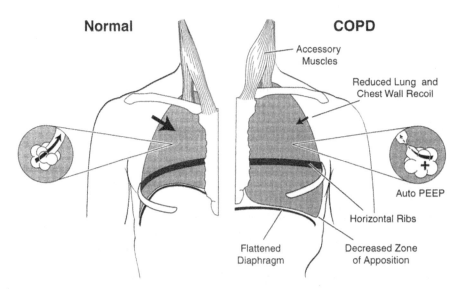

Figure 2 Diagrammatic representation of mechanical dysfunction in severe COPD patients. Hyperinflation leads to diaphragm flattening, decreased zone of apposition between the diaphragm and chest wall, and horizontal positioning of the ribs, all of which decreases respiratory muscle efficiency. The need to use accessory muscles adds to the energy cost of breathing. AutoPEEP results from flow limitation due to decreased elastic recoil and small airway collapse during exhalation. See text for details. (From Ref. 2.)

The greater hyperinflation further exacerbates the mechanical disadvantage of the respiratory muscles. A vicious downward cycle caused by a progressive energy supply/demand imbalance leads to respiratory muscle fatigue and precipitates acute respiratory failure (Fig. 3).

The energy supply/demand imbalance that leads to respiratory muscle fatigue can be predicted by the proportion of maximal respiratory muscle effort used during tidal breathing. Roussos and Macklem (8) have shown that as single indexes, neither the maximal transdiaphragmatic pressure (Pdi_{max}) nor phasic inspiratory swings in transdiaphragmatic pressure (Pdi) during tidal breathing can predict task failure of the diaphragm. Rather, the onset of mechanical failure is a function of the ratio of the Pdi for each breath to the Pdi_{max}. Values of Pdi/Pdi_{max}, or "contraction intensity index" that exceed the threshold value of 40–50% lead progressively to muscle exhaustion. However, if Pdi/Pdi_{max} is below the threshold value, muscle function can be maintained indefinitely.

An increase in inspiratory time as a proportion of the total respiratory cycle or "duty cycle" also predisposes to respiratory muscle fatigue. Bellemare and Grassino (9,10) have shown that an increase in the ratio of diaphragm time of

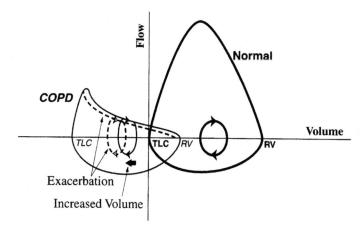

Figure 3 Flow volume loops are shown for normal patients (solid on right), COPD patients (solid on left), and COPD patients during exacerbation (interrupted line on left). Volume is plotted on absolute scale to show hyperinflation in COPD patients, from residual volume (RV) to total lung capacity (TLC) with COPD volumes shown in italics. During a COPD exacerbation, expiratory flows at a given volume fall slightly. Because the COPD patient (in contrast to the normal) uses maximal expiratory flows during tidal breathing (small solid loop on left), the only recourse for maintaining flows is to breathe at higher lung volumes (dark arrow signifying increased volume). (From Ref. 2.)

contraction (Ti) to the total duration of the respiratory cycle (Ttot) potentiates the development of fatigue. When the Pdi/Pdi_{max} and the duty cycle of breathing (Ti/Ttot) are combined as a mathematical product, this index, referred to as the pressure time (PTI) or tension time (TTI) index, is the best predictor of diaphragm fatigue and oxygen consumption by the respiratory muscles (11,12). Using this index, a product exceeding 15–20% reliably predicts the onset of respiratory muscle fatigue. During acute exacerbations of COPD, tidal breathing causes progressive hyperinflation, which increases Pdi during tidal breathing and lowers the Pdi_{max}. Simultaneously, increased respiratory rate tends to raise the Ti/Ttot. These combined alterations eventually push the TTI beyond the fatigue threshold resulting in respiratory failure.

C. Intrinsic Positive End-Expiratory Pressure

Another factor that contributes to ventilatory muscle inefficiency in patients with severe COPD is the phenomenon of auto (or intrinsic) positive end-expiratory pressure (autoPEEP). This refers to positive intra-alveolar pressure that occurs at end expiration, caused by persisting elastic recoil when the lung fails to return to its resting volume. The term ''dynamic hyperinflation'' refers to the increased end-expiratory lung volume caused by delayed gas emptying from the lung that leads to autoPEEP. During mechanical ventilation, autoPEEP is also sometimes referred to as occult PEEP because its presence is not detected by usual pressure-sensing techniques.

In essence, autoPEEP arises when the time needed for the lung to reach its resting volume exceeds the actual expiratory time. This may occur when gas emptying from the lung is delayed, expiratory time is shortened, or both (Table 1). AutoPEEP may also occur without hyperinflation due to persisting expiratory muscle activity at end expiration in both normals (13,14) and asthmatics (15). In normal subjects, persistent expiratory muscle activity increases abdominal pressure at end expiration. The pressure transmitted to the lung increases expiratory flow and reduces end-expiratory lung volume. In severe COPD patients, expiratory flow is already maximal at baseline so that any additional abdominal pressure fails to increase flow or reduce end-expiratory volume and only serves to raise end-expiratory pressure (5). In fact, the high prevalence of this phenomenon is reflected in the common finding that autoPEEP is present in ambulatory patients known to have obstructive disease but no overt respiratory failure (16).

AutoPEEP is most easily measured in mechanically ventilated, paralyzed patients. When an end-expiratory hold is inserted, the airway pressure measured after equilibration is termed ''static'' autoPEEP (17). In spontaneously breathing patients, the measurement of autoPEEP is more complicated. In nonintubated patients, precise measurement of autoPEEP is difficult, but its presence is suspected if expiration is prolonged or expiratory wheezes persist through the onset

Table 1 Factors Contributing to the Development of Auto-PEEP

Prolonged emptying	Reduced exhalation time
Increased airway resistance	Selected respiratory rate set
Bronchospasm	inappropriately high
Airway edema	Tachypnea
Secretions	Prolonged inspiration
Dynamic collapse	Inverse ratio ventilation
Increase lung compliance	
Extrinsic PEEP (without dynamic hyperinflation)	
Extrathoracic obstruction	
Small endotracheal tube	
Laryngeal obstruction or edema	
High tidal volume	
Inspiratory muscle activity during exhalation	
Increased intrathoracic pressure at end expiration	

of the next inspiration. In intubated, spontaneously breathing patients, occlusion pressure measurements at end expiration can be attempted as long as the patient is well sedated or very cooperative. However, the patient must suspend breathing efforts long enough to allow pressure equilibration to occur, and expiratory muscles must be quiescent.

If an esophageal manometry balloon is inserted, autoPEEP can be accurately measured in spontaneously breathing patients (intubated or not). If auto-PEEP is present, inspiratory flow does not begin until esophageal pressure (Pes) "counterbalances" the autoPEEP and alveolar pressure drops below atmospheric pressure. The drop in Pes from the initiation of inspiratory muscle activity to the onset of inspiratory flow is called the "dynamic" autoPEEP (5). This is usually less than the "static" measure of autoPEEP performed in paralyzed patients, presumably because of regional differences in autoPEEP (pendelluft effect) (18). The static measurement represents an average pressure, whereas the dynamic measurement detects the onset of inspiratory flow to lung regions with relatively low levels of autoPEEP. Additionally, the static measurement of autoPEEP can be overestimated if the timing of the occlusion is suboptimal and airflow is interrupted before true completion of exhalation (16).

AutoPEEP adds to the work of breathing in spontaneously breathing subjects, whether mechanically ventilated or not. Inspiratory muscles must isometrically generate sufficient force to overcome autoPEEP and reduce intra-alveolar pressure to subatmospheric levels before inspiratory flow can occur. In patients receiving mechanical ventilation, the inspiratory muscles may be too weak to trigger the ventilator, resulting in patient-ventilator asynchrony. The addition of extrinsic PEEP may reduce the effort required to trigger the inspiratory phase of the ventilator cycle by counterbalancing autoPEEP and raising the pressure threshold for initiating inspiration (3). This may be especially important in the early phases of acute exacerbations of COPD when autoPEEP may be substantially increased over baseline (19). With the addition of extrinsic PEEP, inspiratory workload may be reduced without worsening hyperinflation or changing lung mechanics (20) (Fig. 4).

AutoPEEP may also have adverse hemodynamic effects. During exhalation, increased intrathoracic pressure impedes venous return. With the onset of inspiration, intrathoracic pressure falls leading to abrupt increases in venous return and right ventricular filling. Due to "ventricular interdependence," this may shift the intraventricular septum to the left and compromise left ventricle filling. The net result is reduced cardiac output and systemic hypotension. Although extrinsic PEEP is unlikely to improve this situation, it does not aggravate it as long as the extrinsic PEEP is kept below the level of autoPEEP. In this sense, autoPEEP acts like a waterfall. The extrinsic PEEP resembles the water level below the waterfall in that the level above the waterfall is not affected by that below unless it rises above the upper level (21,22). Likewise, extrinsic PEEP

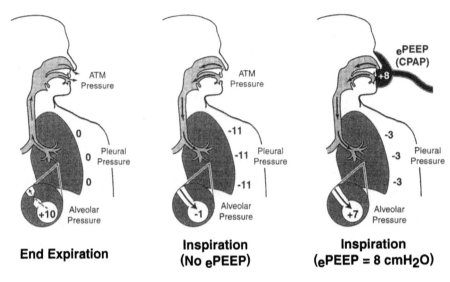

End Expiration   **Inspiration (No ₑPEEP)**   **Inspiration (ₑPEEP = 8 cmH₂O)**

Figure 4 Schematic to illustrate the counterbalancing effect of extrinsic PEEP (ePEEP) or CPAP during unassisted breathing on intrinsic PEEP (iPEEP). Left diagram shows a spontaneously breathing subject with an iPEEP of 10 cm H_2O. The middle diagram shows that in order to initiate the next inspiration, the subject must reduce alveolar pressure to subatmospheric pressure, necessitating an 11 cm H_2O swing in pleural pressure. If 8 cm ePEEP is applied (right diagram), the subject needs only to lower alveolar pressure to +7 cm H_2O to initiate the next inspiration, decreasing the requisite reduction in pleural pressure by 8 cm H_2O. (From Ref. 2.)

does not aggravate hyperinflation or further compromise hemodynamics unless it approaches the level of autoPEEP.

D. Hypoxemia

Patients with severe COPD often have a mild to moderate increase in the alveolar-arterial oxygen difference that has multiple etiologies. The severe oxygenation deficit seen in "blue bloaters" is largely a consequence of the additional burden of hypoventilation. During exacerbations of COPD, however, hypoxemia usually worsens, due in part to increasing hypoventilation. Alveolar-arterial oxygen differences often widen, due to worsening ventilation-perfusion mismatch and increases in shunt caused by retained secretions or additional contributing factors such as superimposed pneumonia, congestive heart failure, pulmonary embolism, or pneumothorax. These latter factors should be sought and promptly treated if clinically warranted.

Clinicians have long been cautioned about the overzealous use of oxygen supplementation in hypoxemic patients with COPD exacerbations. The concern has been that the oxygen will blunt the "hypoxic drive" and cause worsening CO_2 retention, particularly in patients whose chronic CO_2 retention is already substantial. Although this concern is well justified, the mechanism for the increased CO_2 is probably more complicated. Aubier et al. (23) found little evidence for blunting of respiratory drive when COPD patients were administered high concentrations of O_2 but, instead, found increased dead space ratios. This led to reduced alveolar ventilation and increasing CO_2 retention, even without significant changes in drive. Although oxygen should not be withheld in severely hypoxemic patients who are otherwise alert and cooperative, caution should be exercised while supplementing O_2 in patients with COPD exacerbations. Low flow O_2 should be started with close monitoring of ventilatory response and mental status.

E. Impaired Blood Supply to the Respiratory Muscles

Reduced blood flow to the diaphragm also contributes to the development of diaphragmatic fatigue. In addition to the increased muscle tension causing hyperinflation mentioned earlier, diaphragmatic blood flow can be compromised by increased in the Pdi/Pdi_{max} (24). Muscle contractions that raise Pdi more than 20–30% of Pdi_{max} have been shown to reduce blood flow and cause postcontraction hyperemia, which is indicative of oxygen debt (25). A proposed explanation for this observation is that increases in intramuscular pressure mechanically impede phrenic arterial blood flow. If the vascular back pressure increases to the level of upstream vascular pressure, blood flow ceases as observed when contraction intensity reaches 75% of Pdi_{max} (24).

Concomitant congestive heart failure may also predispose to respiratory muscle fatigue in COPD. Animal studies by Supinski et al. (26) have shown that the diaphragmatic muscle in dogs with congestive heart failure produces 10–15% less tension, receives reduced blood flow, and has less endurance than controls without heart failure. McParland et al. (27) found that human subjects with heart failure also have reduced inspiratory and expiratory muscle strength when compared to healthy age- and sex-matched controls. Consistent with the idea that respiratory muscle dysfunction contributes to dyspnea, muscle strength and dyspnea index were correlated when these patients performed normal daily activities (27). Work by Aubier et al. (28) showed that COPD patients with acute respiratory failure could increase diaphragmatic blood flow by 30–50% with administration of intravenous dopamine. Increased diaphragmatic blood flow was associated with a 40% increase in twitch Pdi that returned to baseline when the dopamine infusion was stopped. These experimental data suggest that reductions in blood flow to the diaphragm can compromise muscle function and that augmentation of blood flow can improve muscle function.

F. Effect of Critical Illness

During critical illness requiring either hospitalization or admission to an intensive care unit, multiple factors may impair respiratory muscle function in COPD patients. Experimentally induced sepsis in animal models results in respiratory muscle impairment (29) with large increases in PTI, respiratory muscle oxygen consumption, and lactate production (30). Healthy human volunteers have exhibited respiratory muscle dysfunction several days after the onset of a viral syndrome (31). Malnutrition and electrolyte abnormalities are potentially reversible causes of muscle dysfunction during critical illness that, if left uncorrected, may prolong the need for ventilatory support. Critical illness polyneuropathy, a primary axonal polyneuropathy that is thought to result from the neurotoxic effects of severe sepsis may also compromise respiratory function during bouts of respiratory failure (32). Clearly, multiple factors contribute to respiratory muscle dysfunction in acutely ill COPD patients, only some of whom are amenable to strategies of ventilator management. Clinicians should adopt a global approach in attempting to treat all potentially reversible contributing factors as a complement to optimal ventilator management.

G. Complications of Therapy

Therapeutic interventions for COPD may also contribute to muscle dysfunction. Corticosteroids, routinely used in the treatment of exacerbations of asthma or COPD, may contribute to respiratory muscle weakness (33,34). Use of neuromuscular blocking agents complicated by a postparalysis myopathy has also been linked with respiratory muscle dysfunction (35). The reported association between the use of high-dose steroids and prolonged use of neuromuscular blocking agents with postparalysis weakness (36,37) should discourage their use unless absolutely necessary. Routine monitoring of the depth of neuromuscular blockade using transcutaneous peripheral nerve stimulator devices has been recommended as a way of reducing the risk of this complication (38,39). Either agent alone has been associated with prolonged muscle weakness (35,40). In the management of COPD exacerbation and respiratory failure, the clinician must consider that medication choices can affect respiratory muscle function and consequently contribute to the prolonged need for mechanical ventilatory support.

H. Relevance to Mechanical Ventilation Strategies

The multiple pathophysiological defects described above have direct relevance to the rational provision of mechanical ventilatory assistance in patients with severe COPD. The optimal therapeutic approach is not limited to ventilatory management, but also focuses on the optimization of other aspects of care, such as minimization of bronchoconstriction and airway inflammation, optimization of nutritional status and fluid balance, infection eradication, correction of electrolyte imbalances, and so forth. Attention to these other aspects will speed the resolution of the pathophysiological defects and potentially shorten the duration of need for mechanical ventilatory assistance. In addition, knowledge of the basic pathophysiological defects such as hyperinflation and autoPEEP is critically important to the optimal use of mechanical ventilation in COPD patients with respiratory failure. The remaining sections of this chapter will apply these principles while discussing ventilator strategies.

III. Noninvasive Ventilation for Exacerbations of COPD

Noninvasive ventilation, mechanical ventilatory assistance provided without the need for tracheal intubation, has grown in popularity as a therapy for acute respiratory failure (41). This increasing use has been fueled by the desire to avoid complications of invasive ventilation, including upper airway trauma, nosocomial pneumonia and sinusitis, and the need for heavy sedation that may delay weaning efforts. Also, because the capacity for swallowing and speech are left intact, noninvasive ventilation is usually more acceptable to patients.

From a pathophysiological perspective, noninvasive ventilation may be viewed as a means of providing partial ventilatory support. As airway obstruction and hyperinflation worsen during a COPD exacerbation, noninvasive ventilation serves as a way of interrupting the vicious cycle that leads to respiratory muscle fatigue and ventilatory failure. By providing inspiratory assistance, noninvasive ventilation reduces the Pdi necessary for tidal breathing and lowers the Pdi/Pdi_{max}. Furthermore, by helping to lower the respiratory rate, noninvasive ventilation reduces Ti/Ttot. In this way, the TTI can be reduced below the threshold level for muscle fatigue and a ventilatory crisis is avoided. Theoretically, the reduction in breathing work needs to be only a small proportion of the total breathing effort if the TTI is lowered sufficiently. Carrey et al. (42) have elegantly demonstrated that noninvasive ventilation may be used to provide partial or even complete ventilatory support in COPD patients (Fig. 5). Another benefit of noninvasive ventilation is that by augmenting ventilation, it avoids the hypoventilation resulting from oxygen supplementation (43).

Although various approaches to noninvasive ventilation including negative pressure ventilation have been tried in the past, NPPV has received most of the recent attention in the literature and will be the focus of the following discussion. In addition, some studies suggest that noninvasive applications of continuous positive airway pressure (CPAP) alone may be of some benefit in COPD exacer-

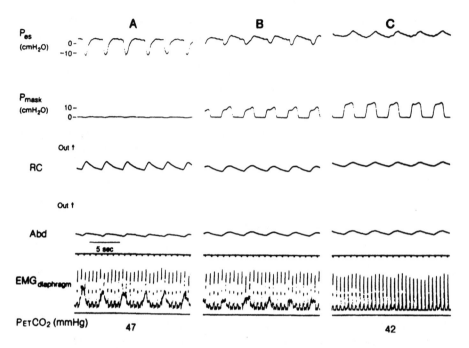

Figure 5 The effect of mask pressure (P_{mask}) on the mean amplitudes of inspiratory surface EMG activity. Tracings from a subject with COPD during spontaneous breathing (A) and during NPPV with P_{mask} of 12 (B) and 15 (C) cm H_2O. Increasing P_{mask} from 12 (B) to 15 (C) cm H_2O was associated with additional reduction in spontaneous inspiratory effort shown by suppression of the phasic surface diaphragmatic EMG ($EMG_{diaphram}$) and only positive inspiratory P_{es} swings. The paradoxic abdominal (Abd) motion seen during spontaneous breathing (A) became synchronous with the ribcage (RC) during NPPV (B and C). $P_{ET}CO_2$ = expired CO_2 tension. (From Ref. 42.)

bations, and its use will be reviewed briefly. Subsequent sections will weigh the evidence for the efficacy of the various noninvasive approaches, provide guidelines for the selection of appropriate patients, and discuss practical applications as they relate to COPD patients.

A. Role of CPAP in COPD Exacerbations

Although it is not truly a mode to assist ventilation, CPAP applied noninvasively may be used to reduce ventilatory effort in COPD patients because of its ability to counterbalance autoPEEP. Petrof et al. (44) observed a dose response relationship between increasing levels of CPAP (from 0 to 15 cm H_2O) and reduced inspiratory effort as determined by Pes or transdiaphragmatic pressure (Fig. 6). Other investigators have reported beneficial responses to CPAP alone in patients with COPD exacerbations. De Lucas et al. (45) administered 5 cm H_2O CPAP via a face mask to 15 COPD patients during an exacerbation and found that after 4 hours, $PaCO_2$ decreased from 73 to 61 mmHg, PaO_2 improved from 57 to 64 mmHg, respiratory rate decreased from 30 to 25 per minute, and the dyspnea index improved. No randomized, controlled trials have been performed, so no conclusions regarding efficacy can be drawn. Nonetheless, the reported studies raise the possibility that CPAP alone could be an effective therapy in the management of COPD exacerbations.

More recent studies demonstrate that the combination of expiratory pressure and inspiratory pressure support (PSV) is more effective than CPAP alone for reducing Pdi. Both Appendini et al. (46) and Nava et al. (47) found that both CPAP and inspiratory pressure support alone reduce inspiratory effort in COPD patients as determined by decreases in esophageal or transdiaphragmatic pressure swings. However, when the two are combined as pressure support with PEEP, decreases in inspiratory effort are even greater. This effect is presumably because extrinsic PEEP reduces the inspiratory effort used to overcome autoPEEP while inspiratory pressure support augments the effort needed for lung inflation.

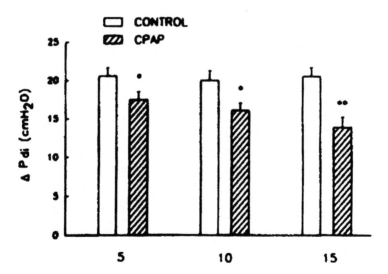

Figure 6 Mean values ($\pm$ SE) for tidal excursions of transdiaphragmatic (P_{di}) pressures in patients with COPD before and during application of CPAP at 5, 10, and 15 cm H_2O. Single asterisk indicates $p < 0.01$; double asterisks indicate $p < 0.001$. (From Ref. 44.)

B. Evidence for the Efficacy of NPPV in COPD Exacerbations

The ability of noninvasive ventilatory assistance to reduce breathing work during
COPD exacerbations has led to the hypothesis that NPPV might be helpful in
averting intubation in such patients. Brochard et al. conducted the first study to
test this hypothesis in any controlled fashion (48). Among their 13 patients with
severe COPD exacerbations treated with PSV via a face mask, only 1 required
intubation. The 13 physiologically matched historical controls required 11 intubations and spent substantially longer periods of time using the ventilator and
occupying the intensive care unit. These findings supported the hypothesis and
stimulated the performance of numerous subsequent uncontrolled trials that reported similar findings (49–53). However, studies using historical controls are
known to bias results in favor of the treated group (54), while uncontrolled trials
are insufficient to prove efficacy.

Since 1993, six randomized controlled trials have been reported to evaluate
the efficacy of noninvasive ventilation in COPD. The first, by Bott et al. (55),
randomized 60 COPD patients to receive volume limited nasal ventilation or
conventional therapy. NPPV-treated patients were less dyspneic and showed significant improvements in pH and $Paco_2$ after one hour compared to controls.
Although there was a strong trend toward improved mortality (10% in NPPV
treated vs. 30% in controls), the difference in 30-day mortality did not reach
statistical significance. However, when four patients, two of whom died, were
excluded because they had randomized to NPPV but did not actually receive
it, the survival advantage of NPPV became statistically significant ($p < 0.05$).
Subsequently, Kramer et al. (56) randomized 31 patients, most of whom had
COPD, to receive NPPV using "bilevel" ventilator versus conventional therapy.
Not only did NPPV-treated patients exhibit improved vital signs and oxygenation,
they also had a statistically significant reduction in intubation rate when compared
to controls (74% vs. 26%, NPPV vs. control, $p < 0.05$).

Brochard et al. (57) performed a larger, multicenter, randomized study in
85 patients, all of whom had COPD exacerbations. Like Kramer et al., these
investigators reported improved vital signs and reduced intubation rates in patients treated with noninvasive ventilation. In addition, NPPV-treated patients
had reductions in complication rates, length of hospital stay, and in-hospital mortality when compared to controls. More recently, Celikel et al. (58) randomized
30 patients to receive NPPV or conventional therapy and observed similar effects
on vital signs, gas exchange, intubation rates, and hospital length of stay as those
reported previously.

Most recently, Plant et al. (58a) randomized 236 patients to receive noninvasive ventilation or conventional therapy in a multicenter trial in England. This
trial was performed in general medical wards and NPPV was implemented by
nurses who had received only a brief training session on the proper application

of NPPV. These authors found a significant reduction in intubation rate (29% to 16%) and in mortality rate (20% to 10%) among the patients treated with NPPV (both $p < 0.05$; controls vs. NPPV).

In contrast to the previous studies, Barbé et al. reported no difference in the outcome of 24 COPD patients who were randomized to either bilevel noninvasive ventilation or usual care consisting of supplemental oxygen, bronchodilators, and intravenous prednisolone (59). Of note, these authors enrolled consecutive patients with COPD exacerbations, none of whom required intubation or died, and who, on average, had less severe respiratory acidosis than patients in the other trials.

Using pooled data from most of the above studies, a recent meta-analysis addressed the effects of noninvasive ventilation on mortality and intubation rates (60). After excluding the Barbé study (59) due to differences in disease severity among enrolled patients compared to the Bott (55), Kramer (56), and Brochard (57) studies, these authors found a significant reduction in hospital mortality (odds ratio 0.22, 95% CI 0.09–0.54) and an even stronger beneficial effect on intubation rate (odds ratio 0.12, 95% CI 0.05–0.29) (49,55,56,49). Based on this convincing evidence, the authors concluded that NPPV reduces intubation rates and hospital mortality in COPD patients and should be considered as first line therapy. None of the studies used in the meta-analysis reported long-term outcome beyond hospital discharge. However, one other prospective study with historical controls reported statistically significant improvements in 6- and 12-month mortality as well as a reduced rates of rehospitalization at one year (61). In addition, a retrospective study (51) reported a trend toward lower one-year mortality and a statistically significant reduction in new ICU admissions within one year. Unfortunately, the lack of randomized controls limits the conclusions that can be drawn from these latter studies.

With the above-listed randomized controlled trials showing improvements in clinical response, avoidance of intubations, and reductions in morbidity and mortality rates, the evidence supporting the use of noninvasive ventilation as the ventilatory mode of first choice for properly selected COPD patients with acute respiratory failure is compelling. Another potential benefit of NPPV is more efficient resource utilization. However, the evidence to demonstrate reductions in resource utilization and time consumption by medical personnel is lacking. In general, shortened ICU or hospital lengths of stay lead to cost savings but studies that have examined finances have not shown statistically significant savings (56,62). In addition, one early study reported patients who had NPPV required a large expenditure of nursing time (52). Human and financial costs of using noninvasive ventilation versus conventional therapy in more recent studies show no significant difference in time expenditure by nurses or respiratory therapists during the first 24 hours of care (53,55,56,62). However, if the first 6–8 hours of hospital care are examined, two of the studies reported that use of respiratory therapist time was greater in the NPPV group, with one study showing a significant decrease by the second 8 hours (56). These findings suggest that management with NPPV initially requires more personnel time than conventional therapy, but after the patient successfully adapts, time requirements for NPPV are no greater. Costs of NPPV have been examined in relatively few studies, but two studies examining total costs found no significant differences between NPPV and conventional care (56,62).

C. Selection of COPD Patients to Receive Noninvasive Ventilation

Predictors of Success or Failure

Noninvasive assisted ventilation is not uniformly successful in improving arterial blood gases or avoiding intubation in patients with acute respiratory failure. Selection of appropriate recipients of NPPV is an important factor in optimizing success rates. As such, knowledge of factors associated with success or failure of NPPV can be useful in proper patient selection and perhaps lead to improved success rates. In particular, rapid identification of poor candidates for noninvasive mechanical ventilation may avoid unnecessary delays in endotracheal intubation and mechanical ventilation. Among several studies attempting to identify useful predictors, unsuccessfully treated patients, defined as those who were intolerant of nasal mechanical ventilation and required intubation, had worsening respiratory acidosis, higher initial severity of illness scores (APACHE II) and more frequently had excessive secretions than successfully treated patients (50,63,64). They also had worse neurological function, which likely interferes with their ability to cooperate with treatment (63). Furthermore, unsuccessfully treated patients were more often edentulous or used pursed-lip breathing; factors that prevented formation of an adequate mouth seal and contributed to greater mouth leaks than in successfully treated patients (63,64) (Table 2).

Compared to failures, successfully treated patients, defined as those whose respiratory acidosis is corrected and who avoid intubation, adapted more rapidly to the nasal mask and ventilator while showing a greater and more rapid improvement (within 1 hour) in respiratory rate, $Paco_2$, and pH (57,63–66) (Table 2). In some studies, patients with a $Paco_2$ greater than 45 mmHg on presentation (Type II respiratory failure) had a greater reduction in the need for endotracheal intubation, length of ICU stay, and mortality (64,67,68) than hypoxemic patients without hypercapnia (Type I respiratory failure).

The above observations indicate that there is a "window of opportunity" for the application of noninvasive ventilation. The findings that patients with markedly elevated $Paco_2$ and APACHE scores fare less well compared to patients with lower values have led some authors to encourage earlier use of NPPV (63). Delays in achieving proper settings and adjustments may permit patient deteriora-

Table 2 Determinants of Success During Noninvasive Positive Pressure Ventilation

Mask (interface) properly fitted and applied
Rapid adaptation and coordination of respiratory efforts with breathing device
Good cognitive/neurological function
Younger age
Lower illness severity score
Presence of teeth
Low volume of oral or airway secretions
No pneumonia
Hypercarbia but not severe (>45, <100 mm Hg)
Acidemia but not severe (pH < 7.35, >7.1)
Increased APACHE II Score, but not too high (i.e., <21)
Improved vital signs and blood gases within 2 hours of NPPV application

tion to the extent that only invasive mechanical ventilation will be successful. In order to maximize success rates, rapid identification of appropriate candidates and prompt application of NPPV is essential (63,64).

Patient Selection Guidelines for Application of Noninvasive Ventilation

Guidelines for the selection of patients with COPD exacerbations to receive NPPV are based on entry criteria used in studies reporting successful application of NPPV. Appropriate candidates are those with respiratory insufficiency who are at risk for requiring endotracheal intubation. Patients should be neither too mildly ill (and thus unlikely to benefit from assisted ventilation) nor too severely ill (and thus in need of immediate intubation). NPPV appears to be most appropriate for those who fall between these extremes and are not placed at risk if noninvasive techniques are applied. In addition to clinical signs of acute respiratory distress (moderate to severe dyspnea, tachypnea, tachycardia, accessory muscle use or paradoxical abdominal motion), patients should have physiological evidence of acute respiratory failure or insufficiency (i.e., acute respiratory acidosis or acute hypoxemia) (Table 3). The patient should be cooperative, but need not be alert; some authors have used NPPV successfully with obtunded patients (50,65,69,70).

The presence of concomitant conditions such as congestive heart failure or pneumonia may be associated with less favorable outcomes than bronchitic exacerbations (63,68,71,72). Although high rates of success have been reported when these conditions are present (58), the reduced benefit with these associated conditions seen in some studies may be attributed to several factors, including less rapid reversibility, inability to handle secretions, high ventilatory and oxy-

Table 3 Suggested Selection Criteria for NPPV in COPD Patients
with Acute Respiratory Failure

Step 1. Identification of patients who need ventilatory assistance
  Clinical Exam
    Increased dyspnea of at least moderate severity
    Tachypnea (>24)
    Use of accessory muscles and/or paradoxical abdominal motion
  Gas Exchange
    $Paco_2 > 45$ mm Hg
    pH < 7.35
    $Pao_2/Fio_2 < 200$
Step 2. Exclusion of patients who would not benefit from NPPV
  Respiratory arrest
  Medically unstable
    Hypotensive shock unresponsive to fluids or low-dose pressors
    Uncontrolled cardiac ischemia or arrhythmias
    Massive upper GI bleed
  Inability to protect airway
    Impaired cough or swallowing reflex
    Excessive secretions
  Uncooperative or agitated
  Facial trauma or deformities that preclude adequate mask fit

---

genation requirements, and reduced lung compliance requiring higher inspiratory pressures. The presence of these other factors should be considered in selecting patients. Finally, NPPV is also useful in patients who have refused or are not believed to be candidates for endotracheal intubation (65,73,74). In such patients, success rates approximating 60% have been reported (65,74), and even when unsuccessful, NPPV may provide adequate time for ethical discussions or completion of personal matters.

An extremely important aspect of proper patient selection for NPPV is to exclude patients who would be more safely managed with invasive ventilation. Poor candidates include those with respiratory or cardiac arrest, compromised upper airway function, high risk for aspiration due to swallowing dysfunction or impaired cough and excessive secretions. Since NPPV affords no direct airway access for secretion removal and frequent expectoration interferes with the delivery of ventilatory assistance, patients with these conditions should have invasive ventilation. NPPV should also be avoided in patients with hemodynamic instability, or uncontrolled life-threatening cardiac arrhythmias, acute ischemic myocardial infarctions or upper gastrointestinal bleeding. Finally, patients who are agitated, unable to cooperate, or have any condition that precludes mask application, such as facial trauma, should not be supported with NPPV (Table 3).

D. Initiation of Noninvasive Ventilation in COPD Patients

Once an appropriate recipient of noninvasive ventilation has been identified, the clinician must promptly select an interface (or mask) and a ventilator to deliver pressurized gas into the upper airway. Selection of a ventilator mode, initial settings, and appropriate adjunctive therapies, such as oxygen or humidification, contribute to the successful application of NPPV. A more detailed discussion of the implementation of noninvasive ventilation is provided in Chapter 6, but considerations that are of particular importance to COPD patients will be briefly discussed here.

Many combinations of interfaces and ventilators have been successfully used in COPD patients with respiratory failure. Little scientific evidence is available to guide equipment selections, so both theoretical and individual biases must guide clinician decisions. The two most commonly used interfaces are nasal and oronasal masks. Proponents of nasal masks tout reduced claustrophobia, greater ease of communication and expectoration, ability for oral intake, and reduced rebreathing of air as factors supporting their preference. Oronasal mask proponents stress reduced oral air leaks and more efficient delivery of respiratory support, especially in COPD patients who are commonly perceived to be "mouth breathers." No randomized, controlled trial comparing the two mask types has been published, although success rates in studies using one mask or the other have been similar.

Scientific evidence supporting ventilator selection is lacking as well, so specific ventilator choice is also influenced by theoretical and practical considerations. Ventilators used in NPPV can be divided into "critical care" or "noninvasive" types. While advances in ventilator technology are blurring the distinction between these types of ventilators, in general, critical care ventilators have more sophisticated monitoring and alarm systems. Factors such as the need to deliver high oxygen concentrations, tolerance for air leaks, and equipment cost all may influence a clinician's selection.

When selecting modes and settings, the clinician should consider several unique characteristics of COPD patients (Table 4). First, two studies comparing volume- and pressure-limited modes in COPD patients suggest that the pressure support mode is perceived as more comfortable (75,76). On the other hand, ventilator asynchrony may occur with the pressure support mode in patients with COPD, either because of a delay in cycling to expiratory pressure after the patient has begun exhalation (77) or because of air leaks. In either case, ventilators that are capable of adjusting inspiratory time may be helpful in improving synchrony.

Table 4 Suggested Initial NPPV Settings for Acute Respiratory Failure
in COPD Patients

Pressure-limited ventilation	
Mode	Assist/control
Inspiratory pressure	8–12 cm H_2O
Expiratory pressure	4–5 cm H_2O
Backup respiratory rate	0–14/minute
Oxygen supplementation	2–4 L/min via mask or ventilator circuit or FIO_2 via blender titrated to O_2 sat > 90%
Volume-limited ventilation	
Mode	Assist/control
Tidal volume	10–15 mL/kg with exhaled V_T = 7 mL/kg
Expiratory pressure	4–5 cm H_2O
Backup respiratory rate	10–14/minute
Oxygen supplementation	24–40% titrated to O_2 sat > 90%

Second, COPD patients may be more comfortable with rapid inspiratory flow rates, so pressure-limited modes with adjustable times for reaching the targeted inspiratory pressure (often referred to as "rise time") may be useful for enhancing comfort. Finally, because patients with COPD exacerbations often have increased levels of autoPEEP, expiratory pressures of at least 4–5 cm H_2O may be useful in facilitating ventilator triggering and patient-ventilator synchrony.

Adjuncts to NPPV can also play a critical role in the rapid and successful adaptation of COPD patients in respiratory failure to NPPV. Oxygen supplementation, air humidification, and inhaled respiratory treatments all can enhance patient comfort and are discussed further in Chapter 6. It is important to keep in mind that the delivery of aerosolized bronchodilators during NPPV via the ventilator tubing has been described (78). Although this practice has not been evaluated in COPD patients, it is probably justifiable during the early period after NPPV initiation when even short-term discontinuation of ventilation to administer nebulizer therapy could worsen respiratory distress.

In both COPD and non-COPD patients, the most common complications associated with NPPV are related to the mask interface. Mask trauma and airway irritation, can be reduced by using a variety of techniques and adjuncts (see Chapter 6). Emesis and aspiration are feared complications of oronasal NPPV but, fortunately, are rare. Delivery of positive pressure ventilation, whether by endotracheal tube or by noninvasive means, may adversely affect hemodynamics in COPD patients, especially those with low fluid volumes. Therefore, careful monitoring of heart rate and blood pressure is recommended in these patients. In addition, barotrauma is a concern in hyperinflated COPD patients. However, because inflation pressures are generally much less than with invasive ventilation, the complications of barotrauma are much less likely to occur with NPPV.

E. Use of NPPV for COPD—A Strategic Approach

The increasing use of NPPV to treat COPD exacerbations represents an advance in therapy that reduces the overall morbidity and mortality of COPD patients. For these reasons, NPPV should be considered the ventilator therapy of first choice in properly selected patients. Respiratory clinicians are encouraged to gain experience and skill in the application of this modality so that patient outcomes can

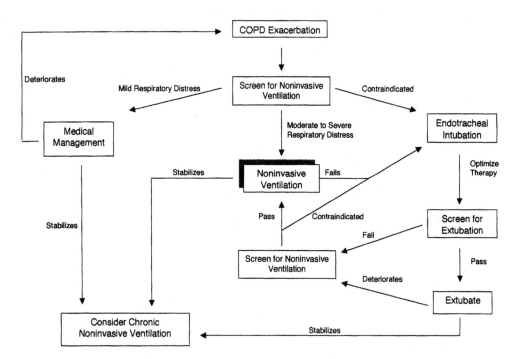

Figure 7 Algorithm for application of noninvasive ventilation to patients with COPD exacerbations. Patients are screened initially and treated with noninvasive ventilation if found to be appropriate candidates. If patients are too ill initially or fail noninvasive ventilation, they should undergo endotracheal intubation. Once stabilized, patients should be screened for extubation and may be considered for early extubation to noninvasive ventilation if they fail a T-piece weaning trial. Noninvasive ventilation should also be considered for patients who fail planned or unplanned extubations. Once patients stabilize, chronic noninvasive ventilation may be considered in patients who remain severely hypercapnic.

be optimized. A suggested strategy for incorporation of NPPV into the routine management of COPD exacerbations is depicted in Figure 7. All patients entering the hospital with respiratory distress due to suspected COPD exacerbations should be screened to determine whether they meet criteria for noninvasive ventilation. If they are too mildly ill they are managed medically, and if they are too severe they are managed invasively. As shown in Figure 7, NPPV can also be considered to facilitate early removal of the endotracheal tube or to avoid reintubation in patients who fail after extubation. These latter applications have not been as thoroughly studied as in patients presenting with acute respiratory failure, so patients should be selected carefully. Patients who recover from their acute exacerbations of COPD, whether treated invasively or not, can be considered for long-term NPPV in the home. Guidelines for selection of such patients have not been established but patients with persisting severe hypercapnia and nocturnal desaturations despite oxygen supplementation are probably the best candidates (79).

IV. Invasive Mechanical Ventilation for Acute Respiratory Failure in COPD

The increasing use of noninvasive ventilation in the therapy of acute COPD exacerbations will reduce the need for invasive mechanical ventilation. Nonetheless, many patients will still require invasive ventilation, either because on presentation they are not candidates for noninvasive ventilation (Table 3) or they fail an initial trial of noninvasive ventilation. Even at experienced centers, up to one third of appropriately selected patients fail noninvasive ventilation. In Brochard's study (57) comparing NPPV versus standard treatment, 26% of COPD patients enrolled in the noninvasive arm failed and required intubation. Overall, when the patients who require immediate intubation upon presentation are added to those who fail NPPV, a substantial proportion (perhaps 30–40%) of patients admitted with an acute deterioration of COPD will eventually require invasive mechanical ventilation. A complete discussion of invasive mechanical ventilation techniques is beyond the scope of this chapter. The following discussion will focus on aspects pertinent to the management of COPD patients requiring mechanical ventilation, particularly with regard to minimizing complications. The discussion will also reflect basic principles outlined in two consensus documents that comment on mechanical ventilation in severe COPD (80,81).

A. Basic Principles of Ventilating COPD Patients

Avoiding Hyperinflation

Patients presenting with acute respiratory failure superimposed on severe underlying COPD usually have an increase in expiratory resistance caused by a viral or bacterial respiratory infection. This increased resistance necessitates further increases in lung volume to maintain airflow (see Fig. 3), worsening the mechanical disadvantage for already dysfunctional respiratory muscles. For reasons discussed earlier (see Sec. II), these alterations may upset the precarious balance that these patients maintain by exceeding the capacity of respiratory muscles to supply breathing work and leading to respiratory failure. The role of mechanical ventilation, whether invasive or noninvasive, is to unload the respiratory muscles, permitting a restoration of the supply/demand balance while medical therapies are given time to reduce airway resistance. In this regard, it is unnecessary to completely eliminate the work of breathing. Noninvasive ventilation usually achieves only a partial unloading, and the relatively low inspiratory pressures used during noninvasive ventilation rarely cause substantial worsening of hyperinflation.

On the other hand, invasive ventilation allows complete control of the airway, enabling the clinician to vary inflation pressure and volume within a wide range of settings. As a consequence, inappropriately high inflation pressures, volumes, and respiratory rates may be selected, particularly if an inexperienced clinician deems these necessary to treat a markedly elevated $Paco_2$. The effect of such a ventilator strategy will be to exacerbate the severity of hyperinflation, increase autoPEEP, and compromise venous return, all of which will contribute to hemodynamic instability and greatly increase the risk of barotrauma. To make matters worse, the clinician may be misled into diagnosing cardiogenic shock in this circumstance, particularly if a pulmonary catheter has been placed to facilitate hemodynamic monitoring. The elevated autoPEEP may affect pulmonary capillary wedge pressure measurements in the compressible pulmonary arteries, causing an overestimation of actual cardiac filling pressures and leading the nonastute clinician to administer cardiotonics and diuretics.

To avoid this scenario, it is essential that clinicians choose ventilator settings that will minimize hyperinflation in patients with COPD. The clinician should also keep in mind that partial support of breathing is usually adequate and that overzealous correction of CO_2 retention is not only unnecessary, but may also cause excessive alkalosis, increasing the risk of seizures and cardiac arrhythmias. Studies on the effect of ventilatory pattern on hyperinflation in patients with severe airway obstruction demonstrate that expiratory volume (V_T), and expiratory time (T_E) are the most important determinants of hyperinflation (82). Since expiratory flow can be increased only by reducing airway resistance (something not easily influenced by manipulation of mechanical ventilator settings) or increasing lung volume (undesirable if hyperinflation is to be avoided), the clinician must pay close attention to V_T and T_E. Although definitive studies determining ideal V_T in COPD patients are lacking, current recommendations are for V_T between 5 and 7 mL/kg (83). As shown in Table 5, excessive V_T should be avoided, so that less air per breath needs to be exhaled.

Table 5 Effect of Ventilator Settings on Expiratory Times

Rate/Min	V_T(L)	IFR (L/Min)	T_I(s)	T_E(s)	I:E
12	0.67	40	1.0	4.0	1:4
12	1.00	40	1.5	3.5	1:2.3
12	0.67	60	0.7	4.3	1:6
20	0.67	40	1.0	2.0	1:2
20	1.00	40	1.5	1.5	1:1
20	0.67	60	0.7	2.3	1:3

V_T = Tidal volume; IFR = inspiratory flow rate; T_I = inspiratory time;
T_E = expiratory time; I:E = inspiratory/expiratory ratio.
Source: Ref. 2.

The main determinants of T_E are respiratory rate and inspiratory: expiratory (I:E) ratio. The most common mistake in selecting ventilator settings is to choose an excessive rate, which has a dramatic shortening effect on T_E (Table 5). Standard initial ventilator rates of 10–14 per minute should not be exceeded in patients with acute respiratory failure due to COPD exacerbations, and to avoid hyperinflation the lowest acceptable rate should be used. An important determinant of I:E ratio is inspiratory flow rate because it determines the inspiratory time necessary to deliver a given tidal volume. Relatively high inspiratory flow rates (>60 L/min) are recommended for patients with COPD on mechanical ventilation because this results in shorter inspiratory times, allowing more time in the respiratory cycle for expiration. Also, some studies have shown better relief of dyspnea and patient-ventilator synchrony when rapid inspiratory flow rates are used for COPD patients (84). In addition, dead space ratios may be reduced and oxygenation improved when patients with airway obstruction are ventilated at higher compared to lower inspiratory flow rates (85). On the other hand, as long as the I:E ratio is no greater than 1:3, further lowering of the ratio (by raising inspiratory flow rate, for instance) results in relatively little lengthening of T_E, and because expiratory flow rates are so low late during the expiratory phase, relatively little additional lung emptying is achieved.

The above observations are based on the use of volume-limited ventilation, using assist/control or intermittent mandatory ventilation (IMV) modes. In recent years, pressure-limited modes have seen increasing use in a variety of forms of respiratory failure, including adult (or acute) respiratory distress syndrome. This approach was discouraged in the past for obstructive lung diseases because of the difficulty in delivering consistent tidal volumes when airway resistance was subject to rapid fluctuations caused by bronchospasm and airway secretions. However, the increased monitoring capabilities of modern critical care ventilators enable clinicians to use pressure-limited modes to ventilate patients with respiratory failure caused by obstructive lung diseases. If a pressure-limited mode is selected, the principles of administration are similar to those for volume-limited ventilation, except that the clinician can be assured that the selected peak pressure will not be exceeded. The peak inspiratory pressures should be selected so that VT is 5–7 mL/kg, respiratory rate and I:E ratio set to allow for an adequate TE, and both delivered VT and autoPEEP are closely monitored.

During use of volume-limited ventilation, the clinician should closely monitor both the patient and ventilator to assure that excessive hyperinflation is avoided. Systemic hypotension, agitation, or difficulty synchronizing with the ventilator should raise immediate suspicion of hyperinflation. Peak inspiratory airway pressure should be monitored and is ideally <40 cm H_2O. However, this may be higher in patients receiving high inspiratory flow rates, as pressure is dissipated to overcome airway resistance. For this reason, plateau pressure should also be monitored and should be <35 cm H_2O (81,83). This is measured by inserting an inspiratory hold, with the pressure stabilization point corresponding to the lung static inflation pressure. AutoPEEP should also be monitored, usually by the end-expiratory occlusion technique described previously in Section II. An earlier study using VT that exceed current recommendations found that average pressures on the first day of mechanical ventilation in eight patients with COPD (mean VT was 0.69 L) were 47 and 26 cm H_2O, respectively, for peak and plateau pressures (19).

Managing autoPEEP

As discussed earlier, autoPEEP is a consequence of dynamic hyperinflation and at least some autoPEEP is detectable in most patients with acute COPD exacerbations (46). Furthermore, autoPEEP can be greatly exacerbated by mechanical ventilation, particularly if initial ventilator settings are inappropriate. Thus, the first step in minimizing autoPEEP is to follow standard recommendations for ventilator settings. However, when these settings are used, autoPEEP can still be substantial, necessitating periodic monitoring, particularly when mechanical ventilation is initiated.

Major adverse consequences of autoPEEP, such as hemodynamic instability, barotrauma, and increased work of breathing, are managed in different ways. If a patient is hypotensive because of increased autoPEEP, the only recourse is to further lower VT and/or respiratory rate (raising inspiratory flow above recommended rates will have little effect). This may necessitate employing permissive hypercapnia, as described below. The eventual settings will be based on the clinician's assessment of risks and benefits; the benefit of the lowered inflation pressure versus the risk of greater metabolic disturbance and the need for more sedation. Adding extrinsic PEEP in this situation is of no value because it does not reduce hyperinflation. In fact, if too much extrinsic PEEP is added, hypotension can be potentiated because extrinsic PEEP greater than autoPEEP exacerbates lung hyperinflation. On the other hand, extrinsic PEEP may be very effective in reducing work of breathing and improving patient-ventilator synchrony. Synchrony is enhanced when autoPEEP reduces the inspiratory effort needed to trigger the ventilator. In this case, the extrinsic PEEP counterbalances the autoPEEP, reducing the inspiratory threshold load, as shown in Figure 5.

The determination of the optimal extrinsic PEEP level to counterbalance autoPEEP has received considerable attention. Values of 75–85% of the static measured autoPEEP are the values most often recommended (20,86). Ideally, the optimal extrinsic PEEP is the level that minimizes work of breathing or triggering effort without increasing lung volume or inflation pressures (i.e., remains below the level of the waterfall). Additional benefit may also derive from the smaller negative pleural pressure swings needed to initiate inspiration. These smaller reductions in intrathoracic pressure may temper the increases in volume of venous blood returning to the right ventricle and consequent leftward shift of the intraventricular septum. The latter effect may reduce LV stroke volumes during inspiration that lead to large swings in blood pressure and contribute to hemodynamic instability. Application of PEEP has been shown to reverse leftward shift in the intraventricular septum in a spontaneously breathing COPD patient (5). In practice, the optimal extrinsic PEEP may be a difficult point to establish for several reasons. AutoPEEP measurements may be inaccurate if the patient's expiratory effort is not completely suppressed or if extrinsic factors such as tubing or humidifier resistance interfere. Thus, for pragmatic purposes, many clinicians titrate extrinsic PEEP in small increments until triggering effort is reduced and patient-ventilator synchrony improves. If indicators of excessive PEEP such as increases in peak inspiratory or plateau pressure occur, the clinician lowers the extrinsic PEEP.

Permissive Hypercapnia

Permissive hypercapnia, the acceptance of hypercapnia in mechanically ventilated patients so that less risky ventilator settings can be used, was first described in 1984 in patients with acute asthma (87). Although the terminology was not used, this approach had been in use for many years prior to 1984 in patients with COPD who had been chronic CO_2 retainers. These patients were intentionally hypoventilated so that they could wean at $Paco_2$ matching their level of chronic CO_2 retention. In COPD patients who are experiencing significant hyperinflation despite the use of standard recommended ventilator settings, the strategy of permissive hypercapnia can be employed to minimize the risk of barotrauma or ventilator-induced lung injury. Smaller tidal volumes and lower respiratory rates are used to minimize hyperinflation, but $Paco_2$ may rise to very high levels. The maximum safe level for $Paco_2$ during use of permissive hypercapnia is unknown. Although definitive studies are lacking, permissive hypercapnia has been advocated in the management of respiratory failure due to other causes (88,89). Most clinicians monitor pH, attempting to keep it above 7.1, and administer intravenous bicarbonate if it falls below this level. Fortunately, most patients with chronic CO_2 retention are very tolerant of severe hypercapnia. No controlled trials have analyzed this approach in COPD patients, but the aim is to use permissive hypercapnia until airway resistance has improved, and then to lower $Paco_2$ until the baseline value has been reached. Use of heavy sedation is usually necessary while the pH is low.

Patient-Ventilator Synchrony

Good synchrony between the patient and ventilator during mechanical ventilation enhances patient comfort and permits the ventilator to unload the breathing muscles. Poor synchrony contributes to patient agitation and respiratory distress sometimes necessitating sedation and/or paralysis to maintain adequate oxygenation and ventilation. The endotracheal tube, ventilator valves, and circuitry may actually increase the work of breathing, especially if the patient is making large asynchronous breathing efforts. For these reasons, the clinician must choose ventilator modes and settings that enhance patient synchrony.

When a controlled ventilator mode is used in a patient who is heavily sedated or paralyzed, asynchrony is not an issue. However, synchrony must be optimized when assisted or spontaneous breathing modes are used. In COPD patients, causes of asynchrony may be related to the patient or ventilator (Table 6) (90). Patient-related factors include pain or discomfort and respiratory factors such as increased dyspnea due to bronchospasm, secretions, or other respiratory complications. Ventilator-related factors include inadequate triggering, an inappropriate inspiratory flow rate or V_T and inability to cycle from inspiration to expiration appropriately. As discussed above, autoPEEP is a common cause of failure to trigger and can be counterbalanced with extrinsic PEEP, but an excessively insensitive trigger setting could also contribute. An inappropriately low or high inspiratory flow rate or V_T could also contribute to respiratory distress. COPD patients, in particular, seem to prefer relatively high inspiratory flow rates, and a common error is to select a flow rate that is too low (i.e., 40 L/min).

Jubran et al. (77) reported that patients with severe COPD may encounter difficulty with cycling from inspiration to expiration when using the pressure support mode. These patients have relatively high inspiratory flow rates and short inspiratory times. The inspiratory flow rates remain high throughout the duration of inspiration, and flow-cycled ventilator modes, like PSV, may have trouble promptly detecting the onset of patient exhalation. Accordingly, the ventilator continues to deliver inspiratory pressure after the patient starts to expire. In order

Table 6 Causes of Patient-Ventilator Asynchrony Among
Invasively Mechanically Ventilated COPD Patients

Ventilator-related causes
  Insensitive or overly sensitive ventilator trigger
  Ventilator failure to detect exhalation
  Inadequate set inspiratory flow rate
  Inadequate extrinsic PEEP in patient with significant autoPEEP
  Ventilator circuit obstruction or malfunction
Patient-related causes
  Pain
  Bronchospasm
  Excessive secretions
  Anxiety
  Pulmonary edema
  Unfavorable body positioning
  Electrolyte imbalance
  Dynamic hyperinflation
  Pneumothorax
  Hypoxia
  Acidosis
  Malpositioned or malfunctioning endotracheal tube

Source: Adapted from Ref. 90.

to cycle the ventilator, the patient must exert a greater expiratory effort that contributes to respiratory distress.

Alternatively, asynchrony may occur if the flow triggering mechanism is
too sensitive. Because of the reduced expiratory flows and prolonged expiratory
times during exhalation, the ventilator may switch to inspiratory flow before the
patient has completed exhalation. Switching to a pressure assist mode with a
relatively low I:E ratio or using a ventilator that has adjustable triggering and
cycling mechanisms in the pressure support mode can help enhance synchrony.
Sedation and analgesia may be helpful in facilitating synchrony but should be
used sparingly and only after the possible contributions of inappropriate ventilator
settings or other factors have been considered. Although paralytics eliminate
problems with patient-ventilator asynchrony very effectively, they should be
avoided in patients treated with high-dose steroids because of the association
with postparalysis myopathy (37,40).

B. Weaning from Invasive Mechanical Ventilation

Traditional Approaches

Weaning from invasive mechanical ventilation is an art that requires optimal
medical therapy, close observation of the patient, and considerable practitioner

judgment and experience. Timely and appropriate removal of the endotracheal tube is desirable so that complications of invasive ventilation are minimized and resource utilization optimized. Although pressure support ventilation and IMV have been touted as modes to facilitate weaning, well-designed controlled trials have failed to consistently show one ventilation mode to be superior in expediting the weaning process (91–93). However, recent studies demonstrate that daily use of a T-piece weaning trial may be helpful in minimizing duration of ventilator use (94,95).

One of the most important aspects of expeditious weaning is prompt initiation of optimal medical therapy, including bronchodilators, corticosteroids, antibiotics, and pulmonary toilet. Theophylline should be considered in patients with refractory bronchospasm resistant to maximal bronchodilator therapy. Sedation and analgesia are also necessary to alleviate patient distress and enhance patient-ventilator synchrony, but excessive sedation must be avoided so as not to delay the weaning process. In this regard, the short-acting sedative propofol may be advantageous because, in addition to possible bronchodilator effects (96), it permits rapid withdrawal of the sedative effect. If the patient is not excessively sedated, has adequate oxygenation ($Pao_2 > 60$ mmHg on $Fio_2 < 40\%$), has an intact cough without excessive secretions, and tolerates a T-piece weaning trial without a significant change in vital signs or blood gases for 30 minutes (97), extubation should be undertaken. Some clinicians use the "rapid shallow breathing" index (the ratio of respiratory rate to V_T during spontaneous breathing, f/V_T) to predict the likelihood of weaning (98). However, some studies evaluating f/V_T have reported high rates of false negatives. For this reason, the negative predictive value may be lower than originally reported (99,100).

Use of Noninvasive Ventilation to Facilitate Weaning

Another application of NPPV in patients with COPD exacerbations is to facilitate weaning from invasive mechanical ventilation. COPD patients with acute respiratory failure may initially require endotracheal intubation but, once stabilized, could be switched to NPPV even before standard weaning criteria are met. In this way, the endotracheal tube can be removed earlier and potential complications of prolonged intubation can be avoided. Nava et al. (101) tested this hypothesis in a recent controlled trial on 50 patients intubated for acute respiratory failure due to COPD (described in more detail in Chapter 11). If the patients failed a T-piece weaning trial after 48 hours of invasive mechanical ventilation, patients were randomized to undergo early extubation followed by face mask ventilation or to remain intubated and undergo routine weaning. NPPV patients had higher overall weaning rates (88 vs. 68%) at 21 days, a shorter duration of mechanical ventilation (10.2 vs. 16.6 days), briefer stays in the intensive care unit (15.1 vs. 24 days), and improved 60-day survival rates (92% vs. 72%, NPPV-treated vs. controls, all

$p < 0.05$). In addition, no NPPV-treated patient had a nosocomial pneumonia, compared to seven of the controls.

More recently, Girault et al. prospectively studied a mixed population of chronic respiratory failure patients requiring acute invasive mechanical ventilation (102). Of the 33 patients who failed a 2-hour T-piece weaning trial after 48 hours, those randomized to NPPV had shorter duration of intubation (4.56 days vs. 7.69 days, $p < 0.004$) with no difference in rate of reintubation. Unlike Nava et al., these investigators found no significant difference in overall weaning rates, length of ICU stay, overall duration of mechanical ventilation (including noninvasive), or 3-month survival. Thus, although available studies support the use of NPPV to expedite extubation in patients intubated for acute respiratory failure, important selection factors such as level of sedation, quantity of secretions, and ability to expectorate have not been systematically evaluated. Further studies are needed to confirm the initial promising findings and to better define patient selection criteria.

Another related potential application of NPPV in the weaning process of COPD patients is to avoid reintubation in patients beginning to deteriorate after extubation. Hilbert et al. (103) studied 30 COPD patients who had hypercapnic respiratory failure within 72 hours of extubation and were treated with NPPV. When compared to 30 historically matched controls, NPPV treated patients had significantly lower rates of reintubation (20% vs. 67%), fewer days of ventilatory assistance (6 vs. 11), and shorter ICU stays (8 vs. 14 days, all $p < 0.01$). A trend toward fewer deaths in the NPPV group was seen (2 vs. 6 deaths), but the difference was not statistically different. Although NPPV is being used routinely for this application at some centers, it is important that additional controlled trials be performed to determine whether NPPV can improve outcomes in this subpopulation of patients with acute respiratory failure.

C. Failure to Wean from Mechanical Ventilation

A small percentage of patients intubated for COPD exacerbations fail to wean despite optimal medical therapy and multiple weaning attempts. Thirty to 40% of patients intubated for acute COPD exacerbations die prior to discharge (104,105), and the majority of survivors eventually wean (104). The small percentage that fail to wean usually undergo tracheostomy placement within 3 weeks of intubation. Nava et al. (106) examined outcomes in 42 COPD patients who were unable to wean after 21 days of mechanical ventilation. These investigators found that 55% eventually weaned after an average of 44 days. The remaining 45% had a poor prognosis, with over half dying within 6 months and 78% within 2 years. Ideally, these patients should be enrolled in rehabilitation programs where their functional capacities can be optimized prior to eventual discharge home. Unfortunately, the reality is that most of these patients are not good candidates for rehabilitation or discharge home, either because of severe debility or insufficient financial or family resources. They often require long hospitalizations in acute care hospitals while they await the opening of limited beds in chronic ventilator facilities.

D. Prognosis of Invasive Mechanical Ventilation in COPD

A number of studies have examined the survival of patients with COPD who are intubated for acute respiratory failure (104,107–109). Among COPD patients ventilated for greater than 24 hours, average survival to hospital discharge ranges from 64 to 74% (104,110). A report on outcomes of COPD patients admitted to ICUs for exacerbations from the Acute Physiology Analysis and Chronic Health Evaluation (APACHE) III database found ICU mortality rates of 16% and 32% for the entire hospital stay (105). In addition, advanced age, poor functional status, low albumin, and difficulty with weaning are all risk factors associated with a poor prognosis (104). In one study (111), 69% of patients with COPD requiring more than 10 days of mechanical ventilation died prior to hospital discharge. These studies also show that after a COPD patient requires invasive mechanical ventilation for acute respiratory failure, the longer-term prognosis is poor. Many patients have recurrent bouts of acute respiratory failure, and only 20–40% of these patients are alive 1 year after the initial hospitalization (104,111).

Outcomes of COPD patients with tracheostomies receiving mechanical ventilation at home have also been reported. Robert et al. (112) reported average survivals of 2–3 years for COPD patients receiving home mechanical ventilation. More recently, improved survivals averaging 4.3 years among more than 259 such patients have been reported (113), with younger and better oxygenated patients having the best survivals. These results show that home invasive mechanical ventilation is a viable option for patients with COPD who are unable to wean. However, success requires well-organized and financed programs such as those found in France. Less well-organized and financed programs (such as those found in the United States) are less likely to have equally favorable outcomes.

E. End-of-Life Decision Making

Initiation of mechanical ventilation, whether invasive or noninvasive, should be performed in accordance with the wishes of the patient or those of the health care proxy if the patient is incompetent. Ideally, patients should be informed about the ventilatory options and possible outcomes well in advance of a crisis, so that they and their loved ones can have discussions and make decisions under less stressful circumstances. This is particularly important if patients do not want life support, although they may reverse their decisions at any time. The increasing use of noninvasive ventilation for acute respiratory failure in COPD patients has changed the ethical decision-making process somewhat. Although the modality is often used for life support, it is much more acceptable to most patients than invasive mechanical ventilation. Many patients will accept a trial of it even if they have decided to forgo endotracheal intubation. In one study, noninvasive ventilation was able to correct gas exchange abnormalities in 7 of 11 patients who had refused endotracheal intubation (74). NPPV should be made available to patients who satisfy criteria for its use, but they should be informed that NPPV is being used as a form of life support. Unless the patient or their health care proxy changes their mind on "Do Not Intubate" status, intubation should not be performed if noninvasive ventilation fails.

V. Summary and Conclusions

Concepts concerning mechanical ventilation in patients with severe COPD have been evolving, with several important advances occurring in recent years. These concepts are based on an understanding of basic pathophysiological defects observed in COPD patients that have been elucidated in recent decades. It has long been known that the fundamental defect in severe COPD is minimally reversible expiratory flow limitation. This limitation and the accompanying loss in lung elasticity predisposes to lung and chest wall hyperinflation, placing the inspiratory muscles at a mechanical disadvantage. In many patients, these muscles are precariously poised near the point of failure so that any additional load can push the system over the edge, precipitating respiratory muscle fatigue and an episode of acute respiratory collapse. Increased awareness of the consequences of expiratory flow limitation, dynamic hyperinflation, and resulting autoPEEP fundamentally alters the approach to mechanical ventilation in COPD patients. Familiarity with the physiological effects of autoPEEP and its potential complications helps the clinician to more effectively manage patients with severe obstructive disease. In addition, the increased understanding of the effects of both critical illness as well as potential side effects of routine therapeutic interventions allow the formulation of a comprehensive patient care plan.

One implication of the advances in basic pathophysiological understanding is that the intervention used to stabilize the ventilatory imbalance may be minimal. Accordingly, NPPV has been very successful in partially assisting ventilation in patients with acute exacerbations of COPD, serving as a "crutch" while medical interventions are given time to reduce airway resistance and restore the precarious balance. Based on studies showing improved morbidity and mortality and shorter ICU stays among NPPV-treated patients, many clinicians now consider NPPV to be the ventilatory modality of first choice for acute respiratory failure in appropriately selected COPD patients. NPPV is also being evaluated as a technique to expedite weaning of COPD patients, although further studies are needed before this can be routinely recommended.

When invasive mechanical ventilation is required, the preferred ventilatory strategy is to avoid excessive $\overset{\prime}{V_T}$ and to use properly selected respiratory and inspiratory flow rates to allow for sufficient expiratory time. The justification of this strategy is to avoid excessive autoPEEP and its associated complications of hypotension and barotrauma at the expense of high $Paco_2$ levels. If autoPEEP is interfering with ventilator triggering or weaning because of increased inspiratory work, extrinsic PEEP may be added to reduce the inspiratory threshold load. The concepts of reducing dynamic hyperinflation and application of extrinsic PEEP to reduce inspiratory work represent important advances in the management of invasive mechanical ventilation in COPD patients.

Implementation of these ventilator strategies should result in the more efficient use of scarce health care resources and improved patient outcomes. The importance of close communication with patients and their families cannot be overemphasized so that technological advances are used according to patient desires. With continued research, we can also expect a better understanding of the pathophysiological mechanisms underlying COPD that will result in more effective, more comfortable, and less complicated therapeutic approaches. Of course, in the long run, continued efforts directed toward cessation of cigarette smoking offer the best hope of eliminating the need for mechanical ventilation in COPD patients.

References

1. Feinlieb M, Rosenberg HM, Collins JG. Trends in COPD morbidity and mortality in the United States. Am Rev Respir Dis 1989; 140:S9–S18.
2. Hill NS. Current concepts in mechanical ventilation for chronic obstructive pulmonary disease. Semin Respir Crit Care Med 1999; 20(4):375–393.
3. Smith TA, Marini JJ. Impact of PEEP on lung mechanics and work of breathing in severe airflow obstruction. J Appl Physiol 1988; 65(4):1488–1499.
4. Leatherman JW. Mechanical ventilation in obstructive lung disease. Clin Chest Med 1996; 17(3):577–590.
5. Ranieri VM, Grasso S, Fiore T, Giuliani R. Auto-positive end-expiratory pressure and dynamic hyperinflation. Clin Chest Med 1996; 17:379–394.
6. Rochester DF, Braun NMT, Arora NS. Respiratory muscle strength in chronic obstructive pulmonary disease. Am Rev Respir Dis 1979; 119:151–154.
7. Roussos C. Function and fatigue of respiratory muscles. Chest 1985; 88:124S–132S.
8. Roussos C, Macklem P. Diaphragmatic fatigue in man. J Appl Physiol Respir Environ Exerc Physiol 1977; 43(2):189–197.
9. Bellemare F, Grassino A. Effect of pressure and timing of contraction on human diaphragm fatigue. J Appl Physiol Respir Environ Exerc Physiol 1982; 53(5):1190–1195.
10. Bellemare F, Grassino A. Evaluation of human diaphragm fatigue. J Appl Physiol Respir Environ Exerc Physiol 1982; 53(5):1196–1206.
11. Field S, Sanci D. Respiratory muscle oxygen consumption estimated by the dia-

phragm pressure-time index. J Appl Physiol Respir Environ Exerc Physiol 1984; 57(1):44–51.

12. Collett P, Perry C, Engel L. Pressure-time product, flow, and oxygen cost of resistive breathing in humans. J Appl Physiol 1985; 58(4):1263–1272.

13. Bishop B, Hirsch J, Thursby M. Volume, flow and timing of each breath during positive-pressure breathing in man. J Appl Physiol 1978; 45:495–501.

14. Road JD, Leevers AM, Goldman E, Grassino A. Respiratory muscle coordination and diaphragm length during expiratory threshold loading. J Appl Physiol 1991; 70(4):1554–1562.

15. Martin JG, Shore S, Engel LA. Effects of continuous positive airway pressure on respiratory mechanics and pattern of breathing in induced asthma. Am Rev Respir Dis 1982; 126:812–817.

16. Aldrich TK, Hendler JM, Vizioli LD, Park M, Multz AS, Shapiro SM. Intrinsic positive end-expiratory pressure in ambulatory patients with airways obstruction. Am Rev Respir Dis 1993; 147:845–849.

17. Marini JJ. Should PEEP be used in airflow obstruction? Am Rev Respir Dis 1989; 140:1–3.

18. Maltais F, Reissmann H, Navalesi P, Hernandez P, Gursahaney A, Ranieri VM, Sovilj M, Gottfried SB. Comparison of static and dynamic measurements of intrinsic PEEP in mechanically ventilated patients. Am J Respir Crit Care Med 1994; 150:1318–1324.

19. Broseghini C, Brandolese R, Poggi R, Polese G, Manzin E, Milic-Emili J, Rossi A. Respiratory mechanics during the first day of mechanical ventilation in patients with pulmonary edema and chronic airway obstruction. Am Rev Respir Dis 1988; 138:355–361.

20. Ranieri VM, Giuliani R, Cinnella G, Pesce C, Brienza N, Ippolito EL, Pomo V, Fiore T, Gottfried SB, Brienza A. Physiologic effects of positive end-expiratory pressure in patients with chronic obstructive pulmonary disease during acute ventilatory failure and controlled mechanical ventilation. Am Rev Respir Dis 1993; 147: 5–13.

21. Permutt S, Bromberger-Barnea B, Bane HN. Alveolar pressure, pulmonary venous pressure, and the vascular waterfall. Med Thorac 1962; 19:239–260.

22. Pride NB, Permutt S, Riley RL, Bromberger-Barnea B. Determinants of maximal expiratory flow from the lungs. J Appl Physiol 1967; 23:646–662.

23. Aubier M, Murciano D, Milic-Emili J, Touaty E, Daghfous J, Pariente R, Derenne JP. Effects of the administration of O_2 on ventilation and blood gases in patients with chronic obstructive pulmonary disease during acute respiratory failure. Am Rev Respir Dis 1980; 122(5):747–54.

24. Bellemare F, Wight D, Lavigne C, Grassino A. Effect of tension and timing of contraction on the blood flow of the diaphragm. J Appl Physiol Respir Environ Exerc Physiol 1983; 54(6):1596–1606.

25. Bark H, Supinski G, Lamanna J, Kelsen S. Relationship of changes in diaphragmatic muscle blood flow to muscle contractile activity. J Appl Physiol 1987; 62(1): 291–299.

26. Supinski G, DiMarco A, Dibner-Dunlap M. Alterations in diaphragm strength and fatiguability in congestive heart failure. J Appl Physiol 1994; 76(6):2707–2713.

27. McParland C, Krishnan B, Wang Y, Gallagher CG. Inspiratory muscle weakness and dyspnea in chronic heart failure. Am Rev Respir Dis 1992; 146:467–472.
28. Aubier M, Murciano D, Menu Y. Dopamine effects on diaphragmatic strength during acute respiratory failure in chronic obstructive pulmonary disease. Ann Intern Med 1989; 110:17–23.
29. Hussain SNA, Simkus G, Roussos C. Respiratory muscle fatigue: a cause of ventilatory failure in septic shock. J Appl Physiol 1985; 58(6):2033–2040.
30. Hussain SNA, Graham R, Rutledge F, Roussos C. Respiratory muscle energetics during endotoxic shock in dogs. J Appl Physiol 1986; 60(2):486–493.
31. Mier-Jedrzejowicz A, Brophy C, Green M. Respiratory muscle weakness during upper respiratory tract infections. Am Rev Respir Dis 1988; 138:5–7.
32. Bolton CF, Gilbert JJ, Hahn AF, Sibbald WJ. Polyneuropathy in critically ill patients. J Neurol Neurosurg Psychiatry 1984; 47:1223–1231.
33. Weiner P, Azgad Y, Weiner M. The effect of corticosteroids on inspiratory muscle performance in humans. Chest 1993; 104:1788–1791.
34. Decramer M, Stas KJ. Corticosteroid-induced myopathy involving respiratory muscles in patients with chronic obstructive pulmonary disease or asthma. Am Rev Respir Dis 1992; 146:800–802.
35. Douglas JA, Tuxen DV, Horne M, Scheinkestel CD, Weinmann M, Czarny D, Bowes G. Myopathy in severe asthma. Am Rev Respir Dis 1992; 146:517–519.
36. Leatherman JW, Fluegel WL, David WS, Davies SF, Iber C. Muscle weakness in mechanically ventilated patients with severe asthma. Am J Respir Crit Care Med 1996; 153:1686–1690.
37. Griffin D, Fairman N, Coursin D, Rawsthorne L, Grossman JE. Acute myopathy during treatment of status asthmaticus with corticosteroids and steroidal muscle relaxants. Chest 1992; 102:510–514.
38. Darrah WC, Johnston JR, Mirakhur RH. Vecuronium infusions for prolonged muscle relaxation in the intensive care unit. Crit Care Med 1987; 17:1297–1300.
39. Frankel H, Jeng J, Tilly E, St. Andre A, Champion H. The impact of implementation of neuromuscular blockade monitoring standards in a surgical intensive care unit. Am Surg 1996; 62:503–506.
40. Giostra E, Magistris MR, Pizzolato G, Cox J, Chevrolet J-C. Neuromuscular disorder in intensive care unit patients treated with pancuronium bromide. Chest 1994; 106:210–220.
41. Meyer TJ, Hill NS. Noninvasive positive pressure ventilation to treat respiratory failure. Ann Intern Med 1994; 120:760–770.
42. Carrey Z, Gottfried SB, Levy RD. Ventilatory muscle support in respiratory failure with nasal positive pressure ventilation. Chest 1990; 97:150–158.
43. Sauret J, Guitart AC, Rodriguez-Frojan G, Comedella R. Intermittent short-term negative pressure ventilation and increased oxygenation in COPD patients with severe hypercapnic respiratory failure. Chest 1991; 100:455–459.
44. Petrof BJ, Legare M, Goldberg P, Milic-Emili J, Gottfried SB. Continuous positive airway pressure reduces work of breathing and dyspnea during weaning from mechanical ventilation in severe chronic obstructive pulmonary disease. Am Rev Respir Dis 1990; 141(2):281–289.

45. de Lucas P, Tarancon C, Puente L, Rodriguez C, Tatay E, Monturiol J. Nasal continuous positive airway pressure in patients with COPD in acute respiratory failure. A study of immediate effects. Chest 1993; 104(6):1694–1697.

46. Appendini L, Patessio A, Zanaboni S, Carone M, Gukov B, Donner CF, Rossi A. Physiologic effects of positive end-expiratory pressure support during exacerbations of chronic obstructive pulmonary disease. Am J Respir Crit Care Med 1994; 149:1069–1076.

47. Nava S, Ambrosino N, Bruschi C, Confaloniere M, Rampulla C. Physiological effects of flow and pressure triggering during non-invasive mechanical ventilation in patients with chronic obstructive pulmonary disease. Thorax 1997; 52(3):249–254.

48. Brochard L, Isabey D, Piquet J, Amaro P, Mancebo J, Messadi A, Brun-Buisson C, Rauss A, Lemaire F, Harf A. Reversal of acute exacerbations of chronic obstructive lung disease by inspiratory assistance with a face mask. N Engl J Med 1990; 323(22):1523–1530.

49. Daskalopoulou E, Teara V, Fekete V, et al. Treatment of acute respiratory failure in COPD patients with positive airway pressure via nasal mask (NIPPV). Chest 1993; 103:S271.

50. Confalonieri M, Aiolfi S, Gandola L, Scartabellati A, Della Porta R, Parigi P. Severe exacerbations of chronic obstructive pulmonary disease treated with BiPAP by nasal mask. Respiration 1994; 61:310–316.

51. Vitacca M, Clini E, Rubini F, Nava S, Foglio K, Ambrosino N. Non-invasive mechanical ventilation in severe chronic obstructive lung disease and acute respiratory failure: short- and long-term prognosis. Intensive Care Med 1996; 22(2):94–100.

52. Chevrolet J, Jolliet P, Abajo B, Toussi A, Louis M. Nasal positive pressure ventilation in patients with acute respiratory failure. Chest 1991; 100:775–782.

53. Conway JH, Hitchcock RA, Godfrey RC, Carroll MP. Nasal intermittent positive pressure ventilation in acute exacerbations of chronic obstructive pulmonary disease: A preliminary study. Respir Med 1993; 87:387–394.

54. Sacks H, Chalmers TC, Smith HJ. Randomized versus historical controls for clinical trials. Am J Med 1982; 72:233–240.

55. Bott J, Carroll MP, Conway JH, et al. Randomized controlled trial of nasal ventilation in acute ventilatory failure due to chronic obstructive airways disease. Lancet 1993; 341:1555–1557.

56. Kramer N, Meyer TJ, Meharg J, Cece RD, Hill NS. Randomized, prospective trial of noninvasive positive pressure ventilation in acute respiratory failure. Am J Respir Crit Care Med 1995; 151:1799–1806.

57. Brochard L, Mancebo J, Wysocki M, Lofaso F, Conti G, Rauss A, Simonneau G, Benito S, Gasparetto A, Lemaire F, Isabey D, Harf A. Noninvasive ventilation for acute exacerbations of chronic obstructive pulmonary disease. N Engl J Med 1995; 333:818–822.

58. Celikel T, Sungur M, Ceyhan B, Karakurt S. Comparison of noninvasive positive pressure ventilation with standard medical therapy in hypercapnic acute respiratory failure. Chest 1998; 114(6):1636–1642.

58a. Plant PK, Owen JL, Elliot MW. Early use of noninvasive ventilation for acute exacerbations of chronic obstructive pulmonary disease on general respiratory wards: a multicenter randomized controlled trial. Lancet 2000; 355:1931–1935.

59. Barbé F, Togores B, Rubí M, Pons S, Maimo A, Agustí AGN. Noninvasive ventilatory support does not facilitate recovery from acute respiratory failure in chronic obstructive disease. Eur Respir J 1996; 9:1240–1245.

60. Keenan SP, Brake D. An evidence-based approach to noninvasive ventilation in acute respiratory failure. Crit Care Clin 1998; 14(3):359–372.

61. Confalonieri M, Parigi P, Scarabellati A, Aiolfi S, Scorsetti S, Nava S, Gandola L. Noninvasive mechanical ventilation improves immediate and long-term outcome of COPD patients with acute respiratory failure. Eur Respir J 1996; 9:422–430.

62. Nava S, Evangelisti I, Rampulla C, Compagnoni ML, Fracchia C, Rubini F. Human and financial cost of noninvasive mechanical ventilation in patients affected by COPD and acute respiratory failure. Chest 1997; 111:1631–1638.

63. Ambrosino N, Foglio K, Rubini F, Cline E, Nava S, Vitacca M. Non-invasive mechanical ventilation in acute respiratory failure due to chronic obstructive pulmonary disease: correlates for success. Thorax 1995; 50:755–757.

64. Soo Hoo GW, Santiago S, Williams A. Nasal mechanical ventilation for hypercapnic respiratory failure in chronic obstructive pulmonary disease: determinants for success and failure. Crit Care Med 1994; 22:1253–1261.

65. Benhamou D, Girault C, Faure C, Portier F, Muir JF. Nasal mask ventilation in acute respiratory failure. Chest 1992; 102:912–917.

66. Meduri GU, Abou-Shala N, Fox RC, Jones CB, Leeper KV, Wunderink RG. Noninvasive face mask mechanical ventilation in patients with acute hypercapnic respiratory failure. Chest 1991; 100:445–454.

67. Wysocki M, Tric L, Wolff MA. Noninvasive pressure support ventilation in patients with acute respiratory failure. Chest 1993; 103:907–913.

68. Wysocki M, Tric L, Wolff MA, Millet H, Herman B. Noninvasive pressure support ventilation in patients with acute respiratory failure. A randomized comparison with conventional therapy. Chest 1995; 107:761–768.

69. Elliot MW, Steven MH, Phillips GD. Non-invasive mechanical ventilation for acute respiratory failure. Br Med J 1990; 300:358–360.

70. Shivaram U, Cash ME, Beal A. Nasal continuous positive airway pressure in decompensated hypercapnic respiratory failure as a complication of sleep apnea. Chest 1993; 104:770–774.

71. Meduri GU, Turner RE, Abou-Shala N, Wunderlink R, Tolley E. Noninvasive positive pressure ventilation via face mask. First-line intervention in patients with acute hypercapnic and hypoxemic respiratory failure. Chest 1996; 109:179–193.

72. Greenbaum DM, Millen JE, Eross B, Snyder JV, Grenvi KA, Safar P. Continuous positive airway pressure without tracheal intubation in spontaneously breathing patients. Chest 1976; 69:615.

73. De Vita MA, Friedman Y, Petrella V. Mask continuous positive airway pressure in AIDS. Crit Care Med 1993; 9:137–151.

74. Meduri GU, Fox RC, Abou-Shala N, Leeper KV, Wunderlink RG. Noninvasive mechanical ventilation via face mask in patients with acute respiratory failure who refused endotracheal intubation. Crit Care Med 1994; 22:1584–1590.

75. Girault C, Richard JC, Chevron V, Tamion F, Pasquis P, Leroy J, Bonmarchard G.

Comparative physiologic effects of noninvasive assist-control and pressure support ventilation in acute hypercapnic respiratory failure. Chest 1997; 111(6):1639–1648.

76. Vitacca M, Rubini F, Foglio K, Scalvini S, Nava S, Ambrosino N. Non-invasive modalities of positive pressure ventilation improve the outcome of acute exacerbations in COLD patients. Intens Care Med 1993; 19:450–455.

77. Jubran A, Van de Graffe WB, Tobin MJ. Variability of patient-ventilator interaction with pressure support ventilation in patients with chronic obstructive pulmonary disease. Am J Respir Crit Care Med 1995; 152:129–136.

78. Pollack CJ, Fleisch K, Dowsey K. Treatment of acute bronchospasm with beta-adrenergic agonist aerosols delivered by a nasal bilevel positive airway pressure circuit. Ann Emerg Med 1995; 26(5):552–557.

79. Make BJ, Hill NS, Goldberg AI, Bach JR, Criner GJ, Dunne PE, Gilmartin ME, Heffner JE, Kacmarek R, Keens TG, McInturff S, O'Donohue WJJ, Oppenheimer EA, Robert D. Mechanical ventilation beyond the intensive care unit. Report of a consensus conference of the American College of Chest Physicians. Chest 1998; 113:S289–S344.

80. ATS. Standards for the diagnosis and care of patients with chronic obstructive pulmonary disease. Am J Respir Crit Care Med 1995; 152:S7–S120.

81. Slutsky AS. ACCP consensus conference. Mechanical ventilation. Chest 1993; 104: 1833–1859.

82. Tuxen DV, Lane S. The effects of ventilatory pattern on hyperinflation, airway pressures, and circulation in mechanical ventilation of patients with severe airflow obstruction. Am Rev Respir Dis 1987; 136:872–879.

83. Tobin M. Mechanical ventilation. N Engl J Med 1994; 330(15):1056–1061.

84. Bonmarchand G, Chevron V, Chopin C, Jusserand D, Girault C, Moritz F, Leroy J, Pasquis P. Increased initial flow rate reduces inspiratory work of breathing during pressure support ventilation in patients with exacerbation of chronic obstructive pulmonary disease. Intens Care Med 1996; 22:1147–1154.

85. Connors AF, McCaffree RD, Gray BA. Effect of inspiratory flow rate on gas exchange during mechanical ventilation. Am Rev Respir Dis 1981; 124:537–543.

86. Crotti S, Pelosi P, Mascheroni D, et al. The effect of extrinsic PEEP on lung inflation and regional compliance in mechanically ventilated patients: A CT scan study. Intens Care Med 1995; 21:S135.

87. Darioloi R, Perret C. Mechanical controlled hypoventilation in status asthmaticus. Am Rev Respir Dis 1984; 129:385–387.

88. Madison J, Irwin R. Status asthmaticus. In: Irwin R, Cerra F, Rippe J, eds. Intensive Care Medicine: 4th ed. New York: Lippincott-Raven, 1999; 601.

89. Foner BJ, Norwood SH, Taylor RW. The acute respiratory distress syndrome. In: Civetta JM, Taylor RW, Kirby RR, eds. Critical Care. 3rd ed. New York: Lippincott-Raven, 1997:1835–1836.

90. Dick P, Sassoon CH. Patient-ventilator synchrony. Clin Chest Med 1996; 17:452–472.

91. Brochard L, Rauss A, Benito S, Conti G, Mancebo J, Rekik N, Gasparetto A, Lemaire F. Comparison of three methods of gradual withdrawal from ventilatory support during weaning from mechanical ventilation. Am J Respir Crit Care Med 1994; 150:896–903.

92. Esteban A, Frutos F, Tobin MJ, Alia I, Solsona JF, Valverdu I, Fernandez R, de la Cal MA, Benito S, Tomas R, Carriedo D, Macias S, Blanco J. A comparison of four methods of weaning patients from mechanical ventilation. N Engl J Med 1995; 332:345–50.

93. Esteban A, Alia I, Gordo F, Fernandes R, Solsona JF, Vallverdu I, Marcias S, Allegue JM, Blanco J, Carriedo D, Leon M, de la Cal MA, Toboada F, Gonzalez de Velasco J, Palazon E, Carrizosa F, Tomas R, Suarez J, Goldwasser RS. Extubation outcome after spontaneous breathing trials with T-tube or pressure support ventilation. Am J Respir Crit Care Med 1997; 156:459–465.

94. Ely E, Baker A, Dunagan D, Burke H, Smith A, Kelly P, Johnson M, Browder R, Bowton D, Haponik E. Effect on the duration of mechanical ventilation of identifying patients capable of breathing spontaneously. N Engl J Med 1996; 335:1864–1869.

95. Kollef MH, Shapiro SD, Silver P, St. John RE, Prentice D, Sauer S, Ahrens TS, Shannon W, Baker-Clinkscale D. A randomized, controlled trial of protocol-directed versus physician-directed weaning from mechanical ventilation. Crit Care Med 1997; 25:567–574.

96. Eames WO, Rooke GA, Wu RS-C, Bishop MJ. Comparison of the effects of etomidate, propofol, and thiopental on the respiratory resistance after tracheal intubation. Anesthesiology 1996; 84:1307–1311.

97. Esteban A, Alia I, Tobin MJ, Gil A, Gordo F, Valverdu I, Blanch L, Bonet A, Vazquez A, de Pablo R, Torres A, de la Cal MA, Macias S. Effect of spontaneous breathing trial duration on outcome of attempts to discontinue mechanical ventilation. The Spanish Lung Failure Collaborative Group. Am J Respir Crit Care Med 1999; 159(2):512–518.

98. Yang KL, Tobin MJ. A prospective study of indexes predicting the outcome of trials of weaning from mechanical ventilation. N Eng J Med 1991; 324:1445–1450.

99. Epstein S. Etiology of extubation failure and the predictive value of the rapid shallow breathing index. Am J Respir Crit Care Med 1995; 152:545–549.

100. Lee K, Hui K, Chan T, Tan W, Lim T. Rapid shallow breathing (frequency-tidal volume ratio) did not predict extubation outcome. Chest 1994; 105:540–543.

101. Nava S, Ambrosino N, Clini E, Prato M, Orlando G, Vitacca M, Brigada P, Fracchia C, Rubini F. Noninvasive mechanical ventilation in the Weaning of patients with respiratory failure due to chronic obstructive pulmonary disease. A randomized, controlled trial. Ann Intern Med 1998; 128:721–728.

102. Girault C, Daudenthun I, Chevron V, Tamion F, Leroy J, Bonmarchand G. Noninvasive ventilation as a systematic extubation and weaning technique in acute-on-chronic respiratory failure. Am J Respir Crit Care Med 1999; 160:86–92.

103. Hilbert G, Gruson D, Portel L, Gbikpi-Benissan G, Cardinaud JP. Noninvasive pressure support ventilation in COPD patients with postextubation hypercapnic respiratory insufficiency. Eur Respir J 1998; 11:1349–1353.

104. Menzies R, Gibbons W, Goldberg P. Determinants of weaning and survival among patients with COPD who require mechanical ventilation for acute respiratory failure. Chest 1989; 95:398–405.

105. Seneff MC, Wagner DP, Wagner RP, et al. Hospital and 1 year survival of patients

admitted to intensive care units with acute exacerbations of chronic obstructive pulmonary disease. JAMA 1995; 274:1852–1857.

106. Nava S, Rubini F, Zanotti E, Ambrosino N, Bruschi C, Vitacca M, Fracchia C, Rampulla C. Survival and prediction of successful ventilator weaning in COPD patients requiring mechanical ventilation for more than 21 days. Eur Respir J 1994; 7:1645–1652.

107. Gillespie DJ, Marsh HMM, Divertie MB, Meadows JA. Clinical outcome of respiratory failure in patients requiring prolonged (>24 hours) mechanical ventilation. Chest 1986; 90:364–369.

108. Kaelin R, Assimacopoulos A, Cheverolet JC. Failure to predict six month survival of patients with COPD requiring mechanical ventilation by analysis of simple indices. A prospective study. Chest 1987; 92:971–978.

109. Petheram IS, Branthwaite MA. Mechanical ventilation for pulmonary disease. A six year study. Anaesthesia 1980; 35:467–473.

110. Stauffer JL, Fayter NA, Graves B, Cromb M, Lynch JC, Goebel P. Survival following mechanical ventilation for acute respiratory failure in adult men. Chest 1993; 104:1222–1229.

111. Spicher JE, White DP. Outcome and function following prolonged mechanical ventilation. Arch Intern Med 1987; 147:421–428.

112. Robert D, Willing TN, Paulus J, et al. Long term nasal ventilation in neuromuscular disorders: report of a consensus conference. Eur Respir Rev 1993; 6:599–606.

113. Muir JF, Cuvelier A, Tengang B, et al. Long term home nasal intermittent positive pressure ventilation (NPPV) + oxygen therapy (LTOT) versus LTOT alone in severe hypercapnic COPD. Preliminary results of a European multicenter trial. Am J Respir Crit Care Med 1997; 155:A408.

13

Strategies of Mechanical Ventilation in Patients with Acute Respiratory Distress Syndrome

JOSEPH V. MEHARG

Roger Williams Hospital
Providence, Rhode Island

JAMES R. KLINGER

Brown University School of Medicine
Rhode Island Hospital
Providence, Rhode Island

I. Introduction

Over the last decade, numerous modalities and strategies have been developed and advocated as improvements in ventilating patients with acute respiratory distress syndrome (ARDS). Virtually every aspect of mechanical ventilation has been examined in an effort to improve gas exchange or to avoid lung damage. Tidal volume (VT), airway pressure (P_{aw}), inspiratory time, mode of mechanical ventilation, position of the patient, even the medium used to ventilate the patient have all been studied in an attempt to improve outcome in patients with acute lung injury. There is evidence to suggest that these efforts are beginning to pay dividends. In some centers, mortality from ARDS appears to be declining (1). Recent studies (2) have demonstrated that a protective lung strategy can improve survival in ARDS, suggesting that how we use the ventilator really does make a difference. In this chapter we will present the evidence for much of the rationale that has been used to design modern strategies for ventilating the ARDS patient. We will review the various modes of mechanical ventilation and discuss their effects on gas exchange, hemodynamics, lung injury, and, where data are available, on outcomes.

II. Background

Broadly defined, ARDS is an acute, diffuse lung injury, manifesting epithelial and endothelial cell damage. This damage leads to depleted or dysfunctional surfactant and increased surface tension, interstitial and alveolar edema, and a reduction in lung volume and compliance. Hypoxemia occurs as the result of reduced ventilation-to-perfusion (V/Q) matching (3) and intrapulmonary shunting. At the same time, the dead space-to-tidal volume ratio (VD/VT) can increase to as much as 65%, and minute volume (VE) requirements may double (4). Resistance to airflow is increased (5) with fewer or narrower airways creating a spectrum of impedance characteristics that result in regional variations in alveolar time constants, unequal distribution of ventilation, and incomplete emptying of some alveoli during expiration. Early in the course of ARDS, much of the lung is recruitable with positive end-expiratory pressure (PEEP) or prone positioning (6–9), but as the disease progresses, alveolar damage can result in substantial atelectasis that becomes increasingly difficult to reverse. It seems unlikely that any one ventilator strategy can be effective across this spectrum of pathophysiology. Rather, ventilatory therapy may need to be adjusted as the patient's disease progresses or as recovery begins.

The goals of mechanical ventilation in ARDS are to assume the work of breathing, recruit collapsed alveoli, and distribute VT in a way that matches lung perfusion. High transpulmonary pressures are often required to reach some of these objectives. Unfortunately, these pressures may result in alveolar overdistension, the release of inflammatory mediators, and hemodynamic compromise. The challenge in ventilating patients with ARDS is achieving adequate gas exchange while avoiding ventilator-induced lung injury (VILI) (9). This chapter begins with a brief review of VILI and alveolar recruitment, as we feel that they constitute the underpinnings of current ventilatory management strategies in ARDS.

III. Ventilator-Induced Lung Injury

Barotrauma is the term commonly used to describe the presence of extra-alveolar gas that occurs when transpulmonary pressures exceed the tensile strength of the alveoli or airways. Examples include pneumothorax, pneumomediastinum, pulmonary interstitial emphysema, pneumoperitoneum, subcutaneous emphysema (10–12), and systemic air embolus (13). Histological findings in barotrauma include tension lung cysts, subpleural air cysts, and bronchiolectasis (14), and these findings have been shown to correlate with high VT, high peak inspiratory pressure (PIP), and an increased incidence of pneumothorax (15). However, the relative importance of high pressure versus excessive tidal excursion in the etiology of barotrauma is unclear, and in several studies of ARDS (16,17) pneumothorax did not appear to correlate with airway pressure or VT.

In 1964, Greenfield and colleagues (18) described a type of VILI that seemed distinct from barotrauma. Dogs ventilated for 2 hours at a PIP of 26–32 cm H_2O demonstrated atelectasis and increased surface tension of lung extracts. Later, Webb and Tierney (19) found that a PIP of 30 cm H_2O caused pulmonary edema in rats after 1 hour of ventilation and that a PIP of 45 cm H_2O produced edema in as little as 13 minutes. Excessive end-inspiratory alveolar volume appears to be the principal determinate of this type of injury (20). Dreyfuss et al. (21) found that pulmonary edema developed in rats receiving high VT (40 mL/kg) via positive or negative pressure ventilation but did not occur in rats ventilated with low VT (13 mL/kg) at high pressure (PIP 45 cm H_2O due to chest wall strapping). Elevated end-inspiratory volume can cause pulmonary edema whether it is achieved by increasing VT or by increasing functional residual capacity (FRC) with PEEP and using low VT (22,23). In fact, recent evidence suggests that mean airway pressure (P_{aw}) contributes more to volutrauma than VT (22). However, high P_{aw} without elevated end-inspiratory volumes generally does not result in lung injury (24,25). Thus, the term volutrauma is used to describe this type of VILI.

In addition to alveolar overdistension, VILI may be caused by repeated opening and collapse of alveoli (23). The high pressures required to open collapsed alveoli causes mechanical stress that injures the alveolar epithelia and increases radial traction on pulmonary microvessels resulting in increased endothelial cell permeability (26). Furthermore, repeated opening and collapse of alveoli reduces the quantity and function of surfactant by increasing loss of surfactant into the airways (27) and by disrupting the surface film upon reinflation (28,29). Increased surface tension greatly contributes to end expiratory collapse in ARDS. Thus, repeated opening and collapse of alveoli can directly injure the lung, a self-perpetuating process due to the adverse effects on surfactant function.

Volutrauma in healthy lung causes the same time-dependent pathological findings as in ARDS; diffuse alveolar damage (21,30,31), increased capillary permeability (24,25,31–33), and altered alveolar epithelial cell function (34). Recent studies are now beginning to link large VT and mechanical stress to the release of inflammatory mediators that may in turn potentiate VILI or even multisystem organ failure (35–39).

Avoiding VILI requires a method of assessing alveolar overdistension. Measurement of static end-inspiratory pressure, commonly known as plateau pressure (P_{plat}), can be used to assess the level of alveolar distension. However, it is not a measure of transpulmonary pressure and can lead to overestimation of alveolar distension when chest wall compliance is reduced (5,40–43). Another approach to evaluating the effect of P_{aw} on alveolar inflation is to evaluate the pressure-volume relationship of the respiratory system.

A. Pressure-Volume Curves

In the normal lung, the pressure-volume (PV) curve has a sigmoidal shape with a low slope at lung volumes well below FRC, followed by an increase in the slope at volumes around FRC, and ending with a decrease in slope at high lung volumes. Hysteresis is demonstrated by higher volumes at any given pressure during expiration than during inspiration (Fig. 1).

The initial change in slope of the inspiratory limb of the PV curve has been referred to as the lower inflection point (LIP) or P_{flex}. In ARDS, the pressure at which LIP occurs is frequently elevated (Fig. 2). It is speculated that the LIP, if present, represents the pressure at which the majority of the atelectatic alveoli are recruited (8,44), although Gattinoni (45) and others (46,47) have demonstrated continued recruitment above LIP. Some investigators have recommended setting PEEP 2 cm H_2O above LIP to prevent alveolar collapse during expiration. The LIP may represent the pressure needed to recruit the majority of collapsed alveoli, but the pressure needed to maintain alveolar inflation may be considerably less and is probably best described by the lower inflection point on the deflation limb of the PV curve (46). Because most techniques for constructing a PV curve only measure the inspiratory limb, this value is often not known.

The decrease in slope of the PV curve at high lung volumes is known as the upper inflection point (UIP) and may represent the point at which alveolar overdistension begins (Fig. 2). Ventilating below the UIP may avoid alveolar

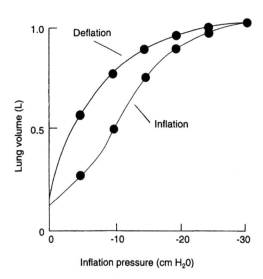

Figure 1 Static pressure-volume curve in the isolated normal lung. Higher pressures are required for each volume during inflation than deflation. (From Ref. 257.)

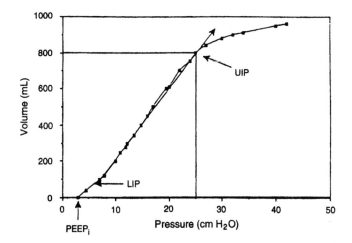

Figure 2 Pressure-volume curve in a patient with ARDS. The lower and upper pressures associated with a change in the slope from the linear portion of the pressure-volume curve are referred to as the upper and lower "inflection" points (LIP and UIP, respectively, PEEPi is intrinsic PEEP). (From Ref. 258.)

overdistension and volutrauma. However, the UIP may simply signal the end of recruitment and not overdistension. Also, if overdistension and recruitment occur simultaneously in different parts of the lung, no UIP may be identifiable on the PV curve (46).

The use of bedside respiratory mechanics to guide our ventilator strategies is far from straightforward. Recent work suggests that the LIP and the UIP can be influenced by deranged chest wall mechanics, necessitating measurement of pleural pressures for accurate assessment of PV relations. Also, global assessment of respiratory mechanics may not be representative of the behavior of individual units subjected to different regional pressures and loads (48). The volume created by PEEP, whether intrinsic (PEEPi) or extrinsic, also needs to be considered when plotting these curves. Failure to do so may lead to erroneous conclusions regarding the PEEP-induced changes in the respiratory system mechanics (47,49,50). Finally, the PV curve for any patient cannot be thought of as a constant measure. Repeated measurements of the PV curve in an individual patient can show substantial changes as lung compliance is affected by the progression or resolution of the underlying lung disease or by changes in lung volume accomplished by changes in the method of ventilatory support (Fig. 3).

Thus, there are several limitations to interpretation of the PV curve that have dampened enthusiasm for this technique with many investigators. Rimensberger et al. (51) recently concluded that the inflation limb of the PV curve is

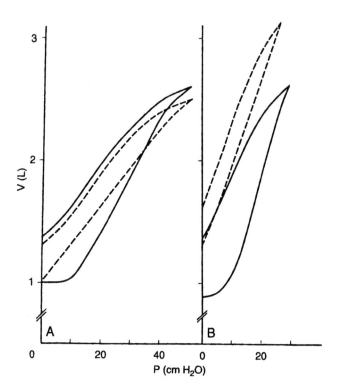

Figure 3 Successive pressure-volume curves in two patients (A and B) with ARDS, early (solid curve) and later (dashed curves) in the course of their disease. Loss of a lower inflection point is demonstrated with disease progression. (From Ref. 44.)

of little significance for positive pressure ventilation and that LIP is irrelevant to the setting of the PEEP, except as it describes the pressure needed to initially open collapsed lung units. Although it is tempting to use PV curves as a map with which to set end inspiratory and end expiratory pressures, there are few data to suggest that operating within the linear portion of the PV curve ensures adequate alveolar recruitment or prevents alveolar overdistension. The limitations of this technique need to be considered when designing ventilation strategies for ARDS.

IV. Alveolar Recruitment

Alveolar recruitment has long been a goal in ventilating patients with ARDS, primarily because it leads to a reduction in the shunt fraction and improved oxygenation. In addition, adequate alveolar recruitment and prevention of repeated alveolar collapse and reopening appear to be vital to the prevention of VILI.

A. Mean Airway Pressure (P_{aw})

The primary determinant of alveolar recruitment is transpulmonary pressure [pulmonary alveolar pressure (P_{alv}) minus pleural pressure]. In the clinical setting, mean P_{aw} may serve as a surrogate of mean P_{alv}, because they are related by the formula:

$$\text{Mean } P_{alv} = \text{Mean } P_{aw} + [(VE/60) \times (R_{exp}-R_{insp})]$$

where VE is minute ventilation and R_{exp} and R_{insp} represent expiratory and inspiratory resistance, respectively (52). In the clinical setting, mean P_{aw} is determined by adjusting PEEP, VT, and the ratio of inspiratory to expiratory time (I:E).

Increasing mean P_{aw} will improve oxygenation, presumably by recruiting collapsed alveoli that are perfused and thereby reducing intrapulmonary shunt or by improving ventilation in alveoli with long time constants and thereby reducing areas of low V/Q. Pesenti et al. (53) investigated mean P_{aw} in acute lung injury induced by saline lavage. PEEP just above LIP improved oxygenation. Raising PEEP further did not improve oxygenation, but raising mean P_{aw} 5 cm H_2O via prolonging the inspiratory time did. While PEEP increased Paco$_2$ and VD/VT, raising the mean P_{aw} decreased VD/VT in this model. At the same PEEP, oxygenation and ventilation were better with the higher mean P_{aw}.

The beneficial effect of increasing mean P_{aw} on oxygenation must be weighed against the increased risk of volutrauma. Broccard et al. (54) found that increased mean P_{aw} correlated with a histologic lung injury score (Fig. 4) and changes in capillary permeability in rabbits and that mean P_{aw} correlated better with lung injury than VT. Ludwigs et al. (34) found that lung injury, as assessed by TcDTPA clearance, was greater in rabbits ventilated with pressure control ventilation (PCV) and an I:E ratio of 4:1 than in rabbits ventilated with VCV and PEEP. PEEP, P_{plat}, and VT were equal in both modes of ventilation, but P_{aw} was higher with PCV and long I:E than with VCV and PEEP. Thus, raising mean P_{aw} appears to be associated with greater lung injury in animals. However, there are no clinical data available that indicate how much the risk of VILI is increased by raising mean P_{aw}.

B. Sighs

Atelectasis develops during positive pressure ventilation with delivery of normal VT. In 1959, Mead and Collier (55) found that lung compliance in dogs decreases after one hour of mechanical ventilation. This decrease was reversed by intermittently providing a large VT breath termed a "sigh." In anesthetized patients, Bendixen et al. (56) demonstrated a gradual 22% fall in oxygenation and 15%

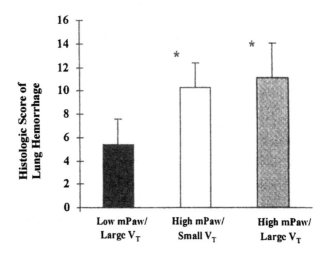

Figure 4   Histological scoring of hemorrhage in isolated rabbit lungs. High mean airway pressure resulted in greater histological evidence of lung hemorrhage than did large tidal excursions. (From Ref. 54.)

drop in compliance after a mean of 76 minutes of positive pressure ventilation with normal VT. These abnormalities could be reversed by the addition of sighs. More recent work by Rothen and colleagues (57) found that atelectasis as measured by CT scans could be diminished in humans receiving general anesthesia by inflating the lung to a pressure of 30 cm H_2O for 15 seconds. Atelectasis could be eliminated altogether by inflating to a pressure of 40 cm H_2O, which was roughly equal to the vital capacity. In another study (58), a sigh to P_{plat} of 30–45 cm H_2O for 20 seconds resulted in significant improvement in oxygenation within 10 minutes (86.9 ± 5.5 to 94.3 ± 2.3% O_2 Hgb saturation). This improvement lasted at least 4 hours in 10 of 14 subjects. All 4 patients with less than 4 hours' improvement were on PEEP < 10, and in 3 of 3 increasing the PEEP led to sustained improvements in postsigh oxygenation.

Ventilatory sighs also appear to be effective in recruiting alveoli in ARDS patients. Pelosi et al. (59) studied the effect of sighs on gas exchange in 10 patients with ARDS. Sighs consisted of a VT that produced a P_{plat} of 45 cm H_2O, delivered three times in a row every minute. Subjects underwent 2 hours of baseline ventilation, followed by one hour of ventilatory sighs, and then were returned to baseline ventilation for one hour. Respiratory rate (RR) was adjusted so that there was no change in VE. Compared to PEEP alone, the addition of sighs increased Pao_2 by 50 ± 22%, lowered Qs/QT by 26 ± 26%, and reduced $Paco_2$ by 7 ± 9%.

Recent work from Toronto suggests that the use of sighs may improve alveolar recruitment enough to lower PEEP and thereby reduce mean P_{aw} (51,60). In these studies, a sigh was an inspiratory hold pressure of 30 cm H_2O for 30 seconds. The VT was 5 mL/kg, I:E 1:1, and PEEP was set at LIP. PEEP was decreased in 2 cm H_2O increments, every 5 minutes, while measuring end-expiratory lung volume (EELV) at each step. A sigh was given after each step. The PEEP level at which EELV and oxygenation deteriorated was called suboptimal PEEP, and optimal PEEP was the PEEP where Pao_2 and EELV did not fall, plus an extra 2 cm H_2O (Fig. 5). Two groups were evaluated over 4 hours: optimal PEEP plus a sigh versus optimal PEEP without a sigh. Immediately after the initial sigh, ventilation occurred on the deflation limb of the PV curve at all three PEEP levels examined (5, 10, and 15 cm H_2O), but fell off the deflation curve with PEEP < optimal, presumably because lung units collapsed and were not reopened on the next breath (Fig. 6). At optimal PEEP, a sigh increased FRC from 8 to 13 mL/kg and improved Pao_2 from 135 to 431 torr. The authors concluded that in the setting of small tidal excursions, a sigh improved alveolar recruitment, and that with the use of sighs, PEEP could be decreased to well below LIP. Decreasing the PEEP moved the ventilatory curve onto the steep part of the deflation limb of the PV curve, improving compliance and decreasing

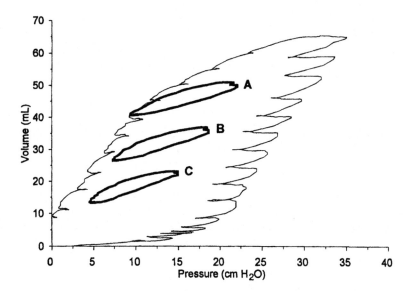

Figure 5 At optimal PEEP (A), the tidal cycle is positioned on the deflation limb of the PV curve, while at suboptimal PEEP (B and C) the tidal loops fall off the deflation limb and compliance and oxygenation (data not shown) are decreased. (From Ref. 51.)

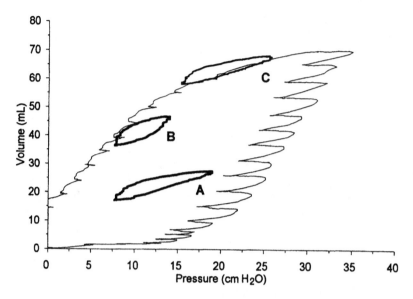

Figure 6 Dynamic pressure-volume loops using a tidal volume of 5 mL/kg during three ventilator strategies: (A) PEEP < P_{flex} without a sigh; (B) PEEP < P_{flex} with a sigh; (C) PEEP > P_{flex} without a sigh. Use of a sigh allows lowering of PEEP and puts the loop on the compliant portion of the expiratory curve. (From Ref. 51.)

PIP. Using a similar strategy in lavaged rats, there was a significant reduction in histological evidence of lung injury when sighs were combined with low V_T and PEEP below LIP compared to low V_T and PEEP below LIP without a sigh. There was also a trend toward less lung injury in this group compared to low V_T with PEEP above P_{flex} (60).

Thus, the addition of a sigh appears capable of recruiting additional lung units that remain collapsed despite the application of PEEP above the LIP of the inspiratory PV curve. The potential advantage of this technique is that additional alveolar recruitment will increase the number of alveoli that are operating on the deflation as opposed to the inflation portion of the PV curve. Hence, ventilation may be achieved at lower P_{aw}. In fact, the use of sighs may allow for a reduction in PEEP, because less PEEP is needed to prevent the collapse of recruited alveoli (on the deflation limb of the PV curve) than is needed to recruit collapsed alveoli (on the inflation limb).

C. Positive End-Expiratory Pressure

Like mean P_{aw} and inspiratory sighs, PEEP can be used to recruit collapsed alveoli. In addition, maintenance of positive airway pressure throughout the respiratory cycle helps to prevent collapse of inflated alveoli. As a result, PEEP is a vital part of ventilating patients with ARDS. The ability of PEEP to recruit alveoli varies from subject to subject. Ranieri et al. (50) evaluated eight patients with ARDS, applying PEEP of 0 (ZEEP), 5, 10, and 15 cm H_2O for 30–35 minutes in random order. They measured change in FRC and recruited lung volume. In some patients, the PV curve with ZEEP was concave and recruitment occurred during application of the tidal excursion (Fig. 7). In these subjects, addition of PEEP recruited collapsed units and improved oxygenation. Other subjects exhibited a convex PV curve on ZEEP, suggesting alveolar overdistension with in-

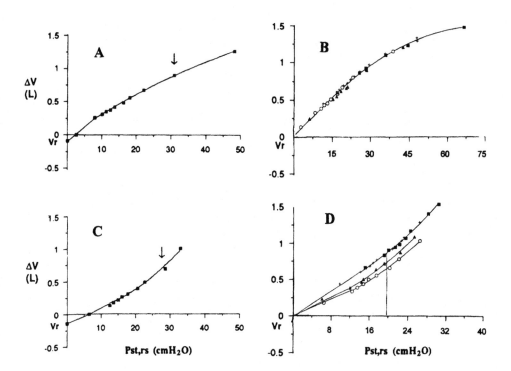

Figure 7 In some patients with ARDS, the pressure-volume (PV) curve at zero end-expiratory pressure (ZEEP) was convex (A). Increasing tidal volume did not recruit alveoli and improve compliance. In these patients, PEEP does not recruit, it simply moves the lung out along the ZEEP PV curve (B). In other patients with ARDS, the ZEEP PV curve is concave and increasing tidal volume recruits lung and improves compliance (C). In these subjects, PEEP recruits alveoli and the lung operates on a more compliant curve (D). The difference between the volume at an end-inspiratory pressure of 20 cm H_2O, ZEEP (open circles) versus PEEP (squares and crosses) is a measure of recruited volume. (From Ref. 50.)

creased volume. In these patients, the addition of PEEP did not recruit collapsed alveoli, it simply moved the lung further out on the PV curve. PEEP did not significantly change static compliance, corrected or uncorrected for PEEPi. Change in PaO_2 correlated with recruited volume, but not with change in compliance.

The immediate benefit of alveolar recruitment from PEEP is improved oxygenation, likely as a result of decreased Qs/Qt. PEEP may also decrease Qs/Qt by lowering CO (61) and by redistributing fluid out of alveoli (62,63). Another benefit of PEEP appears to be the prevention of VILI (64,65). Open-chest dogs develop severe lung injury after 8 hours of positive pressure ventilation between 15 and 55% of TLC, but closed-chest dogs develop no lung injury when ventilated with the same Vt between 45 and 85% of TLC (66). The use of adequate levels of PEEP may prevent this type of lung injury by preventing alveolar collapse at end expiration (21). In other studies, PEEP has been shown to attenuate the development of pulmonary edema during ventilation with high PIP (19), preserve surfactant function (28), and decrease extravascular water in oleic acid–injured lungs (67).

In the injured lung, failure to use enough PEEP may lead to further lung damage. Muscedere et al. (23) found that in saline lavaged lungs, ZEEP or PEEP set below LIP resulted in increased alveolar distension in nondependent lung zones, atelectasis in dependent lung zones, and a progressive decline in total compliance. At a PEEP set above LIP, ventilation appeared to be more evenly distributed, with large areas of atelectesis opening early and smaller more focal areas opening later. There was no change in compliance and less histological evidence of injury.

The ideal level of PEEP in ARDS ventilation has been the topic of intense research and debate for many years, ranging from "least PEEP" to "super PEEP" (68,69). Some investigators have argued that the best PEEP is the level that provides the greatest improvement in oxygenation and compliance without reducing cardiac stroke volume (SV) (70). However, improvements in oxygenation with PEEP may not always correlate with increases in compliance (50), and the benefit of improving oxygenation with PEEP may be offset by the increased risk of VILI. The LIP on the inflation limb of the PV curve has also been advocated as a reference for choosing PEEP in ARDS, and at least one study (71) has shown improvement in mortality in ARDS when this strategy was combined with limiting Vt.

PEEP is not without potential adverse consequences, however. Increasing PEEP almost always increases mean P_{aw} and P_{plat}, which, if great enough, could worsen VILI. High levels of PEEP can impede venous return to the right ventricle and significantly compromise CO. Under some circumstances, such as unilateral lung disease (72), PEEP may redirect perfusion from well-ventilated to poorly ventilated or atelectatic lung regions, thereby worsening V/Q matching or increasing intrapulmonary shunt regions. Failure of PEEP to improve oxygenation may also result from shunting through a patent foramen ovale (73). In one study (74), a PFO was demonstrable in 15% of patients with ARDS, and the application of PEEP led to an increased shunt fraction in 86% of these subjects. Also, PEEP can increase the V/Q ratio, thus decreasing the efficiency of ventilation (75,76).

In summary, the many approaches to alveolar recruitment in patients with ARDS confront us with myriad options. We can operate above the LIP on the PV curve, but should we choose the inflation or deflation limb? We can operate below the UIP, but some portions of the lung may still be overinflated. Should we add sighs to recruit alveoli (59), avoid high inspiratory flows (77), ''open up the lung and keep the lung open'' (78), or leave it closed since attempting to open atelectatic lung results in injury to healthy alveoli (79)? Adding to the confusion is the idea that these variables may assume greater or lesser importance at different stages of the disease process (80). Although specific recommendations for the use of each type of recruitment maneuver are not likely to be made in the near future, ventilating as many alveoli as possible within their physiological range while avoiding regional alveolar collapse and overdistension should be an integral part of strategies for ventilating patients with ARDS.

V. Modes of Mechanical Ventilation in ARDS

Time-cycled, volume-controlled ventilation (VCV) with PEEP added to provide for adequate oxygenation has long been considered the conventional mode of mechanical ventilation for ARDS. Conventional ventilation has been manipulated by making adjustments in the inspiratory flow profile. The resulting modes, pressure control (PC), VC decelerating flow, and inverse ratio ventilation (IRV), are now so frequently used as to be deemed ''conventional.'' The following section will discuss the benefits and pitfalls of these modes.

A. Decelerating Flow

Delivering VT with a decelerating flow waveform is accomplished by rapidly increasing airway pressure and then maintaining that pressure constant throughout inspiration. Maximal inspiratory flow occurs soon after breath initiation, and flow then decelerates rapidly as respiratory system compliance falls during inflation. Decelerating flow is utilized in time-cycled, pressure-limited modalities such as pressure control, and several ventilators can now deliver volume-cycled decelerating flow as well.

Numerous potential benefits have been attributed to the decelerating flow waveform. It may improve oxygenation (81) and decrease dead space (82). In the setting of widespread shunt due to atelectasis or airway obstruction, decelerating flow may improve gas exchange by delivering the VT and the peak pressure early in the inspiration, allowing more time for collateral ventilation, and resulting in a more protracted application of high airway pressure, which may improve alveolar recruitment (83). *Furthermore*, the decelerating flow profile, with flows as high as 200 L/min, may better match the patients inspiratory demands than constant flow modalities that generate flows of 40–100 L/min (84). By reducing the difference between desired and delivered flow, decelerating flow may reduce the work of breathing and improve patient comfort. Another putative benefit of the decelerating flow pattern is lowered PIP. PIP is a function of both airway resistance and thoracic compliance. For a given V_T and inspiratory time, PIP is lower with the decelerating flow pattern compared to constant flow modalities. Warters et al. (85) found that PIP was lower with PCV compared to SIMV, but peak tracheal pressures were the same. Thus, decelerating flow puts less stress on the ventilator circuit and endotracheal tube, but it may not reduce peak alveolar pressures.

B. Pressure-Controlled Decelerating Flow

Pressure-controlled ventilation (PCV) is a patient- or time-triggered mode that delivers a preset level of pressure to the airway opening for a period of time dependent on the I:E ratio and the breathing frequency. The square wave of pressure, in association with decreasing thoracic compliance as inspiration proceeds, creates a decelerating flow wave form. There are conflicting data as to whether PCV offers advantages over VCV in oxygenation, ventilation, and PIP. Abraham and Yoshihara (86) compared PCV to VCV in 10 subjects with ARDS who had "failed" VCV. In this group of patients, changing from VCV to PCV improved Pao_2 (80 ± 9 to 92 ± 8 torr, $p < 0.05$), increased Do_2 (509 ± 75 to 559 ± 67 mL/min, $P < 0.05$), and lowered PIP (62 ± 5 vs. 45 ± 3 mmHg, $p < 0.01$). There was no significant change in mean P_{aw}, PEEPi, $Paco_2$, Qs/QT, CO, or mixed venous saturation. Four years later this same group prospectively randomized 27 patients with acute respiratory failure to PCV or VCV within 24 hours of intubation (84). No significant differences in V_T, PEEP, mean P_{aw}, or I:E ratios were seen between the two groups. PCV resulted in lower PIP, but there were no differences between the two modes of ventilation regarding Pao_2 and Pao_2/Fio_2 or sedation. Cereda et al. (87) compared PCV to VCV at 5, 10, and 15 cm H_2O of PEEP for 30 minutes in eight patients with ARDS. The V_T was 8.5 ± 0.4 mL/kg and inspiratory time was 33%. Ten 1 L breaths normalized volume history in between trials. Again, PIP was lower with PCV. There was no change in oxygenation despite a higher mean P_{aw} with PCV. The V_D/V_T seemed to be reduced with PCV.

PCV is encumbered with several management issues. Variations in the resistance and compliance of the respiratory system during PCV will alter V_T, and thus, a constant VE is not guaranteed. Even when applied pressure, resistance,

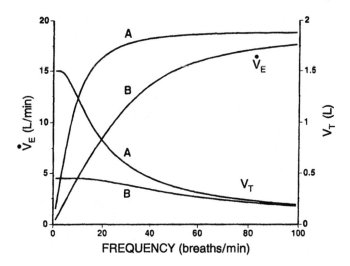

Figure 8 Relationship of minute volume and tidal volume to respiratory rate during pressure control ventilation at a fixed inspiratory time. Conditions A and B refer to models of high and low compliance, respectively. As respiratory rate increases, tidal volume falls due to shorter inspiratory time and minute volume approaches a bounding limit. (From Ref. 259.)

and compliance remain constant, VE does not increase linearly with frequency, but approaches a distinct bounding limit (88) (Fig. 8). As VT falls with increasing RR, the increased VD/VT decreases alveolar ventilation and may result in increased $Paco_2$ even with a stable or increased VE.

C. Volume-Cycled Decelerating Flow

Delivery of a set VT with a decelerating flow pattern has the potential advantages of maintaining a constant VT in the face of changing respiratory compliance as well as any of the advantages that a decelerating flow pattern may have on gas exchange and P_{aw}. Markstrom et al. (89) compared VCV with constant flow to VCV with decelerating flow in a piglet saline lavage model of acute lung injury. The PEEP was set at 4, 9, 13, 17, and 22 cm H_2O, and RR, I:E ratio, and VT were held constant. Measurements were made after 15 minutes of each new setting. Decelerating flow improved alveolar ventilation at all levels of PEEP. There were no differences between the two groups in P_{plat}, lung compliance, hemodynamics, or Pao_2.

Al-Saady and Bennett (90) compared VCV with constant versus decelerating flow in 14 patients with various causes of respiratory failure, 6 of whom had

ARDS. In this 20-minute crossover study, VT, I:E ratio of 1:2, and RR were kept constant. The decelerating flow pattern produced significant reductions in PIP, P_{plat}, and A-a DO_2, with a 14% improvement in PaO_2. Decelerating flow decreased VD/VT by 16%. Mean P_{aw} was higher with decelerating flow, but the difference did not reach statistical significance.

Few studies have directly compared decelerating flow delivered with PCV versus VCV. Munoz et al. (91) compared PCV to VCV with a decelerating wave form in 11 patients with various causes of respiratory failure, none of whom had ARDS. The VT, I:E ratio, FiO_2, and RR were held constant. No subjects received PEEP. No significant differences in mean P_{aw}, P_{plat}, PEEPi, PaO_2, $PaCO_2$, pH, or compliance were found between these two modes.

In summary, decelerating flow ventilation lowers PIP compared to constant flow ventilation, although this may be a function of tubing resistance and may not result in decreased risk of VILI. Oxygenation is either unchanged or slightly improved, but this is often at the cost of an increased mean P_{aw}. A reduction in dead space has often been demonstrated. Cardiac function appears unaltered by the decelerating waveform. Insufficient data exist to determine if PCV or VCV differ in their effects on mortality, days of mechanical ventilation, or other outcome measures in ARDS.

VI. Ventilation Strategies in ARDS

A. Lung Volume Protection

The concept of using PEEP to prevent alveolar collapse and VT small enough to avoid alveolar overdistension is not new. However, only recently have clinical trials been able to demonstrate that the use of such a "protected lung strategy" can improve outcome in patients with ARDS. The finding that survival in ARDS can be significantly affected by the choice of VT may be among the most important discoveries in mechanical ventilation of patients with ARDS and offers strong support to the theory that volutrauma contributes to the mortality of this disease.

In 1990, Hickling et al. (92) reported that limiting VT improves survival in ARDS. Five years later, Amato et al. (93) reported the first prospective, randomized controlled trial (RCT) of low versus high VT in patients with ARDS. They reported better PaO_2/FiO_2 ratio, static compliance, and percentage of patients weaned from mechanical ventilation in 15 patients ventilated with VT of 6 mL/kg and PEEP set above LIP than in 13 patients ventilated with VT of 12 mL/kg and PEEP adjusted to keep $FiO_2 < 0.6$. In a larger follow-up study, Amato et al. (71) reported a mortality rate nearly twofold lower in 29 patients ventilated with VT of 6 mL/kg and PEEP set 2 cm H_2O above LIP compared to 24 patients ventilated with VT of 12 mL/kg and no restriction on airway pressures. In this study, mean PEEP was higher in the low VT than in the control group between days 2 and 7 of the study (13.2 $\pm$ 0.4 and 9.3 $\pm$ 0.5 cm H_2O, respectively, $p <$ 0.05). Although the difference in survival rates between treatment groups in this study was dramatic, mortality in the control group was considerably higher than anticipated (71%) and could not be explained by differences in APACHE II scores at study entry. The high P_{plat} (>38 cm H_2O) and high incidence of barotrauma in the control group raised the concern that the difference in survival rates between experimental groups in this study was due to an increase in VILI in the control group and not a true improvement in survival in the lung protected group. Data from three subsequent RCTs (94–96) found no improvement in any outcome measures using a less aggressive protected lung strategy. In all of these studies, VT and P_{plat} pressures averaged 7 mL/kg and 24–26 cm H_2O in the protected group, similar to the VT of 6 mL/kg and P_{plat} of 24 cm H_2O in the study by Amato et al. (71). However, VT in the control groups of these three studies ranged from 10.2 to 10.8 mL/kg as compared to 12 mL/kg in Amato's study, and P_{plat} ranged from 27 to 32 compared to 38 cm H_2O. Also, the selection of PEEP in the latter three studies was guided by oxygenation criteria for both low VT and control groups, whereas in Amato's study PEEP was set above LIP in the low VT group but guided by oxygenation in the control group. Thus, the survival advantages in Amato's study (71) may have been conveyed by the greater differences between VT and P_{plat} or the use of LIP to guide the choice of PEEP in the low VT group.

More recently, a much larger, multicenter RCT of protected lung strategy was completed by the ARDS Network (2). In this study, 861 patients with acute lung injury or ARDS were randomized to receive mechanical ventilation with a VT of 6 or 12 mL/kg based on ideal body weight. The PEEP was adjusted to oxygenation requirements using the same criteria in both groups and LIP was not measured. The mean VT and P_{plat} in the protected and conventional ventilation groups were 6.2 and 11.8 mL/kg and 25 and 33 cm H_2O, respectively. Enrollment was stopped at 861 patients after interim analysis revealed a 25% reduction in mortality in the lower VT group (31 vs. 38.9%, $p < 0.007$) (Fig. 9) and a 20% reduction in days of mechanical ventilation through day 28 (10 $\pm$ 11 vs. 12 $\pm$ 11, $p < 0.007$). There were also significantly fewer days of other organ failure and lower plasma interleukin-6 levels in the protected lung group, suggesting that the protected lung strategy in this study reduced systemic inflammatory responses. PEEP was significantly higher in the low VT group than in the control group at 1 and 3 days, but the differences were small (mean + SD: 9.4 $\pm$ 3.6 vs. 8.6 $\pm$ 3.6 cm H_2O, day 1 and 9.2 + 3.6 vs. 8.6 $\pm$ 4.2 cm H_2O, day 3, $p <$ 0.05 for both) and by day 7 PEEP was lower in the low VT group (8.1 $\pm$ 3.4 vs. 9.1 $\pm$ 4.2 cm H_2O). Again, the difference in VT between experimental groups was greater in this study than in the three smaller studies that found no impact on outcome with limited VT in ARDS (94–96). However, in the ARDS Network

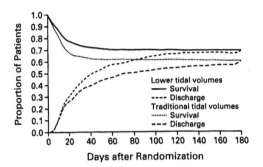

Figure 9   Effect of ventilation with low (6 mL/kg) versus traditional (12 mL/kg) tidal volumes on survival and hospital discharge. (From Ref. 2.)

study, V_T was reported as mL/kg/per body weight predicted from the patient's sex and height. When expressed as mL/kg of measured body weight, V_T in the experimental and controls groups were 5.2 and 9.9 mL/kg, respectively. Also, the P_{plat} and PEEP in the experimental and control groups of the ARDS Network study were comparable to those of the other three studies (Table 1). Thus, the improvement in mortality in the low V_T group of the ARDS Network study appears to have been derived from the use of lower V_T than in previous studies and not from excessive overinflation of the control group. These findings support those of Amato et al. (71) and suggest that reducing V_T to 6 mL/kg of ideal body weight results in a significant improvement in survival in ARDS.

These studies provide evidence that outcome in ARDS is affected by V_T, but it is not known if the relationship between V_T and survival in ARDS is linear or if there is a threshold level of V_T above which mortality is increased. In particular, it is not clear if reducing V_T below 6 mL/kg by techniques such as high-frequency ventilation (HFV) will result in further reductions in mortality. At the present time it appears logical to aim for a V_T of 6 mL/kg in all ARDS patients. Patients who have difficulty maintaining adequate gas exchange or acid base status with this level of ventilation may warrant higher V_T, but aggressive measures including sedation, permissive hypercapnia, and possibly alternative methods of mechanical ventilation should be used to keep V_T at this targeted goal.

B. Permissive Hypercapnia

An extreme form of lung volume protection would be to reduce V_T and/or RR until VE falls below the level needed to maintain normal CO_2 elimination. Hypoxemia could be treated by increasing Fio_2 and respiratory acidosis could be avoided if $Paco_2$ was raised slowly over several days. This strategy, known as permissive

Table 1 Tidal Volumes, Airway Pressures, and Arterial pCO_2 Levels in Randomized Controlled Trials of Mechanical Ventilation with Low Lung Volumes Versus Traditional Lung Volumes

Study (Ref.)	V_T (mL/kg)		P_{plat} (cm H_2O)		PEEP (cm H_2O)		$PaCO_2$ (torr)	
	Low V_T	Controls	Low V_T	Controls	Low V_T	Controls	Low V_T	Controls
Amato et al. (93) (days 2–7)	387 ± 7	738 ± 17*	23.9 ± 0.7	37.8 ± 1.2*	13.2 ± 0.4	9.3 ± 0.5*	50.8 ± 1.1	35.0 ± 0.7*
Stewart et al. (95)	7.2 ± 0.8	10.8 ± 1.0*	22.3 ± 5.4(1) 20.0 ± 4.7(7)	26.8 ± 6.7(1)* 28.6 ± 7.2(7)*	8.6 ± 3.0(1) 9.6 ± 3.9(7)	7.2 ± 3.3*(1) 8.0 ± 3.6(7)	54.4 ± 18.8	45.7 ± 9.8*
Brochard et al. (94)	7.1 ± 1.3	10.3 ± 1.7	59.5 ± 1.5	40.1 ± 1.6*	10.7 ± 2.9	10.7 ± 2.3	41.3 ± 7.6	59.5 ± 15*
Brower et al. (96)	7.3 ± 0.1	10.2 ± 0.1*	50.3 ± 3.5	41.3 ± 7.6*	~9.8(1) ~5.6(5)	~8.7(1) ~6.0(5)	40.1 ± 1.6	50.3 ± 3.5
ARDS Network (2)	6.2 ± 0.8	11.8 ± 0.8*	25 ± 6	33 ± 8*	9.4 ± 3.6(1) 8.1 ± 3.4(7)	8.6 ± 3.6*(1) 9.1 ± 4.2*(7)	40 ± 10(1) 44 ± 12(7)	35 ± 8*(1) 40 ± 10*(7)

Values are mean ± SD for study duration except as noted. (1), (5), and (7) refers to mean values taken on study day 1, 5, or 7. ~ signifies approximate values derived from graphs, data not provided. V_T = tidal volume; P_{plat} = plateau pressure; PEEP = positive end-expiratory pressure; $PaCO_2$ = arterial carbon dioxide tension.

* $p < 0.05$.

hypercapnia (PHY), has been advocated by some investigators in the past, and some degree of hypercapnia occurs in most lung volume protection strategies. However, there are data to suggest that prolonged hypercapnia is associated with significant adverse effects such as alveolar hypoxia, decreased myocardial contractility, cerebral vasodilation, and dyspnea (97). Because PHY alone has not been shown to improve morbidity or mortality in ARDS, it is probably unwise to use this technique without implementation of a specific strategy to limit V_T.

The consequences of hypercarbia and intracellular acidosis have been expertly reviewed by Feihl and Perret (97). Myocardial contractility can be reduced, but there is an associated increase in heart rate and preload and a decrease in systemic vascular resistance, such that CO is maintained. Hypercarbia leads to pulmonary arteriolar constriction and an increased pulmonary vascular resistance. Respiratory acidosis potentiates hypoxic pulmonary vasoconstriction, further augmenting the workload placed on the right heart. Concerns have been raised about organ damage related to decreased splanchnic blood flow during PHY. Stewart et al. (95) found a higher incidence of renal failure that required dialysis in ARDS patients treated with a protected lung strategy ($Paco_2$ 54.4 $\pm$ 18.8 torr) than in controls ($Paco_2$ 45.7 $\pm$ 9.8 torr). On the other hand, Carvalho et al. (98) found no compromise in renal function in a group of patients subjected to PHY for up to 7 days. Hypercarbia can also increase cerebral perfusion pressure and blood flow, and this may cause headache, nausea, drowsiness, and papilledema.

No formal recommendations for the upper limit of $Paco_2$ have been made. Arterial Pco_2 up to 80 torr, with a pH down to 7.15, does not appear to be harmful, provided that oxygenation is preserved and that no contraindications exist. Feihl and Perret (97) suggest raising $Paco_2$ by no more than 10 mmHg per hour and weaning it over 1–3 days if PHY has been used for >24 hours. Arterial pH should not be allowed to fall below 7.15. The possible beneficial and/or adverse effects of intravenous HCO_3 administration to compensate for respiratory acidosis have not been well studied. Of concern, administration of HCO_3 may increase $Paco_2$ and raise intracellular [H^+]. Dead space washout techniques are also being explored as ways to maintain satisfactory $Paco_2$ and pH levels.

Possible contraindications to PHY include left ventricular dysfunction, beta blockers, ongoing cardiac ischemia, splanchnic or renal ischemia, hypovolemia, severe metabolic acidosis, and severe hypoxemia. Most authors agree that permissive hypercapnia should not be instituted in the presence of a significant CNS event.

C. Inverse Ratio Ventilation

An inspiratory phase that is as long or longer than the expiratory phase is referred to as inverse ratio ventilation (IRV). IRV can be achieved in VCV or PCV by decreasing inspiratory flow, prolonging inspiratory flow, or adding an inspiratory pause. Potential benefits of IRV include improved oxygenation, lowered PIPs, and improved efficiency of ventilation (99).

The physiology of any IRV-induced improvement in oxygenation remains uncertain. In a clinical commentary on the use of IRV in ARDS, Shanholtz and Brower (100) argue that improved oxygenation is the result of a decreased shunt fraction and not improved V/Q, but studies specifically designed to evaluate the role of shunt reduction versus improved V/Q are lacking. IRV may decrease intrapulmonary shunt by recruiting additional alveoli due to an increase in mean P_{aw}. IRV may improve V/Q matching by keeping some alveoli open longer during the respiratory cycle, allowing more time for gas distribution and exchange (101).

In a retrospective study, Armstrong and MacIntyre (102) demonstrated improved oxygenation with higher mean P_{aw} using IRV with PCV than with VCV and PEEP. In converting patients from VCV-PEEP they employed an I:E ratio that did not produce PEEPi but did raise mean P_{aw} from 20 to 30 cm H_2O. PEEP was 10 cm H_2O with VCV, 8.2 cm H_2O on IRV (mean I:E of 1.8:1). The Pao_2, Pao_2/Fio_2, and Pao_2/PAo_2 all improved, but the oxygenation index (mean $P_{aw} \times$ [$Fio_2 \times 100/Pao_2$]) was no different with PCV-IRV or VCV-PEEP.

Several studies suggest that IRV has a modest effect on decreasing V_D/V_T (99,103,104). This effect has been attributed to improved distribution of V_T with less alveolar overdistension (105–107), better collateral ventilation, or improved efficiency of expiration (107). Prolonged inspiratory time may allow dead space gas in conducting airways to participate in gas exchange, effectively reducing physiological dead space (34). Armstrong and MacIntyre (102) point out that lowered PIP will reduce the circuit distention volume and thus account for some of the improvement in V_D/V_T. Improved efficiency of ventilation might permit a reduction of operating tidal volumes, reducing the risk of volutrauma.

Does IRV offer any advantage over conventional I:E ratio ventilation with PEEP at an equivalent mean P_{aw}? In several studies, when mean P_{aw} was raised with PEEP versus IRV, shunt fraction and oxygenation were better with PEEP (108–110). Lessard et al. (111) compared the effect of 30 minutes of PCV, PCV-IRV, and VCV, at the same VE and PEEP, on gas exchange and compliance. They found no significant differences in P_{plat}, ventilation, oxygenation, and lung or respiratory system compliance. However, it has been speculated that the effects of IRV are time dependent and may require more than 30 minutes to be realized (99,104). Mercat et al. (112) and Lessard et al. (111) found no IRV benefit at 30 to 60 minutes versus VCV when PEEP was kept constant. Four years later, Mercat et al. (113) compared 6 hours of VCV with I:E ratio of 1:2 to 6 hours of VCV and an I:E ratio of 2:1. The V_T and total PEEP were kept constant. In this study, IRV improved CO_2 elimination, increased mean P_{aw}, decreased PIP and shunt fraction, and decreased CO. IRV produced no change in P_{plat} or oxygenation and exerted no time-dependent effects.

Potential problems when IRV is used with PCV include variable Vt with changing respiratory system mechanics, the development of high levels of intrinsic PEEP, and the potential need for heavy sedation and/or paralysis due to patient discomfort. Cardiac stroke volume is not usually affected at I:E ratios around 1:1 but may decline with a ratio $\geq 2:1$ (114,115). These potential adverse effects may be an acceptable risk if IRV offers protection against VILI. While it has been suggested that IRV may result in greater homogeneity of gas distribution and, therefore, less risk of alveolar overdistension (34), solid data are lacking. Hubmayr et al. (116), using time constants to mathematically model the distribution of ventilation in IRV, concluded that use of IRV might reduce alveolar pressure (stress) slightly, with little effect on the inhomogeneous distribution of alveolar gas. Thus, the potential for overdistension of compliant lung units was not reduced in this model. Furthermore, increased mean P_{aw} and a more prolonged exposure to positive P_{aw} may translate into higher mean alveolar pressures and increased risk of volutrauma (54).

D. Prone Positioning

In normal subjects and in patients with ARDS, the dependent portion of the lung is at a mechanical disadvantage compared to the nondependent lung. Computed tomography of the chest in patients with ARDS shows a vertical distribution of roentgenographic density with increasing atelectasis in the gravity-dependent portions of the lung (6). In the supine position, there is a progressive decrease in the transpulmonary pressure gradient, chest wall compliance, and regional ventilation along the vertical axis, from ventral to dorsal (Table 2). In addition, the weight of the heart and lungs act to compress the dependent parenchyma on which they rest (117,118), and the abdominal contents offer increased resistance to movement of the dorsal portion of the diaphragm. The end result is the development of atelectasis in dependent lung zones and a maldistribution of Vt to the

Table 2 Differences in Transpulmonary Pressures (P_{pl}, cm H_2O) in Prone and Supine Position Before and After Volume Infusion

	Before volume infusion		After volume infusion	
	Supine	Prone	Supine	Prone
Nondependent	-3.0 ± 0.6	$-1.3 \pm 0.2*$	-2.3 ± 0.2	$-0.9 \pm 0.2*$
Dependent	0.7 ± 0.3	$-0.1 \pm 0.2*$	$3.0 \pm 0.5**$	$0.9 \pm 0.3*$

$* p < 0.05$ supine versus prone position, before or after volume infusion.
$** p < 0.05$ before versus after volume infusion, supine or prone position.
Source: Ref. 256.

nondependent portion of the lung that produces regional alveolar overdistension. The prone position may result in improved V/Q matching, recruitment of previously collapsed alveoli and reduction of Qs/QT.

In normal dogs, the prone position increases EELV, presumably by recruiting collapsed dorsal lung, with no change in intrapulmonary shunting (119). In canine lungs injured by oleic acid infusion, Albert and colleagues (120) found that the prone position produced a significant decrease in Qs/QT. Pelosi et al. (121) evaluated ARDS patients on VCV before and during 2 hours of prone positioning. Proning improved Pao_2 (103.2 ± 23.8 vs. 129.3 ± 32.9 torr) in 12 of 16 subjects. There was no change in respiratory system compliance, but chest wall compliance dropped significantly from 205 ± 97 to 136 ± 53 mL/cm H_2O in the prone position. Improved oxygenation correlated with the fall in chest wall compliance in the prone position. The prone position decreases the difference in compliance between ventral and dorsal chest wall, producing a more homogeneous distribution of VT.

Increasing ventilation to the dorsal lung by placing it in a nondependent position would be of less benefit if gravitational forces reduced the blood flow to this lung. However, Beck and Rehder (119) showed that in normal dogs, vascular conductance is greater in dorsal lung regions than in ventral regions, regardless of body position, and that V/Q matching is better in the prone than in the supine position. Lung perfusion is fairly well distributed in patients with ARDS as well, and most of the pulmonary circulation is directed to the dorsal lung, even in the prone position (122,123). Hence, in the prone position, ventilation in the dorsal lung may improve while perfusion is maintained and oxygenation should improve. Albert and colleagues (120) found no change in FRC or regional diaphragm movement and no redistribution of blood flow to the less injured ventral lung after proning lungs injured by oleic acid.

Despite the theoretical advantages, the clinical response to prone positioning has varied considerably. Mure et al. (124) found that proning improved oxygenation in 92%(12/13) of ARDS patients, with a rise in mean Pao_2/Fio_2 from 71 to 178 torr. However, in another study (125), only 57% of patients with ARDS improved their Pao_2 by >10% in the prone position. Chatte and colleagues (126) found that Pao_2 increased >20 mmHg in 19 of 25 patients with ARDS immediately after proning, but Pao_2 returned to preprone levels after 4 hours in 10 patients. The lack of a sustained improvement in oxygenation may be due to alveolar collapse in the ventral portion of the lung that assumes the dependent position after proning. Gattinoni et al. (127) found that, in patients with ARDS, a vertical gradient of increased density on CT scan was reestablished just 10 minutes after proning. Interestingly, improvements in oxygenation caused by proning may persist after returning the patient to the supine position. Fridrich et al. (128) ventilated patients with ARDS for 20 hours in the prone position followed by 4 hours supine. The Pao_2/Fio_2 increased from 127 at baseline to 247 mmHg 19 hours after proning. The P:F ratio fell to 162 3 hours after returning to the supine position, but this was still significantly better than baseline.

Prone positioning does not appear to have significant effects on cardiac output, V_D/V_T, or CO_2 elimination (121,129). Improved alveolar recruitment and a more homogeneous distribution of V_T may help to protect against VILI. Broccard et al. (130) prospectively randomized 12 dogs to 4 hours of supine or prone position ventilation 90 minutes after olelic acid–induced lung injury. They set PEEP at LIP and adjusted V_T to a transpulmonary pressure of 35 cm H_2O. Histological markers of injury were increased in the supine animals. The Pao_2 and venous admixture improved immediately with PEEP, then deteriorated in the supine, but not in the prone, position.

To summarize, the prone position produces a variable improvement in oxygenation, largely due to recruitment of dorsal lung units without a decrease in the perfusion to this region. Ventilation and cardiac stroke volume appear to be unaffected by prone positioning. Limited data suggest that the prone position may be useful in reducing the likelihood of VILI. Problems include pressure ulcers on the face and thorax, the need for careful planning of the move, and reluctance on the part of caregivers to initiate proning.

VII. Alternative Modes of Mechanical Ventilation in ARDS

Conventional modes of mechanical ventilation often fail to attain the goal of adequate gas exchange without increasing the risk of VILI. This has led some investigators to explore unconventional modes of mechanical ventilation to determine if new techniques can oxygenate and ventilate the patient with less injury to the lung.

A. Airway Pressure Release Ventilation

Continuous positive airway pressure (CPAP) applies a constant level of pressure to the airway throughout inspiration and expiration. In airway pressure release ventilation (APRV), the lungs are kept inflated using a set level of CPAP known as inflating pressure (P_{inf}) and released at a fixed time interval to a lower pressure designated as release pressure (P_{rel}). Spontaneous respiration is possible during all phases of APRV. APRV is pressure limited, time cycled, and typically used with a greatly prolonged inspiratory time. If no spontaneous ventilation occurs, APRV is similar to PCV with IRV. If spontaneous respiration occurs, then APRV is a form of partial ventilatory support (131).

Some of the proposed benefits of APRV compared to CMV include lowered PIP, less hemodynamic compromise, unrestricted spontaneous ventilation, reduced work of breathing, and a reduction in V_D/V_T. One potential drawback to APRV is patient discomfort. Chiang et al. (131) found that APRV, when used as a partial support mode, was less comfortable than PSV or IMV in 5 of 16 patients with ARDS. Two patients in that study exhibited significant patient-ventilator asynchrony.

There are limited data on the effectiveness of ARPV in ARDS. Cane et al. (132) compared APRV to CMV in 18 patients with ARDS. CMV consisted of VCV set at a V_T of 10–15 mL/kg. The RR was set to maintain eucapnia, and PEEP was set to keep $Pao_2 > 60$ with $Fio_2 < 0.5$. This was followed by APRV set at $P_{rel} = 5$ cm H_2O, $P_{inf} = P_{rel} + PEEP$ needed on VCV, and an I:E ratio of 1:1 or greater. The $Paco_2$ was kept within normal range by increasing the release rate up to a maximum of 20 cycles/min. If this did not maintain eucapnia, P_{inf} was incrementally increased. The Pao_2 was modified by simultaneous and equal changes in P_{inf} and P_{rel}. Mean values for V_T and airway pressures on VCV versus APRV were: V_T 1050 vs. 790 cc, VE 10.4 vs. 12.0 L/min, PIP 64.6 vs. 38.9 cm H_2O, PEEP vs. P_{rel} 17.9 vs. 17.0 cm H_2O, and mean P_{aw} 34.9 vs. 23.7 cm H_2O. Despite the markedly lower airway pressures in the APRV group, no differences in Fio_2, ABGs, BP, or stroke volume were observed. Six patients failed APRV, five of whom were well ventilated with VCV. In another study, Sydow et al. (133) evaluated APRV and VCV with IRV in 18 patients with severe ARDS. After 24 hours spontaneous VE on APRV constituted $34 \pm 14\%$ of total ventilation. Over a 24-hour period, oxygenation improved on APRV, suggesting that spontaneous breathing and regular pressure release to 5 cm H_2O does not result in significant derecruitment and may in fact be beneficial.

Spontaneous respirations with the use of APRV can reduce operating pressures and the risk of VILI. Also, alveolar recruitment may be enhanced due to the prolonged inspiratory phase used in APRV. These benefits could favorably impact morbidity and mortality. However, there have been no studies that have examined the effect of APRV on outcome variables, and further studies are needed to determine if this mode of ventilation offers benefit over CMV in ARDS.

B. High-Frequency Ventilation

High-frequency ventilation (HFV) was developed in the late 1960s and has been studied in animals and humans with acute lung injury for over 20 years. Initially, improvements in airway pressures and oxygenation were reported in some patients with acute lung injury. However, several randomized trials in the mid-1980s found no effect of HFV on outcome in patients with ARDS, essentially ending much of the interest in this novel mode of ventilation. Unfortunately, these studies may have been flawed by the lack of adequate statistical power and alveolar recruitment maneuvers (134). Recent studies in pediatric patients have shown that HFV may improve outcome in acute respiratory failure (135). In theory, the use of HFV to achieve the lowest possible V_T in a well-recruited lung should offer maximum protection against VILI.

Modes of HFV

HFV typically consists of a V_T that approaches or is less than anatomical dead space, delivered at RRs that are several fold higher than the upper limits of normal by ventilators that are specially designed for this purpose. Several techniques for HFV have been developed. High-frequency "jet" ventilation (HFJV) uses a large bore catheter to deliver high-velocity bursts of air into the endotracheal tube. High-frequency flow interruption (HFFI) operates similar to HFJV but uses a device to interrupt a continuous jet of air at a set frequency. High-frequency oscillatory ventilation (HFOV) employs the reciprocating movement of a diaphragm or piston to set up an oscillating current of air in the respiratory circuit. The oscillatory action does not entrain air well, and adequate gas exchange requires a bias airflow. High-frequency percussive ventilation (HFPV) is a type of HFJV that allows driving pressure to be cycled. As driving pressure increases, the lung is inflated by PEEPi. At a fixed interval, driving pressure is dropped to a lower pressure, allowing deflation of the lung (Fig. 10).

Gas Exchange in HVF

In theory, alveolar ventilation (V_A) should approach zero as V_T approaches anatomical dead space V_D. However, it has long been appreciated that adequate ventilation can be achieved with $V_T < V_D$ (136). In 1915, Henderson and coworkers (137) hypothesized that diffusion of gases from the airway to alveoli could provide adequate alveolar ventilation in patients breathing with very small V_T. This concept of ventilation by gas diffusion (diffusive ventilation) as opposed to bulk movement of a volume of air (convective ventilation) was advanced in 1954 by Taylor (138), who demonstrated that turbulence during convective flow greatly enhanced dispersion of tracer gas molecules in a pipe (Taylor dispersion). Several other mechanisms may facilitate alveolar gas exchange during HFV (see Fig. 11):

1. *Convective ventilation* may contribute to ventilation of alveoli closest to the major airways (139–141).
2. *Pendeluft effect* refers to alveoli with fast time constants assisting movement of air into alveoli with slower filling constants during expiration (142).
3. *Convective dispersion* refers to bulk transport of nondiffusable gases by asymmetrical velocity profiles during oscillation (143,144). Simply stated, differences in the velocities of gas molecules in an oscillating

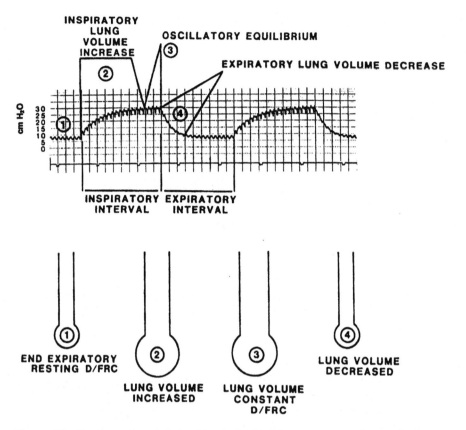

Figure 10 Pressure-volume relationships during high frequency percussive ventilation. (1) Low lung volume at end expiration with oscillatory CPAP between 5 and 10 cm H_2O. (2) Lung inflation occurs from breath stacking due to increasing driving pressure with fixed inspiratory time. (3) Lung inflation reaches equilibrium determined by driving pressure and intrinsic PEEP. (4) Programmed drop in driving pressure results in fall in lung volume to starting level. High-frequency ventilation occurs when lung is inflated. Cyclic drops in lung volume aid in CO_2 elimination. (From Ref. 260.)

wave of air will cause gas molecules that started off close together to disperse.

4. *Molecular diffusion* is dependent on the kinetic energy of individual gas molecules, which presumably is increased in HFV because of the greater velocity of air flow or the high frequency of oscillation.

The relative contribution of each of these mechanisms to VA during HFV is unclear (145).

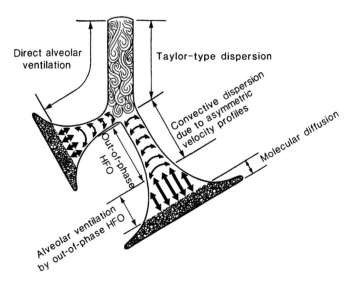

Figure 11 Proposed mechanisms of gas exchange during high-frequency ventilation and the location in the airways where each mechanism is thought to be most active. (From Ref. 45.)

Compared to CMV, HFV may offer several other advantages in ARDS. The attenuated respiratory swings in intrathoracic pressure may decrease PIP and reduce the impedence to venous return during end inspiration. Fredburg et al. (146) postulated that ventilating the lung at its resonance frequency of 5 Hz reduces respiratory impedence. Compared to CMV, HFV has been shown to decrease activation of alveolar neutrophils (147) and lower alveolar levels of inflammatory prostaglandins, platelet-activating factor, and TNF-α (36,148,149). Reducing lung inflammation during mechanical ventilation in ARDS could impact favorably on lung healing and overall survival.

Ventilator Settings in HFV

Few guidelines have been provided for choosing ventilator settings for HFV in patients with ARDS. There is, however, substantial evidence for the need to adequately recruit alveoli. Unlike conventional modes of ventilation that utilize cyclic changes in alveolar volume, HFV attempts to ventilate alveoli near a constant volume and P_{aw}. Although oscillatory pressure amplitude in HFOV can be increased, there is marked attenuation of the change in P_{aw} across the ET tube and proximal airways such that changes in distal airway and alveolar pressure appear to be minuscule (150,151). Thus, alveoli with opening pressures above the mean

P_{aw} are not likely to be recruited at any point in the respiratory cycle during HFV. Several studies have demonstrated that oxygenation with HFV in experimentally induced acute lung injury is closely correlated to mean P_{aw} and lung volume (152–155), and early experiences with HFV in neonates found that recruitment maneuvers were often necessary to maintain adequate oxygenation (156–158). Furthermore, McCulloch et al. (155) found that HFOV produced less VILI in saline lavaged rabbit lungs when mean P_{aw} was maintained at a level to keep $Pao_2 > 350$ torr compared to a level that kept Pao_2 between 70 and 100 torr. Hence, raising mean P_{aw} not only improves oxygenation in HFOV, but appears to reduce VILI by maintaining adequate alveolar recruitment.

Clinical Experience with HFV in ARDS

Case reports between 1977 and 1981 suggested a role for HFV in oxygenating patients with acute lung injury (159–162) and cardiogenic pulmonary edema (161,163). In 1982, Schuster et al. (164) compared HFV to CMV in nine patients with diffuse parenchymal lung injury, including three with ARDS. At the same level of Fio_2 and PEEP, no differences in Pao_2 were seen between HFV and CMV, but PIP was lower on HFV. Throughout the 1980s several investigators reported their experience with different modes of HFV in acute lung injury. Most of these reports were individual cases or small crossover studies that compared the effect of a particular type of HFV on gas exchange in patients who had failed CMV. MacIntyre et al. (101) compared HFFI to CMV in 22 patients with diffuse lung injury. Gas exchange worsened in 10 patients, improved in 4, and remained the same in 8 patients. In patients whose gas exchange was similar on HFV and CMV, PIP was lower with HFV. Cioffi et al. (165) found that HFPV increased Pao_2/Fio_2 and decreased $Paco_2$ in four of five patients with smoke inhalation injury who had failed CMV. Improvements in gas exchange occurred at lower PIP and PEEP than had been used with CMV. However, mean P_{aw} was not measured, and none of the five patients survived. In a larger nonrandomized study, Gluck et al. (166) found that HFJV improved oxygenation at lower PIP in 90 patients with severe ARDS 1 and 24 hours after switching from CMV.

There have been few RCTs of HFV versus CMV in adults with ARDS. Carlon et al. (167) randomized 309 patients with diffuse, noncardiogenic acute respiratory failure to VCV or HFJV. The primary outcome variable was number of patients reaching a predetermined Pao_2 and Fio_2 within 24 hours. More patients in the HFJV group met their endpoint by 24 hours than those in the VCV group (88 vs. 76%). The PIP was lower in the HFJV than in the VCV group. No benefit was seen in survival or length of stay in the ICU. In another study, Hurst et al. (168) randomized 113 patients admitted to a surgical intensive care unit who were at risk of developing ARDS to receive HFPV or CMV. One hundred patients (52 HFPV, 48 CMV) completed the study, and 60 patients developed ARDS.

Patients on HFV reached predetermined endpoints for oxygenation and $Paco_2$ at lower levels of end-expiratory and mean P_{aw}, but no differences in the incidence of ARDS or overall mortality were noted.

Some success with HVOF has been seen in pediatric patients. Arnold et al. (135), randomized 58 patients greater than 40 weeks old and less than 35 kg, with acute lung injury, to HFOV or CMV. Patients who developed circulatory shock, progression of airleak, or respiratory failure ($Pao_2 < 50$ with $Fio_2 - 1.0$ or pH < 7.20 and $PaCO_2 > 60$ for more than 2 hours) were crossed over to the other mode of ventilation. The crossover rate was nearly twice as great in the CMV than in the HFOV group (19 vs. 11). The number of patients surviving without severe lung disease was significantly greater in HFOV- than CMV-treated patients (83 vs. 30%). All 17 patients treated with HFOV throughout the study (not crossed over to CMV) survived, as compared to 6 of 10 patients treated with CMV only. This study used a strategy designed to recruit alveoli and protect against volutrauma. V_T was kept low in both groups and oxygenation was achieved by increasing mean P_{aw} in the HFOV group or PEEP in the CMV group.

Recently, Fort et al. (169) applied a similar strategy of recruiting alveoli by increasing mean P_{aw} to 17 adult patients with ARDS treated with HFOV (169). Patients who had failed CMV were switched to HFOV at a mean P_{aw} 1–2 cm H_2O greater than on CMV, and mean P_{aw} was increased until O_2 sat was >90 and $Fio_2 < 0.6$. Amplitude pressure was adjusted to keep $Paco_2$ less than 60 and pH above 7.25. Significant improvements in oxygenation index were seen within 3 hours and Fio_2 was reduced by 12 hours. Although mean P_{aw} was higher on HFO than on CMV, PIP was less. End-inspiratory pressures and lung volumes were not measured in the studies by Arnold et al. (135) and Fort et al. (169), but the data suggest that HFOV can achieve similar gas exchange with a lower end-inspiratory volume and less cyclic change in alveolar volume than CMV. Additional studies will be needed to determine if HFOV can reduce the incidence of VILI and improve outcome in ARDS.

C. Inhaled Nitric Oxide

Nitric oxide (NO) is a potent vasodilator that rapidly diffuses across cell membranes and is quickly inactivated upon contact with hemoglobin. When administered by inhalation, NO is a selective pulmonary vasodilator that acts preferentially in well-ventilated areas of the lung. The U.S. FDA has recently approved inhaled NO (INO) for neonates with persistent pulmonary hypertension and hypoxic respiratory failure.

In ARDS, INO decreases venous admixture (170) and improves oxygenation by stealing blood flow from intrapulmonary shunts and redirecting it to well ventilated alveoli (Fig. 12). INO has little effect on decreasing blood flow to areas of low V/Q (171,172). The effect of INO on oxygenation is additive to

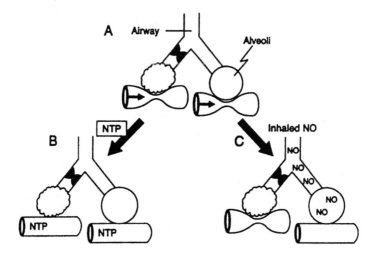

Figure 12 Effect of nitroglycerin and inhaled nitric oxide on ventilation-perfusion relationships in the lung. Like other pulmonary vasodilators, nitroglycerin acts throughout the pulmonary circulation. Inhibition of hypoxic pulmonary vasoconstriction increases blood flow to nonventilated alveoli, thereby increasing Qs/QT. Increasing blood flow to well ventilated alveoli does not offset the increase in Qs/QT because O_2 saturation in blood-perfusing well-ventilated alveoli is already maximal. In contrast, inhaled nitric oxide results in increased perfusion of ventilated alveoli only, resulting in a steal phenomenon from nonventilated alveoli and fall in Qs/QT. (From Ref. 261.)

that of PEEP (173) and can be amplified by concomitant intravenous administration of agents that potentiate hypoxic pulmonary vasoconstriction (174).

Acute improvements in oxygenation with INO have been well demonstrated in patients with ARDS. Overall, some improvement in oxygenation is seen in 80% of ARDS patients and the increase in Pao_2/Fio_2 averages about 35% (175). Criteria that predict a favorable response to INO have not been identified. Although several studies have reported a positive correlation between the degree of improvement in oxygenation and the initial PVR (176–178), other studies (179,180) have found none. The degree of initial venous admixture also does not appear to correlate with the oxygenation response to INO (180). One study (181) reported that the INO response rate may be lower in ARDS patients with septic shock than in ARDS patients who are not septic.

Pulmonary hypertension is a frequent component of ARDS and may correlate with severity of lung injury and overall mortality (182). Numerous studies have shown that INO reduces pulmonary artery pressure (PAP) in ARDS (150,170,173,176,180). On average, mean PAP falls approximately 15% from baseline. INO has little effect on systemic blood pressure or cardiac output, although there is some evidence that INO can improve right ventricular ejection fraction in ARDS (180,161). INO has also been shown to blunt increases in PAP caused by hypercapneic ventilation in ARDS (183).

The effect of INO on oxygenation is dose dependent. The ED_{50} is approximately 1 ppm (184) with a maximal effect between 5 and 10 ppm. At doses >20 ppm INO may worsen oxygenation, probably as the result of diffusion of INO from well-ventilated to poorly ventilated lung regions. In contrast, the pulmonary vasodilator response to INO is nearly linear up to doses of 100 ppm (Fig. 13).

Other possible beneficial effects of INO in ARDS include improved ventilation by relaxing bronchial smooth muscle (185) and decreasing VD/VT due to increasing flow to well-ventilated alveoli (186). Small but significant decreases in $Paco_2$ have been observed in some clinical trials of INO in ARDS (173). NO reduces pulmonary venous tone (187), and one study (188) found that INO reduced pulmonary venous resistance and pulmonary capillary pressure in patients with ARDS. This effect may be partially responsible for the INO-induced reduction in lung fluid filtration (189). INO may also inhibit recruitment of alveolar neutrophils (190), attenuate oxidant-induced increases in pulmonary microvascular permeability (191), and reduce alveolar cytokine levels (192).

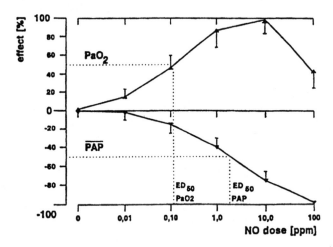

Figure 13 Dose-response of inhaled nitric oxide on Pao_2 and mean pulmonary artery pressure ($\overline{PAP}$). The ED_{50} for oxygenation is less than 1 ppm. The effect of INO on improving oxygenation reaches a maximum effect at 10 ppm and decreases at higher doses. In contrast, the ED_{50} for the effect of INO on lowering $\overline{PAP}$ is nearly 10-fold higher and remains linear up to 100 ppm. (From Ref. 184.)

Adverse Effects

Methemoglobinemia and NO_2 formation are the most serious toxicities of INO. Formation of methemoglobin is dependent on the dose of NO used, whereas production of NO_2 increases with the concentration of both NO and O_2 and the time that these molecules are in contact with each other. Standard practice is to measure NO_2 continuously, to check methemoglobin levels at the beginning of therapy, and to avoid drugs that contribute to methemoglobinemia. Other potential toxicities of INO include free radical injury (193), severe rebound pulmonary hypertension, and hypoxemia during temporary interruption of INO (194).

Clinical Trials

Despite the potential benefits of INO therapy, RCTs have failed to demonstrate improvement in outcome in patients with ARDS (195,196). In a phase II study (197), 177 patients were randomized to receive one of five different doses of INO (1.25, 5, 10, 40, 80 ppm) or placebo (N_2). The oxygenation response during the first 4 hours of study was significantly greater for the INO groups than for placebo. Oxygenation index ($Fio_2 \times$ mean P_{aw}/Pao_2) was lower in INO patients than in controls for the first 4 days of the study. However, there were no differences in survival, days of mechanical ventilation, or ICU days. In a post hoc analysis, the number of days alive and off mechanical ventilation by day 28 was significantly greater in patients that received 5 ppm INO than controls (62 vs. 44%, $p < 0.05$). In a larger phase III trial of INO in ARDS completed in 1998 (198), 385 patients were randomized to receive INO at 5 ppm ($n = 192$) or placebo ($n = 193$). The Pao_2/Fio_2 ratio was higher in the INO patients for the first 2 days of the study, but no differences were seen between treatment groups by day 3. There were no differences in days alive and off assisted ventilation ($10.7 + 9.7$ vs. $10.6 + 9.8$ days) or mortality (23 vs. 20%) between INO and placebo patients, respectively. Similar results have recently been reported in a European trial (199). In this study, only patients that had greater than a 20% increase in Pao_2 were randomized to INO or placebo. No differences in 30 day mortality were seen between INO responders given INO ($n = 93$), INO responders not given INO ($n = 87$), and patients who did not respond to INO ($n = 88$).

At the present time, there are no data that support the routine use of INO in ARDS. Future studies may identify subgroups of patients that benefit from INO therapy. Until that time, INO should be considered investigational and should be reserved for patients that are likely to benefit from acute improvements in oxygenation or RV afterload reduction.

D. Liquid Ventilation

Ventilating the lung with liquid instead of air may sound like the stuff of science fiction, but in reality adequate ventilation with liquid mediums was accomplished in animals as early as the 1960s (200). Over the next decade, several investigators (201–203) confirmed that adequate gas exchange could be accomplished in animals under normoxic conditions using liquid perfluorocarbons. Further refinement in the technique occurred in the early 1990s as investigators discovered that the lung could be partially filled with perfluorocarbon and ventilated with air. This technique, known as partial liquid ventilation (PLV), allowed liquid ventilation to be administered with conventional mechanical ventilators, and ushered liquid ventilation into the ICU (204). Most studies to date have used a perfluorocarbon specifically developed for clinical applications known as perflubron (perfluorooctylbromide, Alliance Pharmaceutical Corp., San Diego, CA). Perflubron is a clear, odorless fluid that has a surface tension that is one fourth that of normal saline. The solubility of O_2 and CO_2 in perflubron is approximately 26- and 3-fold greater than normal saline, respectively.

There are advantages of ventilating ARDS patients with a liquid medium. Alveolar surface tension forces are reduced and more lung is inflated at any given pressure with a liquid medium as compared with air (Fig. 14). A liquid medium also has a vertical pressure gradient. Thus, pressure is greater in the dependent than in the nondependent portions of the lungs. In this regard, PLV has been referred to as "liquid PEEP," preferentially recruiting alveoli in dependent lung zones while sparing nondependent alveoli from elevated pressure (205). Preferential distribution of perflubron to dependent lung zones has been demonstrated in adult sheep with oleic acid–induced lung injury (206). In addition, there is evidence to suggest that PLV redistributes pulmonary blood flow from dependent to nondependent areas of the lung (207), which could improve ventilation perfusion matching.

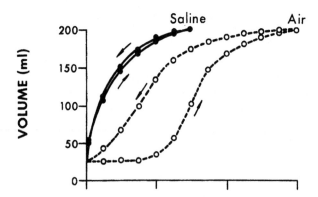

Figure 14 Pressure-volume curves of lungs inflated with saline and with air. Inflation with a liquid medium eliminates surface tension forces at the air liquid interface resulting in the lack of hysteresis and a greater lung volume at any given pressure. (From Ref. 262.)

Many of these potential advantages of liquid ventilation have been demonstrated in animal studies of acute lung injury. In premature lambs delivered by cesarean section, oxygenation, lung compliance, and CO_2 removal were considerably better in animals receiving PLV than CMV (208). Six of seven lambs given PLV survived, whereas six of nine given CMV expired within 3 hours. Similar results were obtained in neonatal pigs (209). Improvements in gas exchange and lung compliance have also been demonstrated in adult animal models of acute lung injury (210–215). In dogs with oleic acid–induced lung injury (215), perflubron improved oxygenation and static respiratory system compliance in a dose-dependent and reversible fashion. In this study, perflubron was equally efficacious when given immediately prior to or 90 minutes after oleic acid. Removal of perflubron resulted in deterioration of oxygenation back to control levels within 30 minutes. Other studies have shown that PLV reduces Qs/QT (206) and increases end-expiratory lung volume and static compliance in isolated perfused, surfactant-deficient lungs (216). Recently (214), addition of perfluobron to acutely injured lungs was shown to reduce the pressure at which the lower inflection point occurs and to return end inspiratory pressure to normal (Fig. 15).

In addition to improved alveolar recruitment, perflubron may have anti-inflammatory effects. Animal studies have shown PLV-related reductions in reactive oxygen species, inflammatory cytokines, and oxidant-induced lung injury (217,218). One study (219) in patients with acute lung injury found that alveoar

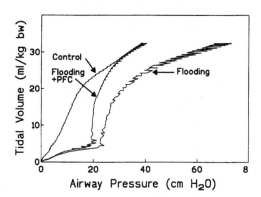

Figure 15 Pressure-volume curves from intact rats ventilated with 33 mL/kg of air before (control) and after instillation of normal saline to mimic acute pulmonary edema (flooding). Ventilating with air after flooding caused a marked shift of the PV curve to the right and the appearance of a distinct inflection point on the lower limb of the curve (LIP). The instillation of perflubron after flooding (flooding + PFC) shifts the LIP to the left, improves compliance, and returns end-inspiratory pressure to normal. (From Ref. 214.)

neutrophil counts, protein levels, and IL-1, IL-6, and IL-10 levels were lower in patients ventilated with PLV than with CMV. Interestingly, animal studies have found that PEEP or HFOV was as effective as PLV in reducing alveolar neutrophil counts, cytokine levels, and myeloperoxidase activity (220–222), suggesting that the anti-inflammatory effect of PLV may be secondary to alveolar recruitment.

Instillation of perflubron into the lung does not appear to significantly affect cardiopulmonary hemodynamics. Some studies (223) have described a drop in cardiac output with the onset of PLV, but others (224) have found no such effect or report that the decrease in cardiac output was easily corrected by volume infusion (225). Early studies (226) found that at the same lung volume, pulmonary vascular resistance was greater in lungs filled with fluorocarbons than in lungs filled with air. However, a recent study (227) found no increase in pulmonary arterial pressure or static or dynamic pulmonary vascular compliance in isolated perfused rabbit lungs filled with 15 mL/kg body weight of perflubron.

Guidelines for ventilator settings in PLV have not been determined. Several studies (228–232) have shown that using PEEP or IRV in PLV improves gas exchange without adversely affecting cardiac output. Some data (229) suggest that PEEP in PLV should be set just above LIP of the PV curve as has been recommended for CMV. A recent study (233) found that when PEEP was set above LIP, neither the mode of mechanical ventilation nor the I:E ratio significantly affected gas exchange or lung mechanics in PLV.

The use of PLV in humans was first reported in the early 1990s when it was used to ventilate several preterm infants with surfactant deficiency and respiratory distress syndrome (234). A larger trial of PLV in premature infants with respiratory distress was published in 1996 (235). In that study, PLV improved Pao_2/Fio_2 from 60 ± 34 to 143 ± 99 mmHg ($p = 0.02$) and dynamic lung compliance from 0.18 ± 0.12 to 0.29 ± 0.12 mL/cm H_2O/kg in 10 of 13 preterm infants with respiratory distress syndrome who had failed surfactant replacement therapy. Infants were given PLV for an average of 2 days, and 8 of 10 survived to 36 weeks gestation. A series of 10 adults, 4 children, and 5 neonates ventilated with PLV while on extracorporeal life support (ECLS) was reported in 1995 (236). Addition of PLV to ECLS decreased the (A-a)Do_2 from 590 ± 25 to 471 ± 42 and increased lung compliance from 0.18 ± 0.04 to 0.29 ± 0.04 12 mL/cm H_2O/kg over the first 3 days of the study. Initial experience in adult patients with ARDS not on ECLS was published in 1998 (237). Gas exchange improved in eight of nine patients given PLV over 4 days. The (A-a)Do_2 decreased from 430 ± 142 to 229 ± 20 mmHg after 48 hours ($p = 0.13$) and Pao_2/Fio_2 increased from 128 ± 20 to 184 ± 34 ($p = NS$). No change in lung compliance was observed. Seven of the nine patients survived beyond 28 days, and five survived to discharge. Data from a phase II RCT of PLV in adult patients with acute hypoxic respiratory failure were published in abstract form in 1997 (238).

Sixty-five patients were randomly assigned to receive PLV with perflubron, and 25 patients were assigned to CMV. PLV was continued for 5 days and patients were followed for 28 days. No difference in ventilator-free days or 28-day mortality were seen (6.3 ± 1 vs. 6.7 ± 2 days and 38.5 vs. 32.0% for PLV vs. conventional ventilation). Interpretation of these results was complicated by an unequal distribution of elderly patients in the PLV limb. Retrospective analysis of patients < 55 years of age revealed trends toward improvement in both days off mechanical ventilation and 28-day mortality in the PLV group (9 ± 1 vs. 4 ± 2 days and 25.6 vs. 36.8% for PLV vs. conventional ventilation) (M. Wedel, personal communication). A phase II–III, multicenter RCT of PLV versus CMV is currently in progress.

VIII. Adjuvants to Mechanical Ventilation in ARDS

The aim of reducing end inspiratory lung volume may inadvertently increase V_D/V_T and raise $Paco_2$. Tracheal gas insufflation (TGI), intratracheal pulmonary ventilation, and aspiration of airway dead space are methods that can reduce V_D/V_T and CO_2 retention when permissive hypercapnia is not desirable.

A. Tracheal Gas Insufflation

In the mid-1980s, Slutsky et al. (239) evaluated TGI of oxygen in paralyzed dogs. With O_2 flows of 2 and 3 L/min delivered to or just beyond the carina, oxygenation was maintained despite a $Paco_2$ of 164 torr after 2 hours. Placing catheters in both mainstem airways allowed maintenance of eucapnea (240). Sznajder et al. (241) evaluated TGI in combination with PEEP and continuous positive pressure ventilation in a canine oleic acid injury model. Flow was delivered 2–5 cm H_2O above the carina. Using equal PEEP and RR, TGI produced a reduction in the P_{plat} from 25.6 to 17.7 cm H_2O and V_T was decreased from 437 to 184 mL, while keeping $Paco_2$ constant. Nakos et al. (242) were also able to reduce V_T, PIP, and mean P_{aw} while keeping $Paco_2$ and oxygenation constant by using TGI with 4–6 L/min of O_2 in seven paralyzed patients with moderate to severe ALI. In addition to improving CO_2 elimination, TGI has been found to improve oxygenation in some models of acute lung injury. This likely occurs from an increase in P_{aw} and additional alveolar recruitment. In dogs with oleic acid–induced lung injury, TGI did not improve oxygenation when EELV was held constant (243).

TGI can be administered as an adjunct to VCV or PCV. In the PCV mode, TGI flow will continue after the ventilator-derived flow has stopped (244). This can raise PIP and V_T prior to expiration, particularly with long inspiratory times. This problem can be avoided by inserting a pressure-relief valve into the circuit (245). TGI has also been used successfully with high-frequency ventilation

(HFV) and airway pressure release ventilation (APRV) to improve oxygenation, reduce $Paco_2$, and lower airway pressures (246–248).

Several types of catheters have been used to administer TGI. Straight catheters direct flow at the carina and reverse thrust catheters direct flow toward the mouth. Other variables include the internal diameter and the distance of the catheter from the carina. Studies in animals suggest that the effect of TGI on CO_2 elimination is not greatly affected by the type of catheter used or the internal diameter of the catheter (249). However, studies in humans (250,251) with various causes of acute respiratory failure found that TGI was more effective with the catheter at 1 cm than at 10 cm from the carina.

In summary, TGI reduces V_T and V_D/V_T by flushing out gas from the anatomic dead space and improves oxygenation, probably by increasing end-expiratory and end-inspiratory lung volumes (252). Several potential adverse effects may occur with TGI, notably overinflation of alveoli with obstruction of expiratory flow and mucosal damage from drying by the air jet, but with further refinements in equipment and technique TGI may be of benefit in low V_T ventilation in ARDS.

B. Intratracheal Pulmonary Ventilation

This form of ventilation may be considered a variant of continuous TGI, modified to function as a stand-alone mode of mechanical ventilation. With intratracheal pulmonary ventilation (ITPV), a continuous flow of gas is delivered through a small catheter placed within but at the end of an endotracheal tube that is 1 cm proximal to the carina (253,254). External controls cycle an expiratory valve, open for expiration, closed for inspiration, at widely variable rates, and with widely variable tidal volumes. As originally described, a diffuser was placed at the end of the catheter, but this resulted in elevated end-expiratory pressures at the level of the carina. Subsequently, the catheter was modified such that the end of the catheter was occluded. Gas exits from side holes in a cephalad direction, creating a venturi effect during expiration that facilitates ventilation and results in PEEP levels of near zero. This arrangement is referred to as the reverse thrust catheter (Fig. 16).

In a sheep model comparing ITPV to pressure-controlled ventilation at constant $Paco_2$ and PEEP, ITPV reduced dead space, V_T, PIP, and VE (253). There were no significant differences in oxygenation or CO. Secretions were watery and scant, and the tracheal mucosa looked intact at autopsy. Rossi et al. (79) evaluated ITPV in 12 tracheostomized sheep with acute lung injury ventilated in the prone position. In the ITPV group carinal PEEP was kept at 3–5 cm H_2O, PIP was <20 cm H_2O, frequency was 30–80 bpm, and V_T was 2.5–6 mL/kg. Control animals were ventilated with square wave flow VCV, V_T was 8–12 mL/kg, and PEEP was titrated to O_2 saturation >90% at an Fio_2 of <0.6 (average

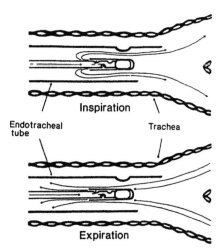

Inspiration

Endotracheal
tube

Trachea

Expiration

Figure 16 The direction of gas flow in the reverse thrust catheter (RTC) system. With the expiratory valve closed, gas emerges from the catheter in a cephalad direction prior to changing direction toward the carina. When the expiratory valve opens, the high-velocity cephalad flow entrains gas (venturi effect) from the surrounding region. (From Ref. 253.)

7.5 ± 2 cm H_2O). The CO was greater in sheep ventilated with ITPV, and they required less volume expansion and lower doses of pressors. Three of six sheep in the ITPV group required ventilatory support, amounting to 40% of the total VT. All six ITPV animals were off supplemental oxygenation in 83 ± 54 hours, whereas all of the control animals were dead in 50 ± 39 hours. Approximately 20% of the lung in the dependent zones was atelectatic in the ITPV group as compared to 50% in the control group. The ITPV group had a lower lung injury score.

C. Aspiration of Dead Space

Instead of flushing the trachea with oxygen during expiration, as occurs in TGI and ITPV, aspiration of dead space (ASPIDS) suctions gas from the trachea 60 mm proximal to the end of the ETT while tubing gas is flushed into the ETT by a stream of fresh oxygen (Fig. 17). De Robertis et al. (254) recently described their experience with ASPIDS. After reducing VT and increasing respiratory frequency to maintain VE, ASPID led to significant reductions in PIP and P_{plat} and no change or a reduction in $Paco_2$.

TGI, ITPV, and ASPIDS are techniques that offer the promise of reduced dead space and hence reduced VE, VT and P_{aw}. ITPV may be able to function as a stand-alone mode of mechanical ventilation (255). More widespread applica-

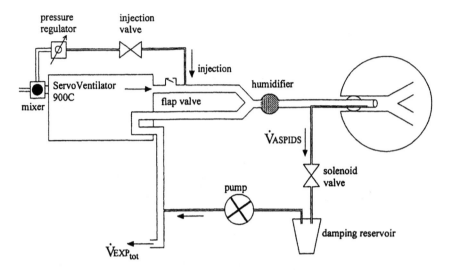

Figure 17 System design for aspiration of dead space. When the solenoid valve opens, gas is aspirated from the tracheal tube, and gas from the oxygen mixer is injected into the inspiratory line, flushing the line from the y-connector down to the end of the endotracheal tube. (From Ref. 254.)

tion of these techniques awaits availability and standardization of the necessary hardware along with outcome-based studies in humans.

IX. Summary and Conclusions

An extensive body of literature regarding the mechanical ventilation of patients with acute lung injury has been generated since the development of intensive care units 3 decades ago. The focus of initial ventilator strategies was optimizing gas exchange. However, experience has taught us that few patients with ARDS die from lack of oxygen or intractable respiratory acidosis and that positive pressure ventilation, when used incorrectly, can do as much harm as good. Although VILI has been well described for many years, only recently have data become available demonstrating that limiting ventilation, even at the expense of elevated $Paco_2$ or increased respiratory rate, can significantly improve survival in ARDS.

Much effort is being expended trying to determine the best strategy to minimize VILI. This continues to be an area of active research that is not likely to offer definitive recommendations for some time. Few investigators today would argue with Lachman's dictum: ''Open up the lung and keep the lung open'' (78), but how this should be accomplished remains to be determined. The clinician should be warned that whatever approach is advocated, it is unlikely to be appropriate for all patients at all stages of their disease. Ventilatory strategies will always need to be tailored to the patient's pathophysiology and reassessed as their disease progresses or their lungs begin to heal. Alternative and adjunct methods of ventilation continue to be attractive to investigators unhappy with the high rate of mortality in ARDS. Although some of these techniques appear promising, we must not forget the lessons learned from HFV and nitric oxide, i.e., improvements in physiologic variables do not always translate into tangible benefits to patients. Preventing alveolar collapse with PEEP and limiting volutrauma with small lung volumes are currently mainstays of modern ventilation strategies for ARDS. Whether further improvement in outcome can be accomplished with more aggressive recruitment maneuvers, prone positioning, high-frequency or liquid ventilation, or adjuvant techniques to decrease dead space remains to be proven.

Acknowledgments

This work was supported in part by National Institutes of Health grant HL-02613 and a grant-in-aid from the American Heart Association—RI Affiliate (J. R. Klinger).

References

1. Milberg JA, Davis DR, Steinberg KP, Hudson LD. Improved survival of patients with acute respiratory distress syndrome (ARDS): 1983–1993. JAMA 1995; 273: 306–309.
2. The Acute Respiratory Distress Syndrome Network. Ventilation with lower tidal volumes as compared with traditional tidal volumes for acute lung injury and the acute respiratory distress syndrome. N Engl J Med 2000; 342:1301–1308.
3. Ralph DD, Robertson HT, Weaver LJ, Hlastala MP, Carrico CJ, Hudson LD. Distribution of ventilation and perfusion during positive end-expiratory pressure in the adult respiratory distress syndrome. Am Rev Respir Dis 1985; 131:54–60.
4. Ravenscraft SA, McArthur CD, Path JM, Iber C. Components of excess ventilation in patients initiated on mechanical ventilation. Crit Care Med 1991; 19:916–925.
5. Pelosi P, Cereda M, Foti G, Giacomino M, Pesenti A. Alterations of lung and chest wall mechanics in patients with acute lung injury: effects of positive end-expiratory pressure. Am J Respir Crit Care 1995; 152:531–537.
6. Gattinoni L, Pesenti A, Bombino M, Baglioni S, Rivolta M, Rossi F, Rossi G, Fumagalli R, Marcolin R, Mascheroni D, Torresin A. Relationship between lung computed tomographic density gas exchange, and PEEP in acute respiratory failure. Anesthesiology 1988; 69:824–832.
7. Maunder RJ, Shuman WP, HcHugh JW, Marglin SI, Butler J. Preservation of normal lung regions in the adult respiratory distress syndrome. JAMA 1986; 255: 2463–2465.

8. Benito S, Lemaire F, Mankikian B, Harf A. Total respiratory compliance as a function of lung volume in patients with mechanical ventilation. Intensive Care Med 1985; 11:76–79.
9. Marini JJ. Tidal volume, PEEP, and barotrauma: an open and shut case. Chest 1996; 109:302–304.
10. Haake R, Schlichtig R, Ulstad DR, Henschen RR. Barotrauma. Pathophysiology, risk factor, and prevention. Chest 1987; 608–613.
11. Pierson DJ. Alveolar rupture during mechanical ventilation: role of PEEP, peak airway pressure, and distending volume. Respir Care 1988; 33:472–486.
12. Tinker J, Vandam L, Cohen LH. Tension lung cyst as a complication of postoperative positive pressure ventilation therapy. Chest 1973; 64:518–520.
13. Weaver LK, Morris A. Venous and arterial gas embolism associated with positive pressure ventilation. Chest 1998; 113:1132–1134.
14. Slavin G, Nunn JF, Crow J, Dore CJ. Bronchiolectasis—a complication of artificial ventilation Br Med J 1982; 285:931–934.
15. Rouby JJ, Lherm T, de Lassale EM, Poete P, Bodin L, Finet JF, Callard P, Viars P. Histologic aspects of pulmonary barotrauma in critically ill patients with acute respiratory failure. Intensive Care Med 1993; 19:383–389.
16. Schnapp LM, Chin DP, Szaflarski N, Matthay MA. Frequency and importance of barotrauma in 100 patients with acute lung injury. Crit Care Med 1995; 23:272–278.
17. Weg JG, Anzueto A, Balk R, Weidemann HP, Pattishall EN, Schork MA, Wagner LA. The relation of pneumothorax and other air leaks to mortality in the acute respiratory distress syndrome. N Eng J Med 1998; 338:341–346.
18. Greenfield LJ, Evert PA, Benson DW. Effect of positive pressure ventilation on surface tension properties of lung extracts. Anesthesiology 1964; 25:312–316.
19. Webb HH, Tierney DF. Experimental pulmonary edema due to intermittent positive pressure ventilation with high inflation pressures. Protection by positive end-expiratory pressure. Am Rev Respir Dis 1974; 110:556–565.
20. Egan EA. Lung inflation, lung solute permeability, and alveolar edema. J Appl Physiol 1982; 53:121–125.
21. Dreyfuss, D, Soler P, Basset G, Saumon G. High inflation pressure pulmonary edema. Respective effects of high airway pressure, high tidal volume, and positive end-expiratory pressure. Am Rev Respir Dis 1988; 137:1159–1164.
22. Dreyfuss D, Saumon G. Role of tidal volume, FRC, and end-inspiratory volume in the development of pulmonary edema following mechanical ventilation. Am Rev Respir Dis 1993; 148:1194–1203.
23. Muscedere JG, Mullen JBM, Gan K, Slutsky AS. Tidal ventilation at low airway pressures can augment lung injury. Am J Respir Crit Care Med 1994; 149:1327–1334.
24. Carlton DP, Cummings JJ, Scheerer RG, Poulain FR, Bland RD. Lung overexpansion increases pulmonary microvascular protein permeability in young lambs. Am Physiol Soc 1990; 161:577–583.
25. Hernandez LA, Peevy KJ, Moise AA, Parker JC. Chest wall restriction limits high airway pressure-induced lung injury in young rabbits. Am Physiol Soc 1989; 161:2364–2368.

26. John J, Taskar V, Evander E, Wollmer P, Jonson B. Additive nature of distension and surfactant perturbation on alveolocapillary permeability. Eur Respir J 1997; 10:192–199.

27. Faridy EE. Effect of ventilation on movement of surfactant in airways. Respir Physiol 1976; 27:323–334.

28. Wyszogrodski I, Kyei-Aboagye K, Taeusch HW, Avery ME. Surfactant inactivation by hyperventilation: conservation by end-expiratory pressure. J Appl Physiol 1975; 3:461–465.

29. Brown ES, Johnson RP, Clements JA. Pulmonary surface tension. J Appl Physiol 1959; 14:717–720.

30. Tsuno K, Miura K, Takeya M, Kolobow T, Morioka T. Histopathologic pulmonary changes from mechanical ventilation at high peak airway pressures. Am Rev Respir Dis 1991; 143:1115–1120.

31. Dreyfuss D, Basset G, Soler G, Saumon G. Intermittent positive-pressure hyperventilation with high inflation pressure produced pulmonary microvascular injury in rats. Am Rev Respir Dis 1985; 132:880–884.

32. Parker JC, Hernandez LA, Longenecker GL, Peevy K, Johnson W. Lung edema caused by high peak inspiratory pressure in dogs. Am Rev Resir Dis 1990; 142: 321–328.

33. Parker JC, Townsley MI, Rippe B, Taylor AE, Thigpen J. Increased microvascular permeability in dog lungs due to high peak airway pressures. J Appl Physiol 1984; 57:1809–1816.

34. Ludwigs U, Philip A, Robertson B, Hendenstierna G. Pulmonary epithelial permeability. An animal study of inverse ratio ventilation and conventional mechanical ventilation. Chest 1996; 110:486–493.

35. Tremblay L, Valenza F, Robeiro SP, Li J, Slutsky AS. Injurious ventilatory strategies increase cytokines and c-fos mRNA expression in an isolated rat lung mode. J Clin Invest 1997; 99:944–952.

36. Takata M, Abe J, Tanaka H, Kitano Y, Dio S, Kohsaka T, Miyasaka K. Intraalveolar expression of tumor necrosis factor-$\propto$ gene during conventional and high-frequency ventilation. Am J Respir Crit Care Med 1997; 156:272–279.

37. Berg JT, Fu Z, Breen EC, Tran H-C, Mathieu-Costello O, West JB. High lung inflation increases mRNA levels of ECM components and growth factors in lung parenchyma. J Appl Physiol 1997; 83:120–128.

38. Parker JC, Breen EC, West JB. High vascular and airway pressures increase interstitial protein mRNA expression in isolated rat lungs. J Appl Physiol 1997; 83:1697–1705.

39. Murphy DB, Cregg N, Tremblay L, Engelberts D, Laffey JG, Slutsky AS, Romaschin A, Kavanagh BP. Adverse ventilatory strategy causes pulmonary-to-systemic translocation of endotoxin. Am J Respir Crit Care Med. 2000; 162:27–33.

40. Jardin F. Chest wall elastance and acute respiratory failure. Crit Care Med 1999; 27:1653–1654.

41. Ranieri VM, Brienza N, Santostasi S, Puntillo F, Mascia L, Vitale N, Giuliani R, Memeo V, Bruno F, Fiore T, Brienza A, Slutsky AS. Impairment of lung and chest wall mechanics in patients with acute respiratory distress syndrome. Role of abdominal distension. Am J Respir Crit Care Med 1997; 156:1082–1091.

42. Mergoni M, Martelli A, Volpi A, Primavera S, Zuccoli P, Rossi A. Impact of positive end-expiratory pressure on chest wall and lung pressure-volume curve in acute respiratory failure. Am J Respir Crit Care Med 1997; 156:846–854.

43. Ranieri VM, Vitale N, Grasso S, Puntillo F, Mascia L, Paparella D, Tunzi P, Guiliani R, de Luca Tupputi L, Fiore T. Time-course of impairment of respiratory mechanics after cardiac surgery and cardiopulmonary bypass. Crit Care Med 1999; 27:1454–1460.

44. Matamis D, Lemaire F, Harf A, run-Buisson C, Ansquer JC, Atlan G. Total respirator pressure-volume curves in the adult respiratory distress syndrome Chest 1984; 86:58–66.

45. Gattinoni L, Pelosi P, Crotti S, Valenza F. Effects of positive end-expiratory pressure on regional distribution of tidal volume and recruitment in adult respiratory distress syndrome. Am J Respir Crit Care Med 1995; 151:1807–1814.

46. Hickling KG. The pressure-volume curve is greatly modified by recruitment. A mathematical model of ARDS lungs. Am J Respir Crit Care Med 1998; 158:194–202.

47. Jonson B, Richard J-C, Straus C, Mancebo J, Lemaire F, Brochard L. Pressure-volume curves and compliance in acute lung injury: evidence of recruitment above the lower inflection point. Am J Respir Crit Care Med 1999; 159:1172–1178.

48. Lemaire F. ARDS and PV curves: the inseparable duet? Intensive Care Med 2000, 26:1–2.

49. Rossi A, Gottfried SB, Zocchi L, Higgs BD, Lennox S, Calverley PMA, Grassino A, Milic-Emili J. Measurement of static compliance of the total respiratory system in patients with acute respiratory failure during mechanical ventilation. Am Rev Respir Dis 1985; 131:672–677.

50. Ranieri VM, Elssa NT, Corbeil C, Chasse M, Braidy J, Matar N, Milic-Emili J. Effects of positive end-expiratory pressure on alveolar recruitment and gas exchange in patients with the adult respiratory distress syndrome. Am Rev Respir Dis 1991; 144:544–551.

51. Rimensberger PC, Cox PN, Frndova H, Bryan C. The open lung during small tidal volume ventilation: concepts of recruitment and "optimal" positive end-expiratory pressure. Crit Care Med 1999; 27:1946–1952.

52. Marini JJ, Ravenscraft SA. Mean airway pressure: physiologic determinants and clinical importance. Part 1: physiologic determinants and measurements. Crit Care Med 1992; 20:1604–1616.

53. Pesenti A, Marcolin R, Prato P, Borelli M, Riboni A, Gattinoni L. Mean airway pressure vs. positive end-expiratory pressure during mechanical ventilation. Crit Care Med 1985; 13:34–37.

54. Broccard AF, Hotchkiss JR, Suzuki S, Olson D, Marini JJ. Effects of mean airway pressure and tidal excursion on lung injury induced by mechanical ventilation in an isolated perfused rabbit lung model. Crit Care Med 1999; 27:1533–1541.

55. Mead J, Collier C. Relation of volume history of lungs to respiratory mechanics in anesthetized dogs. J Appl Physiol 1959; 14:669–678.

56. Bendixen HH, Hedley-Whyte J, Chir B, Laver MB. Impaired oxygenation in surgical patients during general anesthesia with controlled ventilation. N Engl J Med 1963; 269:991–996.

57. Rothen HU, Sporre B, Engberg G, Wegenius G, Hedenstierna G. Re-expansion of atelectasis during general anesthesia: a computed tomography study. Br J Anaesth 1993; 71:788–795.

58. Lapinsky SE, Aubin M, Mehta S, Boiteau P, Slutsky AS. Safety and efficacy of a sustained inflation for alveolar recruitment in adults with respiratory failure. Intensive Care Med 1999; 25:1297–1301.

59. Pelosi P, Cadringher P, Bottino N, Panigada M, Carrieri F, Riva El, Lissoni A, Gattinoni L. Sigh in acute respiratory distress syndrome. Am J Respir Crit Care Med 1999; 159:872–880.

60. Rimensberger PC, Pristine G, Mullen B, Cox PN, Slutsky AS. Lung recruitment during small tidal volume ventilation allows minimal positive end-expiratory pressure without augmenting lung injury. Crit Care Med 1999; 27:1940–1945.

61. Dantzker DR, Lynch JP, Weg JG. Depression of cardiac output is a mechanism of shunt reduction in the therapy of acute respiratory failure. Chest 1980; 77:636–642.

62. Malo J, Ali J, Wood LDH. How does positive end-expiratory pressure reduce intrapulmonary shunt in canine pulmonary edema? J Appl Physiol 1984; 57:1002–1010.

63. Pare PD, Warriner B, Baile EM, Hogg JC. Redistribution of pulmonary extravascular water with positive end-expiratory pressure in canine pulmonary edema. Am Rev Respir Dis 1983; 127:590–593.

64. Taskar V, John HJ, Evander E, Robertson B, Jonson B. Surfactant dysfunction makes lungs vulnerable to repetitive collapse and reexpansion. Am J Respir Crit Care Med 1997; 155:313–320.

65. Sandhar BK, Niblett DJ, Argiras EP, Dunnill MS, Sykes MK. Effects of positive end-expiratory on hyaline membrane formation in a rabbit model of the neonatal respiratory distress syndrome. Intensive Care Med 1988; 14:538–546.

66. Woo SW, Hedley-White J. Macrophage accumulation and pulmonary edema due to thoracotomy and lung overinflation. J Appl Physiol 1972; 33:14–21.

67. Colmenero-Ruiz M, Fernandez-Mondejar E, Fernandez-Sacristan MA, Rivera-Fernandez R, Vazquez-Mata G. PEEP and low tidal volume ventilation reduce lung water in porcine pulmonary edema. Am J Respir Crit Care Med 1997; 155:964–970.

68. Albert RK. Least PEEP: primum non nocere. Chest 1985; 87:2–3.

69. Kirby RR, Downs JB, Civetta JM, Modell JH, Dannemiller FJ, Klein EF, Hodges M. High level positive end expiratory pressure (PEEP) in acute respiratory insufficiency. Chest 1975; 67:156–163.

70. Suter PM, Fairley B, Isenberg MD. Optimum end-expiratory airway pressure in patients with acute pulmonary failure. N Engl J Med 1975; 6:284–289.

71. Amato MBP, Barbas CS, Medeiros DM, Magaldi RB, Schettino GDP, Lorenzi-Filho G, Kairalla RA, Deheinzelin D, Munoz C, Oliveira R, Takagaki TY, Carvalho CR. Effect of a protective-ventilation strategy on mortality in the acute respiratory distress syndrome. N Engl J Med 1998; 338:347–354.

72. Kanarek DJ, Shannon DC. Adverse effect of positive end-expiratory pressure on pulmonary perfusion and arterial oxygenation. Am Rev Respir Dis 1975; 112:457–459.

73. Ravenscraft SA, Marinelli WA, Johnson T, Henke CA. Profound hypoxemia pre-

cipitated by positive end-expiratory pressure: induction of an intracardiac shunt. Crit Care Med 1992; 20:434–436.

74. Cujec B, Polasek P, Mayers I, Johnson D. Positive end-expiratory pressure increases the right-to left shunt in mechanically ventilated patients with patent foramen ovale. Ann Intern Med 1993; 119:887–894.

75. Bindslev L, Hedenstierna G, Santesson J, Gottlieb I, Carvallhas A. Ventilation-perfusion distribution during inhalation anaesthesia. Effects of spontaneous breathing, mechanical ventilation and positive end-expiratory pressure. Acta Anaesth 1981; 25:360–371.

76. Dueck R, Wagner PD, West JB. Effects of positive end-expiratory pressure on gas exchange in dogs with normal and edematous lungs. Anesthesiology 1977; 7:359–366.

77. Peevy JK, Hernandez LA, Moise AA, Parker JC. Barotrauma and microvascular injury in lungs of non-adult rabbits: effect of ventilation pattern. Crit Care Med 1990; 18:634–637.

78. Lachmann B. Open up the lung and keep the lung open. Intensive Care Med 1992; 18:319–321.

79. Rossi N, Kolobow T, Aprigliano M, Tsuno K, Giacomini M. Intratracheal pulmonary ventilation at low airway pressures in a ventilator-induced model of acute respiratory failure improves lung function and survival. Chest 1998; 114:1147–1157.

80. Marini JJ. Inverse ratio ventilation—simply an alternative or something more? Crit Care Med 1995; 80:224–227.

81. Modell IH, Cheney FW. Effects of inspiratory flow pattern on gas exchange in normal and abnormal lungs. J Appl Physiol 1979; 46:1103–1107.

82. Baker AB, Restall R, Clark BW. Effects of varying inspiratory flow waveform and time in intermittent positive pressure ventilation: emphysema. Br J Anaesth 1982; 54:547–554.

83. Ravenscraft SA, Burke WC, Marini JJ. Volume-cycled decelerating flow. An alternative form of mechanical ventilation. Chest 1992; 101:1342–1351.

84. Rappaport SH, Shpiner R, Yoshihara G, Wright J, Chang P, Abraham E. Randomized prospective trial of pressure-limited versus volume-controlled ventilation in severe respiratory failure. Crit Care Med 1994; 22:22–32.

85. Warters RD, Allen SJ, Tonnesen AS. Intratracheal pressure monitoring during synchronized intermittent mandatory ventilation and pressure controlled-inverse ratio ventilation. Crit Care Med 1997; 25:227–230.

86. Abraham E, Yoshihara G. Cardiorespiratory effects of pressure controlled ventilation in severe respiratory failure. Chest 1990; 98:1445–1449.

87. Cereda M, Foti G, Musch G, Sparacino ME, Pesenti A. Positive end-expiratory pressure prevents the loss of respiratory compliance during low tidal volume ventilation in acute lung injury patients. Chest 1996; 109:480–485.

88. Marini JJ, Crooke PS, Truwit JD. Determinants and limits of pressure-preset ventilation: a mathematical model of pressure control. J Appl Physiol 1989; 67:1081–1092.

89. Markstrom AM, Lichtwarck-Aschoff M, Svensson BA, Nordgren KA, Sjostrand UH. Ventilation with constant versus decelerating inspiratory flow in experimentally induced acute respiratory failure. Anesthesiology 1996; 84:882–889.

90. Al-Saady N, Bennett ED. Decelerating inspiratory flow waveform improves lung mechanics and gas exchange in patients on intermittent positive pressure ventilation. Intensive Care Med 1985; 11:68–75.

91. Munoz J, Guerrero JE, Escalante JL, Palomino R, De la Calle B. Pressure-controlled ventilation versus controlled mechanical ventilation with decelerating inspiratory flow. Crit Care Med 1993; 21:1143–1148.

92. Hickling KG, Henderson SJ, Jackson R. Low mortality associated with low volume pressure limited ventilation with permissive hypercapnia in severe adult respiratory distress syndrome. Intensive Care Med 1990; 16:372–377.

93. Amato MBP, Barbas CSV, Medeiros DM, Schettino GDP, Filho GL, Kairalla RA, Deheinzellin D, Morais C, Fernandes ED, Takagaki TY, Carvalho CRR. Beneficial effects of the "open lung approach" with low distending pressures in acute respiratory distress syndrome. Am J Respir Crit Care Med 1995; 152:1835–1846.

94. Brochard L, Roudot-Thoraval F, Roupie E, Delclaux C, Chastre J, Fernandez-Mondejar E, Clementi E, Mancebo J, Factor P, Matamis D, Raniere M, Blanch L, Rodi G, Mentec H, Dreyfuss D, Ferrer M, Brun-Buisson C, Tobin M, Lemaire F, and the Multicenter Trial Group on Tidal Volume Reduction in ARDS. Tidal volume reduction for prevention of ventilator-induced lung injury in acute respiratory distress syndrome. Am J Respir Crit Care Med 1998; 158:1831–1838.

95. Stewart TE, Meade MO, Cook DJ, Granton JT, Hodder RV, Lapinsky ST, Mazer CD, McLean RF, Rogovein TS, Schouten BD, Todd TRJ, Slutsky AS, and the Pressure and Volume Limited Ventilation Strategy Group. Evaluation of a ventilation strategy to prevent barotrauma in patients at high risk for acute respiratory distress syndrome. N Engl J Med 1998; 338:355–361.

96. Brower RG, Shanholts CB, Fessler HE, Shade DM, White P, Wiener CM, Teeter JG, Dodd-o-JM, Almog Y, Piantadosi S. Prospective, randomized controlled clinical trial comparing traditional versus reduced tidal volume ventilation in acute respiratory distress syndrome patients. Crit Care Med 1999; 27:1492–1498.

97. Feihl F, Perret C. Permissive hypercapnia. How permissive should we be? Am J Respir Crit Care Med 1994; 150:1722–1737.

98. Carvalho CRR, Barbas CSV, Medeiros DM, Magaldi RB, Filho GL, Kairalla RA, Deheinzelin D, Munhoz C, Kaufmann M, Ferreira M, Takagaki TY, Amato MBP. Temporal hemodynamic effects of permissive hypercapnia associated with ideal PEEP in ARDS. Am J Respir Crit Care Med 1997; 156:1458–1466.

99. Tharratt RS, Allen RP, Albertson TE. Pressure controlled inverse ratio ventilation in severe adult respiratory failure. Chest 1988; 94:755–762.

100. Shanholtz C, Brower R. Should inverse ratio ventilation be used in adult respiratory distress syndrome? Am J Respir Crit Care Med 1994; 149:1354–1358.

101. MacIntyre NR, Follett JV, Deitz JL, Lawlor BR. Jet ventilation at 100 breaths per minute in adult respiratory failure. Am Rev Respir Dis 1986; 134:897–901.

102. Armstrong BW, MacIntyre NR. Pressure-controlled inverse ratio ventilation that avoids air trapping in the adult respiratory distress syndrome. Crit Care Med 1995; 23:279–285.

103. Gurevitch MJ, Van Dyle J, Young ES, Jackson K. Improved oxygenation and lower peak airway pressure in severe adult respiratory distress syndrome. Chest 1986; 89:211–213.

104. Lain DC, Dibenderto R, Morris SL, Nguyen AV, Saulters R, Causey D. Pressure control inverse ratio ventilation as a method to reduce peak inspiratory pressure and provide adequate ventilation. Chest 1989; 95:1081–1088.

105. Marcy TW, Marini JJ. Inverse ratio ventilation in ARDS. Rationale and implementation. Chest 1991; 100:494–504.

106. Presenti A, Marcolin R, Prato P, Borelli M, Riboni A, Gattinoni L. Mean airway pressure vs. positive end-expiratory pressure during mechanical ventilation Crit Care Med 1985; 13:34–37.

107. Knelson JH, Howatt WF, DeMuth GR. Effect of respiratory pattern on alveolar gas exchange. J Appl Physiol 1970; 29:328–331.

108. Cheney FW, Burnham C. Effect of ventilatory pattern on oxygenation in pulmonary edema. J Appl Physiol 1971; 31:909–912.

109. Berman LS, Downs JB, Van Eeden A, Delhagen D. Inspiration: expiration ratio. Is mean airway pressure the difference? Crit Care Med 1981; 9:775–777.

110. Tyler DC, Cheney FW. Comparison of positive end-expiratory pressure and inspiratory positive pressure plateau in ventilation of rabbits with experimental pulmonary edema. Anesth Analg 1979; 58:288–292.

111. Lessard MR, Guerot E, Lorino H, Lemaire F, Brochard L. Effects of pressure-controlled with different I:E ratios versus volume-controlled ventilation on respiratory mechanics, gas exchange, and hemodynamics in patients with adult respiratory distress syndrome. Anesthesiology 1994; 80:983–991.

112. Mercat A, Graini L, Teboul JL, Lenique F, Richard C. Cardiorespiratory effects of pressure-controlled ventilation with and without inverse ratio in the adult respiratory distress syndrome. Chest 1993; 104:871–875.

113. Mercat A, Titiriga M, Anguel N, Richard C, Teboul JL. Inverse ratio ventilation (I/E = 2/1) in acute respiratory distress syndrome. A six-hour controlled study. Am J Respir Crit Care Med 1997; 155:1637–1642.

114. Abraham E, Oshihara G. Cardiorespiratory effects of pressure controlled inverse ratio ventilation in severe respiratory failure. Chest 1989; 96:1356–1359.

115. Chan K, Abraham E. Effects of inverse ratio ventilation on cardiorespiratory parameters in severe respiratory failure. Chest 1992; 102:1556–1561.

116. Hubmayr RD, Abel MD, Rehder K. Physiologic approach to mechanical ventilation. Crit Care Med 1990; 18:103–113.

117. Hyatt RE, Bar-Yishay E, Abel MD. Influence of the heart on the vertical gradient of transpulmonary pressure in dogs. J Appl Physiol 1985; 58:52–57.

118. Albert RK, Hubmayr RD. The prone position eliminates compression of the lungs by the heart. Am J Respir Crit Care Med 2000; 161:1660–1665.

119. Beck KC, Rehder K. Differences in regional vascular conductances in isolated dog lungs. J Appl Physiol 1986; 61:530–538.

120. Albert RK, Leasa D, Sanderson M, Robertson HT, Hlastala MP. The prone position improves arterial oxygenation and reduces shunt in oleic-acid-induced acute lung injury. Am Rev Respir Dis 1987; 135:628–633.

121. Pelosi P, Tubiolo D, Macheroni D, Vicardi P, Crotti S, Valenza F, Gattinoni L. Effects of the prone position on respiratory mechanics and gas exchange during acute lung injury. Am J Respir Crit Care Med 1998; 157:387–393.

122. Wiener CM, Kirk W, Albert RK. Prone position reverses gravitational distribution

of perfusion in dog lungs with oleic acid-induced injury. J Appl Physiol 1990; 68: 1386–1392.

123. Glenny RW, Lamm WE, Albert RK, Robertson HT. Gravity is a minor determinant of pulmonary blood flow distribution. J Appl Physiol 1991; 71:620–629.

124. Mure M, Marting CR, Lindahl SGE. Dramatic effect on oxygenation in patients with severe acute lung insufficiency treated in the prone position. Crit Care Med 1997; 25:1539–1544.

125. Jolliet P, Bulpa P, Chevrolet JC. Effects of the prone position on gas exchange and hemodynamics in severe acute respiratory distress syndrome. Crit Care Med 1998; 26:1977–1985.

126. Chatte G, Sab JM, Dubois JM, Sirodot M, Gaussorgues P, Robert D. Prone position in mechanically ventilated patients with severe acute respiratory failure. Am J Respir Crit Care Med 1997; 155:473–478.

127. Gattinoni L, Pelosi P, Vitale G, Pesenti A, D'Andrea L, Mascheroni D. Body position changes redistribute lung computed-tomographic density with acute respiratory failure. Anesthesiology 1991; 74:15–23.

128. Fridrich P, Krafft P, Hochleuthner H, Mauritz W. The effects of long-term prone positioning in patients with trauma-induced adult respiratory distress syndrome. Anesth Analg 1996; 83:1206–1211.

129. Lamm WJE, Graham MM, Albert RK. Mechanism by which the prone position improves oxygenation in acute lung injury. Am J Respir Crit Care Med 1994; 150: 184–193.

130. Broccard AF, Shapiro RS, Schmitz LL, Ravenscraft SA, Marini JJ. Influence of prone position on the extent and distribution of lung injury in a high tidal volume oleic acid model of acute respiratory distress syndrome. Crit Care Med 1997; 25: 16–27.

131. Chiang AA, Steinfeld A, Gropper C, MacIntyre N. Demand-flow airway pressure release ventilation as a partial ventilatory support mode: Comparison with synchronized intermittent mandatory ventilation and pressure support ventilation. Crit Care Med 1994; 22:1431–1437.

132. Cane RD, Peruzzi W, Shapiro BA. Airway pressure release ventilation in severe acute respiratory failure. Chest 1991; 100:460–463.

133. Sydow M, Burchardi H, Ephraim E, Zielmann S, Crozier TA. Long-term effects of two different ventilatory modes on oxygenation in acute lung injury. Am J Respir Crit Care Med 1994; 149:1550–1556.

134. Herridge MS, Slutsky AS, Colditz GA. Has high-frequency ventilation been inappropriately discarded in adult acute respiratory distress syndrome? Crit Care Med 1998; 26:2073–2077.

135. Arnold JH, Hanson JH, Toro-Figuero LO, Gutierrez J, Berens RJ, Anglin DL. Prospective randomized comparison of high-frequency oscillatory ventilation and conventional mechanical ventilation in pediatric respiratory failure. Crit Care Med 1994; 22:1530–1539.

136. Briscoe WA, Forster RE, Comroe JH. Alveolar ventilation at very low tidal volumes. J Appl Physiol 1954; 7:27–30.

137. Henderson YH, Chillingworth FP, Whitney JL. The respiratory dead space. Am J Physiol 1915; 38:1–19.

138. Taylor GI. The dispersion of matter in turbulent flow through a pipe. Proc R Soc London 1954; 223:446–468.

139. Brusasco VT, Knopp J, Rehder K. Gas transport during high-frequency ventilation. J Appl Physiol 1983; 55:472–478.

140. Rossing TH, Slutsky AS, Lehr JL, Drinker PA, Kamm R, Drazen JM. Tidal volume and frequency dependence of carbon dioxide elimination by high frequency ventilation. N Engl J Med 1981; 305:1375–1379.

141. Slutsky AS, Kamm RD, Rossing TH, Loring SH, Lehr JL, Shapiro AH, Ingram RH, Drazen JM. Effects of frequency, tidal volume and lung volume on CO_2 elimination in dogs by high frequency (2–30 Hz), low tidal volume ventilation. J Clin Invest 1981; 68:1475–1484.

142. Isabey D, Harf A, Chang HK. Alveolar ventilation during high-frequency oscillation: core dead space concept. J Appl Physiol Respir Environ Exercise Physiol 1984; 56:700–707.

143. Haselton FR, Scherer PW. Flow visualization of steady streaming in oscillatory flow through a bifurcating tube. J Fluid Mech 1982; 123:315–373.

144. Schroter RC, Sudlow MF. Flow patterns in models of the human bronchial airways. Respir Physiol 1969; 7:341–355.

145. Chang HK. Mechanisms of gas transport during ventilation by high-frequency oscillation. J Appl Physiol 1984; 56:553–563.

146. Fredburg JJ, Allen J, Tsuda A. Mechanics of the respiratory system during high frequency ventilation Acta Anaesthesiol Scand 1989; 33:39–45.

147. Matsuoka T, Kawano T, Miyasaka K. Role of high frequency ventilation in surfactant-depleted lung injury as measured by granulocytes. Appl J Physiol 1994; 76:539–544.

148. Imai Y, Kawano T, Miyasaka K, Takata M, Imai T, Okuyama K. Inflammatory chemical mediators during conventional ventilation and during high frequency oscillatory ventilation. Am J Respir Crit Care Med 1994; 150:1550–1554.

149. Nagase T, Fukuchi Y, Shimizu T, Matsuse T, Orimo H. Reduction of 15-hydroxyeicosatetraenoic acid (15-HETE) in tracheal fluid by high frequency oscillatory ventilation. Prostaglandins Leukot Essent Fatty Acids 1990; 40:177–180.

150. Gerstmann DR, Fouke JM, Winter DC, Taylor AF, deLemos RA. Proximal, tracheal, and alveolar pressures during high-frequency oscillatory ventilation in a normal rabbit model. Pediatr Res 1990; 28:367–373.

151. Bryan AC, Slutsky AS. Long volume during high frequency oscillation. Am Rev Respir Dis 1986; 133:928–930.

152. Thompson WK, Marchak BE, Froese AB, Bryan AC. High-frequency oscillation compared with standard ventilation in pulmonary injury model. J Appl Physiol 1982; 52:543–548.

153. Boynton BR, Villanueva D, Hammond MD, Vreeland PN, Buckley B, Frantz ID. Effect of mean airway pressure on gas exchange during high-frequency oscillatory ventilation. J Appl Physiol 1991; 70:701–707.

154. Byford LJ, Finkler JH, Froese AB. Lung volume recruitment during high-frequency oscillation in atelectasis-prong rabbits. Am Physiol Soc 1988; 88:1607–1614.

155. McCulloch PR, Forkert PG, Froese AB. Lung volume maintenance prevents lung

injury during high frequency oscillatory ventilation in surfactant-deficient rabbits. Am Rev Respir Dis 1988; 137:1185–1192.

156. Bell RE, Kuehl TJ, Coalson JJ, Ackerman BB, Null DM, Escobedo MB, Yoder BA, Cornish JD, Nalle L, Skarin RM, Cipiani CA, Montes M, Robotham JL, De-Lemos RA. High frequency ventilation compared to conventional positive-pressure ventilation in the treatment of hyaline membrane disease in primates. Crit Care Med 1984; 12:764–768.

157. Boynton BR, Manino FL Davis RF, Kopotic RJ. Friederichsen. Combined high frequency oscillatory ventilation and intermittent mandatory ventilation in critically ill neonates. J Pediatr 1984; 105:297–302.

158. Froese AB, Butler PO., Fletcher WA Byrord LF. High frequency oscillatory ventilation in premature infants with respiratory failure: a preliminary report. Anesth Analg 1987; 66:814–824.

159. Bjerager K, Sjostrand U, Wattwil M. Long-term treatment of two patients with respiratory insufficiency with IPPV/PEEP and HFPPV/PEEP. Acta Anaesthesiol Scand Suppl 1977; 64:55–68.

160. Butler WJ, Bohn DJ, Bryan AC, Froese AB. Ventilation by high-frequency oscillation in humans. Anesth Analg 1980; 59:577–584.

161. Flatau E, Barzilay E, Kaufmann N, Lev A, Ben-Ami M, Kohn D. Adult respiratory distress syndrome treated with high-frequency positive pressure ventilation. Isr J Med Sci 1981; 17:453–456.

162. Yetson NS, Grasberger, RC, McCormick JR. Severe combined respiratory and myocardial failure treated with high-frequency ventilation. Crit Care Med 1985; 13:208–209.

163. Schuster DP Synder JV, Klain M, Grenvik A. High-frequency jet ventilation during the treatment of acute fulminant pulmonary edema. Chest 1981; 80:682–685.

164. Schuster DP, Klain M, Snyder JV. Comparison of high frequency jet ventilation to conventional ventilation during severe acute respiratory failure in humans. Crit Care Med 1982; 10:625–630.

165. Cioffi WG, Graves TA, McManus WF, Pruitt BA. High-frequency percussive ventilation in patients with inhalation jury. J Trauma 1989; 29:350–354.

166. Gluck E, Heard S, Patel C, Mohr J, Calkins J. Use of ultrahigh frequency ventilation in patients with ARDS. A preliminary report. Chest 1993; 103:1413–1420.

167. Carlon GC, Howland WS, Ray C, Miodownik S, Griffin JP, Groeger JS. High-frequency jet ventilation. A prospective randomized evaluation. Chest 1983; 84: 551–559.

168. Hurst JM, Branson RD, Davis K, Barrette RR, Adams KS. Comparison of conventional mechanical ventilation and high- frequency ventilation. A prospective randomized trial in patients with respiratory failure. Ann Surg 1990; 4:486–491.

169. Fort P, Farmer C, Westerman J, Johanningman J, Beninati W, Dolan S, Derdak S. High-frequency oscillatory ventilation for adult respiratory distress syndrome—a pilot study. Crit Care Med 1997; 25:937–947.

170. Rossaint R, Falke KJ, Lopez, Slama K, Pison U, Zapol WM. Inhaled nitric oxide for the adult respiratory distress syndrome. N Engl J Med 1993; 328:399–405.

171. Hillman S, Neliones JN, Black DR, Craig DM, Cheifetz IM, Smith PK. An acute lung injury, inhaled nitric oxide improves ventilation-perfusion matching pulmo-

nary vascular mechanics transpulmonary vascular efficiency. J Thorac Cardiovasc Surg 1995; 110:563–600.

172. Putensen C, Rasanen J, Downs JB. Effect of endogenous and inhaled nitric oxide on the ventilation-perfusion relationships in oleic-acid lung injury. Am J Respir Crit Care Med 1994; 150:330–336.

173. Puybasset L, Rouby J-J, Mourgeon E, Cluzel P, Souhil Z, Law-Koune J-D, Stewart T, Devilliers C, Lu Q, Roche S, Kalfon P, Vicaut E, Viars P. Factors influencing cardiopulmonary effects of inhaled nitric oxide in acute respiratory failure. Am J Respir Crit Care Med 1995; 152:318–328.

174. Wysocki M, Delclauz C, Poupie E, Additive effect on gas exchange of inhaled nitric oxide and intravenous almitrine bismesylate in the adult respiratory distress syndrome. Intensive Care Med 1994; 20:254–259.

175. Green JH, Klinger JR. The efficacy of inhaled nitric oxide in the treatment of acute respiratory distress syndrome: an evidence-based medicine approach. Crit Care Clin 1998; 14:387–409.

176. Bigatello LM, Hurford WE, Kacmarek RM, Roberts JD, Zapol WM. Prolonger inhaltion of low concentrations of nitric oxide in patients with severe adult respiratory distress syndrome. Anesthesiology 1994; 80:761–770.

177. Frostell CG, Blomqvist H, Hedenstierna G, Lundberg J, Zapol WM. Inhaled nitric oxide selectively reverses human hypoxic pulmonary vasoconstriction without causing systemic vasodilation. Anesthesiology 1993; 78:427–435.

178. Young JD, Brampton WJ, Knighton JD, et al. Inhaled nitric oxide in acute respiratory failure in adults Br J Anaesth 1994; 73:499–502.

179. Fierobe L, Burnet F, Dhainaut F-F, Finfer SR. Effect of inhaled nitric oxide on right ventricular function in adult respiratory distress syndrome. Am J Respir Crit Care Med 1995; 115:1414–1419.

180. Rossaint R, Gerlach H, Schmidt-Ruhnke H, Pappert D, Lewandowski K, Steudel W, Jalke K. Efficacy of inhaled nitric oxide in patients with severe ARDS. Chest 1995; 107:1107–1115.

181. Krafft P, Fridrich P, Fitzgerald RD, Koc D, Steltzer H. Effectiveness of nitric oxide inhalation in septic ARDS. Chest 1996; 109:486–493.

182. Sibbald WJ, Driedger AA, Myers ML, Short IK, Well GA. Biventricular function in the adult respiratory distress syndrome. Chest 1983; 84:126–134.

183. Puybasset L, Rouby J-J, Mourgeon E, Stewart T, Cluzel P, Arthaud M, Poete P, Bodin L, Korinek AM, Viars P. Inhaled nitric oxide in acute respiratory failure: dose-response curves. Intensive Care Med 1994; 20:3189–327.

184. Gerlach H, Rossaint R, Pappert D, Falke KJ. Time-course and dose-response of nitric oxide inhalation for systemic oxygenation and pulmonary hypertension in patients with adult respiratory distress syndrome. Eur J Clin Invest 1993; 23:499.

185. Hogman M, Frostell C, Arnberg H, Hedenstierna G. Bleeding time prolongation and NO inhalation. Lancet 1993; 341:1664–1665.

186. Moinard J, Manier G, Pillet O, Castaing Y. Effect of inhaled nitric oxide on hemodynamics and V_A/Q inequalities in patients with chronic obstructive pulmonary disease. Am J Respir Crit Care Med 1994; 149:1482–1487.

187. Rimar S, Gillis CN. Site of pulmonary vasodilation by inhaled nitric oxide in the perfused lung. J Appl Physiol 1995; 78:1745–1749.

188. Rossetti M, Geunard H, Gabinski C. Effects of nitric oxide inhalations on pulmonary serial vascular resistance in ARDS. Am J Respir Crit Care Med 1996; 154: 1375–1381.

189. Benzing A, Geiger K. Inhaled nitric oxide lowers pulmonary vascular pressure and changes longitudinal distribution of pulmonary vascular resistance in patients with acute lung injury. Acta Aneasesh Scand 1994; 34:640–645.

190. Bloomfield GL, Sweeney LB, Fisher BJ, Blocher CR, Sholley MM, Sugerman HJ, Fowler AA. Delayed administration of inhaled nitric oxide preserves alveolar capillary membrane integrity in porcine gram negative sepsis. Arch Surg 1997; 132:65–75.

191. Poss WB, Timmons OD, Farrukh IS, Hoidal JR, Michael JR. Inhaled nitric oxide prevents the increase in pulmonary vascular permeability caused by hydrogen peroxide. J Appl Physiol 1995; 79:886–891.

192. Chollet-Martin S, Gatecel C, Kermarrec N, Gougerot-Pocidalo M-A, Payen DM. Alveolar neutrophil functions and cytokine levels in patients with the adult respiratory distress syndrome during nitric oxide inhalation. Am J Respir Crit Care Med 1996; 153:985–990.

193. Freeman BA. The free radical chemistry of nitric oxide: Looking at the dark side. Chest 1994; 105(3):79S–84S.

194. Lavoie A, Hall JB, Olson DM, Wylam ME. Life-threatening effects of discontinuing inhaled nitric oxide in severe respiratory failure. Am J Respir Crit Care Med 1996; 153:1985–1987.

195. Michael JR, Barton RG, Saffle JR, Mone M, Markewitz BA, Hillier K, Esltad MR, Campbell EJ, Troyer BE, Whatley RE, Liou TG, Samuelson WM, Carveth HJ, Hinson DM, Morris SE, Davis BL, Day RW. Inhaled nitric oxide versus conventional therapy: effect on oxygenation in ARDS. Am J Respir Crit Care Med 1998; 157:1372–1380.

196. Troncy E, Collet J-P, Shapiro S, Guimond J-G, Blair L, Ducruet T, Francoeur M, Charbonneau M, Blaise G. Inhaled nitric oxide in acute respiratory distress syndrome: a pilot randomized controlled study. Am J Respir Crit Care Med 1998; 157: 1483–1488.

197. Dellinger RP, Zimmerman JL, Taylor RW, Straube RC, Hauser DL, Criner GJ, Davis K, Hyers TM, Papadakos P. Effect of inhaled nitric oxide in patients with acute respiratory distress syndrome: results of a randomized phase II trial. Crit Care Med 1998; 26:15–23.

198. Taylor RW, Zimmerman JL, Dellinger RP, Straube RC. A double-blind randomized, placebo controlled study of 5 ppm inhaled nitric oxide in acute respiratory distress syndrome. 29th Educational and scientific symposium. Society of Critical Care Medicine, February 2000, Orlando, FL.

199. Lundin S, Mang H, Smithies M, Stenquvist O, Frostell C. Inhalation of nitric oxide in acute lung injury: results of a European multicentre study. Intensive Care Med 1999; 25:911–919.

200. Kylstra JA, Paganelli CV, Lanphier EH. Pulmnary gas exchange in dogs ventilated with hyperbarically oxygenated liquid. J Appl Physiol 1966; 21:177–184.

201. Matthews WH, Balzer RH, Shelburne JD, Pratt PC, Kylstra JA. Steady-steady gas exchange in normothermic, anesthetized, liquid-ventilated dogs. Undersea Biomed Res 1978; 5:341–354.

202. Modell JH, Hood CI, Kuck EJ, Ruiz BC. Oxygenation by ventilation with fluoro-carbon liquid (FX-80). Anesthesiology 1971; 34:312–320.

203. Modell JH, Calderwood HW, Ruiz BC, Tham MK, Hood CI. Liquid ventilation of primates. Chest 1976; 69:79–81.

204. Fuhrman BP, Paczan PR, DeFrancisis M. Perfluorocarbon-associated gas exchange. Crit Care Med 1991; 19:712–722.

205. Hirschl RB, Overbeck MC, Parent A, Hernandez R, Schwartz S, Dosanjh A, Johnson K, Bartlett RH. Liquid ventilation provides uniform distribution of perfluorocarbon in the setting of respiratory failure. Surgery 1994; 116:159–167.

206. Quintel M, Hirschl RB, Roth H, Loose R, van Ackern K. Computer tomographic assessment of perfluorocarbon and gas distribution during partial liquid ventilation for acute respiratory failure. Am J Respir Crit Care Med 1998; 158:249–255.

207. Enrione MA, Papo MC, Leach CL, Holm BA, Hernan LJ, Fuhrman BP, Dowhy MS, Rath MG, Frisicaro PE. Regional pulmonary blood flow during partial liquid ventilation in normal and acute oleic acid-induced lung-injured piglets. Crit Care Med 1999; 27:2716–2723.

208. Wolfson MR, Greenspan JS, Deoras KS, Rubenstein SD, Shaffer TH. Comparison of gas and liquid ventilation: Clinical, physiological and histological correlates. J Appl Physiol 1992; 72:1024–1031.

209. Papo MC, Paczan PR, Fuhrman BP, Steinhorn DM, Hernan LJ, Leach CL, Holm BA, Fisher JE, Kahn BA. Perfluorocarbon-associated gas exchange improves oxygenation, lung mechanics, and survival in a model of adult respiratory distress syndrome. Crit Care Med 1996; 24:466–474.

210. Hernan LJ, Fuhrman BP, Kaiser RE, Penfil S, Foley C, Papo MC, Leach CL. Perfluorocarbon-associated gas exchange in normal and acid-injured large sheep. Crit Care Med 1996; 24:475–481.

211. Hirschl RB, Tooley R, Parent A, Johnson K, Bartlett RH. Evaluation of gas exchange, pulmonary compliance and lung injury during total and partial liquid ventilation in the acute respiratory distress syndrome. Crit Care Med 1996; 24:1001–1008.

212. Overbeck MC, Pranikoff T, Yadao CM, Hirschi RB. Efficacy of perfluorocarbon partial liquid ventilation in a large animal model of acute respiratory failure Crit Care Med 1996; 24:1208–1214.

213. Tutuneu AS, Faithful NS, Lachmann B. Comparison of ventilatory support with intratracheal perfluorocarbon administration and conventional mechanical ventilation in animals with acute respiratory failure. Am Rev Respir Dis 1993; 148:785–792.

214. Dreyfuss D, Martin-Lefevre L, Saumon G. Hyperinflation-induced lung injury during alveolar flooding in rats. Effect of perfluorocarbon instillation. Am J Respir Crit Care Med 1999; 159:1752–1757.

215. Curtis SE, Peek JT, Kelly DR. Partial liquid breathing with perflubron improves arterial oxygenation in acute canine lung injury. J Appl Physiol 1993; 75:2696–2702.

216. Tooley R, Hirschl RB, Parent A, Bartlett RH. Total liquid ventilation with perfluorocarbons increases pulmonary end-expiratory volume and compliance in the setting of lung atelectasis. Crit Care Med 1996; 24:268–273.

217. Smith TM, Steinhorn DM. Thusu K, Fuhrman BP, Dandona P. A liquid perfluorochemical decreases the in vitro production of reactive oxygen species by alveolar macrophages. Crit Care Med 1995; 23:1533–1539.

218. Rotta AT, Gunnarsson B, Hernan IJ, Fuhrman BP, Steinhorn DM. Partial liquid ventilation influences pulmonary histopathology in an animal model of acute lung injury. J Crit Care 1999; 14:84–92.

219. Croce MA, Fabian TC, Patton JH Jr, Melton SM, Moore M, Trenthem LL. Partial liquid ventilation decreases the inflammatory response in the alveolar environment of trauma patients. J Trauma 1998; 45:273–282.

220. Rotta AT, Steinhorn DM. Partial liquid ventilation reduces pulmonary neutrophil accumulation in an experimental model of systemic endotoxemia and acute lung injury. Crit Care Med 1998; 26:1702–1715.

221. Colton DM, Till GO, Johnson KJ, Dean SB, Bartlett RH, Hirschi RB. Neutrophil accumulation is reduced during partial liquid ventilation. Crit Care Med 1998; 26: 1716–1724.

222. Kawamae K, Pristine G, Chiumello D, Tremblay LN, Slutsky AS. Partial liquid ventilation decreases serum tumor necrosis factor-alpha concentrations in a rat acid aspiration lung injury model. Crit Care Med 2000; 28:479–483.

223. Lowe C, Tuma RF, Sivieri EM, Shaffer TH. Liquid ventilation: cardiovascular adjustments with secondary hyperlactatemia and acidosis. J Appl Physiol 1979; 47: 1051–1057.

224. Houmes RJ, Verbrugge SJ, Hendrik ER, Lachmann B. Hemodynamic effects of partial liquid ventilation with perfluorocarbon in acute lung injury. Intensive Care Med 1995; 21:963–965.

225. Curtis SE, Fuhrman BP, Howland DF, DeFrancisis M, Motoyama EK. Cardiac output during liquid (perfluorocarbon) breathing in newborn piglets. Crit Care Med 1991; 19(2):225–230.

226. Lowe CA, Shaffer TH. Pulmonary vascular resistance in the fluorocarbon-filled lung. J Appl Physiol 1986; 60:154–159.

227. Loer SA, Tarnow J. Effects of partial liquid ventilation with perfluorocarbons on pressure-flow relationships, vascular compliance, and filtration coefficients of isolated blood-perfused rabbit lungs. Crit Care Med 1998; 26:2037–2041.

228. Manaligod JM, Bednel-Stenzel EM, Meyers PA, Ding DR, Connett JE, Mammel Variations in end-expiratory pressure during partial liquid ventilation. Impact on gas exchange, lung compliance and end-expiratory lung volume. Chest 2000; 117: 184–190.

229. Ferreyra G, Goddon S, Fujino Y, Kacmarek RM. The relationship between gas delivery patterns and the lower inflection point of the pressure-volume curve during partial liquid ventilation. Chest 2000; 117:191–198.

230. Kirmse M, Fujino Y, Hess D, Kacmarek RM. Positive end-expiratory pressure improves gas exchange and pulmonary mechanics during partial liquid ventilation. Am J Respir Crit Care Med 1998; 158:1550–1556.

231. Zobel G, Rodl S, Urlesberger B, Dacer D, Trafojer U, Trantina A. The effect of positive end-expiratory pressure during partial liquid ventilation in acute lung injury in piglets. Crit Care Med 1999; 27:1934–1939.

232. Lim C-M, Koh Y, Shim TS, Lee SD, Kim WS, Kim DS, Kim WD. The effect of

varying inspiratory to expiratory ratio on gas exchange in partial liquid ventilation. Chest 1999; 116:1032–1038.

233. Fujino Y, Kirmse M, Hess D, Kacmarek R. The effect of mode, inspiratory time, and positive end-expiratory pressure on partial liquid ventilation. Am J Respir Crit Care Med 1999; 159:1087–1095.

234. Greenspan JS, Wolfson MR, Rubinstein SD, Shaffer TH. Liquid ventilation of human preterm neonates. J Pediatr 1990; 117:106–111.

235. Leach CL, Greenspan JS, Rubenstein SD, Shaffer TH, Wolfson MR, Jackson JC, DeLemos R, Fuhrman BP. Partial liquid ventilation with perflubron in premature infants with severe respiratory distress syndrome. N Engl J Med 1996; 335:761–767.

236. Hirschl RB, Pranikoff T, Gauger P, Schreiner RJ, Dechert R, Bartlett RH. Liquid ventilation in adults, children and full-term neonates. Lancet 1995; 346:1201–1202.

237. Hirschl RB, Conrad S, Kaiser R, Zwischenberger JB, Bartlett RH, Booth F, Cardenas V. Partial liquid ventilation in adult patients with ARDS: a multicenter phase I-II trial. Adult PLV Study Group. Ann Surg 1998; 228:692–700.

238. Bartlett R, Croce M, Hirschi R, Gore D, Wiedermann H, Davis K, Zwischenberger J. A phase II randomized, controlled trial of partial liquid ventilation (PLV) in adult patients with acute hypoxemic respiratory failure (AHRF). Crit Care Med 1997; 25:A35.

239. Slutsky AS, Watson J, Leith D, Brown R. Tracheal insufflation of O_2 (TRIO) at low flow rates sustains life for several hours. Anesthesiology 1985; 63:278–286.

240. Watson JW, Burwen DR, Kamm RD, Brown R, Slutsky AS. Effect of flow rate on blood gases during constant flow ventilation in dogs. Am Rev Respir Dis 1986; 133:626–629.

241. Sznajder JI, Becker CJ, Crawford GP, Wood LDH. Combination of constant-flow and continuous positive-pressure ventilation in canine pulmonary edema. J Appl Physiol 1989; 67:817–823.

242. Nakos G, Zakinthinos S, Kotanidou A, Tsagaris H, Roussos C. Tracheal gas insufflation reduces the tidal volume while $PaCO_2$ is maintained constant. Intensive Care Med 1994; 20:407–413.

243. Nahum A, Chandra A, Niknam J, Ravenscraft SA, Adams AB, Marini JJ. Effect of tracheal gas insufflation on gas exchange in canine oleic acid-induced lung injury. Crit Care Med 1995; 23:348–356.

244. Gowski DT, Delgado E, Miro AM, Tasota FJ, Hoffman LA, Pinsky MR. Tracheal gas insufflation during pressure-control ventilation: Effect of using a pressure relief valve. Crit Care Med 1997; 25:145–152.

245. Kirmse M, Fujino Y, Hromi J, Mang H, Hess D, Kacmarek RM. Pressure-release tracheal gas insufflation reduces airway pressures in lung-injured sheep maintaining eucapnia. Am J Respir Crit Care Med 1999; 160:1462–1467.

246. Dolan S, Derdak S, Solomon D, Farmer C, Johanningman J, Gelineau J. Tracheal gas insufflation combined with high-frequency oscillatory ventilation. Crit Care Med 1996; 24:458–465.

247. Wei H, Jin SA, Ma Z, Bi H, Ba X. Experimental study of high-frequency two-way jet ventilation. Crit Care Med 1992; 20:420–423.

248. Okamoto K, Kishi H, Choi H, Sato T. Combination of tracheal gas insufflation and airway pressure release ventilation. Chest 1997; 111:1366–1374.

249. Nahum A, Burke WC, Ravenscraft SA, Marcy TW, Adams AB, Crooke PS, Marini JJ. Lung mechanics and gas exchange during pressure-control ventilation in dogs. Augmentation of CO_2 elimination by an intratracheal catheter. Am Rev Respir Dis 1992; 146:965–973.

250. Cereda MF, Sparacino ME, Frank AR, Trawoger R, Kolobow T. Efficacy of tracheal gas insufflation in spontaneously breathing sheep with lung injury. Am J Respir Crit Care Med 1999; 159:845–850.

251. Ravenscraft SA, Burke WC, Nahum A, Adams AB, Nakos G, Marcy TW, Marini JJ. Tracheal gas insufflation augments CO_2 clearance during mechanical ventilation. Am Rev Respir Dis 1993; 148:345–351.

252. Belghith M, Fierobe L, Bunet F, Monchi M, Mira JP. Is tracheal gas insufflation an alternative to extrapulmonary gas exchangers in severe ARDS? Chest 1995; 107:1416–1419.

253. Kolobow T, Powers T, Mandava S, Aprigliano M, Kawaguchi A, Tsuno K, Mueller E. Intratracheal pulmonary ventilation (ITPV): control of positive end-expiratory pressure at the level of the carina through the use of a novel ITPV catheter design. Anesth Analg 1994; 78:455–461.

254. De Robertis E, Sigurdsson SE, Drefeldt B, Jonson B. Aspiration of airway dead space. Am J Respir Crit Care Med 1999; 159:728–732.

255. Perez CA, Bui KC, Bustorff-Silva J, Atkinson JB. Comparison of intratracheal pulmonary ventilation and hybrid intratracheal pulmonary ventilation with conventional mechanical ventilation in a rabbit model of acute respiratory distress syndrome by saline lavage. Crit Care Med 2000; 28(3):774–781.

256. Mutoh, T, Guest RJ, Lamm WJ, Albert RK. Prone position alters the effect of volume overload on regional pleural press improves hypoxemia in pigs in vivo. Am Rev Respir Dis 1992; 146(2):300–306.

257. Grippe M. Respiratory mechanics. In: Pulmonary Pathophysiology. Philadelphia: Lippincott, 1995:21.

258. Roupie E, Dambrosio M, Servillo G, Mentec H, el Atrous S, Beydon L, Brun-Buisson C, Lemaire F, Brochard L. Titration of tidal volume and induced hypercapnia in acute respiratory distress. Am J Respir Crit Care Med 1995; 152(1):121–128.

259. Marini JJ. Evolving concepts in the ventilatory management of acute respiratory distress. Clin Chest Med 1996; 17(3):555–575.

260. Bird FM. The diffuse/connective mechanical ventilation of the lung: the state of the art as we enter the 1990s. Sandpoint, ID: Percussionaire Corp.

261. Lunn RJ. Inhaled nitric oxide therapy. Mayo Clin Proc 1995; 70(3):247–255.

262. Murray J. Ventilation. In: The Normal Lung. Philadelphia: W.B. Saunders, 1986: 89.

14

Noninvasive Positive-Pressure Ventilation in Acute Respiratory Failure Not Related to Chronic Obstructive Pulmonary Disease

G. UMBERTO MEDURI

University of Tennessee
Memphis, Tennessee

MASSIMO ANTONELLI and GIORGIO CONTI

Università "La Sapienza" Policlinico
Umberto I
Rome, Italy

I. Introduction

The term acute respiratory failure (ARF) refers to a severe deterioration in gas exchange that may require mechanical ventilation (MV) for life support. Instituted when conservative treatment fails, MV aims to correct the pathophysiology of ARF, reduce the work of breathing, and ameliorate dyspnea, while concomitant pharmacological intervention is directed at correcting the condition that resulted in ARF. Traditionally, an endotracheal tube (ET) is inserted into the trachea to deliver positive pressure to the patient's lungs. Placing this artificial airway is an invasive procedure associated with potential complications and discomfort and has confined the use of MV to the most severe forms of ARF.

Complications can result from insertion of the tube during mechanical ventilation. Injury to the upper airways can occur at the point of contact between the mucosa and the endotracheal tube or cuff and can result in ulceration, edema, and hemorrhage, with potential stenosis. More importantly, however, the ET directly places the patient at significant risk for developing life-threatening nosocomial infections, mainly ventilator-associated pneumonia and sinusitis (1). Noninvasive ventilation (NIV) includes various techniques for augmenting alveolar ventilation without an endotracheal airway. The theoretical advantages of this

Table 1 Studies on Mask CPAP in Patients with Hypoxemic Respiratory Failure

Study	Number	Mask	Pao₂:Fio₂	CPAP (cm H₂O)	Duration	Intubation	Complications	Mortality	Type
Greenbaum, 1976	14	F[a]	68	4–14	NA	6 (43%)	1 VF, 1 PNM, 1 GD	NA	CPE, PO, PN, TR
Smith, 1980	44	F[a]	171 ± 42	9 ± 3	3–71 h	1 (2%)	1 Pco₂R	NA	PO, TR
Suter, 1981	98	F[b]	≤200	5–10	3.4 ± 0.3 days	38 (39%)	33 INT	17%	CPE, PO, PN, TR
Covelli, 1982	40	F	133 ± 47	5–15	45 ± 5 h	5 (12%)	2 INT, 1 FSN	NA	ARDS, AT
Linton, 1982	13	F	NA	≥5	3–21 days	1 (8%)	0	0	TR
Räsänen, 1985	20/R	F	248 ± 48	10	3 h	6 (30%)	0	NA	CPE
Hurst, 1985	33	F	131 ± 10	5–15	28 ± 19 h	2 (6%)	0	NA	TR
DeHaven, 1985	27	F	130 ± 17	8.3 ± 2.8	23 ± 14 h	2 (7%)	0	NA	PO
Branson, 1985	135	F	126 ± 12	9.2 ± 2.7	39.8 ± 2.7 h	10 (7%)	1 FSN	NA	PO, TR
Väisänen, 1987	40	F	187 ± 30	10	NA	4 (10%)	0	NA	CPE
Gregg, 1990	18	F	75 (33–183)	5–10	4.5 days	1 (10%)[c]	1 PTX, 4 FSN, 2 GD	55%	PCP
Miller, 1991	8	F	84 (59–131)	10–20	4 days	1 (14%)	0	14%	PCP
Bersten, 1991	19/R	F	138 ± 32	10	9.3 ± 4.9 h	0	0	0	CPE
Gachot, 1992	36	F	<150	5–12	8 days	9 (36%)	0	26%	PCP
DeVita, 1993	25	F	<350	NA	2.2 days	11 (44%)	(NA) FSN	36%	PCP
Lin, 1995	50/R	F	<350	2.5–12.5	≥3 h	8 (16%)	NA	4%	CPE
Boix, 1995	15	F	≤200	5–12	3 days	4 (26%)	NA	26%	PCP
Lenique, 1997	9	F	NA	5–10	NA	0	0	NA	CPE
Takeda, 1997	15/R	N	163 ± 70	4–10	11.9 ± 8.4	1 (7%)	0	7%	CPE
L'HerE, 1998	64	F	≤200	5–10	NA	10 (16%)	0	NA	CPE, PN

[a] Nasogastric tube inserted.
[b] Intermittent application.
[c] 1 of 10 patients not refusing intubation.

ATE = Atelectasis; CPE = cardiogenic pulmonary edema; FSN = facial skin necrosis; GD = gastric distention; INT = intolerance of the mask; PCP = *Pneumocystis carinii* pneumonia in AIDS; Pco₂R = retention of carbon dioxide; PN = pneumonia; PNM = pneumomediastinum; PO = postoperative; TR = trauma; VF = ventricular fibrillation; R = randomized study; F = facial; N = nasal; NA = not reported.

approach include avoiding the complications associated with endotracheal intuba- tion, improving patient comfort, preserving airway defense mechanisms, and pre- serving speech and swallowing (2). Furthermore, NIV provides greater flexibility in instituting and removing MV. Noninvasive methods include external negative pressure, chest wall oscillation, and positive-pressure ventilation administered through a mask, which are the subject of this chapter.

It was not until 1935 that Alvin Barach reported a series of studies involving a powered mechanical ventilator to deliver continuous positive airway pressure (CPAP) through a face mask to patients with pulmonary edema and other forms of respiratory failure (3–7). With the evolution of aeronautical engineering during the Second World War, technical knowledge was gained that led to the develop- ment of modern mechanical ventilators. By the early 1960s, the endotracheal tube was widely accepted as the preferred interface to deliver mechanical tidal breaths to patients with ARF.

In the late 1970s and early 1980s, two methods of noninvasive positive- pressure ventilation, using a facial or nasal mask, were introduced into clinical practice. These modalities included CPAP to improve oxygen exchange in pa- tients with hypoxemic ARF (Table 1) (8–26). and intermittent positive pressure ventilation (IPPV) to augment ventilation and rest the respiratory muscles of patients with chronic respiratory failure due to neuromuscular disease and chronic obstructive pulmonary disease (COPD). In the early 1990s, the encouraging re- sults of a pilot study in patients with hypercapnic or hypoxemic ARF (27) stimu- lated investigation of NIV with IPPV in patients with ARF (Table 2) (27–70). In this chapter, clinical application of NIV using CPAP alone is referred to as mask CPAP and NIV using IPPV with or without CPAP as noninvasive (intermit- tent) positive-pressure ventilation (NPPV).

The aim of this chapter is to provide readers with a systematic review of the literature about applying noninvasive ventilation in various forms of ARF in patients without COPD. The use of NPPV in patients with COPD is discussed in another chapter. In the ensuing discussion for each disease state causing ARF, a description of the underlying pathophysiology is followed by a review of physi- ological data (when available) explaining the mechanisms of action of NIV. A critical review of clinical studies is followed by specific suggestions.

II. Hypercapnic Respiratory Failure

Hypoventilation as a result of pump failure leads to hypercapnic ARF (71). ARF in patients with exacerbation of obstructive airway disease (OAD) is associated with significant expiratory obstruction, dynamic hyperinflation, and respiratory muscle fatigue (72). Dynamic hyperinflation causes substantial shortening of the diaphragm and the inspiratory intercostal and accessory muscles, thereby reduc-

Table 2 Studies Using Noninvasive Positive-Pressure Ventilation in Adult Patients with Acute Respiratory Failure

Study	No.	Type of hyperc.	RF hypox.	Type of face		Mode of ventilation	Duration (h/d)	MV days	Success		Mask intolerance	Complications
				Face	Nasal				(No.)	(%)		
Meduri, 1989	10	6	4	+		CPAP/PSV	24	≤4	7	70	1	2 FSN
Brochard, 1990	13	13	–	+		IPAP	7.5 for	3	12	92	NA	0
Elliott, 1990	6	4	2		+	AC	NA		5	83	1	1 secretions ret.
Meduri, 1991	18	18			+	CPAP/PSV	24	<4	13	72	2	1 FSN, 1 PN
Marino, 1991	13	10	3	+	+	AC		1–3	9	69	4	NA
Chevrolet, 1991	6	6	–			AC	5–10	5–13	3	50	0	NA
Pennock, 1991	29	8	21		+	BiPAP	24	6	22	76	3	0
Hodson, 1991	6	–	6		+	AC		14	5	83	NA	NA
Benhamou, 1992a	30	30	–	+		AC		<14	18	60	7	2 FSN, 5 conj.
Wysocki, 1993	17	6	11	+		PSV		4	8	47	1	1 FSN
Vitacca, 1993	29	29	–	+		PSV, AC^d	4	9	24	83	0	6 FSN, 1GD
Fernandez, 1993	12	12	–	+		CPAP/PSV	8 ± 4		9	75	0	2 secretions ret.
Bott, 1993b	30	30	–		+	AC	>16	8	26	86	NA	NA
Pennock, 1994c	110	NA	NA		+	BiPAP		1–6	84	76	NA	NA
Meduri, 1994c	11	9	2	+		CPAP/PSV	24	<4	7	64	1	1 FSN
Soo Hoo, 1994a	12	12	–		+	AC	8	2.3	5	42	NA	NA
Tognet, 1994f	15	–	15	+		PSV	12 ± 7	1–16	6	40	5	2 GD
Confalonieri, 1994	28	28	–	+		BiPAP	24	8	18	64	2	2 FSN, 4 conj.
Wysocki, 1995b	21	–	21	+		CPAP/PSV	NA	NA	12	62	NA	NA
Kramer, 1995b	16	12	4		+	BiPAP	14 ± 2	4 ± 1	27	93	2	2 FSN
Sacchetti, 1995	22	–	22		+	BiPAP	NA	≤2	20	91	NA	NA
Brochard, 1995b	43	43	–	–	+	IPAP	>6	4 ± 4	32	74	NA	1FSN, 2PN
Ambrosino, 1995	59	59	–	+	+	PSV or AC	NA	NA	46	78	NA	NA
Meduri, 1996	158	92	49	+	+	CPAP/PSV	25 ± 24		112	65	6	20FSN/,3 GD,1PN

Study	n					Mode			n	%		
Patrick, 1996	11	5	6	+	+	PAV	3–48		8	73	2	0
Pollack, 1996	50	24	26	+	+	BiPAP	NA	2.6 ± 2	43	86	2	NA
Vitacca, 1996	30	30	–	+	+	PSV or IMV	NA	1	22	74	NA	NA
Antonelli, 1996	8	–	8	+	–	CPAP/PSV	2	<5	8	100	0	0
Confalonieri, 1996	24	24	–	–	+	BiPAP	22	3	22	91	NA	4FSN,1GD,6Conj.
Barbe F., 1996	14	14	–	–	–	BiPAP	6	6	10	71	7	0
Hilbert, 1998	30	30	–	+	–	CPAP/PSV	3	7	24	80	NA	NA
Hilbert, 1997	42	42	–	+	+	BiPAP sequential	4	7	31	73	0	0
Corbetta, 1997	40	40	–	+	+	BiPAP sequential	4	1	31	73	0	0
Aguilo, 1997	10	–	10	–	+	BiPAP	1		NA	NA	0	0
Antonelli, 1998	32	–	32	+	+	CPAP/PSV	24	3 ± 3	22	69	2	3FSN,1PN
Gregoretti, 1998	22	–	22	+	–	CPAP/PSV	6–144	<6	13	59	3	NA
Celikel, 1998	15	15	15	+	+	CPAP/PSV	24	<3	14	93.4	0	7FSN,1GD
Conti, 1998	16	–	16	–	+	BiPAP	24	<4	11	69	0	NA
Varon, 1998	60	7	53	–	+	BiPAP	NA	1–5	42	70	NA	0
Wood	16	2	14	–	+	BiPAP	NA	5.9 ± 5.2	9	56	NA	0
Rocker, 1999	10	–	10	+	+	CPAP/PSV	24	1–4	7	66	2	NA
Rusterholtz, 1999	26	–	26	+	–	CPAP/PSV	NA	NA	21	79	0	0
Hoffman, 1999	29	–	29	+	+	CPAP/PSV	1–24		28	96	0	0
Alsous, 1999	75	44	31	–	+	BiPAP	3.5 ± 6.7		47	62	NA	NA
Confalonieri, 1999	28/R	–	28	+	–	CPAP/PSV	15 ± 1.7	1.8 ± 0.7	22	79	0	IGD
Antonelli, 2000	20/R	–	20	+	–	CPAP/PSV	24 h	2	16	80	0	0

a It includes patients from Pennock et al., 1991.

b Randomized studies comparing NPPV to conventional treatment.

c Studies in patients with advanced disease or refusing endotracheal intubation.

d Comparison study between PSV and AC, all patients received CPAP 5 cm H_2O.

Hyperc. = hypercapnic; Hypox. = hypoxemic; NA = not available; AC = assist control; IPAP = inspiratory positive airway pressure; PSV = pressure support ventilation; BiPAP® = bilevel positive airway pressure (Respironics); h/d = hours/days; FSN = facial skin necrosis; ret. = retention; GD = gastric distention; PN = pneumonia by clinical criteria; conj. = [ ].

ing their mechanical efficiency and endurance (73). In addition, the presence of intrinsic positive end-expiratory pressure (PEEPi) results in an inspiratory threshold load (74). When the load on the respiratory muscle pump becomes excessive, muscle fatigue can develop. Respiratory muscle fatigue is defined as a condition in which the respiratory muscle fibers repeatedly contracting under load cannot generate enough force and velocity; the condition is reversible with rest (71,75). Patients with exacerbation of OAD (COPD and asthma) present with dyspnea and a high respiratory frequency. However, most of the breaths are shallow, and much of the tidal volume is wasted as dead space ventilation, a situation resulting in retention of carbon dioxide and respiratory acidosis (76). Hypercapnia correlates with hyperinflation (77). Furthermore, acute respiratory acidosis itself impairs the contractility of the diaphragm in humans (78).

In patients with OAD and acute exacerbation, the inspiratory effort is divided into two components: an isometric contraction of the inspiratory muscles to counterbalance PEEPi (inspiratory threshold load) followed by an isotonic contraction to generate inspiratory flow and tidal volume (79). Studies evaluating the effects of mechanical ventilation delivered by mask on the work of breathing and gas exchange in patients with OAD indicate that low-level CPAP (5 cm H_2O) can offset one of the detrimental effects of PEEPi. CPAP can reduce the magnitude of the inspiratory effort to resume spontaneous breathing (alveolar pressure needs to be lowered to the CPAP pressure rather than to ambient pressure to begin inspiration) (79–81), while IPPV improves tidal volume, gas exchange, respiratory rate, and diaphragmatic activity in proportion to the amount of pressure applied (28,79,82–84).

A. Asthma

The incidence and severity of asthma has increased in recent years. As a result, the number of asthmatic patients developing ARF and requiring ICU admission has increased. Respiratory failure in asthma is referred to as status asthmaticus (SA) (85). The pathophysiology of SA includes airflow obstruction of both large and small airways, inhomogeneous lung inflation, considerable dynamic hyperinflation (PEEPi = 9–19 cm H_2O), ventilation/perfusion mismatch, and respiratory muscle fatigue (73,86,87). The pathogenesis of airflow obstruction involves airway wall inflammation, smooth muscle–mediated bronchoconstriction, and intraluminal mucus (85). Mucous plugs consisting of mucus, fibrin, desquamated epithelium, and inflammatory cells may lead to occlusion of peripheral airways and may be difficult to remove. Yet the alveolar units distal to these obstructed airways may be slightly ventilated through collateral pathways from relatively less affected neighboring lung units (86). For a more detailed analysis of the pathophysiology and ventilation management of asthma, see Chapter 11.

In spontaneously breathing asthmatics, progressive reductions in FEV_1 are associated with proportional increments in the inspiratory work of breathing (WOBi) (73). A fall in FEV_1 to 50% of baseline is associated with a 10.7-fold increase in inspiratory muscle work (73). At any level of bronchoconstriction, increased inspiratory muscle work is largely the result of hyperinflation and, to a lesser extent, increased airway resistance (73). As airway obstruction becomes more severe (FEV_1 < 25% of predicted) and the WOBi becomes excessive, carbon dioxide production is greater than can be eliminated by alveolar ventilation, so that Pco_2 begins to increase (88). Furthermore, with progression of asthma, mean pleural pressure becomes more negative as patients breathe against increased airway resistance and increased intrathoracic pressure. When pleural pressures drop to oppose airway closure, interstitial pressures are also lowered, but vascular pressure is maintained, promoting pulmonary interstitial edema and peribronchial cuffing, which may further increase airway resistance (89). In severe asthma, large negative swings in intrapleural pressure can significantly impair right ventricular function (90).

ETI and MV are required for a minority of patients with asthma and hypercapnia but are rarely needed in patients without hypercapnia (91). In assessing the need for MV, changes in response to therapy appear to be as important as absolute values (92). Mountain and Sahn (91) found that among 61 patients with SA presenting with hypercarbia (46% with pH < 7.30), only 5 (8%) required MV. Because intubation is an invasive procedure resulting in increased airflow resistance (93,94) and a high rate of complications (95), ETI is used only as a last resort in SA, when patients develop exhaustion of the ventilatory muscles or life-threatening complications (e.g., hypotension, arrhythmias, decreased level of consciousness) (92).

In intubated patients, ventilatory strategies that avoid overdistention have been shown to reduce barotrauma and mortality (96). Although several case reports suggest that externally applied positive end-expiratory pressure (PEEP) may offset PEEPi (97–100), one study of four asthmatic patients (using a Vt of 15 ± 3 mL/kg) did not confirm this finding (94). Applying PSV has been shown to decrease PEEPi by increasing expiratory time (101). Neuromuscular paralysis and corticosteroids place the intubated asthmatic patient at significant risk for developing muscle weakness (102).

Physiological Response to Mask Ventilation

The pathophysiology of SA can be improved by applying mask CPAP. Mask CPAP (1) causes bronchodilation and decreases airway resistance, (2) reexpands atelectasis and promotes removal of secretions, (3) rests the inspiratory muscles and offsets PEEPi, and (4) decreases the adverse hemodynamic effects of large negative peak and mean inspiratory pleural pressures.

In 1939, Barach and Swenson (6) documented with bronchography bronchial dilation during CPAP. In seven asthmatic patients, CPAP (7 cm H_2O) increased the diameter of smaller bronchi by 1 mm and moderate-sized bronchi by 2 mm. Three recent studies have shown that applying mask CPAP (8–12 cm H_2O) in exercise or induced (histamine or methacholine) asthma significantly decreases airflow obstruction (102–105).

Mask CPAP is also useful for reexpanding atelectasis and promoting the removal of secretions by increasing collateral flow (through collateral channels) to obstructed lung region (106) (see Sec. III.G).

In acute asthma, mask CPAP reduces Pdi, pressure-time product for the inspiratory muscles and diaphragm, and fractional inspiratory time (TI/TTOT) (81,104). When increasing levels of CPAP (0, 5, 7.5, 10, and 12 cm H_2O) were applied by face mask in severe acute asthma (peak flow < 200 L/min), patients were most comfortable at a CPAP level of 5.3 ± 2.8 cm H_2O, which corresponded to a significant reduction (by 8.65%; $p < 0.01$) in TI/TTOT (8).

In asthma, CPAP also decreases the adverse hemodynamic effects of large negative swings in mean inspiratory pleural pressures, which compromise right and left ventricular ejection (89,90,98).

Clinical Application of Mask Positive Pressure

Mask CPAP

The use of positive pressure as an aid to breathing in the treatment of severe asthma was first reported by Oertel in 1878 (107). In 1936, the clinical efficacy of mask CPAP for acute asthmatic exacerbation was reported by two groups (108,109). In 1981, the work of Wilson et al. (103). In subjects with exercise-induced asthma stimulated a reappraisal of this technique in acute asthma. Recently, Shivaram et al. (110) studied (nasal mask) CPAP in 27 patients presenting to the emergency room with severe (peak flow < 150 L/min) asthmatic exacerbation, with 6 serving as controls. CPAP was applied for 30-minute intervals at the levels (5 and 7.5 cm H_2O) previously found to produce maximal improvement in dyspnea (81). CPAP resulted in a significant reduction in dyspnea, cough, and respiratory rate without changes in Pao_2, $Paco_2$, or end-tidal Pco_2. The magnitude of improvement was proportional to the degree of initial abnormality. Two patients left the study because their dyspnea worsened with CPAP. Seventeen (81%) patients were observed to sleep while on CPAP therapy and awakened when CPAP was removed. None of the six control patients improved dyspnea, respiratory rate, or was observed to sleep. Similarly, Mansel et al. (111) reported a patient with acute, severe asthma and metabolic acidosis who was able to forgo intubation by using face mask CPAP (5 cm H_2O) and continuous sodium bicarbonate infusion. Nocturnal nasal CPAP may benefit asthmatic patients with coexisting sleep apnea (112,113) but is associated with disrupted sleep architecture in nonapneic asthmatics (114).

NPPV

In 1935, Barach first described in asthmatic patients receiving a helium-oxygen mixture a method to increase pressure during inspiration by using a blower in synchrony with the patient's respiration (3). Relief was felt after 6–10 breaths, and use of the accessory muscles diminished. In three patients who were refractory to adrenalin and had mental obtundation, treatment for 1–2 hours was followed by resolution of asthma and return of consciousness.

The recent experience with NPPV (PEEP + IPPV) in status asthmaticus is limited but encouraging (35,50–52). We (50) recently reported on 17 patients with SA (pH 7.25 $\pm$ 0.01, $Paco_2$ 65 $\pm$ 2) in whom NPPV with PEEP (4 $\pm$ 2 cm H_2O) and PSV (14 $\pm$ 5 cm H_2O) achieved rapid correction of gas exchange abnormalities. The mean ($\pm$SD) peak inspiratory pressure to ventilate in the NPPV-treated patients was 18 $\pm$ 5 cm H_2O and always <25 cm H_2O. Oral patency for intake (liquid diet) or expectoration was preserved. There was no problem with secretion retention. The (previously described) effects of positive pressure (106) in nonsedated patients with patent upper airways and intact cough reflex may have facilitated removal of secretions. Only one patient necessitated some sedation during NPPV. Two patients required intubation (35 min and 89 h into NPPV) for worsening $Paco_2$. All patients survived; duration of NPPV was 16 $\pm$ 21 hours and length of hospital stay was 5 $\pm$ 4 days.

NPPV was also evaluated as a modality to deliver aerosolized β_2-agonist in the emergency room (115). Patients with mild-to-moderate asthma exacerbation were randomized to receive two doses of aerosolized albuterol delivered via small-volume nebulizer (40 patients) or nasal BiPAP® set at IPAP 10 cm H_2O and EPAP at 5 cm H_2O (60 patients). Treatment with BiPAP® was associated with a greater increase in percentage of peak expiratory flow rate (69% $\pm$ 19% vs. 57% $\pm$ 21%; $p = 0.002$) (115).

Conclusion

Physiological studies indicate a beneficial effect for low level mask CPAP in acute asthma. Similar to patients with COPD and ARF, short-term application of mask CPAP does not improve gas exchange. However, when IPPV is added to mask CPAP, gas exchange rapidly improves. Contrary to the COPD experience, however, randomized studies are not available to compare mask CPAP or NPPV to conventional treatment in patients with acute, life-threatening exacerbations of this disease.

B. Sleep Apnea

Cardiopulmonary failure resulting from progression of obstructive sleep apnea (OSA) may lead to hypercapnic or hypoxemic ARF (110). Many of these patients are obese, and intubation is difficult and frequently associated with complications (116). Recent studies have reported encouraging results with mask CPAP (110) and NPPV (117). Physiological studies are not available for this patient population.

Mask CPAP

Shivaram et al. (110) evaluated nasal CPAP in six patients with OSA and acute hypercapnic respiratory failure. CPAP was adjusted (7.5–12 cm H_2O) to obtain an oxygen saturation of >85% by pulse oximetry (delivered Fio_2 was 0.28–0.30). Arterial pH increased from 7.23 ± 0.03 to 7.35 ± 0.01 ($p < 0.01$), while Pao_2 increased from 55 ± 6 mm Hg to 69 ± 7 mm Hg (NS). All patients presented with either lethargy or stupor, which rapidly reversed with CPAP treatment. Improvement in cardiopulmonary function resulted in a large, spontaneous diuresis. None of these patients required intubation.

NPPV

Patel et al. (117) reported five patients with OSA who had failed CPAP and in whom salvage therapy with BiPAP® was attempted before resorting to tracheostomy. BiPAP® levels were adjusted during polysomnography to eliminate 95% of obstructive apnea. Patients had better compliance, and only one patient failed and required surgery. Piper et al. (118) reported the use of nocturnal NPPV with BiPAP® in 13 CPAP-treated patients with severe OSA and persistent CO_2 retention. After 7–18 days of nocturnal NPPV, daytime Pao_2 increased from 50 ± 2.6 mmHg to 66 ± 3 mmHg ($p < 0.001$), and $Paco_2$ decreased from 62 ± 2.5 mmHg to 46 ± 1 mmHg ($p < 0.0001$). Improvements were attributed to improved central ventilatory drive. NPPV was also investigated in 18 obese patients with respiratory failure and a body mass index equal to or greater than 40 kg/m². BiPAP® ventilation reduced inspiratory muscle activity by at least 40%, without decreasing end-tidal CO_2 (119).

Conclusion

The results of these clinical studies are encouraging but insufficient to reach firm conclusions.

C. Cystic Fibrosis and Bridge-to-Lung Transplantation

Using conventional ventilation with an invasive artificial airway (endotracheal tube or tracheostomy) is associated with significant risk in patients with cystic fibrosis (CF) who are heavily colonized with *Pseudomonas aeruginosa* and have severe airflow obstruction (32,120). Among eight patients with cystic fibrosis and end-stage respiratory failure who received conventional ventilation via intubation as a bridge to transplantation, control of hypercarbia was difficult because of high peak inspiratory pressure. All patients developed septic shock within a few days of intubation (mean 1.3 days), suggesting that intubation may be associated with early dissemination of pulmonary infections. Three patients underwent heart-lung transplantation, and only one survived (prior intubation was only 20 h). Physiological studies are not available for this patient population.

Clinical Application of Mask NPPV

Four studies have described the successful implementation of NPPV in cystic fibrosis patients with advanced disease who suffered from acute on chronic respiratory failure (29,34,121,122). Some of these patients had previously failed to respond to nasal CPAP (122). Ventilation was delivered using either pressure support (121) or assist control (29,34,122). After stabilization in the hospital, patients were discharged home on nocturnal ventilation delivered via a nasal mask for up to 18 months. NPPV frequently succeeded (12 out of 16 patients) in keeping the patient alive until transplantation (29,24,122). Irrespective of final outcome, NPPV improved quality of life as well as respiratory muscle strength, cough efficiency, clearing of secretions, quality of sleep, and daytime function (122).

In children with CF, NPPV has been applied successfully to improve respiratory muscle fatigue and O_2 saturation during chest physiotherapy (123). In one study, the short-term application (20 min) of nasal NPPV in patients with CF and stable chronic hypercapnic respiratory failure led to an increase in O_2 saturation and a significant reduction in respiratory rate and transcutaneous CO_2 (124). Caloric conservation from respiratory muscle rest and increased oral intake improves nutritional status (personal observation). The nighttime application of nasal NPPV in patients with CF and stable chronic respiratory failure was found to improve alveolar ventilation during all sleep states without affecting sleep architecture and arousals and was superior to low flow O_2 administration alone (125). No complications have been reported in the literature from prolonged NPPV in cystic fibrosis patients (122). We observed nasal bridge necrosis in one patient, who eventually received successful transplantation (unpublished data). The duration of intubation (6–48 h) and intensive care unit (ICU) stay after transplantation were much shorter in cystic fibrosis patients supported preoperatively with NPPV than in those supported with conventional ventilation (34).

In COPD patients awaiting lung transplantation or volume reduction surgery, NPPV was found effective in improving gas exchange, functional status, sleep quality, and avoiding intubation during acute exacerbation (126). Small uncontrolled reports have described the successful implementation of NPPV in lung transplantation recipients developing acute respiratory failure (127,129). Antonelli et al. recently completed a randomized trial evaluating 40 consecutive solid organ transplant recipients with acute hypoxemic respiratory failure (personal communication of unpublished data). The study compared NPPV delivered through a facial mask to standard treatment with supplemental oxygen administration. NPPV was well tolerated and associated with a significant reduction in rate of endotracheal intubation (20% vs. 70%; $p = 0.002$), rate of severe sepsis (5% vs. 30%; $p = 0.04$), rate of complication leading to death (20% vs. 50%; $p = 0.05$), and intensive care unit mortality (20% vs. 50%; $p = 0.05$).

Conclusion

The results of these studies and the high risk associated with intubation strongly support using NPPV in patients with cystic fibrosis and ARF. In our centers and others (120), NPPV has become a first-line intervention in patients with cystic fibrosis who require ventilatory support prior to transplantation. The ventilatory strategy should be similar to the one described for patients with asthma.

III. Hypoxemic Respiratory Failure

Oxygenation failure results from a severe impairment in matching of ventilation and perfusion or shunt. Such failure can develop from abnormalities in the pulmonary circulation (increased hydrostatic pressure, e.g., increased vascular permeability, or vascular occlusion) or loss of gas exchange surface area (edema, pneumonia, infarction, atelectasis, hemorrhage, fibrosis). Lung diseases culminating in hypoxemic ARF are commonly associated with reduced functional residual capacity and decreased lung compliance. A large body of literature has described the successful application of mask CPAP (Table 1) (8–26) and NPPV (Table 2) (27–70) in hypoxemic ARF of varied etiologies.

Positive end-expiratory pressure maintains airway pressure above atmospheric pressure at end expiration, while CPAP refers to positive airway pressure being maintained throughout the whole respiratory cycle (130,131). In hypoxemic patients, PEEP and CPAP are used for recruiting underventilated alveoli by increasing lung volume at end expiration, resulting in improved gas exchange. Both modes may be used during spontaneous or mechanical ventilation and may be applied (continuously or intermittently) by an endotracheal tube, mask, or mouthpiece (131). The first report of positive pressure applied by face mask was by Bunnell in 1912 to maintain lung expansion during thoracic surgery (132). The first use outside of the operating room was described by Poulton and Oxon in 1936; they used a vacuum cleaner (Hoover or Electrolux) to generate gas flow and a spring-loaded valve to oppose expiration (109).

When mask CPAP is applied in healthy individuals, passive lung inflation is resisted, expiratory flow is facilitated, and expiratory time is shortened by active reflex mechanisms (133). Increments of CPAP levels (5, 10, and 15 cm H_2O) cause a proportional increase in minute ventilation, resulting primarily from an increase in Vt at 5 cm H_2O and an increase in respiratory rate at 15 cm H_2O

(from a shortening of expiratory time [TE] irrespective of any alteration in inspiratory time [TI]). In normal patients, CPAP causes a dose-dependent reduction in cardiac stroke volume starting at 5 cm H_2O with a facial mask and 10 cm H_2O with a nasal mask (134). The heart rate is not affected and cardiac output drops. Mouth opening during nasal mask ventilation negates the hemodynamic effects of positive pressure (134). The effects of mask CPAP in patients with hypoxemia are discussed under each described condition. Retention of carbon dioxide has occasionally been a limiting factor for this technique (8–10). Mean positive airway pressure (mPAP) is the most important determinant of blood oxygenation (135). During pressure-preset ventilation (i.e., pressure support ventilation), mPAP can be estimated by the simple formula: PSET $\times$ TI/TTOT + PEEP $\times$ TE/TT, where PSET corresponds to the amount of pressure applied, and TI, TE, and TT are inspiratory, expiratory, and total cycle times (136). By adding IPPV to a preset level of CPAP, mPAP increases proportionally to increments in applied pressure.

Two studies compared applying CPAP and CPAP with PSV in hypoxemic patients before (breathing through an endotracheal tube) and after extubation (breathing through a face mask) (62,137). In postthoracotomy patients receiving CPAP (10 cm H_2O), transfer to face mask resulted in higher Sao_2 and no differences in hemodynamic parameters (137). In 22 trauma patients, transfer from endotracheal tube to face mask during application of a similar PEEP (5.8 $\pm$ 2.5 and 5.2 $\pm$ 2.2 cm H_2O) and PSV (13 $\pm$ 5 vs. 12.8 $\pm$ 1.7 cm H_2O) resulted in similar blood gases and respiratory pattern (62).

A. Randomized Studies in Patients with Hypoxemic Respiratory Failure of Varied Etiology

Randomized studies of noninvasive ventilation in hypoxemic respiratory failure have investigated either homogeneous populations of patients with a single diagnosis or heterogeneous populations of patients with a wide variety of lung pathologies. Randomized studies of homogeneous populations have included mask CPAP for cardiogenic pulmonary edema (13,20,23,138) and postoperative atelectasis (139) and NPPV for severe community-acquired pneumonia (140), and following solid organ transplantation (70b). These studies are reviewed later under each specific topic. Randomized studies of heterogeneous groups of patients with hypoxemic respiratory failure are reviewed in this section.

Wysocki et al. (41) randomized 41 non-COPD patients with ARF to NPPV via face mask versus conventional medical therapy. NPPV reduced the need for endotracheal intubation (36 vs. 100%; $p = 0.02$), the duration of ICU stay (13 + 15 days vs. 32 + 30 days; $p = 0.04$) and mortality rate (9% vs. 66%; $p = 0.06$) only in those patients with hypercapnia ($Paco_2 > 45$ mmHg). NPPV had no significant advantages in the hypoxemic group without concomitant hypercarbia. On the basis of these results, the authors concluded that NPPV may not be beneficial in all forms of ARF not related to COPD.

Antonelli et al. (61) conducted a prospective, randomized study comparing NPPV via a face mask to endotracheal intubation with conventional mechanical ventilation in patients with hypoxemic acute respiratory failure who met preselected criteria for mechanical ventilation after failure to improve with aggressive medical therapy (61). Sixty-four consecutive patients (32 in each arm) were enrolled in this study. The two groups were similar at study entry. After 1 hour of mechanical ventilation, both groups had a significant ($p < 0.05$) improvement in Pao_2:Fio_2. Ten (31%) patients randomized to noninvasive ventilation required endotracheal intubation. Patients randomized to conventional ventilation developed more frequent and serious complications (38% vs. 66%; $p = 0.02$), and complications (pneumonia or sinusitis) related to the endotracheal tube (3% vs. 31%; $p = 0.004$). Among survivors, patients randomized to noninvasive ventilation had a lower duration of mechanical ventilation ($p = 0.006$) and a shorter intensive care unit stay ($p = 0.002$). Patients with higher simplified acute physiological scores had a worse outcome irrespective of randomization group. Among less severe patients (post hoc analysis of the 45 patients with a simplified acute physiological score <16), the NPPV group had a lower duration of mechanical ventilation ($p = 0.027$) and intensive care unit stay ($p = 0.024$), a lower incidence of septic complications ($p = 0.012$), and improved survival ($p = 0.045$). Factors that may have been involved in shortening the duration of mechanical ventilation in the NPPV group included avoiding sedation, eliminating the imposed work by the endotracheal tube, lower rate of ventilator-associated pneumonia, and earlier removal from ventilation.

In conclusion, NPPV in patients with acute hypoxemic respiratory failure was found to be as effective as conventional ventilation in improving gas exchange abnormalities, and when endotracheal intubation was avoided, the development of ventilator associated pneumonia was also avoided (61). A recent prospective epidemiological survey of 320 consecutive patients with ARF receiving mechanical ventilation also reported a lower ($p = 0.004$) rate of ventilator-associated pneumonia in patients supported noninvasively (0.16 per 100 days of noninvasive ventilation) versus those on conventional ventilation (0.85 per 100 days of tracheal intubation) (142).

Wood et al. (66) randomized 27 patients presenting to an emergency department with acute hypoxemic respiratory failure to receive conventional medical therapy versus early NPPV. NPPV was delivered by a nasal mask and a BiPAP® ventilator. A chin strap was used in patients breathing through their mouths. The rate of intubation was high and similar in both groups (44% and 45%). Among patients requiring intubation, those randomized to NPPV had a longer delay to intubation (26 ± 27 h vs. 4.8 ± 6.9 h; $p = 0.055$). Patients randomized to NPPV had a disturbing trend toward a greater rate of hospital mortality (25% vs. 0%;

$p = 0.123$). However, several confounding variables may have influenced the results of this study. The group randomized to NPPV had a lower Pao_2 (60 ± 21 vs. 71 ± 22), fewer patients with COPD (12% vs. 36%), and more patients with pneumonia (44% vs. 18%), ARDS (1 vs. 0), and interstitial lung disease (1 vs. 0). The NPPV group had a higher APACHE II score (18 ± 7 vs. 16 ± 4; $p = 0.4$), and predicted mortality (26 ± 16 vs. 19 ± 8; $p = 0.4$), and more required admission to an ICU (81% vs. 64%). Hence, it is possible that the worse outcome in the NPPV group was related to inclusion of sicker patients.

B. Cardiogenic Pulmonary Edema

In patients with cardiogenic pulmonary edema (CPE), the work of breathing is increased by reduced lung compliance and increased airway resistance (interstitial and bronchial edema) (72). The reduction in lung compliance correlates with derangements in pulmonary gas exchange (72). In patients with CPE, the inspiratory muscles have to generate large negative swings in pleural pressure (high Pes amplitude), which increase left ventricular transmural pressure (LVPtm) and afterload (143,144). Reduction in cardiac output compromises oxygen delivery to the respiratory muscles and may create a vicious cycle. Increased sympathetic nervous activity (SNA) and catecholamine levels are important acute compensatory mechanisms to maintaining cardiac output and perfusion pressure in patients with CPE (144). Prolonged increases in SNA, however, may actually contribute to progression of CPE by causing cardiac myocyte hypertrophy and necrosis, a reduction in β_1-adrenergic receptors, patchy destruction and depletion of the sympathetic nerve terminals, and impairment in systolic and diastolic function (144).

In patients with stable chronic heart failure, inspiratory and expiratory muscle strength are impaired, and inspiratory muscle weakness significantly correlates with dyspnea during activity (145). Respiratory muscle fatigue with retention of carbon dioxide is frequently observed in patients presenting with CPE (20,146). Of clinical importance, respiratory distress in CPE is not directly related to hypoxemia and cannot be reversed with oxygen administration alone (17,147).

Physiologic Response to Mask Ventilation

Several studies indicate that respiratory and cardiovascular manifestations of severe CPE can significantly benefit from administration of positive-pressure ventilation (23,108,148,155). Haven Emerson in 1909 showed that experimental (epinephrine-induced) pulmonary edema was consistently improved by applying artificial ventilation (149). A series of animal and human studies published from 1936 to 1947 showed that positive-pressure breathing (CPAP and IPPV) applied to a failing heart decreases mean intrapleural negative pressure during inspiration, decreases net filling pressure of the right ventricle, and prevents pulmonary congestion and edema (3,5,156).

The single most important hemodynamic influence of IPPV, with or without PEEP, is to reduce venous return (154). On the normal ventricle (sensitive to preload changes), a reduction in venous return may lead to a decrease in left ventricular preload and cardiac output with a dilated, failing left ventricle (LV) operating on the flat (depressed) portion (insensitive to preload changes and sensitive to afterload changes), a reduction in preload may not affect LV output (148). Applying PPV in zone III conditions (CPE) may also increase LV preload by "squeezing" blood from the lungs into the LV during inspiration (diastole) (154). Finally, during PPV, a portion of the airway pressure is transmitted to the LV and thoracic aorta, reducing the tension that the heart has to develop (LVPtm) in order to eject blood (decreased afterload) (108,148,150,151). The reduction in LVPtm results from increases in Pes (offsetting the exaggerated negative intrapleural swings) rather than decreases in blood pressure (vasodilator therapy) (148). Afterload reduction with CPAP augments that achieved by vasodilator agents (148).

Applying mask CPAP in severe CPE is associated with immediate and marked improvements in hemodynamics and respiratory mechanics (13,138, 152,157,160). In patients with impaired myocardial contractility and undergoing cardiac catheterization, applying (nasal mask) CPAP (5 cm H_2O) in those with a pulmonary wedge pressure (PWP) above 12 mmHg was associated with a significant improvement in cardiac index (from 2.48 ± 0.26 to 2.81 ± 0.26 L/min/ m^2; $p < 0.01$) and stroke volume index (from 52.6 ± 7 to 64.1 ± 8; $p < 0.001$) without change in oxygenation (157). Additional improvement is observed by increasing CPAP from 5 to 10 cm H_2O (159). In a similar study, Baratz et al. (152) found that 7 of 13 patients improved hemodynamic parameters with CPAP irrespective of PWP values. After discontinuing CPAP, the hemodynamic parameters returned to baseline (134,152).

Enhancing left ventricular performance is seen in patients with predominantly systolic dysfunction (158) and is not observed in patients with atrial fibrillation (161). In CPE, mask CPAP causes a significant fall in heart rate (HR) (13,148,157) likely resulting from increased parasympathetic tone from CPAP-induced lung inflation (162). In CPE, mask CPAP also causes a significant reduction in airway resistance (0.57 ± 0.10 to 0.34 ± 0.10 kPa.s/L; $p < 0.05$), lung compliance, and work of breathing (0.80 ± 0.10 to 0.51 ± 0.05 J; $p < 0.05$) (160). Reduced myocardial (LVPtm $\times$ HR) and inspiratory muscle (Pes $\times$ respiratory rate [RR]) energy demands (148) allow greater oxygen availability to other tissues (163). In a randomized study of 30 patients with CPE, nasal CPAP was superior to oxygen supplementation alone in improving hemodynamics and gas exchange was associated with a significant reduction in plasma endothelin-1 levels at 6 and 24 hours (138).

Clinical Application of Mask Positive Pressure

Mask CPAP

Applying mask CPAP in patients with CPE was first reported in the 1930s by Poulton and Oxon (109) and by Barach and associates (4,5). Observational studies (8,10,17,26) (Table 1) and anecdotal reports (150,168–170) describe a positive response to mask CPAP in CPE. The efficacy of mask CPAP in this patient population was proven by three randomized studies (13,20,23). Rasanen et al. (13) randomly assigned 40 patients with CPE (19 with acute myocardial infarction) to either ambient airway pressure or 10 cm H_2O CPAP while Fio_2 was kept constant at 28–30%. In contrast to controls, CPAP rapidly improved Pao_2 ($p < 0.001$) while simultaneously decreasing respiratory rate ($p < 0.001$) and $Paco_2$ ($p < 0.01$). Furthermore, CPAP resulted in rapid and significant improvements in heart rate ($p < 0.001$), blood pressure ($p < 0.05$), and rate-pressure product ($p < 0.01$). During the study period (3 h), 12 patients in the control group and 6 in the CPAP group required intubation ($p = 0.07$). Reasons for intubation included hypoxemia (4 patients), CO_2 retention (1 patient), and need for cardiac resuscitation (1 patient). The study design did not allow for correction of hypoxemia by increasing Fio_2 or CPAP, which may have prevented four intubations in the CPAP-treated group.

Bersten et al. (20) randomized 39 patients with CPE and severe ARF to receive oxygen supplementation alone or in combination with CPAP (10 cm H_2O) by face mask. The CPAP-treated group had a rapid (<30 min) improvement in respiratory rate (35 ± 8 to 27 ± 6; $p = 0.008$), $Paco_2$ (58 ± 8 to 46 ± 4; $p < 0.001$), pH (7.18 ± 0.08 to 7.28 ± 0.06; $p < 0.001$), Pao_2: Fio_2 (138 ± 31 to 206 ± 126; $p = 0.01$), and heart rate (113 ± 21 to 104 ± 19; $p = 0.04$). Seven patients in the control group required intubation versus none among the CPAP-treated patients ($p = 0.005$). In the latter group, length of ICU stay was significantly shorter (1.2 ± 0.4 days vs. 2.7 ± 2.0 days; $p = 0.006$) with tangible cost savings (167).

Lin et al. (23) randomized 100 patients admitted with CPE to either oxygen by nonrebreathing mask or (face) mask CPAP with oxygen (increased every 30 min by 2.5 cm H_2O up to 12.5 cm H_2O). Patients had similar physiological characteristics at study entry, and respiratory acidosis was uncommon. When compared to conventional treatment, mask CPAP therapy was associated with a significant improvement in stroke volume index, heart rate, Pao_2, Qs/Qt, and a lower rate of intubation (16% vs. 36%; $p < 0.01$). In-hospital mortality was similar (8% vs. 12%).

In addition to these reports of successful application of CPAP to patients with acute pulmonary edema, the technique has also been successfully applied to patients with chronic congestive heart failure. When nasal CPAP (8–12 cm H_2O) was applied during sleep in patients with chronic heart failure and recurrent apneas in association with Cheyne-Stokes respiration (144,153,168) the number of apneas fell from 60 ± 12/h to 9 ± 7/h ($p < 0.01$), and symptoms of sleep apnea resolved (153). Inspiratory muscle strength and dyspnea improved (168). Furthermore, resting left ventricular ejection fraction (LVEF) as measured by radionuclide angiography rose from 31 ± 8% to 38 ± 10% ($p < 0.05$), and all patients experienced marked improvement in symptoms of heart failure from functional classes III and IV (New York Heart Association Classification) to class II (after CPAP) (153). Nocturnal nasal CPAP was found to reduce sympathetic nervous activity both while asleep and awake (144). Reduction in sympathetic stimulation (decreased afterload) may have contributed to improved LVEF (144).

NPPV

In his classic work on the effects of positive pressure on the circulation, Werko (156) evaluated three patients in heart failure and found IPPV to increase stroke volume in two. He recommended using IPPV instead of CPAP or PEEP in patients with CPE, because it placed "less strain on the patient" and allowed them to achieve higher inspiratory pressure. In 1959, Miller and Sproule (147) reported a dramatic response to intermittent positive pressure breathing (IPPB) in 35 patients with CPE who did not respond to conventional treatment, including 100% inspired oxygen.

Several recent series have reported good results in CPE patients treated with NPPV (27,33,35,47,68,168,173). Mehta et al. (173a) have compared bilevel versus continuous positive airway pressure delivered by nasal mask in patients with cardiogenic pulmonary edema. Bilevel pressure was found to be more effective in improving a similar rate (7%) of intubation, but was associated with an unexplained higher rate of acute myocardial infarction (71 vs. 31%; $p < 0.05$). Rusterholtz et al. (170) applied CPAP 5 cm H_2O and PSV 20 H_2O by facial mask to eight patients with ischemic cardiomyopathy and ARF (Pao_2:Fio_2 127 ± 8 mmHg, $Paco_2$ 64 ± 4 mmHg). NPPV was associated with rapid and sustained improvement in gas exchange. The mean duration of NPPV was 5 ± 1.5 hours, and no patient required intubation (170). This group later expanded their experience to 26 consecutive patients and observed 5 failures (defined as the need of intubation) and 21 successes. Patients that failed had significantly lower $Paco_2$ (32 ± 2 vs. 54.2 ± 15 mmHg) and higher creatine kinase (CK) values related to acute myocardial infarction (4 of 5 in the failure group vs. 2 of 21 in the success group) (68). Bollaert et al. (172) compared 15 consecutive patients with severe CPE and acute respiratory acidosis treated with NPPV to a matched historical control group. NPPV was associated with a rapid and significant improvement in gas exchange, a lower rate of intubation (13% vs. 87%; $p < 0.01$) and shorter duration of MV (2.8 ± 3.5 h vs. 66 ± 24 h; $p < 0.01$). Hoffmann and Welte (174) reported on the use of NPPV (CPAP 2–8 cm H_2O, IPAP 13–24 cm H_2O) delivered with a facial mask in 29 patients with CPE. NPPV was well tolerated, associated with rapid improvement in gas exchange, and a low intubation rate (3%) (174).

In our experience, applying NPPV in eight patients with severe CPE (pH 7.31 ± 0.01, $Pao_2:Fio_2$ 157 ± 115 mmHg) was effective in improving gas exchange in all but one patient, who required intubation (175). The development of hemodynamic instability, however, led to intubating two additional patients. In patients with CPE, duration of NPPV is usually shorter than with other forms of ARF (33,35,175). Three studies have reported a favorable response (>90% success rate in avoiding ETI) to NPPV with nasal BiPAP (47,171,176).

In a randomized, controlled trial comparing CPAP (10 cm H_2O) to BiPAP (15 cm H_2O inspiratory, 5 cm H_2O expiratory pressures) in patients with acute pulmonary edema, Mehta et al. found more rapid reductions in $Paco_2$ and blood pressure during the first 30 minutes in the 14 BiPAP patients than in the 13 CPAP patients. Of concern, they also found a much higher percentage of completed myocardial infarctions in the BiPAP compared to the CPAP group (71 vs. 31%, $p = 0.05$). Other outcome variables including length of device use, need for intubation, mortality, and hospital stay were similar between the groups. The study was stopped early because of the high infarction rate in the BiPAP group, so optimal randomization of all variables could not be assured. Nonetheless, the authors advised caution during use of bilevel ventilation in the setting of acute myocardial infarction or ischemia.

Conclusion

Physiological data and the results of randomized clinical studies support the continuous (not intermittent) application of mask CPAP in patients with CPE, particularly those with hypercarbia. Improvement in hemodynamic parameters, respiratory rate, dyspnea, and gas exchange abnormality is rapid. If the underlying condition has not improved, however, hemodynamic parameters may return to baseline soon after discontinuing mask CPAP. In patients failing to improve with CPAP alone, consideration should be given to adding IPPV. In patients with acute myocardial infarction, NPPV should be used with caution. A nasal mask is quite effective as long as the mouth opening is minimized.

C. Acute Respiratory Distress Syndrome

Physiological studies with mask CPAP or NPPV are not available for patients with acute respiratory distress syndrome (ARDS).

Clinical Application of Positive Pressure

Mask CPAP

Applying mask CPAP in patients with increased permeability pulmonary edema was first reported by Barach et al. in 1938 (5). In 1982, Covelli et al. (11) evaluated the application of (face) mask CPAP in 33 patients with severe ARDS (Pao_2: Fio_2 of 133 $\pm$ 7 mmHg) of varied etiologies. Most required CPAP application of only 5 cm H_2O. Significant improvement in Pao_2:Fio_2 ($p < 0.001$) was seen within 1 hr of therapy. In seven patients who required $\geq$10 cm H_2O, the shunt fraction decreased from 44 $\pm$ 4 to 28 $\pm$ 4. Five patients ultimately required intubation: two from mask discomfort and three from a change in mental status and uncooperation. After intubation these patients required CPAP >15 cm H_2O to improve hypoxemia. Their initial Pao_2:Fio_2 was 102 $\pm$ 4 mmHg, whereas patients not requiring intubation had a baseline Pao_2:Fio_2 of 138 $\pm$ 8 mmHg. Successful applications of CPAP have also been reported in patients with fat embolism and sepsis (178,179).

NPPV

Relatively few studies have applied NPPV in patients with ARDS (27,33, 61,67,169,175). In a recent study of patients with acute hypoxemic respiratory failure requiring mechanical ventilation, Antonelli et al. (61) reported that 7 of the 32 (22%) patients randomized to NPPV had ARDS of varied etiology. NPPV was associated with a significant improvement in Pao_2:Fio_2 ($p = 0.01$). Four patients randomized to NPPV avoided intubation and survived, while three patients required intubation and died. Rocker et al. (67) reported the use of NPPV via facial mask during 12 episodes of hypoxemic ARF (all but one episode with Pao_2:$Fio_2 < 200$) occurring in hemodynamically stable patients with acute lung injury. Pao_2:Fio_2 improved by 25% in 9 episodes. Intubation was avoided in 66% of the episodes, and ICU survival was 70%. Duration of successful NPPV ranged from 23 to 80 hours. Two anecdotal reports have described the successful application of NPPV in two patients with hematological malignancies who developed ARDS after blood stem cell transplantation (184,185).

Insufficient data are available to evaluate the clinical usefulness of NPPV in ARDS, and its use is discouraged unless ARDS is mild or the patient is not a candidate for intubation (see Sec. IV).

D. Postoperative Respiratory Failure

Thoracic and upper abdominal surgery are associated with a marked and prolonged postoperative reduction in functional reserve (or residual) capacity (FRC), Pao_2, and forced vital capacity (FVC) (182,183).

Physiological Response to Mask Positive Pressure

Following upper abdominal surgery, applying mask CPAP improves FVC (187), FRC (183,184), and gas exchange (185,186). CPAP is superior to incentive spirometry or a regimen of coughing and deep breathing (184). In one study, applying CPAP (12 cm H_2O) through a mouthpiece postoperatively increased FVC from 870 to 2083 mL and FRC from 2030 to 2410 mL (183).

Following coronary artery bypass graft (CABG) surgery, applying mask CPAP improves FEV_1 (187), FVC (187), FRC (184,188), and gas exchange (137,189,191). Mask CPAP is superior to IPPB and incentive spirometry in improving FRC (184,188). Improvements in FRC are not sustained after removing mask CPAP, and deterioration can be seen within 10–30 minutes (188,191). Improvements in gas exchange, however, are more protracted. In one study, nasal CPAP (7.5 cm H_2O) administered for 12 hours postextubation significantly improved $Pao_2:Fio_2$ for 24 hours (190).

Clinical Application of Mask Positive Pressure

Mask CPAP

The use of mask CPAP to maintain lung expansion was first described by Bunnell in 1912 in patients undergoing thoracic surgery (132). Mask CPAP has been evaluated in the postoperative state as a modality to reduce pulmonary complications. Meaningful results are obtained when CPAP is applied at a pressure of 7.5–10 cm H_2O early after surgery and continued intermittently for several days (183). Mask CPAP has also been described for treating postoperative hypoxemia (15,192). The first report of mask CPAP for treating postoperative hypoxemic ARF was by Boothby et al. in 1940 (192). In a postcholecystectomy patient with hypoxemia refractory to 1.0 Fio_2, marked improvement was observed after a 20-minute application of CPAP (6 cm H_2O). In a study of surgical patients with postextubation hypoxemia and who failed to improve with aggressive respiratory therapy, mask CPAP (8.3 $\pm$ 2.8 cm H_2O) was effective in improving gas exchange ($Pao_2:Fio_2$ from 130 $\pm$ 17 to 337 $\pm$ 59; $p < 0.001$) and avoided reintubation in 25 of 27 patients (15). One large study found no difference in postoperative pulmonary complications between the following forms of mask treatment: CPAP, positive expiratory pressure, and inspiratory resistance-positive expiratory pressure (193).

NPPV

Pennock et al. (33) first reported on the use of nasal BiPAP® in 22 postsurgical patients (10 post-CABG) who developed hypoxemic and/or hypercapnic respiratory failure. Patients were hemodynamically stable and without multisystem failure. Initial ventilatory settings were EPAP (5 cm H_2O) and IPAP (10 cm H_2O). One hour into NPPV there was a significant improvement in gas exchange and a reduction in respiratory rate. Only 4 of the 22 patients required intubation. NPPV lasted from 2 hours to 6 days. These investigators later expanded their experience to a total of 97 postoperative patients, with an 80% successful outcome of therapy (defined as withdrawal of ventilatory support for >48 h) (40).

Wysocki et al. (36) applied NPPV (PSV alone) by face mask in seven patients with postoperative respiratory failure. NPPV was unsuccessful in three patients, two of whom had pneumonia. Day et al. (194) randomly applied NPPV with IPAP set at 10 cm H_2O (BiPAP® via a nasal mask) to 467 postoperative patients. The only benefit of the unselected use of postoperative NPPV was a faster radiographic improvement in patients (199) receiving BiPAP® (45% vs. 33%; $p < 0.05$). Among 51 patients considered at higher risk for postoperative respiratory failure, reintubation was lower in the BiPAP®-treated group (1 vs. 3).

Two more recent observational studies involving 85 patients with postoperative respiratory failure reported a 70% success rate in avoiding intubation (195,196). In a prospective study, 19 patients were randomized following lung resection to receive either nasal BiPAP® ventilatory support or standard medical treatment (60). Patients randomized to NPPV had a significant increase in Pao_2, while no change was observed in the control group. NPPV did not increase dead space–to–tidal volume ratio or worsen pleural air leaks. In 76 patients following coronary artery by pass grafting bilevel positive airway pressure or CPAP applied after endotracheal extubation prevented the increase in extravascular lung water during weaning from mechanical ventilation. The effect lasted for at least 1 hour after discontinuation of CPAP or BiPAP® treatment (197).

Conclusion

Mask CPAP is useful for restoring FRC and improving gas exchange postoperatively. To be most effective, treatment should be initiated soon after extubation and applied (intermittently) for several days. The advantages of mask CPAP over other postoperative interventions include increased effectiveness, the need for no effort from the patient, and therapy is not painful (184). Randomized studies are not available for patients with postoperative ARF, and effects on outcomes such as complication rates, lengths of stay, and mortality rates are unknown. In stable patients, however, mask CPAP or NPPV could be tried to avoid intubation.

E. Trauma

Pulmonary function disorders are common in traumatized patients. These disorders lead to reduced FRC, compliance, and subsequent restrictive defects precipitating impaired gas exchange (14). During World War II, as a result of a series of studies published by Barach on CPE and pneumonia, mask CPAP was introduced to treat "traumatic wet lung" (198,199). Since then, several investigators have described the successful application of mask CPAP in posttraumatic hypoxemic ARF (Table 1) (9,10,12,14,16). Physiological data in this patient population are not available.

Mask CPAP

In 1980, Smith et al. (9) described using CPAP by face mask in 44 patients with moderate to severe posttraumatic or postsurgical hypoxemic failure ($Pao_2:Fio_2 = 171 \pm 42$). All patients improved their oxygenation ($Pao_2:Fio_2 = 300 \pm 68$; $p < 0.005$), but one patient developed acidemia and was intubated. In 1981 Suter and Kobel (10) described the intermittent (continuous application for <3 h) use of CPAP (5–10 cm H_2O) for up to 10 days in 15 trauma patients; 67% successfully avoided intubation. In the researchers' experience, trauma patients did better than patients with other forms of ARF. In 1982, Linton and Potgieter (12) reported their experience with 26 patients with blunt chest trauma (21 flail chest); 13 received face mask CPAP (5 cm H_2O) and 13 were intubated and received intermittent mandatory ventilation (IMV). The study was not randomized, but patients were similar in terms of severity of injuries and other clinical features. The mask CPAP–treated group had a shorter ICU stay (7 days vs. 12 days) and a significantly lower rate of complications (2 vs. 10; $p < 0.005$), especially nosocomial infections (0 vs. 5). The only failure, in the CPAP group, was attributed to a seizure in a patient with epilepsy. In 1985, Hurst et al. (14) applied face mask CPAP to 33 trauma patients with $Pao_2:Fio_2 < 150$ with a therapeutic endpoint of achieving a $Pao_2:Fio_2 > 300$. To achieve the treatment goal, 11 patients required 5 cm H_2O and 22 required 10 cm H_2O. Two patients were intubated for worsening hypoxemia and management of secretions. Only one of six patients with obvious flail chest required intubation. These investigators later expanded their experience to 135 patients and reported a similar success rate (16). In the above reports, which include 240 patients, only one complication (nasal bridge nose necrosis) was reported (16). CPAP, however, must be used with caution in patients with gastric anastomosis and with severe maxillofacial injuries (basilar skull fractures) (14). A case of pneumocephalus was reported in trauma patients with unrecognized basilar skull fracture (200).

NPPV

In 22 trauma patients, transfer from an endotracheal tube to a face mask during application of similar PEEP (5.8 ± 2.5 and 5.2 ± 2.2 cm H_2O) and PSV (13 ± 5 vs. 12.8 ± 1.7 cm H_2O) resulted in similar improvement in gas exchange and respiratory pattern (62). The median duration of NPPV was 47 hours (range 6–144). All patients tolerated NPPV, but 9 patients (40.9%) required reintubation after an average of 54 hours of NPPV. Six of these died after 36 ± 13 days while still on mechanical ventilation. There was no statistically significant difference in compliance score between the two techniques. In a recent study of patients with acute hypoxemic respiratory failure requiring mechanical ventilation, Antonelli et al. (61) reported that 7 of the 32 (22%) patients randomized to NPPV had trauma with pulmonary contusion or atelectasis. NPPV was associated with a rapid and significant improvement in $Pao_2:Fio_2$, and all seven patients avoided intubation and survived (61).

Conclusion

A large body of uncontrolled literature has reported favorable results with mask CPAP in posttraumatic ARF. Patients with basilar skull fractures are at risk for complications. Randomized studies are necessary before final recommendations can be made.

F. Acquired Immunodeficiency Syndrome

Respiratory failure due to *Pneumocystis carinii* pneumonia (PCP) remains the most common reason for ICU admission among patients with AIDS (201,202). ICU use for AIDS patients with ARF increased in the late 1980s, following several reports of improved hospital survival (about 40%) when compared to earlier reports (mortality 84–100%) (203). Recent data on outcome and ICU cost, however, are forcing a reevaluation of admission policies to the ICU for patients with AIDS and ARF (202). In a large municipal hospital, among patients admitted from 1989–91, hospital survival was 24%, length of ICU stay was 6.4 days in survivors and 12 days in nonsurvivors, and the mean survival time after discharge was 16 months (202). The cost per average ICU day was $4,128, the hospital cost for nonsurvivors was $30,289 and for survivors $80,948, and the cost per year of life saved was $215,233 (202). A low CD4 count was the strongest predictor of hospital mortality (202). In AIDS patients with ARF, NIV with either mask CPAP or NPPV has shown promising results and may decrease ICU cost when compared to conventional ventilation via intubation.

Mask CPAP

Six reports have described a significant improvement in gas exchange, respiratory rate, and dyspnea in 104 AIDS patients with hypoxemic ARF treated with mask CPAP (18,19,20,21,22,204). Treatment was well tolerated. Only one study (18 patients) reported complications, including one pneumothorax, four facial skin necrosis, and two gastric distention (18). Response to CPAP may identify less severe disease, because patients requiring higher levels of CPAP were more likely to be intubated ($p < 0.01$) (21). Hospital mortality was 9% in the 77 patients who avoided intubation and 81% in the 27 patients who failed CPAP and required mechanical ventilation (patients requiring intubations for bronchoscopy or open-lung biopsy were excluded). Failure of CPAP to avoid intubation was the only variable that predicted mortality (18).

Outcome may also be affected by the low rate of complications in patients responsive to CPAP. In one study, patients responsive to mask CPAP had a shorter duration of mechanical ventilation (6.9 ± 1.6 vs. 24.8 ± 6.7 days; $p <$ 0.05) and a lower incidence of nosocomial infections (12% vs. 60%) and pneumothoraces (0% vs. 30%) (21). In an additional report, CPAP (10 cm H_2O) via nasal mask was very effective for rapid improvement in gas exchange in PCP with milder forms of hypoxemia (209). CPAP delivered with a facial mask was evaluated in 15 AIDS patients with PCP and ARF (24). Eleven patients had a significant improvement in Pao_2:Fio_2 ($p < 0.001$) and clinical parameters and were discharged alive after a mean ICU stay of 8.5 days. Four patients had no improvement, required intubation, and died after a mean ICU stay of 14 days (24).

NPPV

Two groups have reported the use of NPPV (CPAP + PSV) in patients with AIDS and hypoxemic ARF (27,175,206). In our experience of 12 patients, NPPV improved gas exchange and avoided intubation in 10 (27,175). $Pao_2:Fio_2$ increased from a baseline of 132 ± 71 to 222 ± 116 at 1 hour and 285 ± 80 at 2–6 hours. One of three patients failing to improve refused intubation and died. Overall, ICU survival was 67% (8 of 12), and hospital survival was 58%. Duration of NPPV was longer (39 ± 28 h) than in other conditions causing hypoxemic ARF but still safe (only two facial skin necrosis) and well tolerated. Rabbat et al. (205) reported on 18 patients, 5 of whom failed and required ETI (4 patients died).

Conclusion

Mask CPAP and NPPV are highly effective in AIDS patients with PCP and ARF. In patients failing to improve, however, mortality rate is high. Only two (22,175) of five studies have reported any survivors among intubated patients. It is important to recognize that NPPV is highly effective in ameliorating dyspnea even when it fails to improve gas exchange. The role of NPPV in patients with AIDS and respiratory failure should be evaluated prospectively, taking into consideration cost factors and impact on short- and long-term outcome.

G. Severe Community-Acquired Pneumonia

Severe community-acquired pneumonia requiring admission to an ICU is a distinct clinical entity from non–ICU managed pneumonia in terms of clinical presentation, therapeutic intervention, and mortality (207). Mortality of community-acquired pneumonia requiring ICU admission ranges from 22 to 54%. Nearly 58–87% of patients with severe community-acquired pneumonia develop respiratory failure and require mechanical ventilation. In several studies need for conventional ventilatory support was associated with a higher mortality, particularly in the ones requiring PEEP and high Fio_2 (≥ 0.6) (207). A few studies have reported the use of mask CPAP or NPPV in patients with pneumonia and respiratory failure. The effect of CPAP in removing secretions is discussed later under atelectasis. Mask CPAP or NPPV do not impair coughing.

Mask CPAP

In 1936 Bullowa described in his textbook on the management of pneumonia the use of face mask positive airway pressure with oxygen to treat patients with pneumonia (208). Barach et al. (5,7) in 1938 and 1942 reported rapid improvements in respiratory function after applying mask CPAP in patients with life-threatening pneumonia. In 1981 Suter and Kobel (10) described intermittent application of CPAP (5–10 cm H_2O) by face mask in 19 patients with pneumonia and ARF. Mean duration of treatment was 4.5 ± 1.4 days, and intubation was avoided in nine (47%) patients. In the Suter and Kobel experience, patients with thick bronchial secretions had a high rate of failure (66%). Successful application of CPAP in nine patients with pneumonia and ARDS was reported by Covelli et al. (11). Brett and Sinclair (209) reported continuous application of CPAP (10 cm H_2O) by face mask in three patients with severe CAP. CPAP treatment was well tolerated and associated with rapid improvement in gas exchange and clinical signs. Following 12–18 hours of treatment, two patients went on to full recovery, whereas one patients developed ARDS and was intubated; all survived (209). Mask CPAP was found useful in improving gas exchange in patients with pneumonia and ARF admitted to an emergency room (26). Successful applications of mask CPAP have also been described in case reports of severe varicella and influenza pneumonia (210,211).

NPPV

In the literature, the response to NPPV in patients with pneumonia is not uniform (33,35,42,52,169,175). Among 30 patients with ARF receiving NPPV by nasal mask, Benhamou et al. (35) found no difference in response (60% success) in patients with or without pneumonia as the cause of ARF. A similar, but smaller, experience was reported by Pennock et al. (33). In our experience of 41 patients with severe CAP with (27 patients) or without COPD (14 patients), NPPV improved gas exchange in more than 75% and avoided intubation in 62% (175). Only three patients required intubation for an inability to clear secretions. Actual mortality (17%) was lower than predicted (36%). Confalonieri et al. (212) and Pollack et al. (115) reported a high (60–90%) success rate in treating 20 patients with pneumonia and ARF with nasal BiPAP®. Contrary to these results, one group has consistently reported a high (90%) failure rate in patients (12) with pneumonia and ARF (36,169). The reasons for this higher failure rate are not clear.

Confalonieri et al. (140) recently completed a multicenter, prospective, randomized trial to compare the efficacy of NPPV delivered through a face mask with the efficacy of standard medical treatment with supplemental oxygen administration in patients with severe community-acquired pneumonia and acute respiratory failure. Fifty-six consecutive patients (28 in each arm) were enrolled, and the two groups were similar at study entry. The use of NPPV was well tolerated, safe, and associated with a significant reduction in respiratory rate, need for endotracheal intubation (21% vs. 50%; $p = 0.03$), and duration of ICU stay (1.8 ± 0.7 days vs. 6 ± 1.8 days; $p = 0.04$). The two groups had a similar intensity of nursing care workload, time interval from study entry to endotracheal intubation, duration of hospitalization, and hospital mortality. Among patients with COPD, those randomized to NPPV had a lower intensity of nursing care workload ($p = 0.04$) and improved 2-month survival (88.9% vs. 37.5%; $p = 0.05$).

Conclusion

Pneumonia as a cause of ARF is not by itself a contraindication to implementing mask CPAP or NPPV if the patient is capable of expectorating secretions effectively. A recent randomized study supports its application in patients with COPD complicated by pneumonia.

H. NPPV-Assisted Bronchoscopy

The most frequent indication for fiberoptic bronchoscopy (FOB) in an immunosuppressed host is the need to determine the cause of diffuse infiltrates that often occur in association with fever and the new onset of respiratory symptoms (61). Pulmonary disease in the immunosuppressed patient can progress rapidly and has a high associated mortality, often exceeding 50%. Early and accurate diagnosis simplifies management and may improve outcome. In nonintubated patients, severe hypoxemia (defined as requiring continuous positive airway pressure [CPAP] or an inspired oxygen concentration greater than 50% to maintain an arterial oxygen tension of at least 75 mmHg) is an accepted contraindication to bronchoscopy. Since the arterial oxygen tension routinely decreases by 10–20 mmHg after uncomplicated bronchoscopy, these patients are at high risk for developing respiratory failure or serious cardiac arrhythmias. In these high-risk patients, the caring physician has two options: intubate with mechanical ventilation to ensure adequate gas exchange during FOB or avoid FOB and institute empirical treatment.

We recently reported on a new technique to perform FOB with BAL in severely hypoxemic, nonintubated patients utilizing NPPV administered through a facial mask (61). We reported on eight consecutive immunosuppressed patients with suspected pneumonia and a $Pao_2:Fio_2 \leq 100$. After routine application of topical anesthesia to the nasopharynx, a full-face mask was connected to a ventilator set to deliver PEEP (4 cm H_2O), PSV (17 cm H_2O), and 1.0 Fio_2. The mask was secured to the patient with head straps. NPPV began 10 minutes before starting FOB and continued for ≥ 90 minutes after the procedure was completed. The bronchoscope was passed through a T-adapter and advanced through the nose. BAL was obtained by sequential instillation and aspiration of 5–25 cc aliquots of sterile saline through a bronchoscope wedged in a radiographically involved subsegment. Oxygen saturation, heart rate, respiratory rate, and arterial blood gases were monitored during the study. NPPV significantly improved Pao_2: Fio_2 and O_2 saturation. FOB with NPPV was well tolerated, and no patient required endotracheal intubation. A causative pathogen was identified by BAL in all patients. Six patients responded to treatment and survived hospital admission. Two patients died 5–7 days after FOB from unrelated complications of the underlying illness. Our group's experience at La Sapienza University now exceeds 60 episodes of NPPV-assisted FOB.

I. Atelectasis

Atelectasis is a commonly encountered problem following upper abdominal and thoracic surgery and in patients with neuromuscular diseases. Reduction in FRC and retention of secretions are important risk factors. Incentive spirometry as well as cough and deep breathing therapy are frequently applied but require an alert, cooperative, and motivated patient. In spontaneously breathing patients, intermittent application of mask CPAP has been investigated for both prevention and treatment of atelectasis.

Physiological Response to Mask Positive Pressure

In excised human lungs, experimentally collapsed lung regions can be recruited by CPAP through collateral channels with pressures less than or equal to those needed for reinflation through the ordinary bronchial route (106). Collateral reinflation also has a potential secretion clearing effect; that is, the pressure behind the obstruction rises, forcing secretions centrally to larger bronchi where they are more easily removed (106).

Clinical Application of Mask Positive Pressure

Stock et al. (84) demonstrated that postoperative patients receiving intermittent CPAP (7.5 cm H_2O) by face mask had a more rapid recovery in FRC and a lower incidence of atelectasis than did those receiving incentive spirometry or a cough and deep breathing regimen. A nonsignificant reduction in postoperative atelectasis was reported by Knodel et al. (217).

CPAP has also been used for treating established atelectasis (10,11,16, 139,213,214). In experimental work, CPAP is more effective in reexpanding collapsed lung than deep breathing and mechanical ventilation with or without PEEP (106). On the basis of these experimental data, a prospective randomized study evaluated hourly application of CPAP (median 15 cm H_2O) y face mask (25–35 consecutive breaths) in patients with postoperative atelectasis (139). CPAP was superior to standard treatment in improving radiographic and physiological manifestations of atelectasis, implying that collateral ventilation is an important "therapeutic tool" that can be used in patients with atelectasis (139). Duncan et al. (214) described the successful application of nasal CPAP (10–15 cm H_2O)in treating refractory atelectasis. Covelli et al. (11) reported five patients with postoperative atelectasis and hypoxemia who were treated with continuous CPAP (10 cm H_2O) by face mask. Gas exchange improved in all, and three had significant radiographic clearance. In patients with postoperative atelectasis and hypoxemic respiratory failure, mask CPAP was highly effective in improving gas exchange and avoiding intubation (10,16).

The above data support applying mask CPAP to hasten resolution of postoperative atelectasis. A study comparing the efficacy of mask CPAP versus NPPV would be useful.

J. Pediatric Hypoxemic Respiratory Failure

The principles and pathophysiology of noninvasive ventilation in pediatric respiratory failure are the subject of two recent comprehensive reviews (215,216).

Mask CPAP

Gregory et al. first applied CPAP in 20 infants with idiopathic respiratory distress syndrome, in two of them via a pressure chamber around the infant's head (217). Successful application of CPAP via a short nasal cannula was reported by Beasley (218) in infants with bronchiolitis and CO_2 retention.

NPPV

NPPV has been described in pediatric patients with hypoxemic ARF (219–221). Fortenberry et al. (221) treated 28 children (mean age 8 years) with acute respiratory distress and ARF with continuous nasal NPPV (BiPAP®). Significant improvements in Pao_2:Fio_2 (from 141 ± 54 mmHg to 280 ± 146 mmHg; $p < 0.001$) and respiratory rate (from 45 ± 18 to 33 ± 11; $p = 0.002$) were observed within 1 hour of treatment. The median duration of NPPV was 72 hours. Only three children required intubation. Nasal skin necrosis was reported in three patients. Akingbola et al. (220) reported nine patients (14 ± 6 years) with hypoxemic ARF who were treated with facial NPPV (BiPAP®). Gas exchange markedly improved within 1 hour of treatment (Pao_2:Fio_2 from 97 ± 45 mmHg to 289 ± 137 mmHg; $p = 0.03$), and none required intubation. Recently, Padman et al. (222) evaluated the efficacy of bilevel positive airway pressure support in 34 critically ill children (mean age 11 ± 0.9) with respiratory failure of varied origin. NPPV was associated with a reduction in dyspnea score, heart rate ($p < 0.001$), respiratory rate ($p < 0.04$), bicarbonate concentration ($p < 0.01$) and an increase in O_2 saturation (from $85 \pm 2\%$ to $97 \pm 1\%$) (222). Successful NPPV application has also been reported in pediatric patients with primarily neuromuscular ventilatory impairment (223). The use of a face mask applied with a head harness in premature infants has been linked to intracerebral hemorrhage (224), although this finding has subsequently been disputed (225,226).

Conclusion

Noninvasive positive pressure techniques show great promise in pediatric patients of all age groups with a variety of causes of respiratory failure including hypercapnic and hypoxemic types. Unfortunately, the lack of controlled trials precludes the provision of firm recommendations.

IV. Patients with Advanced Disease

Death from respiratory failure is the common endpoint of many diseases. In cases of end-stage pulmonary disease (e.g., severe chronic obstructive lung disease, pulmonary fibrosis, lung cancer), lung function will eventually deteriorate to a point where mechanical support may only prolong the inevitable. Often, however, respiratory failure is due to a reversible condition (e.g., congestive heart failure, bronchospasm, pneumonia) that can be corrected if the patient is supported with mechanical ventilation during treatment of an acute event. Patients with advanced disease who develop respiratory failure are often reluctant to undergo endotracheal intubation and mechanical ventilation even when respiratory failure is acute, potentially reversible, and not a direct manifestation of the disease. They have an understandable fear of spending their final days attached to a machine that deprives them of autonomy and the ability to communicate with others. Not surprisingly, many patients who have been previously intubated often refuse to repeat this experience. For these patients, NIV is the only ventilatory option.

NPPV

Seven reports have described applying NPPV in patients with ARF who are poor candidates for endotracheal intubation for a variety of reasons: advanced age or poor physiological condition ($n = 42$) (35,42), patients with advanced disease ($n = 80$) (1,43,64,65,175), and those with advanced directives (do not resuscitate status, $n = 8$) (227). The overall success rate was 63%, i.e., of these patients with advanced disease, 92 of 146 would likely have died had they not been placed on noninvasive ventilation. Successfully treated patients had rapid improvement in gas exchange (1,42). Even when respiratory failure did not resolve, NPPV was effective in providing symptomatic relief of dyspnea (1). NPPV was well tolerated, more comfortable than ETI (as reported by patients with prior intubation), allowed patients to maintain autonomy and verbal communication, and facilitated withdrawal of life support when ARF did not improve (1). Among successfully treated patients, many survived for years with good a quality life after hospital discharge (175).

Conti et al. (64) evaluated NPPV delivered via a nasal mask utilizing Bi-PAP® ventilator (Respironics, USA) in 16 consecutive patients with hematological malignancies and ARF (64). Fifteen of 16 individuals had an early and sustained improvement in gas exchange, the $Pao_2:FIo_2$ after 1 hour of treatment increased from 87 ± 22 to 175 ± 64 and continued to improve in the following 24 hours ($p < 0.01$). One patient failed to improve, was intubated, and later died from sepsis. One additional patient became intolerant of NPPV, was intubated, and later died from sepsis. Three additional patients died from complications unrelated to respiratory failure. Eleven patients were discharged in stable condition after a mean ICU stay of 4.3 ± 2.4 days (64).

NPPV has also been described for patients with terminal respiratory failure (228). This modality was well tolerated and prolonged life a few extra days, thus allowing life closure tasks to be completed. An editorial accompanied this publication warning of the potential ethical and economic cost of delaying the inevitable in patients with terminal respiratory failure (228). The authors estimated that if only 10% of patients dying with lung cancer and COPD each year used NPPV for only 2 days, the added cost would exceed $300 million per year (229).

Conclusion

Although indiscriminate use of NPPV in patients with advanced disease is not justifiable, individual needs should be carefully taken into consideration by the caring physician. We frequently implement NPPV in those patients who appear to have a reversible cause of respiratory failure, and we have found this approach to be dignified and comfortable for the patient. In the immunocompromised host or those with severe thrombocytopenia, NPPV may avoid potential serious (infectious and hemorrhagic) complications of intubation.

V. Postextubation Respiratory Failure and Difficult Weaning

Nonintubation techniques may prove advantageous during weaning from respiratory support. This topic is covered in more detail in Chapter 17. The benefits of CPAP and IPPV can be maintained after loss of direct access to the airway (following extubation), allowing staged withdrawal of respiratory support while laryngeal function returns (130). Two studies have shown that in patients with postextubation ARF, a face mask is as effective as an endotracheal tube for delivering positive pressure and correcting gas exchange abnormality (30,230).

A. Clinical Application of Mask Ventilation

Seven studies (30,36,37,169,173a,230,232) have reported applying NPPV in 90 patients with postextubation respiratory failure resulting from either respiratory muscle fatigue, reversible upper airway obstruction, or severe hypoxemia. The overall success rate in avoiding reintubation was 79%. None of the patients developed nosocomial pneumonia, which occurs with increased frequency in reintubated patients (233). In one study, three patients had (partial) upper airway obstruction and were supported with NPPV for a mean of 18 hours while receiving treatment with racemic epinephrine and systemic corticosteroids (175).

Recent reports indicate that NPPV may also have a role for patients who are difficult to wean (234–236). Udwadia et al. (237) used NPPV as a weaning modality in difficult-to-extubate patients. Criteria for instituting NPPV consisted of intact bulbar function with preserved cough reflex, minimal airway secretions, hemodynamic stability, functioning gastrointestinal tract, low Fio$_2$, and ability to breath spontaneously for 10–15 minute. Twenty-two patients with prolonged respiratory failure (median 31 days, range 2–219) who failed at least one attempt at extubation were switched to NPPV via nasal mask after extubation. In the patients with a tracheostomy, the cuff was deflated and the tube occluded. If NPPV was well tolerated, decannulation was performed within 36 hours. Transfer to NPPV was unsuccessful in only two patients, both of whom had pulmonary fibrosis. Of the 20 patients tolerating NPPV, only two required reintubation. The remaining patients were discharged home after a median of 11 days (range 8–13). Ten (60%) required continuous domiciliary nocturnal noninvasive ventilation.

A similar study by Restick et al. (234) described 14 patients (10 with endotracheal tube, 4 with tracheostomies) who were weaned by nasal NPPV once they were stable on a synchronous intermittent mandatory ventilation (SIMV) rate of <5 breaths/min or pressure support of 10 cm H$_2$O. Median duration on mechanical ventilation was 14 days. Weaning was successful in 13 patients (success rate 87%), and all left the hospital. Weaning was achieved in all patients with COPD ($n = 8$). Three patients with chest wall disease later required home noninvasive ventilatory support.

Laier-Groeneveld et al. (236) transferred 26 patients (15 chest wall disorders and 11 COPD) to a customized nasal mask when they could not be weaned after 68 ± 42 days of invasive ventilation. Twenty-one patients had a tracheostomy in place. Twenty-two patients were discharged home on intermittent NPPV and two on IPPV via tracheostomy. In another study, Scherzer and Apprusezze (234) reported on six intubated patients successfully transferred to NPPV with nasal BiPAP®.

Recently, Nava et al. (238) conducted a multicenter randomized study evaluating the efficacy of NPPV in accelerating weaning from MV in 50 patients with COPD and ARF intubated for less than 48 hours and failing a T-piece trial. Patients with pneumonia were excluded. Compared to patients who remained intubated, those randomized to NPPV had a higher weaning success rate at day 15 (88% vs. 70%), lower duration of ICU stay (15.1 $\pm$ 5.4 days vs. 24 $\pm$ 13 days; $p = 0.005$), lower rate of pneumonia (0 vs. 7; $p < 0.05$), and improved survival at 60 days (92% vs. 72%; $p < 0.01$).

B. Conclusion

The use of NPPV in patients with postextubation ARF is justified, particularly if the condition precipitating ARF has improved or resolved. NPPV as a modality to accelerate weaning in COPD patients appears promising, and its application in other forms of ARF is being investigated. Additional studies are needed to assess the role of NPPV for early extubation of patients with prolonged respiratory failure who fail conventional weaning.

VI. Conclusions

We have presented a systematic review of the literature of noninvasive mechanical ventilation in patients without COPD and acute respiratory failure. Noninvasive ventilation with either mask CPAP or NPPV was frequently found to be a safe and effective means of recruiting alveoli and augmenting ventilation in patients with acute respiratory failure of varied etiology. Patient selection and familiarity with the technique are essential to avoid complications. Although most patients improve with noninvasive ventilation, the response to treatment and duration of mechanical ventilation cannot be clearly predicted by the severity of the underlying lung disease or by the arterial blood gas values obtained before initiating mechanical ventilation. Mortality from acute respiratory failure is decreased when endotracheal intubation is avoided. Noninvasive ventilation, however, is not uniformly successful. Therefore, patients with ARF placed on noninvasive ventilation should be closely monitored to avoid dangerous delays if intubation becomes necessary.

Acknowledgment

The author wishes to recognize the assistance of Gail Spake for editorial revision of this manuscript.

References

1. Meduri GU, Mauldin GL, Wunderink RG, Leeper KV, Jones C, Tolley E. Causes of fever and pulmonary densities in patients with clinical manifestations of ventilator-associated pneumonia. Chest 1994; 106:221–235.
2. Hill NS. Noninvasive ventilation. Does it work, for whom, and how? Am Rev Respir Dis 1993; 147:1050–1055.
3. Barach AL. The use of helium in the treatment of asthma and obstructive lesions in the larynx and trachea. Ann Intern Med 1935; 9:739–765.
4. Barach AL. Recent advantages in inhalation therapy in the treatment of cardiac and respiratory disease: principles and methods. NY J Med 1937; 37:1095–1110.

5. Barach AL, Martin J, Eckman M. Positive pressure respiration and its application to the treatment of acute pulmonary edema. Ann Intern Med 1938; 12:754–795.

6. Barach AL, Swenson P. Effect of breathing gases under positive pressure on lumens of small and medium sized bronchi. Arch Intern Med 1939; 63:946–948.

7. Barach AL. Physiologically directed therapy in pneumonia. Ann Intern Med 1942; 17:812–819.

8. Greenbaum DM, Miller JE, Eross B, Snyder JV, Grenvik A, Safar P. Continuous positive airway pressure without tracheal intubation in spontaneously breathing patients. Chest 1976; 69:615–620.

9. Smith RA, Kirby RR, Gooding JM, Civetta JM. Continuous positive airway pressure (CPAP) by face mask. Crit Care Med 1980; 8:483–485.

10. Suter PM, Kobel N. Treatment of acute pulmonary failure by CPAP via face mask: When can intubation be avoided? Klin Wochenschr 1981; 59:613–616.

11. Covelli HD, Weled BJ, Beekman JF. Efficacy of continuous positive airway pressure administered by face mask. Chest 1982; 81:147–150.

12. Linton DM, Potgieter PD. Conservative management of blunt chest trauma. S Afr Med J 1982; 61:917–919.

13. Rasanen J, Heikkila J, Downs J, Nikki P, Vaisanen I, Viitanen A. Continuous positive airway pressure by face mask in acute cardiogenic pulmonary edema. Am J Cardiol 1985; 55:296–300.

14. Hurst JM, DeHaven CB, Branson RD. Use of CPAP mask as the sole mode of ventilatory support in trauma patients with mild to moderate respiratory insufficiency. J Trauma 1985; 25(11):1065–1068.

15. DeHaven CB, Hurst JM, Branson RD. Postextubation hypoxemia treated with a continuous positive airway pressure mask. Crit Care Med 1985; 13:46–48.

16. Branson RD, Hurst JM, DeHaven CB. Mask CPAP: State of the art. Respir Care 1985; 30:846–857.

17. Vaisanen IT, Rasanen J. Continuous positive airway pressure and supplemental oxygen in the treatment of cardiogenic pulmonary edema. Chest 1987; 92:481–485.

18. Gregg RW, Friedman BC, Williams JF, McGrath BJ, Zimmerman JE. Continuous positive airway pressure by face mask in *Pneumocystis carinii* pneumonia. Crit Care Med 1990; 18:21–24.

19. Miller RF, Semple SJ. Continuous positive airway pressure ventilation for respiratory failure associated with *Pneumocystis carinii* pneumonia. Respir Med 1991; 85:133–138.

20. Bersten AD, Holt AW, Vedic AE, Skowronski GA, Baggoley CJ. Treatment of severe cardiogenic pulmonary edema with continuous positive airway pressure delivered by face mask. N Engl J Med 1991; 325:1825–1830.

21. Gachot B, Clair B, Wolff M, Regnier B, Vachon F. Continuous positive airway pressure by face mask or mechanical ventilation in patients with human immunodeficiency virus infection and severe *Pneumocystis carinii* pneumonia. Intens Care Med 1992; 18:155–159.

22. DeVita MA, Friedman V, Petrella V. Mask continuous positive airway pressure in AIDS. Crit Care Clin 1993; 9:137–151.

23. Lenique F, Habis M, Lofaso F, Touchard D, Saal JP, Dubois-Randé JL, Gueret P, Brochard L, Harf A. Ventilatory and hemodynamic effects of continuous positive airway pressure (CPAP) in congestive heart failure (CHF). Am J Respir Crit Care Med 1994; 149:A644.

24. Lin M, Yang Y, Chiany H, Chang M, Chiany BN, Chitlin MD. Reappraisal of continuous positive airway pressure therapy in acute cardiogenic pulmonary edema: short-term results and long-term follow-up. Chest 1995; 107:1379–1386.

25. Boix JH, Miguel V, Aznar O, Alvarez F, Tejeda M, Gonzalez E, Monferrer J, Kuret E. [Airway continuous positive pressure in acute respiratory failure caused by *Pneumocystis carinii* pneumonia (see comments)]. Rev Clin Esp 1995; 195:69–73.

25a. Takeda S, Takano T, Ogawa R. The effect of nasal continuous positive airway pressure on plasma endothelin-1 concentrations in patients with severe cardiogenic pulmonary edema. Anesth Analg 1997; 84:1091–1096.

26. L'HerE, Moriconi M, Texier F, Bouquin V, Kaba L, Renault A, Garo B, Boles JM. Non-invasive continuous positive airway pressure in acute hypoxaemic respiratory failure—experience of an emergency department. Eur J Emerg Med 1998; 5:313–318.

27. Meduri GU, Conoscenti CC, Menashe P, Nair S. Noninvasive face mask ventilation in patients with acute respiratory failure. Chest 1989; 95:865–870.

28. Brochard L, Isabey D, Piquet J, Amaro P, Mancebo J, Messadi AA, Brun-Buisson C, Rauss A, Lemaire F, Harf A. Reversal of acute exacerbations of chronic obstructive lung disease by inspiratory assistance with a face mask. N Engl J Med 1990; 323:1523–1530.

29. Elliott MW, Steven MH, Phillips GD, Branthwaite MA. Non-invasive mechanical ventilation for acute respiratory failure. Br Med 1990; 300:358–360.

30. Meduri GU, Abou-Shala N, Fox RC, Jones CB, Leeper KV, Wunderink RG. Noninvasive face mask mechanical ventilation in patients with acute hypercapnic respiratory failure. Chest 1991; 100:445–454.

31. Marino W. Intermittent volume cycled mechanical ventilation via nasal mask in patients with respiratory failure due to COPD. Chest 1991; 99:681–684.

32. Chevrolet JC, Jolliet P, Abajo B, Toussi A, Louis M. Nasal positive pressure ventilation in patients with acute respiratory failure. Difficult and time-consuming procedure for nurses. Chest 1991; 100:775–782.

33. Pennock BE, Kaplan PD, Carlin BW, Sabangan JS, Magovern JA. Pressure support ventilation with a simplified ventilatory support system administered with a nasal mask in patients with respiratory failure. Chest 1991; 100:1371–1376.

34. Hodson ME, Madden BP, Steven MH, Tsang VT, Yacoub MH. Non-invasive mechanical ventilation for cystic fibrosis patients—a potential bridge to transplantation. Eur Resp J 1991; 4:524–527.

35. Benhamou D, Girault C, Faure C, Portier F, Muir JF. Nasal mask ventilation in acute respiratory failure. Experience in elderly patients. Chest 1992; 102:912–917.

36. Wysocki M, Tric L, Wolff MA, Gertner J, Millet H, Herman B. Noninvasive pressure support ventilation in patients with acute respiratory failure. Chest 1993; 103:907–913.

37. Vitacca M, Rubini F, Foglio K, Scalvini S, Nava S, Ambrosino N. Non-invasive

modalities of positive pressure ventilation improve the outcome of acute exacerbations in COLD patients. Intens Care Med 1993; 19:450–455.

38. Fernandez R, Blanch LI, Valles J, Baigorri F, Artigas A. Pressure support ventilation via face mask in acute respiratory failure in hypercapnic COPD patients. Intens Care Med 1993; 19:456–461.

39. Bott J, Carroll MP, Conway JH, Keilty SEK, Ward EM, Brown AM, Paul EA, Elliott MW, Godfrey RC, Wedzicha JA, Moxham J. Randomized controlled trial of nasal ventilation in acute ventilatory failure due to chronic obstructive airways disease. Lancet 1993; 341:1555–1558.

40. Pennock BE, Crawshaw L, Kaplan PD. Noninvasive nasal mask ventilation for acute respiratory failure. Chest 1994; 105:441–444.

41. Meduri GU, Fox RC, Abou-Shala N, Leeper KV, Wunderink RG. Noninvasive mechanical ventilation via face mask in patients with acute respiratory failure who refused endotracheal intubation. Crit Care Med 1994; 22:1584–1590.

42. Soo Hoo GW, Santiago S, Williams AJ. Nasal mechanical ventilation for hypercapnic respiratory failure in chronic obstructive pulmonary disease: determinants of success and failure. Crit Care Med 1994; 22:1253–1261.

43. Tognet E, Mercatello A, Polo P, Coronel B, Bret M, Archimbaud E, Moskovtchenko JF. Treatment of acute respiratory failure with non-invasive intermittent positive pressure ventilation in hematological patients. Clin Intens Care 1994; 5: 282–288.

44. Confalonieri M, Aiolfi S, Gandola L, Scartabellati A, Della Porta R, Parigi P. Severe exacerbations of chronic obstructive pulmonary disease treated with BiPAP by nasal mask. Respiration 1994; 61:310–316.

45. Wysocki M, Girard T, Chevret S, Wolff MA, Millet H, Herman B. Noninvasive ventilation in acute exacerbation of COPD: Which patients have high probability of failure? Intens Care Med 1995; 21:S48.

46. Kramer N, Meyer TJ, Meharg J, Cece RD, Hill NS. Randomized, prospective trial of noninvasive positive pressure ventilation in acute respiratory failure. Am J Respir Crit Care Med 1995; 151:1799–1806.

47. Sacchetti AD, Harris RH, Paston C, Hernandez Z. Bi-level positive airway pressure support system use in acute congestive heart failure: preliminary case series. Acad Emerg Med 1995; 2:714–718.

48. Brochard L, Mancebo J, Wysocki M, Lofaso F, Conti G, Rauss A, Simonneau G, Benito S, Gasparetto A, Lemaire F, Isabey D, Harf A. Noninvasive ventilation for acute exacerbations of chronic obstructive pulmonary disease. N Engl J Med 1995; 333:817–822.

49. Ambrosino N, Foglio K, Rubini F, Clini E, Nava S, Vitacca M. Non-invasive mechanical ventilation in acute respiratory failure due to chronic obstructive pulmonary disease: correlates for success. Thorax 1995; 50:755–757.

50. Meduri GU, Cook TR, Turner RE, Cohen M, Leeper KV. Noninvasive positive pressure ventilation in status asthmaticus. Chest 1996; 110:767–774.

51. Patrick W, Webster K, Ludwig L, Roberts D, Wiebe P, Younes M. Noninvasive positive-pressure ventilation in acute respiratory distress without prior chronic respiratory failure. Am J Respir Crit Care Med 1996; 153:1005–1011.

52. Pollack CV, Jr., Torres MT, Alexander L. Feasibility study of the use of bilevel

positive airway pressure for respiratory support in the emergency department. Ann Emerg Med 1996; 27:189–192.

53. Vitacca M, Clini E, Rubini F, Nava S, Foglio K, Ambrosino N. Non-invasive mechanical ventilation in severe chronic obstructive lung disease and acute respiratory failure: short- and long-term prognosis. Intens Care Med 1996; 22:94–100.

54. Antonelli M, Conti G, Riccioni L, Meduri GU. Noninvasive positive-pressure ventilation via face mask during bronchoscopy with BAL in high-risk hypoxemic patients. Chest 1996; 110:724–728.

55. Confalonieri M, Parigi P, Scartabellati A, Aiolfi S, Scorsetti S, Nava S, Gandola L. Noninvasive mechanical ventilation improves the immediate and long-term outcome of COPD patients with acute respiratory failure. Eur Respir J 1996; 9:422–430.

56. Barbe F, Togores B, Rubi M, Pons S, Maimo A, Agusti AG. Noninvasive ventilatory support does not facilitate recovery from acute respiratory failure in chronic obstructive pulmonary disease. Eur Respir J 1996; 9:1240–1245.

57. Hilbert G, Gruson D, Portel L, Gbikpi-Benissan G, Cardinaud JP. Noninvasive pressure support ventilation in COPD patients with postextubation hypercapnic respiratory insufficiency. Eur Respir J 1998; 11:1349–1353.

58. Hilbert G, Gruson D, Gbikpi-Benissan G, Cardinaud JP. Sequential use of noninvasive pressure support ventilation for acute exacerbations of COPD. Intens Care Med 1997; 23:955–961.

59. Corbetta L, Ballerin L, Putinati S, Potena A. Efficacy of noninvasive positive pressure ventilation by facial and nasal mask in hypercapnic acute respiratory failure: experience in a respiratory ward under usual care. Monaldi Arch Chest Dis 1997; 52:421–428.

60. Aguilo R, Togores B, Pons S, Rubi M, Barbe F, Agusti AG. Noninvasive ventilatory support after lung resectional surgery. Chest 1997; 112:117–121.

61. Antonelli M, Conti G, Rocco M, Bufi M, De Blasi RA, Vivino G, Gasparetto A, Meduri GU. A comparison of noninvasive positive-pressure ventilation and conventional mechanical ventilation in patients with acute respiratory failure. N Engl J Med 1998; 339:429–435.

62. Gregoretti C, Beltrame F, Lucangelo U, Burbi L, Conti G, Turello M, Gregori D. Physiologic evaluation of non-invasive pressure support ventilation in trauma patients with acute respiratory failure. Intens Care Med 1998; 24:785–790.

63. Celikel T, Sungur M, Ceyhan B, Karakurt S. Comparison of noninvasive positive pressure ventilation with standard medical therapy in hypercapnic acute respiratory failure. Chest 1998; 114:1636–1642.

64. Conti G, Marino P, Cogliati A, Dell'Utri D, Lappa A, Rosa G, Gasparetto A. Noninvasive ventilation for the treatment of acute respiratory failure in patients with hematologic malignancies: a pilot study. Intens Care Med 1998; 24:1283–1288.

65. Varon F, Fromm RE, Polansky M, Sukumaran AV, Supkis E. Non-invasive mechanical ventilation in cancer patients with acute respiratory failure. Am J Respir Crit Care Med 1996; 153(4):A613.

66. Wood KA, Lewis L, Von Harz B, Kollef MH. The use of noninvasive positive pressure ventilation in the emergency department: results of a randomized clinical trial. Chest 1998; 113:1339–1346.

67. Rocker GM, Mackenzie MG, Williams B, Logan PM. Noninvasive positive pressure ventilation: successful outcome in patients with acute lung injury/ARDS. Chest 1999; 115:173–177.

68. Rusterholtz T, Kempf J, Berton C, Gayol S, Tournoud C, Zaehringer M, Jaeger A, Sauder P. Noninvasive pressure support ventilation (NIPSV) with face mask in patients with acute cardiogenic pulmonary edema (ACPE). Intens Care Med 1999; 25:21–28.

69. Hoffman B, Goebel G, Jepsen M, Huth C, Welte T. The influence of non-invasive positive pressure ventilation (NIPPV) on cardiac output—first results of a controlled, prospective study. Am J Respir Crit Care Med 1999; 159:A367.

70. Alsous F, Amoanteg-Adjepong Y, Manthous CA. Noninvasive ventilation: experience at a community teaching hospital. Intens Care Med 1999; 25:458–463.

70a. Confalonieri M, Potena A, Carbone G, Porta RD, Tolley EA, Meduri GU. Acute respiratory failure in patients with severe community-acquired pneumonia. A prospective randomized evaluation of noninvasive ventilation. Am J Respir Crit Care Med 1999; 160:1585–1591.

70b. Antonelli M, Conti G, Bufi M, Costa MG, Lappa A, Rocco M, Gasparetto A, Meduri GU. Noninvasive ventilation for treatment of acute respiratory failure in patients undergoing solid organ transplantation: a randomized trial. JAMA 2000; 283:235–241.

71. Roussos C, Macklem PT. The respiratory muscles. N Engl J Med 1982; 307:786–797.

72. Broseghini C, Brandolese R, Poggi R, Polese G, Manzin E, Milic-Emili J, Rossi A. Respiratory mechanics during the first day of mechanical ventilation in patients with pulmonary edema and chronic airway obstruction. Am Rev Respir Dis 1988; 138:355–361.

73. Martin JG, Shore SA, Engel LA. Mechanical load and inspiratory muscle action during induced asthma. Am Rev Respir Dis 1983; 128:455–460.

74. Smith T, Marini J. Impact of PEEP on lung mechanics and work of breathing in severe airflow obstruction. J Appl Physiol 1988; 65:1488–1499.

75. NHLBI WS. Respiratory muscle fatigue—report of the respiratory muscle fatigue workshop group. Am Rev Respir Dis 1990; 142:474–480.

76. Derenne JP, Fleury B, Pariente R. Acute respiratory failure of chronic obstructive pulmonary disease. Am Rev Respir Dis 1988; 138:1006–1033.

77. Pitcher WD, Cunningham HS. Oxygen cost of increasing tidal volume and diaphragmatic flattening in obstructive pulmonary disease. J Appl Physiol 1993; 74:2750–2756.

78. Juan G, Calverey P, Talamo C, Schnader J, Roussos C. Effect of carbon dioxide on diaphragmatic function in human beings. N Engl J Med 1985; 310:874–879.

79. Appendini L, Patessio A, Zanaboni S, Carone M, Gukov B, Donner CF, Rossi A. Physiologic effects of positive end-expiratory pressure and mask pressure support during exacerbations of chronic obstructive pulmonary disease. Am J Respir Crit Care Med 1994; 149:1069–1076.

80. de Lucas P, Taranco'n C, Puente L, Rodriquez C, Tatay E, Monturiol JM. Nasal continuous positive airway pressure in patients with COPD in acute respiratory failure. Chest 1993; 104:1694–1697.

81. Shivaram U, Donath J, Khan FA, Juliano J. Effects of continuous positive airway pressure in acute asthma. Respiration 1987; 52:157–162.
82. Carrey Z, Gottfried SB, Levy RD. Ventilatory muscle support in respiratory failure with nasal positive pressure ventilation. Chest 1990; 97:150–158.
83. Ambrosino N, Nava S, Bertone P, Fracchia C, Rampulla C. Physiologic evaluation of pressure support ventilation by nasal mask in patients with stable COPD. Chest 1992; 101:385–391.
84. Elliott MW, Aquilina R, Green M, Moxham J, Simonds AK. A comparison of different modes of noninvasive ventilatory support: effects on ventilation and inspiratory muscle effort. Anaesthesia 1994; 49:279–283.
85. Corbridge TC, Hall JB. The assessment and management of adults with status asthmaticus. Am J Respir Crit Care Med 1995; 151:1296–1316.
86. Rodriguez-Roisin R, Ballester E, Roca J, al. ae. Mechanisms of hypoxemia in patients with status asthmaticus requiring mechanical ventilation. Am Rev Respir Dis 1989; 139:732–739.
87. Roca J, Ramis L, Rodriquez-Roisin R, et al. Serial relationships between ventilation perfusion inequality and spirometry in acute severe asthma requiring hospitalization. Am Rev Respir Dis 1988; 137:1055–1061.
88. Nowak RM, Tomlanovich MC, Sarker DD, Kvale PA, Anderson JA. Arterial blood gases an pulmonary function testing in acute bronchial asthma: predicting patient outcomes. JAMA 1983; 249:2043–2046.
89. Stalcup S, Mellins RB. Mechanical forces producing pulmonary edema in acute asthma. N Engl J Med 1977; 297:592–596.
90. Jardin F, Dubourg O, Margairaz A, et al. Inspiratory impairment in right ventricular performance during acute asthma. Chest 1987; 92:789–795.
91. Mountain RD, Sahn SA. Clinical features and outcome in patients with acute asthma presenting with hypercapnia. Am Rev Respir Dis 1988; 138:535–539.
92. Finfer SR, Garrard CS. Ventilatory support in asthma. Br J Hosp Med 1993; 49: 357–360.
93. Shnider SM, Papper EM. Anesthesia for the asthmatic patient. Anesthesiology 1961;22:886–889.
94. Tuxen DV. Detrimental effects of positive end-expiratory pressure during controlled mechanical ventilation of patients with severe airflow obstruction. Am Rev Respir Dis 1989; 40:5–9.
95. Zimmerman JL, Dellinger RP, Shah AN, Taylor RW. Endotracheal intubation and mechanical ventilation in severe asthma. Crit Care Med 1993; 21:1727–1730.
96. Darioli R, Perret C. Mechanical controlled hypoventilation in status asthmaticus. Am Rev Respir Dis 1984; 129:385–387.
97. Qvist J, Anderson JB, Pemberton M, Bennike KA. High-level PEEP in severe asthma. N Engl J Med 1982; 307:1347–1348.
98. Tenaillon A, Salmona JP, Burdin M. Continuous positive airway pressure in asthma. Am Rev Respir Dis 1983; 127:658.
99. Mathieu M, Tonneau MC, Zarka D, Sartene R. Effect of positive end-expiratory pressure in severe acute asthma. Crit Care Med 1987; 15:1164.
100. Maltais F, Sovilj M, Goldberg P, Gottfried SB. Respiratory mechanics in status asthmaticus. Chest 1994; 106:1401–1406.

101. Tokioka H, Saito S, Saeki S, Kinjo M, Kosaka F. The effect of pressure support ventilation on auto-PEEP in a patient with asthma. Chest 1992; 101:285–286.

102. Leatherman JW, Fluegel WL, David WS, Davies SF, Iber C. Muscle weakness in mechanically ventilated patients with severe asthma. Am J Respir Crit Care Med 1996; 153:1686–1690.

103. Wilson BA, Jackson PJ, Evans J. Effects of positive end-expiratory breathing on exercise-induced asthma. Int J Sports Med 1981; 2:27–30.

104. Martin JG, Shore S, Engel LA. Effect of continuous positive airway pressure on respiratory mechanics and pattern of breathing in induced asthma. Am Rev Respir Dis 1982; 126:812–817.

105. Horng-Chyuan L, Chun-Hua W, Cheng-Ta Y, Tung-Jung H, chih-Teng Y, Wen-Bin S, Han-Pin K. Effect of nasal continuous positive airway pressure on methacholine-induced bronchoconstriction. Am J Respir Crit Care Med 1995; 151:A398.

106. Anderson JB, Qvist J, Kann T. Recruiting collapsed lung through collateral channels with positive end expiratory pressure. Scand J Respir Dis 1979; 60:260–266.

107. Oertel MJ. Von Ziemssen's Handbook of Therapeutics. In: Yeo JB, ed. Wm. Wood & Co, 1885: 547.

108. Barach AL. The therapeutic use of helium. JAMA 1936; 107:1273.

109. Poulton EP, Oxon DM. Left-sided heart failure with pulmonary edema—its treatment with the "pulmonary plus pressure machine." Lancet 1936; 231:981–983.

110. Shivaram U, Cash ME, Beal A. Nasal continuous positive airway pressure in decompensated hypercapnic respiratory failure as a complication of sleep apnea. Chest 1993; 104:770–774.

111. Mansel JK, Stogner SW, Norman JR. Face-mask CPAP and sodium bicarbonate infusion in acute, severe asthma and metabolic acidosis. Chest 1989; 96:943–944.

112. Chan CS, Woolcock AJ, Sullivan CE. Nocturnal asthma: role of snoring and obstructive sleep apnea. Am Rev Respir Dis 1988; 137:1502–1504.

113. Guilleminault C, Quera-Salva MA, Powell N, Romaker A, Partinen M, Baldwin R. Nocturnal asthma: snoring, small pharynx and nasal CPAP. Eur Respir J 1988; 1:1902–1907.

114. Martin RJ, Pak J. Nasal CPAP in nonapneic nocturnal asthma. Chest 1991; 100: 1024–1027.

115. Pollack CV, Fleisch KB, Dowsey K. Treatment of acute bronchospasm with beta-adrenergic agonist aerosols delivered bys a nasal bilevel positive airway pressure circuit. Ann Emerg Med 1995; 26:552–557.

116. Esclamado RM, Glenn MG, McCulloch TM, Cummings CW. Perioperative complications and risk factors in the surgical treatment of obstructive sleep apnea syndrome. Laryngoscope 1989; 99:1125–1129.

117. Patel SR, Stelmach K, Golish J. BiPAP as salvage in CPAP failures for obstructive sleep apnea. Chest 1993; 104(2):135S.

118. Piper AJ, Sullivan CE. Effects of short-term NIPPV in the treatment of patients with severe obstructive sleep apnea and hypercapnia. Chest 1994; 105:434–440.

119. Pankow W, Hijjeh N, Schuttler F, Penzel T, Becker HF, Peter JH, von Wichert P. Influence of noninvasive positive pressure ventilation on inspiratory muscle activity in obese subjects. Eur Respir J 1997; 10:2847–2852.

120. Swami A, Evans TW, Morgan CJ, Hodson ME, Keogh BF. Conventional ventila-

tion as a bridge to heart-lung transplantation in cystic fibrosis. Eur Respir J 1991; 4:188S.

121. Padman R, Nadkarni VM, Von Nessen S, Goodill J. Noninvasive positive pressure ventilation in end-stage cystic fibrosis: a report of seven cases. Respir Care 1994; 39:736–739.

122. Piper AJ, Parker S, Torzillo PJ, Sullivan CE, Bye PTP. Nocturnal nasal IPPV stabilizes patients with cystic fibrosis and hypercapnic respiratory failure. Chest 1992; 102:846–850.

123. Fauroux B, Boule M, Lofaso F, Zerah F, Clement A, Harf A, Isabey D. Chest physiotherapy in cystic fybrosis: improved tolerance with nasal pressure support ventilation. Pediatrics 1999; 103:E32.

124. Granton JT, Kesten S. The acute effects of nasal positive pressure ventilation in patients with advanced cystic fibrosis. Chest 1998; 113:1013–1018.

125. Gozal D, Costance S, Kaufman. Pediatric ventilatory support in patients with cystic fibrosis: comparison with supplemental oxygen. Eur Respir J 1997; 10:1999–2003.

126. Quaranta AJ, Roy B, O'Brien G, Kreimer DT, Krachman S, Criner GJ. Noninvasive positive pressure ventilation as bridge therapy to lung transplantation or volume reduction surgery. Am J Respir Crit Care Med 1996; 153(4):A608.

127. Ambrosino N, Nava S, Bertone P, Fracchia C, Rampulla C. Noninvasive mechanical ventilation in the treatment of acute respiratory failure due to infectious complications of lung transplantation. Monaldi Arch Chest Dis 1994; 49:311–314.

128. Kilger E, Briegel J, Haller M, Hummel T, Groh J, Dienemann H, Welz A, Forst H. [Noninvasive ventilation after lung transplantation]. Med Klin 1995; 90:26–28.

129. Rubini F, Nava S, Callegari G, Fracchia C, Ambrosino N. [Nasal pressure support ventilation (NPSV) in a case of *Pneumocystis carinii* pneumonia in single-lung transplantation]. Minerva Anestesiol 1994; 60:139–142.

130. Duncan AW, Oh TE, Hillman DR. PEEP and CPAP. Anaesth Intens Care 1986; 14:236–250.

131. Branson RD. PEEP without endotracheal intubation. Respir Care 1988; 33:598–610.

132. Bunnell S. The use of nitrous oxide and oxygen to maintain anesthesia and positive pressure for thoracic surgery. JAMA 1912; 58:835.

133. Bishop B, Hirsch J, Thursby M. Volume, flow, and timing of each breath during positive-pressure breathing in man. J Appl Physiol 1978; 45:495–501.

134. Montner PK, Greene ER, Murata GH, Stark DM, Timms M, Chick TW. Hemodynamic effects of nasal and face mask continuous positive airway pressure. Am J Respir Crit Care Med 1994; 149:1614–1618.

135. Pesenti A, Marcolin R, Prato P, Borelli M, Riboni A, Gattinoni L. Mean airway pressure vs. positive end-expiratory pressure during mechanical ventilation. Crit Care Med 1985; 13:34–37.

136. Marini JJ, Ravenscraft SA. Mean airway pressure: Physiologic determinants and clinical importance—Part 1: physiologic determinants and measurements. Crit Care Med 1992; 20:1461–1472.

137. Jousela I. Endotracheal tube versus face mask with and without continuous positive airway pressure (CPAP). Anaesth Scand 1993; 37:381–385.

138. Takeda S, Takano T, Ogawa R. The effect of nasal continuous positive airway

pressure on plasma endothelin-1 concentrations in patients with severe cardiogenic pulmonary edema. Anesth Analg 1997; 84:1091–1096.

139. Andersen JB, Olesen KP, Eikard B, Jansen E, Qvist J. Periodic continuous positive airway pressure, CPAP, by mask in the treatment of atelectasis. Eur J Respir Dis 1980; 61:20–25.

140. Confalonieri M, Della Porta R, Potena A, Carbone G, Gregoretti C, Gandola L, Tolley EA, Meduri GU. Acute respiratory failure in patients with severe community-acquired pneumonia: a prospective randomized evaluation of noninvasive ventilation. Am J Respir Crit Care Med 1999; 160:1585–1591.

141. Wysocki M, Tric L, Wolff MA, Millet H, Herman B. Noninvasive pressure support ventilation in patients with acute respiratory failure. A randomized comparison with conventional therapy. Chest 1995; 107:761–768.

142. Guerin C, Girard R, Chemorin C, De Varax R, Fournier G. Facial mask noninvasive mechanical ventilation reduces the incidence of nosocomial pneumonia. A prospective epidemiological survey from a single ICU. Intens Care Med 1998; 24:27.

143. Buda AJ, Pinsky MR, Ingles NB, Daughters GT, Stinson EB, Alderman EL. Effect of intrathoracic pressure on left ventricular performance. N Engl J Med 1979; 301: 453–459.

144. Naughton MT, Benard DC, Liu PP, Rutherford R, Rankin F, Bradley TD. Effects of nasal CPAP on sympathetic activity in patients with heart failure and central sleep apnea. Am J Respir Crit Care Med 1995; 152:473–479.

145. McParland C, Krishnan B, Wang Y, Gallagher CG. Inspiratory muscle weakness and dyspnea in chronic heart failure. Am Rev Respir Dis 1992; 146:467–472.

146. Perel A, Williamson DC, Modell JH. Effectiveness of CPAP by mask for pulmonary edema associated with hypercarbia. Intens Care Med 1983; 9:17–19.

147. Miller WF, Sproule BJ. Studies on the role of intermittent inspiratory positive pressure oxygen breathing (IPPB/I-Oz) in the treatment of pulmonary edema. Dis Chest 1959; 5:469–479.

148. Naughton MT, Rahman MA, Hara K, Floras JS, Bradley TD. Effects of continuous positive airway pressure on intrathoracic and left ventricular transmural pressure in congestive heart failure. Circulation 1995; 91:1725–1731.

149. Emerson H. Artificial respiration in the treatment of edema of the lungs. Arch Intern Med 1909; 3:368–371.

150. Pinsky MR, Summer WR. Cardiac augmentation by phasic high intrathoracic pressure support in man. Chest 1983; 84:370–375.

151. Rasanen J, Vaisanen IT, Heikkila J, Nikki P. Acute myocardial infarction complicated by left ventricular dusfunction and respiratory failure—the effects of continuous positive airway pressure. Chest 1985; 87:158–162.

152. Baratz DM, Westbrook PR, Shah PK, Mohsenifar Z. Effect of nasal continuous positive airway pressure on cardiac output and oxygen delivery in patients with congestive heart failure. Chest 1992; 102:1397–1401.

153. Takasaki Y, Orr D, Popkin J, Rutherford R, Liu P, Bradley TD. Effect of nasal continous positive airway pressure on sleep apnea in congestive heart failure. Am Rev Respir Dis 1989; 140:1578–1584.

154. Robotham JL, Peters J, Takata M. Cardiorespiratory interactions. In: Bone RC, ed. Pulmonary and Critical Care Medicine. St. Louis: Mosby, 1995:1.

155. Genovese J, Huberfeld W, Tarasiuk A, Moskowitz M, Scharf SM. Effects of CPAP on cardiac output in pigs with pacing-induced congestive heart failure. Am J Respir Crit Care Med 1995; 152:1847–1853.

156. Werko L. The influence of positive pressure breathing on the circulation in man. Acta M Scan 1947; 193:1–125.

157. Bradley TD, Holloway RM, McLaughlin PR, Ross BL, Walters J, Lui PP. Cardiac output response to continuous positive airway pressure on congestive heart failure. Am Rev Respir Dis 1992; 145:377–382.

158. Thong H, Cuadra O, DiBenedetto RJ. Noninvasive positive ventilation and cardiac output in heart failure. Chest 1995; 108:S108.

159. De Hoyos A, Liu PP, Benard DC, Bradley TD. Haemodynamic effects of continuous positive airway pressure in humans with normal and impaired left ventricular function. Clin Sci 1994; 87.

160. Lenique F, Habis M, Lofaso F, Dubois-Rande JL, Harf A, Brochard L. Ventilatory and hemodynamic effects of continuous positive airway pressure in left heart failure. Am J Respir Crit Care Med 1997; 155:500–505.

161. Liston R, Deegan PC, McCreery C, Costello R, Maurer B, McNicholas WT. Haemodynamic effects of nasal continuous positive airway pressure in severe congestive heart failure. Eur Resp J 1995; 8:430–435.

162. Seals DR, Suwarno O, Dempsey JA. Influence of lung volume on sympathetic nerve activity in normal humans. Circ Res 1990; 67:130–141.

163. Pery N, Payen D, Pinsky MR. Monitoring the effect of CPAP on left ventricular function using continuous mixed-blood saturation. Chest 1991; 99:512–513.

164. Hoff BH, Flemming DC, Sasse F. Use of positive airway pressure without endotracheal intubation. Crit Care Med 1979; 7:559–562.

165. Huff JS, Whelan TV. CPAP as adjunctive treatment of severe pulmonary edema in patients with ESRD. Am J Emerg Med 1994; 12:388.

166. Feinberg AN, Shabino CL. Acute pulmonary edema complicating tonsillectomony and adenoidectomy. Pediatrics 1985; 75:112–114.

167. Holt AW, Bersten AD, Fuller S, Piper RK, Worthley LKG, Vedig AE. Intensive care costing methodology: cost benefit analysis of mask continuous positive airway pressure for severe cardiogenic pulmonary edema. Anaesth Intens Care 1994; 22:170–174.

168. Granton JT, Naughton MT, Benard DC, Liu PP, Goldstein RS, Bradley TD. CPAP improves inspiratory muscle strength in patients with heart failure and central sleep apnea. Am J Respir Crit Care Med 1996; 153:277–282.

169. Wysocki M, Tric L, Mazeyrac C, Wolff M, Gertner J, Millet H, Herman B. Non invasive pressure support ventilation (NIPSV) in acute respiratory failure (ARF). Am Rev Respir Dis 1992; 145:A527.

170. Rusterholtz T, Kempf J, Berton C, Gayol S, Kopferschmitt J, Jaeger A, Sauder P. Efficacy of facial mask pressure support ventilation (FMPSV) during acute cardiogenic pulmonary edema: a descriptive study. Am J Respir Crit Care Med 1995; 151:A422.

171. Ward WL, Pennock BE, Kaplan PD, Crawshaw LM, Lucid EJ. BIPAP ventilatory support in the emergency room (ER) as an adjunct to therapy for acute left ventricular failure. Am J Respir Crit Care Med 1995; 151:A426.

172. Bollaert PE, Weber M, Lucchelli JP, Boes P, Nace L, Maire B, Aussedat M, Larcan A. Non invasive pressure support ventilation (NIPSV) for acute cardiogenic pulmonary edema: a case control study. Am J Respir Crit Care Med 1996; 153(4):A609.

173. Hoffmann BS, Welte T. Experiences with non-invasive bilevel positive airways pressure (NI-BIPAP) ventilation for acute respiratory failure. Am J Respir Crit Care Med 1996; 153(4):A613.

173a. Mehta S, Jay GD, Woolard RH, Hipona RA, Connolly EM, Cimini DM, Drinkwine JH, Hill NS. Randomized, prospective trial of bilevel versus continuous positive airway pressure in acute pulmonary edema. Crit Care Med 1997; 25:620–628.

174. Hoffmann B, Welte T. The use of noninvasive pressure support ventilation for severe respiratory insufficiency due to pulmonary oedema [see comments]. Intens Care Med 1999; 25:15–20.

175. Meduri GU, Turner RE, Abou-Shala N, Tolley E, Wunderink RG. Noninvasive positive pressure ventilation via face mask: first-line intervention in patients with acute hypercapnic and hypoxemic respiratory failure. Chest 1996; 109:179–193.

176. Lapinsky SE, Mount DB, Mackey D, Grossman RF. Management of acute respiratory failure due to pulmonary edema with nasal positive pressure support. Chest 1994; 105:229–231.

177. Mehta S, Jay G, Woolard RH, Hipona RA, Connolly EM, Cimini DM, Drinkwine JH, Hill, NS. Randomized, prospective trial of bilevel versus continuous positive airway pressure in acute pulmonary edema. Crit Care Med 1997, 25:620.

178. Sen N, Dhanraj P. Use of facemask continuous positive airway pressure (CPAP) in patients with refractory hypoxaemia caused by burn sepsis. Burns 1994; 20(3): 271–272.

179. Naver L, Walter S, Glowinski J. Pulmonary fat embolism treated by intermittent continuous positive airway pressure given by face mask. Br Med J 1980:1413–1414.

180. Rabitsch W, Staudinger T, Brugger SA, Reiter E, Keil F, Herold C, Lechner K, Greinix HT, Kalhs P. Successful management of adult respiratory distress syndrome (ARDS) after high-dose chemotherapy and peripheral blood progenitor cell rescue by non-invasive ventilatory support. Bone Marrow Transplant 1998; 21: 1067–1069.

181. Marin D, Gonzalez-Barca E, Domingo E, Berlanga J, Granena A. Noninvasive mechanical ventilation in a patient with respiratory failure after hematopoietic progenitor transplantation. Bone Marrow Transplant 1998; 22:1123–1124.

182. Craig DB. Postoperative recovery of pulmonary function. Anesth Analg 1981; 60: 46–52.

183. Linder KH, Lotz P, Ahnefeld FW. Continuous positive airway pressure effect on functional residual capacity, vital capacity and its subdivisions. Chest 1987; 92: 66–70.

184. Stock MC, Downs JB, Guaer PK, Alster JM, Imrey PB. Prevention of postoperative pulmonary complications with CPAP, incentive spirometry, and conservative therapy. Chest 1985; 87:151–157.

185. Richsten SE, Bengtsson A, Soderberg C, Thorden M, Kvist H. Effects of periodic positive airway pressure by mask on postoperative pulmonary function. Chest 1986; 89:774–781.

186. Carlsson C, Sonden B, Thylen U. Can postoperative continuous positive airway pressure (CPAP) prevent pulmonary complications after abdominal surgery? Intens Care Med 1981; 7:225–229.

187. Matte P, Jacquet L, Goenen M. CPAP effects on pulmonary function tests after CABG. Intens Care Med 1995; 21:S44.

188. Paul WL, Downs JB. Postoperative atelectasis—intermittent positive pressure breathing, incentive spirometry, and face-mark positive end-expiratory pressure. Arch Surg 1981; 116:861–863.

189. Thomas AN, Ryan JP, Doran BRH, Pollard BJ. Nasal CPAP after coronary artery surgery. Anaesthesia 1992; 47:316–319.

190. Pinilla J, Oleniuk FH, Tan L, Rebeyka I, Tanna N, Wilkinson A, Bharadway B. Use of a nasal continuous positive airway pressure mask in the treatment of post-operative atelectasis in aortocoronary bypass surgery. Crit Care Med 1990; 18:836.

191. Stock MC, Downs JB, Corkran ML. Pulmonary function before and after prolonged continuous positive airway pressure by mask. Crit Care Med 1984; 12:973–974.

192. Boothby WM, Mayo Cw, Lovelace WR, II. The use of oxygen and oxygen-helium, with special reference to surgery. Surg Clin North Am 1940; 20:1107–1168.

193. Ingwersen UM, Larsen KR, Bertelsen MT, Kiil-Nielsen K, Laub M, Sandermann J, Back K, Hansen H. Three different mask physiotherapy regimens for prevention of post-operative pulmonary complications after heart and pulmonary surgery. Intens Care Med 1993; 19:294–298.

194. Day S, Griffis M, Macintyre NR, Hidinger C, Robbins P, Whitfield S. Routine nasal mask pressure support ventilation in recently extubated postoperative patients. Respir Care 1992; 37(11):1310.

195. Karg O, Bullemer F, Thetter O. [Perioperative use of noninvasive ventilation]. Med Klin 1996; 91 (suppl 2):38–40.

196. Varon J, Walsh GL, Fromm RE, Jr. Feasibility of noninvasive mechanical ventilation in the treatment of acute respiratory failure in postoperative cancer patients. J Crit Care 1998; 13:55–57.

197. Gust R, Gottschalk A, Schmidt H, Bottiger BW, Bohrer H, Martin E. Effects of continuous (CPAP) and bi-level positive airway pressure (BiPAP) on extravascular lung water after extubation of the trachea in patients following coronary artery bypass grafting. Intens Care Med 1996; 22:1345–1350.

198. Brewer LA, III, Samson PC, Burbank B, Schiff C. The wet lung in war casualties. Ann Surg 1946; 123:343–361.

199. Buford TH, Burbank B. Traumatic wet lung. Observations on certain physiologic fundamentals of thoracic trauma. J Thorac Surg 1945; 14:415–424.

200. Klopfenstein CE, Foster A, Suter PM. Pneumocephalus. A complication of CPAP after trauma. Chest 1980; 78:656–657.

201. Meduri GU, Stein DS. Pulmonary manifestations of acquired immunodeficiency syndrome. Clin Infect Dis 1992; 14:98–113.

202. Wachter RM, Luce JM, Safrin S, Berrios DC, Charlebois E, Scitovsky AA. Cost and outcome of intensive care for patients with AIDS, *Pneumocystis carinii* pneumonia, and severe respiratory failure. JAMA 1995; 273:230–235.

203. Friedman Y, Franklin C, Rackow EC, Weil MH. Improved survival in patients

with AIDS, *Pneumocystis carinii* pneumonia, and severe respiratory failure. Chest 1989; 96:862–866.

204. Miller WC, Mason JW. Nasal CPAP for severe hypoxia. Chest 1990; 98:1542–1543.

205. Kesten S, Rebuck AS. Nasal continuous positive airway pressure in pneumocystis carinii pneumonia. Lancet 1988:1414–1415.

206. Rabbat A, Leleu G, Bekka F, Leroy F, Schlemmer B, Laaban JP, Le Gall JR, Rochemaure J. Non invasive ventilation in HIV patients with severe *Pneumocystis carinii* pneumonia. Am J Respir Crit Care Med 1995; 151:427.

207. Leeper KV, Torres A. Community-acquired pneumonia in the intensive care unit. Clin Chest Med 1995; 16:155–172.

208. Bullowa JGH. The management of pneumonias. New York: Oxford University Press, 1936:192–195.

209. Brett A, Sinclair DG. Use of continuous positive airway pressure in the management of community acquired pneumonia. Thorax 1993; 48:1280–1281.

210. Sadovnikoff N, Varon J. CPAP mask management of varicella-induced respiratory failure. Chest 1993; 103:1894–1895.

211. Taylor GJ, Brenner W, Summer WR. Severe viral pneumonia in young adults—therapy with continuous positive airway pressure. Chest 1976; 69:722–728.

212. Confalonieri M, Aiolfi S, Scartabellati A, Parigi P, Patrini G, Ghio L, Gandola L. Use of noninvasive positive pressure ventilation in severe community acquired pneumonia. Am J Respir Crit Care Med 1995; 151:A424.

213. Knodel AR, Covelli HD, O'Reilly M. The role of mask CPAP in preventing post-operative atelectasis. Am Rev Respir Dis 1984; 126:A110.

214. Duncan SR, Negrin RS, Mihn FG, Guilleminault C, Raffin TA. Nasal continuous positive airway pressure in atelectasis. Chest 1987; 92:621–624.

215. Teague WG, Fortenberry JD. Noninvasive ventilatory support in pediatric respiratory failure. Respir Care 1995; 40:86–96.

216. Birnkrant DJ, Pope JF, Eiben RM. Management of the respiratory complications of neuromuscular diseases in the pediatric intensive care unit. J Child Neurol 1999; 14:139–143.

217. Gregory GA, Kitterman JA, Phibbs RH, Tooley WH, Hamilton WK. Treatment of the idiopathic respiratory distress syndrome with continuous positive airway pressure. N Engl J Med 1971; 284:1332–1340.

218. Beasley JM, Jones SEF. CPAP in bronchiolitis. Br Med J 1980; 282:1506–1508.

219. Fortenberry JD, Del Toro J, Evey L, Haase D, Jefferson LS. Nasal mask bi-level positive ventilation (BiPAP) in children with mild to moderate hypoxemic respiratory failure. Chest 1993; 104:133S.

220. Akingbola Q, Palmisano J, Servant G, Custer J, Moler F. Bi-PAP mask ventilation in pediatric patients with acute respiratory failure. Crit Care Med 1994; 22:A144.

221. Fortenberry JD, Del Toro J, Jefferson LS, Evey L, Haase D. Management of pediatric acute hypoxemic respiratory insufficiency with bilevel positive pressure (BI-PAP) nasal mask ventilation. Chest 1995; 108:1059–1064.

222. Padman R, Lawless ST, Kettrick RG. Noninvasive ventilation via bilevel positive airway pressure support in pediatric practice. Crit Care Med 1998; 26:169–173.

223. Niranjan V, Bach JR. Noninvasive management of pediatric neuromuscular ventilatory failure [see comments]. Crit Care Med 1998; 26:2061–2065.

224. Pape KE, Armstrong DL, Fitzhardinge PM. Central nervous system pathology associated with mask ventilation in the very low birthweight infant: a new etiology for intracerebellar hemorrhages. Pediatrics 1976; 58:473–483.

225. Shuman RM, Oliver TK. Face masks defended. Pediatrics 1976; 58:621–623.

226. Tuck S, Ment LR. A follow-up study of very low-birthweight infants receiving ventilatory support. Devel Med Child Neurol 1980; 22:633–641.

227. Averill FJ, Adkins G. Use of bilevel positive airway pressure (BIPAP) in patients with acute respiratory failure. Chest 1993; 104:143S.

228. Freichels TA. Palliative ventilatory support: use of noninvasive positive pressure ventilation in terminal respiratory insufficiency. Am J Crit Care 1994; 3:5–9.

229. Clarke DE, Vaughan L, Raffin TA. Noninvasive positive pressure ventilation for patients with terminal respiratory failure: the ethical and economic costs of delaying the inevitable are too great. Am J Crit Care 1994; 3:4–5.

230. Gregoretti C, Burbi L, Berardino M, Biolino P, Giagiaro PM, Della Valle A, Turello M. Non invasive mask ventilation (NIMV) in trauma and major burn patients. Am Rev Respir Dis 1992; 145:A75.

231. Chiang AA, Lee KC. Use of nasal mask BiPAP in patients with respiratory distress after extubation. Chest 1993; 104(2):135S.

232. Maldonado OA, Cevallos S, Elizalde J, Franco J, Martinez SJ. Unplanned extubation (UE): Is there a role for mechanical ventilation? Chest 1995; 108:186S.

233. Torres A, Gatell JM, Aznar E, El-Ebiary M, De La Bellacasa JP, Gonzalez J, Ferrer M, Rodriguez-Roisin R. Re-intubation increases the risk of nosocomial pneumonia in patients needing mechanical ventilation. Am J Respir Crit Care Med 1995; 152: 137–141.

234. Scherzer HH, Apprusezze N. Bi-level, nasal positive pressure ventilation for acute respiratory failure. Chest 1993; 104(2):135S.

235. Restrick LJ, Scott AD, Ward EM, Feneck RO, Cornwell WE, Wedzicha JA. Nasal intermittent positive-pressure ventilation in weaning intubated patients with chronic respiratory disease from assisted intermittent, positive-pressure ventilation. Respir Med 1993; 87:199–204.

236. Laier-Groeneveld G, Kupfer J, Hüttemann U, Criée C-P. Weaning from invasive mechanical ventilation. Am Rev Respir Dis 1992; 145:A518.

237. Udwadia ZF, Santis GK, Steven MH, Simonds AK. Nasal ventilation to facilitate weaning in patients with chronic respiratory insufficiency. Thorax 1992; 47:715–718.

238. Nava S, Ambrosino N, Clini E, Prato M, Orlando A, Vitacca M, Brigada P, Fracchia C, Rubini F. Non-invasive mechanical ventilation in the weaning of patients with respiratory failure due to chronic obstructive pulmonary disease. Ann Intern Med 1998; 128:721–728.

15

Strategies for Predicting Successful Weaning from Mechanical Ventilation

G. R. SCOTT BUDINGER and MARTIN J. TOBIN

Loyola University of Chicago Stritch School of Medicine
Maywood
and Hines Veterans Administration Hospital
Hines, Illinois

I. Introduction

While often life-saving, mechanical ventilation is an invasive, costly therapy with well-documented complications (1–3). Accordingly, the intensive care physician wishes to wean patients from mechanical ventilation and extubate them at the earliest possible point in their course. Unfortunately, the gestalt derived during clinical examination has limited accuracy in identifying patients who are likely to tolerate weaning (4). Several physiological tests, so-called weaning predictors, have been developed with the goal of improving clinical prediction. A growing body of evidence suggests that the use of these predictors can shorten the duration of mechanical ventilation and prevent the development of complications during weaning, such as respiratory muscle fatigue.

This chapter will first review the role of weaning predictors in clinical practice followed by our current understanding of the causes of weaning failure and reintubation. The methodology used in the evaluation of weaning predictors and their predictive power will then be discussed. Controversial topics and areas of active investigation will be highlighted throughout the chapter.

II. Why Obtain Weaning Predictors?

A major challenge in the management of the ventilator-supported patient is identifying the point in time at which a patient is ready to be weaned. The decision to commence weaning is usually made on clinical grounds. Stroetz and Hubmayr, however, showed that clinical judgment alone had positive and negative predictive values for weaning success of only 50 and 67%, respectively (4). Accordingly, although clinical examination remains a necessary component of patient assessment, it is not sufficient in deciding the time to discontinue ventilator support.

Substantial evidence suggests that physicians are more likely to procrastinate in weaning than to carry it out prematurely. Two large prospective series of mechanically ventilated patients found that 75% of medical patients could be extubated following their first trial of spontaneous breathing (5,6). When compared with physician-directed weaning, respiratory therapy–driven protocols have been shown to decrease the duration of mechanical ventilation and costs and to improve the rate of successful weaning (7,8).

Ely et al. (9) investigated whether the systematic use of objective predictors of weaning outcome might be superior to clinical judgment in reducing the duration of mechanical ventilation. They randomized 300 patients to receive either standard management or daily objective measurements by nurses and respiratory therapists. Eligibility for weaning was determined by (1) the ratio of the arterial partial pressure of oxygen to the inspired oxygen concentration (Pao_2/Fio_2) > 200 mmHg, (2) positive end-expiratory pressure (PEEP) ≤ 5 cm H_2O, (3) no infusions of vasopressor agents or sedatives, (4) cough with suctioning, and (5) a frequency-to-tidal volume ratio (f/V_T) < 105 breaths/mm/L. Patients in the intervention arm who satisfied these criteria underwent a 2-hour spontaneous-breathing trial without obtaining permission from the attending physician. If the patient tolerated this trial without developing respiratory distress, the attending physician was notified of its outcome. Patients in the control group were managed according to their physicians' customary manner. The median duration of mechanical ventilation was 4.5 days in the intervention group compared with 6 days in the control group ($p < 0.001$), despite higher severity of illness scores in the intervention group.

Weaning predictors may also be helpful in the avoidance of weaning complications. For example, patients who fail a weaning trial are at risk for the development of respiratory muscle fatigue, and the associated muscle injury could prolong the duration of mechanical ventilation (see below). The detection of incipient fatigue through the use of diaphragmatic twitch pressure generation, electromyography, or phonomyography (10) might be helpful in foreshortening spontaneous breathing trials that will ultimately be unsuccessful. None of these diagnostic modalities, however, has been evaluated satisfactorily in patients undergoing weaning trials.

III. Pathophysiology of Weaning Failure

Recent studies have improved our understanding of the pathophysiology of weaning failure, and this knowledge provides an important background for the evaluation of weaning predictors. Weaning refers to the process of discontinuing mechanical ventilation (11). At the point when patients are able to sustain spontaneous ventilation without distress, they can be extubated unless there is a concern about their ability to protect their upper airway. Despite being able to sustain spontaneous ventilation, 10–20% of patients require reintubation (5,6,12). Clinical problems related to reintubation will be discussed separately from the pathophysiology of weaning failure.

In recent prospective studies, Jubran and Tobin (13,14) investigated the pathophysiology of weaning failure. During failed weaning trials, patients developed rapid shallow breathing, a progressive worsening of lung mechanics, and a substantial increase in the respiratory muscle load as measured by the pressure-time product. These findings were confirmed by Vassilakopoulos et al. in a subsequent study (15). The methodology employed by these two groups of investigators was not sufficient to conclusively determine whether, or not, patients developed respiratory muscle fatigue. In both studies, however, circumstantial evidence suggested that the level of respiratory work was sufficient to cause fatigue in some patients by the end of the trial (Fig. 1).

Given the magnitude of the respiratory muscle load in patients who fail a weaning trial, the respiratory controller might be expected to decrease its output in an attempt to circumvent contractile muscle fatigue while accepting decreased ventilation and hypercapnia. This strategy, known as the central wisdom hypothesis, is theoretically attractive (16–18), but available evidence suggests it rarely occurs in patients who fail a weaning trial (19–24). Indeed, patients who fail weaning trials display normal or supranormal respiratory drive, as assessed by airway occlusion pressure ($P_{0.1}$)(25–34) and mean inspiratory flow rate (V_T/T_I) (35). Moreover, Jubran and Tobin demonstrated increased respiratory muscle power generation at the end of unsuccessful weaning trials (14), suggesting that respiratory controller output had not decreased. This observation was confirmed by Vassilakopoulos et al. (15). Respiratory center depression may be responsible for hypercapnia in some patients; Jubran and Tobin noted that 2 of the 17 patients who failed a weaning trial developed severe hypercapnia, while

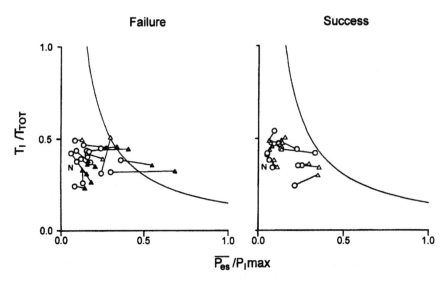

Figure 1 The relationship between mean esophageal pressure/maximum inspiratory pressure ratio and duty cycle (T_I/T_{TOT}) in 17 ventilator-supported patients with COPD who failed a weaning trial and 14 patients who tolerated the trial. The isopleth corresponds to a tension-time index of 0.15. Circles and triangles represent values at the start and end of the trial, respectively; closed symbols represent patients whose P_aco_2 increased during the trial. Of the 17 patients in the failure group, 5 developed a tension-time index of >0.15 (indicated by the isopleth), suggesting respiratory muscle fatigue. (From Ref. 14.)

their pulmonary mechanics were similar to those in patients who were successfully weaned (14).

The above data suggest that weaning failure may be associated with impending or actual respiratory muscle fatigue. Extensive evidence from animals and humans indicates that fatigue has prolonged and serious consequences (17,18). Skeletal muscle fatigue appears to result from increased generation of reactive oxygen species. Reactive oxygen species are capable of inducing nonspecific lipid peroxidation, oxidizing cellular proteins, and disrupting sarcomeres (36–40). Indeed, studies in animals reveal that breathing to fatigue through an inspiratory load results in histological evidence of diaphragmatic myocyte injury. (Fig. 2) (37). Diaphragmatic fatigue results in prolonged (>24 hour) significant decrements in diaphragmatic force generation, as assessed by diaphragmatic twitch pressures (Fig. 3) (17). If fatigue actually develops in patients who fail a weaning trial, the associated structural injury is likely to prolong the duration of mechanical ventilation.

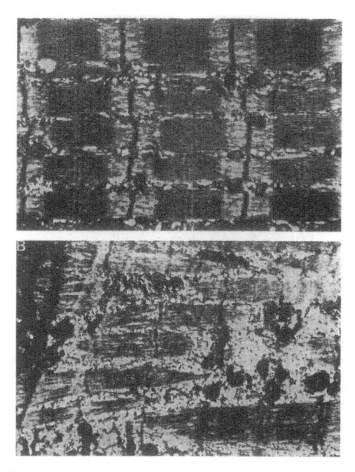

Figure 2 Electron micrograph of a diaphragm in a control hamster (top) and a hamster that had breathed through a resistive load for 6 days (bottom). Loading was achieved by tightening a polyvinyl band around the trachea until swings in esophageal pressure were about 20% of maximal pressure; pulmonary resistance was increased 6.5-fold. Compared with the normal structure, the loaded animal developed sarcomeric disruption with loss of distinct A and I bands and the development of Z line streaming. (From Ref. 37.)

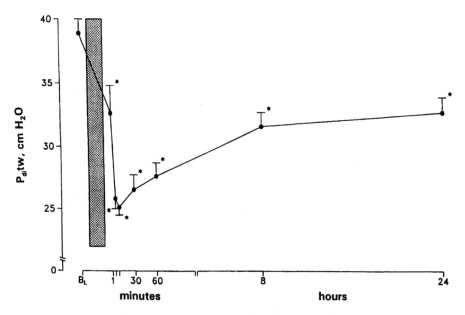

Figure 3 Induction of diaphragmatic fatigue (stippled bar) produced a significant fall in transdiaphragmatic pressure (Pdi) elicited by twitch stimulation of both phrenic nerves. Significant recovery of transdiaphragmatic twitch pressure was noted in the first 8 hours following completion of the fatigue protocol, but no further change was observed between 8 and 24 hours; the 24-hour value was significantly lower than baseline. The delay in reaching the nadir of twitch transdiaphragmatic pressure probably resulted from twitch potentiation, induced by repeated contractions, which was present at the termination of the protocol. Values are mean $\pm$ SE* significant difference compared with baseline value, $p < 0.01$. (From Ref. 17.)

IV. Reintubation

About 10–20% of successfully weaned patients require reintubation within 48 hours of extubation (5,6,12,41,42). Reintubated patients have a much higher mortality (30–40%) than successfully extubated patients (3–5%) (12,43). Studies have not been conducted to define the pathophysiology in patients who require reintubation. To date, investigations have simply defined the clinical characteristics of patients requiring reintubation and evaluated the likelihood that markers might be able to identify which patients will need reintubation.

In a cohort of 72 patients requiring reintubation, Epstein and Ciubarto recorded the patient characteristics and reasons for reintubation (44). They found that a bedside diagnosis of recurrent respiratory failure was the most common reason for reintubation. Other common reasons included clinical diagnoses of retained secretions, laryngeal edema, congestive heart failure, and encephalopathy. In patients reintubated for laryngeal edema or "aspiration or excess secretions," the mortality was significantly less (11–18%) than that in patients reintubated for other causes (36–53%) (Table 1).

The clinical course of 526 ventilator-supported patients was prospectively evaluated by Esteban et al. (12) during the first 48 hours after extubation. Reintubation was required in 13.5% of patients, and it was associated with a higher mortality (32.8%) than in that of patients who tolerated extubation (4.6%). The reasons for reintubation were similar to those reported by Epstein and Ciubarto (44) (Table 1). Weaning predictors were measured before the spontaneous breathing trial, and serial measurements of oxygen saturation, respiratory rate, heart rate, and systolic blood pressure were made during the spontaneous breathing trial. Disappointingly, none of these measurements distinguished patients who were successfully extubated from those requiring reintubation (12).

Patients who require reintubation have higher severity of illness scores, are older, and have a longer duration of mechanical ventilation than successfully extubated patients (12,44). It is not clear whether reintubation per se contributes to mortality or is simply a marker of disease severity. Sorting out this "chicken or egg" situation is important because identification of patients at risk for reintubation will result in improved outcomes only if the act of reintubation and the subsequent period of mechanical ventilation are the cause of the increased mortality. Epstein and Ciubarto found that reintubation was associated with ventilator-associated pneumonia, arrhythmias, atelectasis, myocardial infarction, and cerebrovascular accidents. This observation led them to speculate that these complications, which are associated with reintubation, were responsible for the excess mortality. In that study, however, the mortality rate in patients reintubated

Table 1 Conditions Necessitating Reintubation Within 48 Hours of Extubation in Patients in Medical Intensive Care Units

Cause	% of Patients	
	(n = 72)[a]	(n = 61)[b]
Upper airway obstruction	15	15
Excess secretions	16	28
Respiratory failure	28	19
Congestive heart failure	23	7
Encephalopathy	9	18
Other	9	13

[a] From Ref. 44.
[b] From Ref. 12.

for airway causes was similar to that of successfully extubated patients (44). That the act of reintubation per se is unlikely to explain the excess mortality seen in reintubated patients is further suggested by the observation of Schwartz et al. that only two deaths occurred in 230 consecutive intubations performed in an emergent setting for reasons other than cardiopulmonary arrest (45).

V. General Principles in the Evaluation of Weaning Predictors

Weaning predictors are used to minimize the duration of mechanical ventilation by identifying patients who are able to resume spontaneous breathing; they can also prevent cardiorespiratory distress by identifying patients in whom a trial of weaning is likely to fail (46). To evaluate the usefulness of weaning predictors, it is useful to review the methodology involved in their development. Of particular value are the standards developed by Wasson et al. for the design of research studies that evaluate predictors of clinical outcomes (Table 2) (47).

1. The outcome variable of interest needs to be clearly defined. In the case of weaning predictors, the outcome variable is either weaning outcome or extubation. For example, in a prospective study Yang and Tobin demonstrated that measurement of the f/V_T ratio predicted which patients could tolerate a trial of spontaneous breathing. In patients who tolerate a spontaneous breathing trial, however, the f/V_T ratio does not reliably discriminate between patients who tolerate extubation and those who need reintubation (12,48).
2. When investigators assess the accuracy of a previously described weaning predictor, the methodology of the original report should be precisely followed. For example, Yang and Tobin measured the f/V_T

Table 2 Methodological Standards for Evaluating Clinical Predictors

1. The outcome measure is clearly defined.
2. The methodology of the predictive finding is clearly defined.
3. The study site and population are clearly defined, and predictive power is reported both as sensitivity and specificity and positive and negative predictive values.
4. The misclassification rate is prospectively tested in a population separate from the one in which it was initially determined, and appropriate statistical tests are employed to determine the predictive power of the test.
5. The test is sufficiently simple or useful to justify its use in clinical practice.
6. Data dredging is avoided.

Source: Ref. 47.

ratio using a hand-held spirometer connected to an endotracheal tube while the patient was disconnected from the ventilator (46). In a subsequent study, Lee et al. showed that the f/V_T ratio had poor predictive power when measured during pressure support ventilation, probably because pressure support ventilation is known to increase the tidal volume and decrease the respiratory frequency (49).

3. The study site and population need to be clearly defined, and the predictive power of the weaning predictor should be reported both as sensitivity and specificity and positive and negative predictive values. The pretest probability of weaning success has a profound impact on the predictive value of a weaning predictor. This point is illustrated by the difference between the sensitivity and specificity of a weaning predictor and its positive and negative predictive value. The sensitivity and specificity of a weaning predictor are relatively independent of the prevalence of weaning failure in the population studied provided the sample is sufficiently large to include adequate numbers of patients in each outcome group. In contrast, the positive and negative predictive values of a weaning predictor depend heavily on the pretest probability of weaning failure. When a weaning predictor is studied in a population with a very low rate of weaning failure, such as postoperative patients, the small number of true negatives will lower the negative predictive value of the test. The basis of this modulation is a necessary consequence of Bayes' theorem (50).

4. Appropriate statistical tests should be employed in evaluating weaning predictors. In general, threshold values for weaning predictors should be obtained from the post hoc analysis of prospectively collected data in a population of patients undergoing weaning trials. These threshold values should then be evaluated prospectively in another group of patients. Weaning predictors are almost always less accurate in the prospectively tested population than in the population from which the threshold values were determined. Hence, failure to test the predictor in a separate population will likely overestimate its accuracy. The strength of the association between the predictor and weaning outcome can be evaluated statistically using receiver operating characteristic (ROC) curves (51–54). ROC curves are plots of the false-positive rate against the true-positive rate at different threshold values. The accuracy of the test in predicting weaning outcome is quantified by the area under the ROC curve (Fig. 4). These curves have the advantage of assessing the overall accuracy of a predictor independently of the threshold value. Moreover, the ROC curve can be used to select the optimal threshold value. Such statistical tests should only be employed if the sample size includes at least five patients for each index under

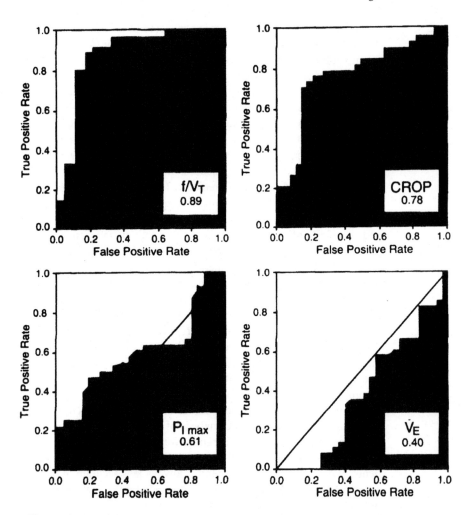

Figure 4   Receiving operator characteristic (ROC) curves for the f/V_T ratio, CROP index, maximal inspiratory pressure (P_{Imax}) and minute ventilation (VE) in 36 patients who were successfully weaned and 28 patients who failed a weaning trial. The ROC curve is generated by plotting the proportion of true-positive results against the proportion of false-positive results for each value of a test. The curve for an arbitrary test that is expected a priori to have no discriminatory value appears as a diagonal line, while a useful test has an ROC curve that rises rapidly and reaches a plateau. The area under the curve (shaded) is expressed (in boxes) as a proportion of the total area. (From Ref. 46.)

evaluation. Accordingly, it is necessary to include very large numbers of patients when evaluating predictors in populations with a very low or very high rate of weaning failure.

5. The logistics involved in the measurement of any weaning predictor should be considered. Predictors that require invasive measurements or complex calculations are unlikely to gain acceptance in clinical practice unless their accuracy is exceptional. For this reason, measurements such as the tension-time index or pressure-time product are unlikely to be useful weaning predictors unless their performance is markedly superior to simple measurements.

6. As in the case of all investigations, it is important to identify an a priori research question before conducting the study. Dredging through data collected for a question other than the one currently addressed is likely to result in considerable observer bias.

VI. Specific Weaning Predictors

A. Frequency-to-Tidal Volume Ratio

Tobin et al. described a pattern of rapid shallow breathing after disconnection of mechanical ventilation in patients who went on to fail weaning trials (Fig. 5). In a subsequent study, Yang and Tobin (46) prospectively measured eight traditional weaning predictors and two new indices in 100 patients undergoing weaning trials. The new indices were the f/V_T ratio and the CROP index—the latter is an integrative index that includes dynamic compliance, respiratory rate, the ratio of arterial to alveolar oxygen tension (P_aO_2/P_AO_2), and the maximal inspiratory pressure. The threshold value with the lowest misclassification rate was determined for all 10 predictors in a training set of 36 patients and subsequently tested in a validation set of 64 patients. The area under the ROC curve was highest for the f/V_T ratio (threshold $\leq$ 105) followed by the tidal volume, CROP index, and respiratory frequency. The maximal inspiratory pressure (P_{Imax}), minute ventilation, static and dynamic compliance, and the P_aO_2/P_AO_2 ratio had areas under the ROC curve that were not significantly greater than that of an arbitrary test that is expected a priori to have no discriminating value (Table 3).

In the study by Yang and Tobin, the f/V_T ratio was measured by attaching a hand-held spirometer to the endotracheal tube while the patient was disconnected from the ventilator (46). Several studies have reported poor predictive power of the f/V_T ratio when it is measured during pressure support ventilation (4,49,55). This is not surprising since pressure support ventilation is known to increase tidal volume and decrease respiratory frequency (56). The predictive power of the f/V_T ratio in patients receiving continuous positive airway pressure from the ventilator has not been rigorously examined.

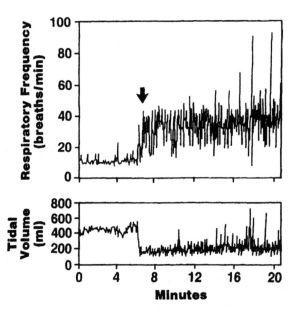

Figure 5 Rapid shallow breathing. Time-series, breath-by-breath plot of respiratory frequency and tidal volume in a patient who failed a weaning trial. Each vertical line represents the volume of a single breath. The arrow indicates the point of resumption of spontaneous breathing after discontinuation of ventilatory support. (From Ref. 35.)

Table 3 Accuracy of Weaning Predictors

Index	Threshold	Positive predictive value	Negative predictive value
Minute ventilation	≤15	0.55	0.38
Respiratory frequency	≤38	0.65	0.77
Tidal volume	≥325	0.73	0.94
Tidal volume/patient weight	≥4	0.67	0.85
Maximal inspiratory pressure	≤−15	0.59	1.00
Dynamic compliance	≥22	0.65	0.58
Static compliance	≥33	0.60	0.53
P_aO_2/P_AO_2 ratio	≥0.35	0.59	0.53
Frequency/tidal volume	≤105	0.78	0.95
CROP index	≥13	0.71	0.70

Source: Modified from Ref. 46.

The predictive power of the f/V_T ratio has been confirmed in a number of studies (14,15,33,48,57–60). Some investigators have found patient characteristics that influence the interpretation of the f/V_T ratio in specific populations. In 100 medical patients with cardiac disease who were being weaned from mechanical ventilation, Chatila et al. measured the f/V_T ratio in the first minute of a spontaneous breathing trial and after another 30–60 minutes (57). The predictive power of the f/V_T ratio, assessed again as the area under the ROC curve, was superior when it was measured after 30–60 minutes of spontaneous breathing than during the first minute. The area under the ROC curve at 30–60 minutes was remarkably similar to that reported by Yang and Tobin (46). In 14 patients, Jubran et al. reported that the value of the f/V_T ratio was 20% higher in the first minute of a spontaneous breathing trial than after 3–6 minutes of spontaneous breathing, and the latter value was similar to that at 30 minutes (61). These data suggest that 3 or more minutes should probably elapse following disconnection from the ventilator before measuring the f/V_T ratio.

In 218 medical patients, Epstein et al. determined the accuracy of the f/V_T ratio for determination of extubation outcome. The negative predictive value of an f/V_T ratio ≥ 100 was lower in women and in patients with small endotracheal tubes (≤ 7.0 mm) (62).

In a prospective study of 49 patients undergoing a weaning trial, Krieger et al. assessed the predictive power of the f/V_T ratio in patients more than 70 years old. They concluded the optimal threshold for the f/V_T ratio may need to be set at a higher level in these patients (59,60). Their results, however, should be interpreted with caution because the investigators did not determine the optimal threshold value in a training set of patients before it was prospectively tested.

In patients who had already tolerated a weaning trial, Epstein found that the positive predictive value of the f/V_T ratio in predicting the need for reintubation was 0.83 but the negative predictive value was only 0.40 (48). The positive predictive value in Epstein's study was similar to that reported by Yang and Tobin (0.78), but the negative predictive value was substantially higher in the latter report (0.95) (48). This difference between these two studies highlights the importance of defining the outcome variable when interpreting studies of weaning predictors. The f/V_T ratio performs better when used according to its original purpose: the identification of the earliest time for the discontinuation of mechanical ventilation. In patients who have already tolerated a trial of spontaneous breathing, the f/V_T ratio does not discriminate between patients who successfully sustain spontaneous ventilation following extubation and patients who require reintubation. Based on this observation, some commentators conclude that the measurement of the f/V_T ratio does not help in predicting the need for reintubation. To justify such a conclusion, however, it would be necessary to measure the f/V_T ratio and then extubate all patients, irrespective of whether or not they are likely to develop respiratory distress during a weaning trial. Such a trial design is not feasible from an ethical standpoint. Nonetheless, it is clear that in patients who have already tolerated a trial of spontaneous breathing, measurement of the f/V_T ratio does not predict the need for reintubation. Conceptually, of course, weaning predictors, as originally described (46,63), were measured before undertaking a spontaneous breathing trial or other approaches to weaning.

In 183 postoperative patients, Jacob et al. demonstrated a higher positive predictive value (0.94) but lower negative predictive value (0.5) for the f/V_T ratio than those reported by Yang and Tobin (0.78 and 0.95, respectively) (58). These findings likely reflect the high pretest probability of weaning success in postoperative patients (see Fig. 4 and above).

Likelihood ratios provide a means of accounting for pretest probability in the clinical application of weaning predictors. The likelihood of an outcome in the presence or absence of a predictor is calculated from the sensitivity and specificity of the test. Based on the original data of Yang and Tobin, Jaeschke et al. determined that the likelihood ratio for an f/V_T ratio <80 breaths/min/L is 7.53 and >100 breaths/min/L is 0.04 (64). The likelihood ratio is combined with the pretest probability (the percentage of patients in the population expected to fail a weaning trial) to give a posttest probability using a simple nomogram (Fig. 6). In the case of clinical equipoise (i.e., pretest probability of 50%), if the f/V_T ratio is >100 breaths/min/L, then a straight line is drawn connecting a pretest probability of 50% with a likelihood ratio of 0.04 and continued to determine the posttest probability. In this example, the posttest probability of weaning success is only 2%. For the same clinical assessment, a f/V_T ratio of <80 breaths/min/L yields a posttest probability of weaning success of 80%. Unlike the situation of clinical equipoise, general surgical patients have a low pretest probability of weaning failure (9% in the study of Jacob et al.). In this population, an f/V_T ratio of >100 breaths/min/L yields a posttest probability for weaning failure of only 45%. Conversely, over 95% of patients receiving prolonged mechanical ventilation (>30 days) will fail a weaning trial on a given day (65). The posttest probability of a low f/V_T ratio in this patient population is less than 20%.

B. Maximum Inspiratory Pressure

The maximum inspiratory pressure (P_{Imax}) is the most negative pressure generated by the respiratory muscles during a maximal inspiratory effort against an occluded valve (10,66–70). In healthy volunteers, P_{Imax} is similar to pressure measurements obtained from direct phrenic nerve stimulation (16,71–74). In 20 patients receiving mechanical ventilation, Marini et al. developed a method for measuring P_{Imax} that does not require patient cooperation (75,76). While the patient is disconnected from the ventilator for 30 seconds, a unidirectional valve is placed in the ventilator circuit that allows expiration but not inspiration. P_{Imax} is therefore measured near residual volume, where it is expected to be maximal

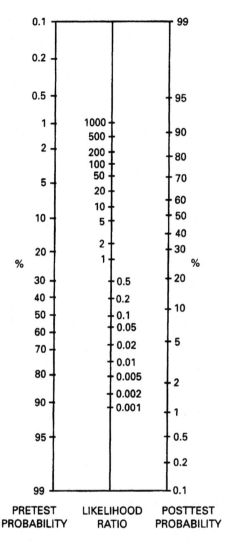

Figure 6 A nomogram for applying likelihood ratios. The pretest probability of weaning success is determined from clinical assessment. The likelihood ratio of the test is then calculated based on its known sensitivity and specificity; the likelihood ratio for a f/V_T ratio of >100 breaths/min/L is 0.04 and for a f/V_T ratio of <80 breaths/min/L it is 7.53. See text for details. (From Ref. 143.)

(77). The reproducibility of this method was evaluated by Multz et al., who asked one to five experienced investigators to perform triplicate measurements of P_{Imax} (78). Little variation was noted between the three measurements obtained by one investigator at one time; however, the coefficient of variation between different investigators studying the same patient in the same day was substantial—resulting in an average difference of 12.6 ± 1.3 cm H_2O among the recorded values of P_{Imax}.

Sahn and Lakshminarayan reported that all patients with a P_{Imax} more negative than -30 cm H_2O tolerated a weaning trial, but all patients with a P_{Imax} less negative than -20 cm H_2O failed the trial; values between these thresholds were not accurate in predicting outcome (63). Other investigators have failed to confirm the usefulness of the P_{Imax} as a weaning predictor (43,46,79,80). Using the methodology described by Marini et al. (75). Yang and Tobin prospectively demonstrated that the P_{Imax} was no better than chance in predicting the outcome of a weaning trial (46).

C. Vital Capacity

The vital capacity is normally 65–75 mL/kg, and a value of 10 mL/kg or more has been suggested to predict weaning outcome (81,82). However, several studies have demonstrated that the vital capacity is not useful in predicting weaning outcome (43,80,83).

D. Respiratory System Compliance

Respiratory system compliance is calculated as the delivered tidal volume/(plateau pressure minus positive end-expiratory pressure) (84). Respiratory compliance is a poor predictor of weaning success (Table 3) with positive and negative predictive values of only 0.6 and 0.53 (46).

E. Minute Ventilation and Maximum Voluntary Ventilation

Maximum voluntary ventilation (MVV) is the minute ventilation during a 1-minute maximal effort (usually measured over 15 seconds). It requires an unusual degree of patient cooperation for its measurement (84). Minute ventilation is normally <6 L/min, and MVV is normally 50–250 L/min. Sahn and Lakshiminaryan found that the combination of a minute ventilation <10 L/min with the ability to double this value during an MVV maneuver was able to predict 100% of weaning successes and 71% of weaning failures (63). Tahvanainen et al. found that a minute ventilation of 10 L/min had a sensitivity of 75% and specificity of 90% for weaning success, and the sensitivity and specificity of the MVV were 24% and 86%, respectively (43). Yang and Tobin found a minute ventilation of

<10 L/min to be a poor predictor of weaning outcome, with positive and negative predictive values of 0.55 and 0.38, respectively (Table 3) (46).

F. Airway Occlusion Pressure

The negative pressure generated during contraction of the inspiratory muscles against an occluded airway is directly related to its neural stimulus, as reflected by the diaphragmatic EMG or integrated phrenic nerve activity (85–87). An index of respiratory motor output, the airway occlusion pressure ($P_{0.1}$), is obtained by performing inspiratory occlusions without warning at irregular intervals and measuring the change in airway pressure at a point (typically 0.1 s) before the patient recognizes the occlusion and reacts to it (88,89). In a typical circuit (88–90), an airway adapter or mouthpiece is attached to a one-way valve to facilitate independent control over the inspiratory and expiratory limbs of the circuit. During expiration, a shutter or valve is activated in the inspiratory limb. The occlusion is maintained during the subsequent inspiration for less than 0.25–0.3 s, and the airway pressure generated at 0.1 s is measured. A pneumotachograph is usually included in the circuit to provide simultaneous measurement of airflow. Although intrinsically negative, the result is expressed as a positive number, with a normal value of 0.5–1.5 cm H_2O.

In ventilated patients, it is possible to measure $P_{0.1}$ using the demand valve in the ventilator circuit. Since these valves usually take substantially longer than 100 ms to open, the $P_{0.1}$ can be obtained from airway pressure measurements during ventilator triggering. Such measurements have been shown to correlate well with conventional methods for measuring $P_{0.1}$ (91,92). Some newer ventilators include software that provides a calculation of $P_{0.1}$ values (93).

The presence of intrinsic PEEP posses a potential problem in the measurement of $P_{0.1}$ since in this setting the inspiratory muscles become active long before airway pressure begins to fall. In a careful study of this issue, Conti et al. demonstrated that $P_{0.1}$ measured at the airway opening correlated well with the change in esophageal pressure during the first 100 ms after the initiation of inspiration (94).

Several investigators have evaluated $P_{0.1}$ as a predictor of weaning outcome (25–34). With one exception (32), these studies have demonstrated higher values of $P_{0.1}$ in patients failing a weaning trial than in patients who were successfully weaned. At first glance, it might seem surprising that a supranormal respiratory drive predisposes to ventilatory failure. However, the increased $P_{0.1}$ values likely reflect respiratory distress and signify the response of the respiratory centers to increased ventilatory loads. In these studies, the threshold value of $P_{0.1}$ discriminating between weaning success and weaning failure ranged from 3.4 to 6.0 cm H_2O. Since the studies varied in the definition of weaning success and failure, prevalence of different outcomes, method of weaning (T-piece trials, intermittent mandatory ventilation, or pressure support ventilation), and threshold value of $P_{0.1}$, it is not surprising the accuracy of $P_{0.1}$ differed among the studies. In general, $P_{0.1}$ was good at predicting weaning success (sensitivity >0.8) but less reliable in predicting weaning failure (95).

Most of these studies were based on relatively small patient populations, and the threshold value of $P_{0.1}$ was selected in a post hoc manner—a step known to overestimate the accuracy of a predictive index (47). To date, the only prospective study of $P_{0.1}$ as a weaning predictor is that undertaken by Sassoon and Mahutte (33). A $P_{0.1}$ of ≤ 5.5 cm H_2O had a sensitivity of 0.95 for predicting weaning success but a specificity of only 0.40. Combining $P_{0.1}$ with the f/V_T ratio ($P_{0.1} \times f/V_T$) improved the specificity to 0.60 without a change in sensitivity. ROC analysis revealed no difference in the area under the curves for the $P_{0.1} \times f/V_T$ product and the f/V_T ratio alone.

G. Estimates of the Work of Breathing

Failed weaning trials are usually accompanied by a deterioration in respiratory mechanics, with a consequent increase in the load imposed on the respiratory muscles (14,15). Accordingly, measurements of the work of breathing might be predictive of weaning outcome.

Mechanical work is performed when a force moves its point of application through a distance. In the case of a three-dimensional system, like the respiratory system, work is done when a pressure changes the volume of the system. Work can be described as work per liter (mechanical work) or work per minute (power). Measurements of mechanical work fail to include the expenditure of energy that occurs during isometric muscle contractions (96–98).

A number of investigators have evaluated the measurements of respiratory work as weaning predictors (79,99–101). In all of these studies, the work of breathing was greater in patients who failed a weaning trial than in those who succeeded. Fiastro et al. found that both work per liter and work per minute values predicted weaning outcome, but that neither index on its own was as accurate as the combination of the two (79). With the exception of the study by Proctor and Woolson (657 measurements in 168 patients) (101), all of these studies were small. Also, the threshold values of work under evaluation as weaning predictors were determined on a post hoc basis instead of being prospectively defined—a process known to overestimate the accuracy of a predictor.

Commercial systems for measuring the work of breathing have recently come on the market, such as the Bicore CP-100 (Bicore Monitoring Systems, Irvine, CA) and Ventrak (Novametrix Medical Systems, Wallingford, CT). Of these, the Bicore system has undergone more detailed evaluation (4,102–105). The device includes a pneumotachograph connected between the endotracheal tube and the ventilator circuit and an esophageal balloon.

In a study designed to evaluate the Bicore system as a weaning predictor, Kirton et al. selected 28 patients with a respiratory frequency of >30/min who otherwise were considered likely to tolerate discontinuation of mechanical ventilation (106). Employing the Bicore system, six patients had work per liter values within the manufacturer's normal range (<0.8 J/L), and all six were successfully extubated. In 22 patients with elevated work of breathing, the investigators recorded pressure at the carinal end of the endotracheal tube and calculated imposed work. When imposed work was subtracted from total work, the resulting value was <0.8 J/L in 21 patients. The latter were extubated and two required intubation. The investigators concluded that direct measurements of work of breathing expedited the weaning process. Although possibly correct, the reported data do not provide sufficient proof for this conclusion. Preexisting reports indicate that patients with respiratory frequencies >30 breaths per minute can be safely extubated without invasive measurements (46). Also, the study population was weighted toward patients who were successfully extubated; to prove that work measurements help in clinical decision making, it is necessary to show that high values preclude successful weaning. Levy et al. addressed this last point (107). They measured work of breathing in 24 patients using the Bicore system, 14 of whom were successfully extubated despite values of work per liter above the manufacturer's normal range.

In 23 patients being weaned from mechanical ventilation by progressive reductions in the amount of ventilator support during intermittent mandatory ventilation or pressure support, Gluck et al. used the Bicore system to determine readiness to wean (108). They then compared the estimated rate of weaning using conventional weaning predictors (respiratory frequency, tidal volume, minute ventilation, respiratory resistance, static compliance, and maximal inspiratory pressure) with the rate of weaning using Bicore data, the f/V_T ratio, and $P_{0.1}$. They estimated that the duration of mechanical ventilation decreased from 7.8 ± 2.8 days to 5.3 ± 2.5 days using the Bicore system. Several problems exist with this study. First, the investigators failed to distinguish between less invasive measurements, such as the f/V_T ratio and $P_{0.1}$ and the Bicore data. Second, the trial was not adequately controlled since the rate of weaning in the absence of the f/V_T ratio, $P_{0.1}$, and Bicore data was only estimated. Finally, the selection of intermittent mandatory ventilation as the weaning modality was unfortunate, since this method has been shown to be the most inefficient method of weaning (5,6).

A particular weakness of the above studies employing the Bicore system is the use of the manufacturer's upper limit of normal as the target value (106–110) for decision making. The manufacturer's normal range is arbitrary because a satisfactory study to define the normal range for work of breathing has never been conducted. Moreover, there is no reason to presuppose that the upper limit of the normal range—even if rigorously determined—should serve as an appropriate target for clinical decision making. Studies need to be performed prospectively to define threshold values of the work of breathing that can forecast relevant outcome events such as successful weaning (47).

In summary, an appropriately designed study to evaluate the real worth of work measurements in clinical management has yet to be performed. For example, it would be helpful to have a study in which the primary management team is blinded to work-of-breathing measurements. The predictive power of the work measurements could then be compared with conventional assessment methods using a predefined outcome event. The limitations in the preexisting studies do not mean that measurements of work of breathing are not helpful. Indeed, they furnish some clues that they might be helpful and cost effective, but definite proof of efficacy is awaited.

H. Pressure-Time Product and Tension-Time Index

Measurement of mechanical work does not necessarily take into account the duration of a muscle contraction. Two breaths may have the same tidal volume and intrathoracic pressure excursion but differ in the duration of inspiratory time. Since the pressure-volume relationships are the same, work of breathing will be identical. However, energy requirements will be greater for the breath with the longer inspiratory time. Measurements of the pressure-time product and tension-time index circumvent this problem. Both the pressure-time product and tension-time index take into account respiratory muscle pressure generation and inspiratory time (97,98). Bellemare and Grassino found that healthy volunteers were able to breathe against inspiratory loads indefinitely if the tension-time index was less than 0.15, whereas respiratory muscle fatigue developed when the tension-time index exceeded 0.15 (111). Field et al. found that oxygen consumption by the respiratory muscles in healthy volunteers was closely related to the tension-time index but bore only a weak relationship to the mechanical work of breathing (112).

Jubran and Tobin found that patients who fail a weaning trial had significantly higher values of the pressure-time product than those who successfully weaned (14,112). Employing a multiple logistic regression analysis, Vassilakopoulos et al. found that the tension-time index and the f/V_T ratio were the only significant predictors of weaning outcome (15,112). Neither of these studies was designed to evaluate the utility of the pressure-time product or the tension-time index as a predictor of weaning outcome.

I. Oxygen Cost of Breathing

The metabolic work of the respiratory muscles, i.e., the oxygen cost of breathing, is estimated as the difference in whole body oxygen consumption between spontaneous breathing and complete relaxation during mechanical ventilation. Although estimates vary considerably, the oxygen cost of breathing is usually <1–2% of total oxygen consumption in normal subjects; the value can be markedly elevated in critically ill patients (97,113). Theoretically, the oxygen cost of breathing might be a better estimate of the true metabolic cost of breathing than other measures of work of breathing because it combines the energy expended by respiratory muscle contractions that result in mechanical work with those that do not. Unfortunately, the accuracy of the oxygen cost of breathing as an estimate of respiratory work is compromised by changes in nonrespiratory muscle oxygen consumption during weaning (114–116) and technical problems with its measurement (113,117,118).

The results of investigations of the oxygen cost of breathing during weaning trials are conflicting. Nishimura et al. found that the oxygen cost of breathing was higher in patients who failed a weaning trial (21%) than in patients successfully weaned (8%) (119). Lewis et al. studied 16 patients who were successfully weaned and 14 patients who continued to receive ventilator support (120). They measured oxygen consumption during mechanical ventilation and estimated it when the patient was able to assume "the greatest degree of spontaneous ventilation." As the latter state included some patients who were receiving up to 6 breaths/min of intermittent mechanical ventilation, the investigators extrapolated the oxygen consumption for total spontaneous ventilation. The extrapolated oxygen cost of breathing was 9% (range −3 to 18%) in the success group and 39% (8–120%) in the failure group. In contrast to those studies, Hubmayr et al. found no significant difference in the oxygen cost of breathing in patients who were successfully weaned (13%) compared with those who failed a weaning trial (20%) (117). Likewise, Kemper et al. found that oxygen consumption increased similarly in weaning success (10%) and weaning failure (7%) (121).

J. Gastric Tonometry

Because the gut is particularly susceptible to ischemia (122), monitoring of gut perfusion using gastric tonometry has been advocated for the early detection of hypoperfused states (123–126). Gastric tonometers are saline or air filled balloons placed in contact with the wall of the gastric mucosa. After allowing time for equilibration, the P_{CO_2} in the balloon approximates gastric mucosal P_{CO_2} (127). Anaerobic metabolism in the gut mucosa causes gastric mucosal P_{CO_2} to increase, gastric mucosal pH (pH_i) to decrease, and the difference between gastric mucosal P_{CO_2} and arterial P_{CO_2} to increase. These findings have been associated with poor outcomes in critically ill patients with sepsis syndrome, trauma, post–cardiac surgery, and other postoperative patients (81). During a weaning trial, a fall in gastric P_{CO_2} might result from abnormalities in systemic perfusion (e.g., occult sepsis, cardiovascular dysfunction) or gut hypoperfusion as a result of increased respiratory muscle oxygen consumption and blood flow.

Gastric tonometry has been evaluated as a weaning predictor in two investigations. In 29 patients undergoing spontaneous breathing trials, Mohsenifar et al. compared pH_i with other weaning predictors (55). After 20–30 minutes of spontaneous breathing, all 11 patients who failed the weaning trial either decreased their pH_i by >0.09 or had a $pH_i < 7.30$. Patients who tolerated the spontaneous trial and were extubated had no significant change in pH_i. Based on post hoc analysis, the investigators concluded that a gastric mucosal pH < 7.30 after 20–30 minutes of spontaneous breathing was superior to other weaning predictors (f/V_T, tidal volume, respiratory frequency, and P_{Imax}). Bouachour et al. evaluated gastric tonometry in 26 patients with COPD during spontaneous breathing trials (128). Patients who failed weaning had a higher gastric Pco_2 and lower pH_i at the start of the trial and 20 minutes after its commencement than patients who were successfully weaned. Using ROC analysis, the investigators determined the optimal threshold values at 20 minutes to be a gastric $Pco_2 > 60$ mmHg and gastric $pH_i < 7.30$. Gastric tonometry was found to have superior predictive power when compared with other weaning predictors (f/V_T, tidal volume, respiratory frequency, and the P_aO_2/PAO_2).

Significant problems arise in the interpretation of these studies. Both groups of investigators determined the threshold values for gastric tonometry derived indices in a post hoc manner rather than testing them prospectively in a group of patients distinct from those in which the threshold values were determined; the former method is known to overestimate the accuracy of a predictor (47). Mohensifar et al. measured the f/V_T ratio during pressure support ventilation, a factor that markedly confounds its interpretation (see above). While gastric mucosal Pco_2 increases and gastric mucosal pH falls during failed weaning trials, it is not known whether such measures are superior in predicting weaning failure than more easily obtained measurements.

K. Cardiac Ischemia

Patients undergoing weaning trials are susceptible to myocardial ischemia resulting from increases in plasma catecholamine levels, the added oxygen cost of breathing, and increases in left ventricular afterload. Evidence of myocardial ischemia has been reported in 8–50% of patients undergoing weaning trials (129–134). The large variation in the prevalence of ischemia in these studies may have resulted from variability in the methods used to detect ischemia and in the study populations. Most investigators have employed continuous ECG recordings to detect ischemia, but lead placement and definitions of ischemia differ among the studies (129–131,134). Myocardial thallium-201 scintigraphy was employed by Hurford et al. (132) in 15 mechanically ventilated patients to determine the incidence of myocardial ischemia during spontaneous breathing trials. At baseline, all but one of the patients had abnormal thallium images, but only a single patient demonstrated redistribution of thallium on delayed images. During spontaneous ventilation, 7 of the 15 patients developed changes in the thallium images (alterations of thallium distribution or transient left ventricular dilatation or both). Four of these patients developed new regional decreases of thallium concentration with redistribution on delayed images. The authors concluded that myocardial ischemia may be a significant contributor to weaning failure (132). In a subsequent study, Hurford and Favorito prospectively obtained 24-hour Holter recordings in 17 patients requiring prolonged mechanical ventilation *before* a weaning trial. Six patients exhibited electrocardiographic features of ischemia before the trial, which was associated with an increased risk of weaning failure (131). These findings support the notion that myocardial ischemia may contribute to weaning failure in some patients. Further prospective studies with larger numbers of patients demonstrating improvements in weaning rates after interventions for myocardial ischemia are needed before such monitoring can be recommended for routine use.

L.   Leak Volume on Cuff Deflation

Following extubation, about 5% of patients develop laryngeal edema and stridor—factors that account for about 1% of reintubations (2,135–137). If the cuff of the endotracheal tube is deflated before extubation, a leak is normally audible; the absence of such a leak predicts postextubation stridor (138–142). Before extubating 100 consecutive adult patients, Marik recorded the presence or absence of an audible cuff leak during both spontaneous breathing and positive-pressure ventilation (141). Of 12 patients who did not have a leak in either circumstance, two developed postextubation stridor; of the patients with an audible leak, none developed stridor. These data indicate that the absence of an audible leak after cuff deflation predicts postextubation stridor with a specificity of 33% and a sensitivity of 100%. During mechanical ventilation, Miller and Cole quantified the leak volume on deflation of the cuff (142). To determine the leak, the cuff was deflated for 6 breaths and the average of the three lowest values of exhaled tidal volume was subtracted from the inhaled tidal volume. Using ROC analysis, they found that a cuff leak volume of 110 mL had the greatest discriminatory power; this value predicted postextubation stridor with a sensitivity of 0.67 and specificity of 0.98. A limitation of the cuff leak test is that only a small number of patients develop stridor after extubation.

VII.   Summary

Clinical examination remains a necessary part of patient assessment, but it is not sufficient in the prediction of weaning outcome. Routine measurements of weaning predictors have been shown to decrease the duration of mechanical ventilation, probably through the earlier identification of patients who can tolerate discontinuation of mechanical ventilation. Of the weaning predictors that have been evaluated, the f/V_T ratio appears to be the most useful. The f/V_T ratio is a reasonably accurate predictor of weaning outcome, it is easy to measure, and it has a threshold value that is easy to remember, namely 100 breaths/min/L. In patients whose underlying disease has significantly resolved and whose f/V_T ratio suggests that weaning has a high likelihood of being successful, a 30-minute trial of spontaneous breathing is the most expeditious approach to weaning.

References

1. Kollef MH. The prevention of ventilator-associated pneumonia. N Engl J Med 1999; 340:627–634.
2. Stauffer JL, Olson DE, Petty TL. Complications and consequences of endotracheal intubation and tracheotomy. A prospective study of 150 critically ill adult patients. Am J Med 1981; 70:65–76.
3. Weg JG, Anzueto A, Balk RA, Wiedemann HP, Pattishall EN, Schork MA, et al. The relation of pneumothorax and other air leaks to mortality in the acute respiratory distress syndrome. N Engl J Med 1998; 338:341–346.
4. Stroetz RW, Hubmayr RD. Tidal volume maintenance during weaning with pressure support. Am J Respir Crit Care Med 1995; 152:1034–1040.
5. Brochard L, Rauss A, Benito S, Conti G, Mancebo J, Rekik N, et al. Comparison of three methods of gradual withdrawal from ventilatory support during weaning from mechanical ventilation. Am J Respir Crit Care Med 1994; 150:896–903.
6. Esteban A, Frutos F, Tobin MJ, Alia I, Solsona JF, Valverdu I, et al. A comparison of four methods of weaning patients from mechanical ventilation. N Engl J Med 1995; 332:345–350.
7. Kollef MH, Shapiro SD, Silver P, St, John RE, Prentice D, et al. A randomized, controlled trial of protocol-directed versus physician-directed weaning from mechanical ventilation. Crit Care Med 1997; 25:567–574.
8. Horst HM, Mouro D, Hall-Jenssens RA, Pamukov N. Decrease in ventilation time with a standardized weaning process. Arch Surg 1998; 133:483–489.
9. Ely EW, Baker AM, Dunagan DP, Burke HL, Smith AC, Kelly PT, et al. Effect on the duration of mechanical ventilation of identifying patients capable of breathing spontaneously. N Engl J Med 1996; 335:1864–1869.
10. Tobin MJ, Laghi F. Monitoring of respiratory muscle function. In: Tobin MJ, ed. Principles and Practice of Intensive Care Monitoring. New York: McGraw-Hill, Inc., 1998:497–544.
11. Slutsky AS. Mechanical ventilation. American College of Chest Physicians' Consensus Conference. Chest 1993; 104:1833–1859.
12. Esteban A, Alia I, Tobin MJ, Gil A, Gordo F, Vallverdu I, et al. Effect of spontaneous breathing trial duration on outcome of attempts to discontinue mechanical ventilation. Am J Respir Crit Care Med 1999; 159:512–518.
13. Jubran A, Tobin MJ. Passive mechanics of lung and chest wall in patients who

failed or succeeded in trials of weaning. Am J Respir Crit Care Med 1997; 155: 916–921.

14. Jubran A, Tobin MJ. Pathophysiologic basis of acute respiratory distress in patients who fail a trial of weaning from mechanical ventilation. Am J Respir Crit Care Med 1997; 155:906–915.

15. Vassilakopoulos T, Zakynthinos S, Roussos C. The tension-time index and the frequency/tidal volume ratio are the major pathophysiologic determinants of weaning failure and success. Am J Respir Crit Care Med 1998; 158:378–385.

16. Bellemare F, Bigland-Ritchie B. Central components of diaphragmatic fatigue assessed by phrenic nerve stimulation. J Appl Physiol 1987; 62:1307–1316.

17. Laghi F, D'Alfonso N, Tobin MJ. Pattern of recovery from diaphragmatic fatigue over 24 hours. J Appl Physiol 1995; 79:539–546.

18. Roussos C, Moxham J, Bellemare F. Respiratory muscle fatigue. In: Roussos C, ed. The Thorax. 2d ed. New York: Marcel Dekker, 1995:1405–1461.

19. Banzett RB, Lansing RW, Brown R, Topulos GP, Yager D, Steele SM, et al. 'Air hunger' from increased PCO_2 persists after complete neuromuscular block in humans. Respir Physiol 1990; 81:1–17.

20. Dunn WF, Nelson SB, Hubmayr RD. The control of breathing during weaning from mechanical ventilation. Chest 1991; 100:754–761.

21. Gallagher CG, Hof VI, Younes M. Effect of inspiratory muscle fatigue on breathing pattern. J Appl Physiol 1985; 59:1152–1158.

22. Mador MJ, Tobin MJ. The effect of inspiratory muscle fatigue on breathing pattern and ventilatory response to CO_2. J Physiol 1992; 455:17–32.

23. Mador MJ, Acevedo FA. Effect of respiratory muscle fatigue on subsequent exercise performance. J Appl Physiol 1991; 70:2059–2065.

24. Yan S, Lichros I, Zakynthinos S, Macklem PT. Effect of diaphragmatic fatigue on control of respiratory muscles and ventilation during CO_2 rebreathing. J Appl Physiol 1993; 75:1364–1370.

25. Capdevila XJ, Perrigault PF, Perey PJ, Roustan JP, d'Athis F. Occlusion pressure and its ratio to maximum inspiratory pressure are useful predictors for successful extubation following T-piece weaning trial. Chest 1995; 108:482–489.

26. Conti G, De Blasi R, Pelaia P, Benito S, Rocco M, Antonelli M, et al. Early prediction of successful weaning during pressure support ventilation in chronic obstructive pulmonary disease patients. Crit Care Med 1992; 20:366–371.

27. Fernandez R, Cabrera J, Calaf N, Benito S. P 0.1/PIMax: an index for assessing respiratory capacity in acute respiratory failure. Intens Care Med 1990; 16:175–179.

28. Gandia F, Blanco J. Evaluation of indexes predicting the outcome of ventilator weaning and value of adding supplemental inspiratory load. Intens Care Med 1992; 18:327–333.

29. Herrera M, Blasco J, Venegas J, Barba R, Doblas A, Marquez E. Mouth occlusion pressure (P0.1) in acute respiratory failure. Intens Care Med 1985; 11:134–139.

30. Montgomery AB, Holle RH, Neagley SR, Pierson DJ, Schoene RB. Prediction of successful ventilator weaning using airway occlusion pressure and hypercapnic challenge. Chest 1987; 91:496–499.

31. Murciano D, Boczkowski J, Lecocguic Y, Emili JM, Pariente R, Aubier M. Tra-

cheal occlusion pressure: a simple index to monitor respiratory muscle fatigue during acute respiratory failure in patients with chronic obstructive pulmonary disease. Ann Intern Med 1988; 108:800–805.

32. Pourriat JL, Baud M, Lamberto C, Fosse JP, Cupa M. Effects of doxapram on hypercapnic response during weaning from mechanical ventilation in COPD patients. Chest 1992; 101:1639–1643.

33. Sassoon CS, Mahutte CK. Airway occlusion pressure and breathing pattern as predictors of weaning outcome. Am Rev Respir Dis 1993; 148:860–866.

34. Sassoon CS, Te TT, Mahutte CK, Light RW. Airway occlusion pressure. An important indicator for successful weaning in patients with chronic obstructive pulmonary disease. Am Rev Respir Dis 1987; 135:107–113.

35. Tobin MJ, Perez W, Guenther SM, Semmes BJ, Mador MJ, Allen SJ, et al. The pattern of breathing during successful and unsuccessful trials of weaning from mechanical ventilation. Am Rev Respir Dis 1986; 134:1111–1118.

36. Anzueto A, Supinski GS, Levine SM, Jenkinson SG. Mechanisms of disease: are oxygen-derived free radicals involved in diaphragmatic dysfunction? Am J Respir Crit Care Med 1994; 149:1048–1052.

37. Reid WD, Huang J, Bryson S, Walker DC, Belcastro AN. Diaphragm injury and myofibrillar structure induced by resistive loading. J Appl Physiol 1994; 76:176–184.

38. Sen CK. Oxidants and antioxidants in exercise. J Appl Physiol 1995; 79:675–686.

39. Vollestad NK, Sejersted OM. Biochemical correlates of fatigue. A brief review. Eur J Appl Physiol 1988; 57:336–347.

40. Zhu E, Petrof BJ, Gea J, Comtois N, Grassino AE. Diaphragm muscle fiber injury after inspiratory resistive breathing. Am J Respir Crit Care Med 1997; 155:1110–1116.

41. Esteban A, Alia I, Gordo F, Fernandez R, Solsona JF, Vallverdu I, et al. Extubation outcome after spontaneous breathing trials with T-tube or pressure support ventilation. The Spanish Lung Failure Collaborative Group. Am J Respir Crit Care Med 1997; 156:459–465.

42. Epstein SK, Ciubotaru RL, Wong JB. Effect of failed extubation on the outcome of mechanical ventilation. Chest 1997; 112:186–192.

43. Tahvanainen J, Salmenpera M, Nikki P. Extubation criteria after weaning from intermittent mandatory ventilation and continuous positive airway pressure. Crit Care Med 1983; 11:702–707.

44. Epstein SK, Ciubotaru RL. Independent effects of etiology of failure and time to reintubation on outcome for patients failing extubation. Am J Respir Crit Care Med 1998; 158:489–493.

45. Schwartz DE, Matthay MA, Cohen NH. Death and other complications of emergency airway management in critically ill adults. A prospective investigation of 297 tracheal intubations. Anesthesiology 1995; 82:367–376.

46. Yang KL, Tobin MJ. A prospective study of indexes predicting the outcome of trials of weaning from mechanical ventilation. N Engl J Med 1991; 324:1445–1450.

47. Wasson JH, Sox HC, Neff RK, Goldman L. Clinical prediction rules. Applications and methodological standards. N Engl J Med 1985; 313:793–799.

48. Epstein SK. Etiology of extubation failure and the predictive value of the rapid shallow breathing index. Am J Respir Crit Care Med 1995; 152:545–549.

49. Lee KH, Hui KP, Chan TB, Tan WC, Lim TK. Rapid shallow breathing (frequency-tidal volume ratio) did not predict extubation outcome. Chest 1994; 105:540–543.

50. Jekel JF, Elmore JG, Katz DL. Improving decisions in clinical medicine. In: Jekel JF, Elmore JG, Katz DL, eds. Epidemiology Biostatistics and Preventive Medicine. Philadelphia: W.B. Saunders, 1996; 98–106.

51. Centor RM. Signal detectability: the use of ROC curves and their analyses. Med Decis Making 1991; 11:102–106.

52. Metz CE. ROC methodology in radiologic imaging. Invest Radiol 1986; 21:720–733.

53. Metz CE. Basic principles of ROC analysis. Semin Nucl Med 1978; 8:283–298.

54. Zweig MH. Evaluation of the clinical accuracy of laboratory tests. Arch Pathol Lab Med 1988; 112:383–386.

55. Mohsenifar Z, Hay A, Hay J, Lewis MI, Koerner SK. Gastric intramural pH as a predictor of success or failure in weaning patients from mechanical ventilation. Ann Intern Med 1993; 119:794–798.

56. Jubran A, Van de Graaff WB, Tobin MJ. Variability of patient-ventilator interaction with pressure support ventilation in patients with chronic obstructive pulmonary disease. Am J Respir Crit Care Med 1995; 152:129–136.

57. Chatila W, Jacob B, Guaglionone D, Manthous CA. The unassisted respiratory rate-tidal volume ratio accurately predicts weaning outcome. Am J Med 1996; 101:61–67.

58. Jacob B, Chatila W, Manthous CA. The unassisted respiratory rate/tidal volume ratio accurately predicts weaning outcome in postoperative patients. Crit Care Med 1997; 25:253–257.

59. Krieger BP, Isber J, Breitenbucher A, Throop G, Ershowsky P. Serial measurements of the rapid-shallow-breathing index as a predictor of weaning outcome in elderly medical patients. Chest 1997; 112:1029–1034.

60. Krieger BP, Ershowsky PF, Becker DA, Gazeroglu HB. Evaluation of conventional criteria for predicting successful weaning from mechanical ventilatory support in elderly patients. Crit Care Med 1989; 17:858–861.

61. Jubran A, Leung P, Mullner C, Tobin MJ. Temporal alteration in frequency-to-tidal volume ratio during a weaning trial. Am J Respir Crit Care Med 1997; 155: A525.

62. Epstein SK, Ciubotaru RL. Influence of gender and endotracheal tube size on preextubation breathing pattern. Am J Respir Crit Care Med 1996; 154:1647–1652.

63. Sahn SA, Lakshminarayan S. Bedside criteria for discontinuation of mechanical ventilation. Chest 1973; 63:1002–1005.

64. Jaeschke RZ, Meade MO, Guyatt GH, Keenan SP, Cook DJ. How to use diagnostic test articles in the intensive care unit: diagnosing weanability using f/Vt. Crit Care Med 1997; 25:1514–1521.

65. Scheinhorn DJ, Chao DC, Stearn-Hassenpflug M, LaBree LD, Heltsley DJ. Post-ICU mechanical ventilation: treatment of 1,123 patients at a regional weaning center. Chest 1997; 111:1654–1659.

66. Bellemare F. Strength of the respiratory muscles. In: Roussos C, ed. The Thorax. 2d ed. New York: Marcel Dekker, 1995; 1161–1197.

67. Clanton TL, Diaz PT. Clinical assessment of the respiratory muscles. Phys Ther 1995; 75:983–995.

68. Gibson GJ. Measurement of respiratory muscle strength. Respir Med 1995; 89: 529–535.

69. Larson JL, Covey MK, Vitalo CA, Alex CG, Patel M, Kim M. Maximal inspiratory pressure. Learning effect and test-retest reliability in patients with chronic obstructive pulmonary disease. Chest 1993; 104:448–453.

70. Rochester DF. Tests of respiratory muscle function. Clin Chest Med 1988; 9:249–261.

71. Gandevia SC, McKenzie DK. Activation of human muscles at short muscle lengths during maximal static efforts. J Physiol 1988; 407:599–613.

72. Similowski T, Duguet A, Straus C, Attali V, Boisteanu D, Derenne JP. Assessment of the voluntary activation of the diaphragm using cervical and cortical magnetic stimulation. Eur Respir J 1996; 9:1224–1231.

73. Similowski T, Gauthier AP, Yan S, Macklem PT, Bellemare F. Assessment of diaphragm function using mouth pressure twitches in chronic obstructive pulmonary disease patients. Am Rev Respir Dis 1993; 147:850–856.

74. Similowski T, Yan S, Gauthier AP, Macklem PT, Bellemare F. Contractile properties of the human diaphragm during chronic hyperinflation. N Engl J Med 1991; 325:917–923.

75. Marini JJ, Smith TC, Lamb V. Estimation of inspiratory muscle strength in mechanically ventilated patients: the measurement of inspiratory pressure. J Crit Care 1986; 1:32–38.

76. Truwit JD, Marini JJ. Validation of a technique to assess maximal inspiratory pressure in poorly cooperative patients. Chest 1992; 102:1216–1219.

77. Rahn H, Otis AB, Chadwick LE, Fenn WO. The pressure-volume diagram of the thorax and lung. Am J Physiol 1946; 146:161–178.

78. Multz AS, Aldrich TK, Prezant DJ, Karpel JP, Hendler J. Maximal inspiratory pressure is not a reliable test of inspiratory muscle strength in mechanically ventilated patients. Am Rev Respir Dis 1990; 142:529–532.

79. Fiastro JF, Habib MP, Shon BY, Campbell SC. Comparison of standard weaning parameters and the mechanical work of breathing in mechanically ventilated patients. Chest 1988; 94:232–238.

80. Morganroth ML, Morganroth JL, Nett LM, Petty TL. Criteria for weaning from prolonged mechanical ventilation. Arch Intern Med 1984; 144:1012–1016.

81. Feeley TW, Hedley-Whyte J. Weaning from controlled ventilation and supplemental oxygen. N Engl J Med 1975; 292:903–906.

82. Scoggin CH. Weaning respiratory patients from mechanical support. J Respir Dis 1980; 1:13–23.

83. Millbern SM, Downs JB, Jumper LC, Modell JH. Evaluation of criteria for discontinuing mechanical ventilatory support. Arch Surg 1978; 113:1441–1443.

84. Tobin MJ. Respiratory monitoring in the intensive care unit. Am Rev Respir Dis 1988; 138:1625–1642.

85. Eldridge FL. Relationship between respiratory nerve and muscle activity and muscle force output. J Appl Physiol 1975; 39:567–574.

86. Evanich MJ, Franco MJ, Lourenco RV. Force output of the diaphragm as a function of phrenic nerve firing rate and lung volume. J Appl Physiol 1973; 35:208–212.
87. Lopata M, Lourenco RV. Evaluation of respiratory control. Clin Chest Med 1980; 1:33–45.
88. Whitelaw WA, Derenne JP. Airway occlusion pressure. J Appl Physiol 1993; 74: 1475–1483.
89. Whitelaw WA, Derenne JP, Milic-Emili J. Occlusion pressure as a measure of respiratory center output in conscious man. Respir Physiol 1975; 23:181–199.
90. Lind FG, Truve AB, Lindborg BP. Microcomputer-assisted on-line measurement of breathing pattern and occlusion pressure. J Appl Physiol 1984; 56:235–239.
91. Brenner M, Mukai DS, Russell JE, Spiritus EM, Wilson A. A new method for measurement of airway occlusion pressure. Chest 1990; 98:421–427.
92. Fernandez R, Benito S, Sanchis J, Milic-Emili J, Net A. Inspiratory effort and occlusion pressure in triggered mechanical ventilation. Intens Care Med 1988; 14: 650–653.
93. Kuhlen R, Hausmann S, Pappert D, Slama K, Rossaint R, Falke K. A new method for P0.1 measurement using standard respiratory equipment. Intens Care Med 1995; 21:554–560.
94. Conti G, Cinnella G, Barboni E, Lemaire F, Harf A, Brochard L. Estimation of occlusion pressure during assisted ventilation in patients with intrinsic PEEP. Am J Respir Crit Care Med 1996; 154:907–912.
95. Tobin MJ, Gardner WN. Monitoring of the control of breathing. In: Tobin MJ, ed. Principles and Practice of Intensive Care Monitoring. New York: McGraw-Hill, 1998:415–464.
96. Agostoni E, Campbell EJM, Freedman S Energetics. In: Campbell EJM, Agostoni E, Newsom-Davis J, ed. The Respiratory Muscles. Philadelphia: Saunders, 1970: 115–137.
97. Tobin MJ. Monitoring respiratory mechanics in spontaneously breathing patients. In: Tobin MJ, ed. Principles and Practice of Intensive Care Monitoring. New York: McGraw-Hill, 1998:617–654.
98. Tobin MJ, Van de Graff WB. Monitoring of lung mechanics and work of breathing. In: Tobin MJ, ed. Principles and Practice of Mechanical Ventilation. New York: McGraw-Hill, 1994:967–1003.
99. Henning RJ, Shubin H, Weil MH. The measurement of the work of breathing for the clinical assessment of ventilator dependence. Crit Care Med 1977; 5:264–268.
100. Peters RM, Hilberman M, Hogan JS, Crawford DA. Objective indications for respirator therapy in post-trauma and postoperative patients. Am J Surg 1972; 124:262–269.
101. Proctor HJ, Woolson R. Prediction of respiratory muscle fatigue by measurements of the work of breathing. Surg Gynecol Obstet 1973; 136:367–370.
102. Bates JHT. Report of tests carried out on the Bicore CP-100 pulmonary model validation. Riverside, CA: Bicore Monitoring Systems, 1992.
103. Blanch PB, Banner M. A new respiratory monitor that enables accurate measurement of work of breathing. Respir Care 1994; 39:897–905.
104. Nathan SD, Ishaaya AM, Koerner SK, Belman MJ. Prediction of minimal pressure support during weaning from mechanical ventilation. Chest 1993; 103:1215–1219.

105. Petros AJ, Lamond CT, Bennett D. The Bicore pulmonary monitor. A device to assess the work of breathing while weaning from mechanical ventilation. Anaesthesia 1993; 48:985–988.

106. Kirton OC, DeHaven CB, Morgan JP, Windsor J, Civetta J. Elevated imposed work of breathing masquerading as ventilator weaning intolerance. Chest 1995; 108: 1021–1025.

107. Levy MM, Miyasaki A, Langston D. Work of breathing as a weaning parameter in mechanically ventilated patients. Chest 1995; 108:1018–1020.

108. Gluck EH, Barkoviak MJ, Balk RA, Casey LC, Silver MR, Bone RC. Medical effectiveness of esophageal balloon pressure manometry in weaning patients from mechanical ventilation. Crit Care Med 1995; 23:504–509.

109. Banner MJ, Kirby RR, Kirton OC, DeHaven CB, Blanch PB. Breathing frequency and pattern are poor predictors of work of breathing in patients receiving pressure support ventilation. Chest 1995; 108:1338–1344.

110. Banner MJ, Kirby RR, Gabrielli A, Blanch PB, Layon AJ. Partially and totally unloading respiratory muscles based on real-time measurements of work of breathing. A clinical approach. Chest 1994; 106:1835–1842.

111. Bellemare F, Grassino A. Effect of pressure and timing of contraction on human diaphragm fatigue. J Appl Physiol 1982; 53:1190–1195.

112. Field S, Sanci S, Grassino A. Respiratory muscle oxygen consumption estimated by the diaphragm pressure-time index. J Appl Physiol 1984; 57:44–51.

113. Armaganidis A, Roussos C. Measurement of the work of breathing in the critically ill patient. In: Roussos C, ed. The Thorax. 2d ed. New York: Marcel Dekker, 1995: 1231–1274.

114. Karetzky MS, Cain SM. Effect of carbon dioxide on oxygen uptake during hyperventilation in normal man. J Appl Physiol 1970; 28:8–12.

115. Kennedy SK, Weintraub RM, Skillman JJ. Cardiorespiratory and sympathoadrenal responses during weaning from controlled ventilation. Surgery 1977; 82:233–240.

116. Oh TE, Bhatt S, Lin ES, Hutchinson RC, Low JM. Plasma catecholamines and oxygen consumption during weaning from mechanical ventilation. Intens Care Med 1991; 17:199–203.

117. Hubmayr RD, Loosbrock LM, Gillespie DJ, Rodarte JR. Oxygen uptake during weaning from mechanical ventilation. Chest 1988; 94:1148–1155.

118. Ultman JS, Bursztein S. Analysis of error in the determination of respiratory gas exchange at varying FIO_2. J Appl Physiol 1981; 50:210–216.

119. Nishimura M, Taenaka N, Takezawa J. Oxygen cost of breathing and inspiratory work of ventilation as weaning monitor in critically ill (abstr). Crit Care Med 1984; 12:258.

120. Lewis WD, Chwals W, Benotti PN, Lakshman K, O'Donnell C, Blackburn GL, et al. Bedside assessment of the work of breathing. Crit Care Med 1988; 16:117–122.

121. Kemper M, Weissman C, Askanazi J, Hyman AI, Kinney JM. Metabolic and respiratory changes during weaning from mechanical ventilation. Chest 1987; 92:979–983.

122. Shepherd AP, Kiel JW. A model of countercurrent shunting of oxygen in the intestinal villus. Am J Physiol 1992; 262:H1136–1142.

123. Brown SD, Gutierrez G. Gut mucosal pH monitoring. In: Tobin MJ, ed. Principles and Practice of Intensive Care Monitoring. New York: McGraw-Hill, 1998:351–368.

124. Desai MII, Herndon DN, Rutan RL, Abston S, Linares HA. Ischemic intestinal complications in patients with burns. Surg Gynecol Obstet 1991; 172:257–261.

125. Fink MP. Adequacy of gut oxygenation in endotoxemia and sepsis. Crit Care Med 1993; 21:S4–8.

126. Ivatury RR, Simon RJ, Havriliak D, Garcia C, Greenbarg J, Stahl WM. Gastric mucosal pH and oxygen delivery and oxygen consumption indices in the assessment of adequacy of resuscitation after trauma: a prospective, randomized study. J Trauma 1995; 39:128–34.

127. Grum CM, Fiddian-Green RG, Pittenger GL, Grant BJ, Rothman ED, Dantzker DR. Adequacy of tissue oxygenation in intact dog intestine. J Appl Physiol 1984; 56:1065–1069.

128. Bouachour G, Guiraud MP, Gouello JP, Roy PM, Alquier P. Gastric intramucosal pH: an indicator of weaning outcome from mechanical ventilation in COPD patients. Eur Respir J 1996; 9:1868–1873.

129. Abalos A, Leibowitz AB, Distefano D, Halpern N, Iberti T. Myocardial ischemia during the weaning period. Am J Crit Care 1992; 1:32–36.

130. Chatila W, Ani S, Guaglianone D, Jacob B, Amoateng-Adjepong Y, Manthous CA. Cardiac ischemia during weaning from mechanical ventilation. Chest 1996; 109:1577–1583.

131. Hurford WE, Favorito F. Association of myocardial ischemia with failure to wean from mechanical ventilation. Crit Care Med 1995; 23:1475–1480.

132. Hurford WE, Lynch KE, Strauss HW, Lowenstein E, Zapol W. Myocardial perfusion as assessed by thallium-201 scintigraphy during the discontinuation of mechanical ventilation in ventilator-dependent patients. Anesthesiology 1991; 74:1007–1016.

133. Lemaire F, Teboul JL, Cinotti L, Giotto G, Abrouk F, Steg G, et al. Acute left ventricular dysfunction during unsuccessful weaning from mechanical ventilation. Anesthesiology 1988; 69:171–179.

134. Rasanen J, Nikki P, Heikkila J. Acute myocardial infarction complicated by respiratory failure. The effects of mechanical ventilation. Chest 1984; 85:21–28.

135. Colice GL, Stukel TA, Dain B. Laryngeal complications of prolonged intubation. Chest 1989; 96:877–884.

136. Darmon JY, Rauss A, Dreyfuss D, Bleichner G, Elkharrat D, Schlemmer B, et al. Evaluation of risk factors for laryngeal edema after tracheal extubation in adults and its prevention by dexamethasone. A placebo-controlled, double-blind, multicenter study. Anesthesiology 1992; 77:245–251.

137. Whited RE. A prospective study of laryngotracheal sequelae in long-term intubation. Laryngoscope 1984; 94:367–377.

138. Adderley RJ, Mullins GC. When to extubate the croup patient: the ''leak'' test. Can J Anaesth 1987; 34:304–306.

139. Fisher MM, Raper RF. The 'cuff-leak' test for extubation. Anaesthesia 1992; 47:10–12.

140. Kemper KJ, Benson MS, Bishop MJ. Predictors of postextubation stridor in pediatric trauma patients. Crit Care Med 1991; 19:352–355.
141. Marik PE. The cuff leak test as a predictor of postextubation stridor: a prospective study. Respir Care 1996; 41:509–511.
142. Miller RL, Cole RP. Association between reduced cuff leak volume and postextubation stridor. Chest 1996; 110:1035–1040.
143. Fagan TJ. Letter: Nomogram for Bayes theorem. N Engl J Med 1975; 293:257.

16

Optimizing the Efficiency of Weaning from Mechanical Ventilation

E. WESLEY ELY

Vanderbilt University Medical Center
Nashville, Tennessee

DAVID L. BOWTON

Wake Forest University School of Medicine
Winston-Salem, North Carolina

EDWARD F. HAPONIK

The Johns Hopkins Medical Center
Baltimore, Maryland

I. Introduction

Exciting advances have been made in our understanding of the optimal methods of managing patients receiving mechanical ventilation (MV). During the past two decades, a widely held view regarding the discontinuation of MV has been that a gradual reduction in ventilatory support is important, reflected in ubiquitously applied, but varying forms of "weaning." In just the past 5 years, over 500 articles have been written on weaning from artificial respiration, underscoring the interest, importance, and uncertainties surrounding this clinical issue. Despite the popularity of the term "weaning," one of the most important concepts to arise from recent prospective, randomized, controlled trials (RCTs) is that a gradual reduction in ventilator support may unnecessarily delay extubation of patients who have recovered from respiratory failure (1). With increasing recognition of the complications of MV and growing attention to resources consumed in the care of patients with respiratory failure, a change in the clinical paradigm is warranted. Evidence supports the concept that the rapid identification of patients who have recovered from respiratory failure is more important than manipulation of "weaning" modes in an attempt to accelerate recovery (2–5).

With this in mind, several groups have investigated the utility of protocols in liberating patients from MV. Economic and organizational pressures have encouraged physicians to be even more efficient in the management of patients. We have spent the past 5 years studying the development, implementation, and efficacy of ventilator management protocols for patients with respiratory failure. We have shown that one can improve upon the best practices of board-certified intensivists and cardiologists with the use of a simple two-step protocol incorporating daily screening followed by spontaneous breathing trials in patients who have recovered sufficiently to pass the daily screen. Patient safety is not jeopardized, and complication rates may actually be reduced.

In this chapter, we use an evidence-based review to discuss the salient aspects of establishing a protocolized approach to mechanically ventilated patients. While each institution must make its own adjustments in incorporating these protocols, we present important general concepts that may ease the process of implementation and enhance success.

II. Prospective Randomized Controlled Trials—What Have We Learned?

An early investigation of weaning parameters (6) noted that the weaning process is often arbitrary, "based on judgment and experience." A survey of MV in Spain determined that "weaning time" accounted for over 40% of total ventilator time (7), demonstrating a considerable opportunity for improvement. Despite numerous efforts to determine the best method of weaning patients from MV, it was not until 1994 that any randomized controlled trial (RCT) showed one method (pressure support ventilation, or PSV) to be superior to others (8). Yet, within a year, another well-performed RCT showed seemingly conflicting results, with spontaneous breathing trials leading to earlier extubation among mechanically ventilated patients (4) (Fig. 1). Although these investigations reached contradictory conclusions, these trials showed that (1) weaning strategies influence the duration of MV; (2) the specific criteria used to initiate changes in ventilatory support influence outcome; and (3) the most ineffective approach was intermittent mandatory ventilation, a previously widely used strategy.

Several lines of evidence suggest that physicians do not discontinue MV efficiently. In the above-cited studies (4,8), 69–76% of patients evaluated for enrollment were judged ready for immediate extubation. In addition, as many as half of patients who extubate themselves prematurely do not require reintubation within 24 hours (9,10). Physicians' predictions of whether patients can have MV successfully discontinued are inaccurate, with positive and negative predictive values of only 50% and 67%, respectively (11).

Neither of the above-mentioned studies included a nonprotocol "control" group, which left clinicians without assurance that protocols were superior to their

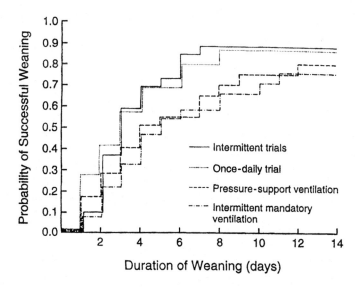

Figure 1 Kaplan-Meier curves of the probability of successful weaning with four different techniques. After adjustment for baseline characteristics in a Cox proportional-hazards model, the rate of successful weaning with a once-daily trial of spontaneous breathing was 2.83 times higher than that with intermittent mandatory ventilation ($p < 0.006$) and 2.05 times higher than that with pressure support ventilation ($p < 0.04$). (From Ref. 4.)

individual decision-making at the bedside. In order to answer this question, we enrolled 300 mechanically ventilated medical and nonsurgical cardiac patients into a RCT in which the treatment group was "weaned" to extubation using a two-step process of screening by respiratory care practitioners followed by spontaneous breathing trial when recovery was sufficient to "pass" the daily screening (5). The daily screening and spontaneous breathing trial are defined in Appendix 1. Because of the difficulty in having busy clinicians change practice patterns, we also incorporated a written and verbal physician prompt into the treatment arm, which notified them when a patient had successfully passed a spontaneous breathing trial.

Importantly, the physicians involved in our investigations were all board-certified intensivists or cardiologists operating in "closed" intensive care units. A survey taken prior to initiating the investigation indicated that the majority (68%) doubted that their practice style could be improved by routine objective measurements along with increased input from respiratory care practitioners. They felt confident in their level of efficiency in removing patients from MV and that the protocol would not lead to improved outcomes. However, the outcomes of the investigation included removal from MV 2 days earlier in the protocol-directed group despite a higher severity of illness, 50% fewer complications, and a reduction in the cost of intensive care unit stay by $5,000 per patient (5).

Kaplan-Meier survival analysis (Fig. 2), and Cox proportional-hazards model demonstrated that subjects assigned to the intervention group had MV success-fully discontinued earlier (relative rate of successful extubation = 2.13, 95% confidence interval, 1.58–2.86; $p < 0.0001$).

The protocol encouraged extubation as soon as recovery was documented, and we expected a higher rate of complications (particularly reintubation) in the intervention group. In fact, the risk of nonlethal complications was lower in the intervention group. The reintubation rate in our institution prior to the initiation of this investigation was 8%, comparable to that seen in our controls. The inter-vention group experienced a lower rate of reintubation (4%), perhaps because of careful objective screening prior to extubation. Because reintubation is associated with an increased risk of nosocomial pneumonia (12), this finding may prove especially important if confirmed. The reintubation rates in this trial compare favorably to those observed in two recent large weaning trials, 7.3% (8) and 17.7% (4). Subsequent implementation of this protocol in 530 patients at another large medical center was associated with a similar reintubation rate (i.e., 6%) and no increased risk of mortality (13).

Because the techniques and measurements require no special monitoring or equipment, no additional expenditures beyond staffing, and no laboratory studies

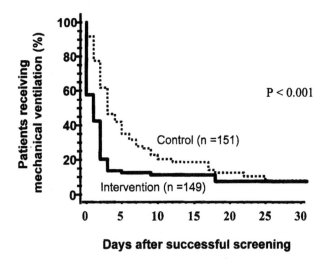

Figure 2 Kaplan-Meier curves of the risk of remaining mechanically ventilated in proto-col vs. control groups. After adjusting for baseline characteristics using covariates that described severity of illness (APACHE II), age, gender, race, ICU location, and duration of intubation prior to enrollment, a Cox proportional-hazards analysis demonstrated that subjects in the protocol groups were removed from mechanical ventilation more rapidly than controls (relative rate of successful extubation = 2.13, 95% confidence interval, 1.55–2.92; $p < 0.001$). (From Ref. 5.)

(arterial blood gases were optional), we believe this protocol to be broadly applicable in university and community hospital settings alike. It has been recommended that ICUs either adopt or adapt the methods of this validated protocol or establish their own protocols with similar goals (14). Use of the protocol to manage just four patients would result in one individual being off MV after 48 hours who otherwise would not have been. In addition, if the protocol were used in six patients, one less complication would be expected.

Simultaneously, Kollef and colleagues (15) were conducting another RCT ($n = 357$) of protocol-directed versus physician-directed weaning in four ICUs (two medical and two surgical). This investigation incorporated three separate "weaning" protocols because of difficulty in achieving consensus among different units, underscoring the practical challenges facing implementation of protocols. The protocol-directed group incorporated an amalgam of spontaneous breaths trial, PSV, and synchronized intermittent mandatory ventilation protocols, and demonstrated an earlier initiation of weaning efforts and a median duration of MV of 35 hours versus 44 hours in the physician-directed group (Fig. 3).

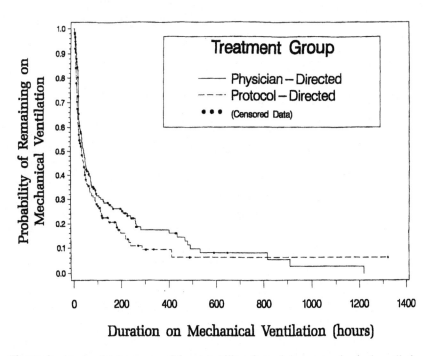

Figure 3 Kaplan-Meier curves of the probability of remaining on mechanical ventilation according to protocol group (dashed line) and control group (solid line). Cox-proportional hazards analysis, adjusting for covariates including severity of illness, showed that the rate of successful weaning was significantly higher in the protocol-directed group than in the control group (risk ratio 1.31, 95% CI 1.15–1.50). (From Ref. 15.)

Prospective investigations of strategies to reduce the cost of intensive care are few. In our study, the total cost of ICU care throughout the study period for the control group was $4,297,024 and for the intervention group was $3,855,001, representing a savings of $442,023. The 25% reduction in the cost of ICU care associated with the use of this protocol presents the opportunity for sizable financial savings when applied throughout an institution or health care system. If applied only to medical and nonsurgical cardiac patients within our institution, the annualized cost savings for ICU care were estimated at greater than $700,000. Kollef et al. (15) reported a savings of $42,960 in their protocol-directed weaning group.

During implementation of our protocol, physician time commitment appeared to be minimal, since respiratory therapists and nurses who were already caring for the patients did most of the monitoring. Personnel expenses are thought to account for more than 50% of the cost of MV (16). While we did not formally assess time spent by the respiratory therapists and nurses instituting the protocol, the daily screen generally required only a few minutes per patient per day and was incorporated readily into respiratory therapists' routines. Some investigators have advocated the use of a weaning team (17), though RCTs of this strategy are lacking. Future RCTs demonstrating the superiority of protocolized care being delivered via a weaning team versus physicians, nurses, and therapists will help elucidate the optimal approach.

III. Daily Screening Techniques

It has been suspected (but not proven) that a daily screening tool could, if applied from the day of initiation of MV, greatly accelerate progress toward extubation. Physicians often fail to identify patients who can be successfully extubated and tend to underestimate the probability of successful discontinuation of MV (18). In one investigation, physicians' clinical judgement had a specificity of 35% and a likelihood ratio of 1.5 (11), values that indicate little clinical utility without the use of objective monitoring parameters. We hypothesized that the busy clinician was unable to systematically accomplish the appropriate screening of patients while burdened with so many other individual patient concerns and professional duties.

Many weaning parameters have been proposed to identify patients ready for extubation (18–30), and range from simple maneuvers [e.g., counting and measuring breaths (19)] to more complicated techniques requiring the insertion of esophageal or gastric balloons (20,21), or use of computerized decision support models (18). Eloquently performed investigations of difficult-to-wean patients have determined that in addition to the frequency/tidal volume ratio (f/V_t) (19), physiological measurements including an airway occlusion pressure at 0.1 second ($P_{0.1}$) above 4.5 cm H_2O (9,23,31) and a tension-time index above 0.15 (30,32) are helpful determinants of diaphragmatic fatigue and weaning failure. In general, these tests indicate that the load imposed on the inspiratory muscles is in excess of the neuromuscular capacity. Reliance on such measures is appealing because of their physiological basis. However, in the majority of patients these technically demanding tests are neither necessary nor practical for widespread use within the confines of a protocol. Until recently, no RCT had documented that application of any tools produced better outcomes than physician judgment alone (5).

Manthous et al. (2) arrived at the following summary statements regarding three commonly used weaning parameters: (1) maximal inspiratory pressure or NIF—the area under a receiver-operating-characteristic (ROC) curve (i.e., sensitivity vs. 1-specificity) was 0.61 to 0.68; (2) spontaneous minute ventilation—shows even poorer predictive combination, with ROC curve area of 0.40–0.54; and (3) f/V_t or rapid shallow breathing index—yielded an ROC curve area of 0.75–0.89. Jaeschke et al. (33) eloquently discussed a process to determine whether these parameters are useful clinically to diagnose weanability. The f/V_t threshold level of 105 breaths/min/L chosen by Yang and Tobin (19) has a relatively high ROC curve area and appeared useful in our screening at least in part because it is followed by a second step—spontaneous breathing trials. In fact, many patients with a ratio between 80 and 105 may fail spontaneous breathing trials (31,33). While alterations in the diagnostic thresholds for different components of the daily screening (e.g., the best "cut-off" for the f/V_t) may be appropriate, this will be discussed below in Sec. XII.

After review of the literature, we chose a set of five simple parameters to use as a daily screen to be obtained on all patients. In the original investigation, a daily screening test was obtained on all 300 enrolled patients each morning between 06:00 and 07:00 by the units' respiratory therapist. In order to "pass" the daily screen, all of the following criteria had to be met:

1. $Pao_2/F_iO_2 \geq 200$ (P/F ratio)—e.g., Pao_2 of 100/F_iO_2 of 0.5 = 200.
2. Positive end-expiratory pressure (PEEP) ≤ 5 cm H_2O.
3. Adequate cough during suctioning (i.e., intact airway reflexes).
4. Patient could not be receiving any vasopressor drips or sedatives by continuous infusion. Dopamine was allowed if dosed <5 μg/kg/min, and intermittent dosing of sedatives was allowed.
5. Frequency/tidal volume ratio (f/V_t) ≤ 105—also known as the rapid shallow breathing index (RSBI). Measured after 1 minute of spontaneous breathing with ventilator rate set to 0 and pressure support set to 0. Average V_t calculated by dividing f into V_e ($V_t = V_e/f$), alternatively: $f/V_t = f^2/V_e$; e.g., rate (f) of 20, V_e of 10 L/min: (20 × 20) divided by 10 = f/V_t of 40. To measure the f/V_t, the patient was placed on continuous positive airway pressure with no mandatory ventilator breaths and with pressure support removed for one minute (19). Minute

ventilation and respiratory rate were recorded as measured by the Puritan-Bennett 7200 or Siemens 900 mechanical ventilator, and tidal volume (V_T) was obtained by dividing the minute ventilation by respiratory frequency (f).

In our original investigation, it took these MICU and CCU patients an average of 2–3 days to pass the daily screening (5). While 75% of our patients eventually passed the screening, another recent report found that 290 of 537 (54%) of patients passed the same screening tool (13). During daily screening assessments in over 1500 patients, there were no complications detected (e.g., during f/V_t) such as temporally associated self-extubation, prolonged desaturation, or hemodynamic instability. During our hospital-wide implementation of the protocol, once patients passed the daily screening ($n = 722$), 41% ($n = 298$) consistently passed the daily screening while 59% ($n = 424$) fluctuated between passing and not passing (34). When the daily screening was passed, patients passed the subsequent spontaneous breathing trial 75.4% of the time, a rate that did not vary over the 12-month period of implementation or among services and units ($p = 0.297$). Overly rigid interpretation of the "rules" of the protocol seemed counterproductive. For example, determining on consecutive days that a patient failed the daily screening because the Pao_2/F_1o_2 ratio was 198 (rather than being > 200) or their f/V_T was 107 (rather than being <105) was felt to be inappropriate because some patients do not fit within the confines of specified "cut-offs" or thresholds (26,33,35,36). Continuing to advance patients through the protocol at this point and assessing their ability to breathe with a spontaneous breathing trial proved to be successful in many of these circumstances.

IV. Spontaneous Breathing Trials

Because of the heterogeneity of patients with respiratory failure and the dynamic interplay of multiple factors determining their need for ventilatory support, we believe there are inherent limitations of any current measures used to determine whether the patient can be liberated. Rather, allowing the patient to breathe spontaneously for a predetermined time trial during close monitoring (i.e., an SBT) is the optimum confirmation of the patient's readiness for extubation.

A. What Is a Spontaneous Breathing Trial and Who Receives One?

- Trials of spontaneous breathing are conducted for 30–120 minutes using "flow-by" mode or T-piece, with ventilator rate set to 0 and pressure support set to 0.
- Patients who pass the daily screening are candidates for a spontaneous breathing trial.

B. Who Performs the Spontaneous Trial?

- Respiratory care practitioners or nurses perform daily screening and either initiate or prompt a physician to order an spontaneous breathing trial.
- Respiratory care practitioners or nurses initiate the spontaneous breathing trial, monitor the patient during the trial (in conjunction with the nurse), and reinitiates MV if criteria for trial termination are met.
- ICU nurses monitor the patient during the trial and notify the respiratory care practitioner if termination criteria are met.

C. When Is a Spontaneous Trial Terminated?

- If the patient successfully tolerates the spontaneous breathing trial for up to 2 hours, or when one of the following conditions is met:
- Respiratory rate > 35 for more than 5 minutes.
- $Sao_2 < 90\%$ during more than 30 seconds of good quality measurement despite O_2 supplementation.
- 20% increase or decrease in heart rate for >5 minutes.
- SBP > 180 or SBP < 90 during at least one minute of continuous recording or repeated measurements.
- Agitation, anxiety, or diaphoresis confirmed as a change from baseline and present for more than 5 minutes.
- Some investigators have repeated the f/V_T after 30 minutes to 3 hours of spontaneous breathing and found that this approach raised the accuracy by about 10% (36).

D. What Does It Mean if a Patient Passes a Spontaneous Breathing Trial?

- Successful completion of a 2-hour spontaneous breathing trial in non-neurologically impaired patients indicates a 90% chance of successfully staying off of MV for 48 hours (5).
- After passing a spontaneous breathing trial, the median length of time a patient remained on the ventilator was 1 day, a rate that did not vary among different patient populations or ICUs (34). This time on the ventilator *after* passing the SBT represents an opportunity to *further* improve the efficiency of liberation from mechanical ventilation.

The spontaneous breathing trial described above was used in the aforementioned investigations (4,5) and further validated by other investigators (31). In a preliminary report, Wood and colleagues (13) found that of 275 patients passing the daily screening who were selected for an spontaneous breathing trial, 264 (96%) passed, with 232 of 264 (88%) extubated, and 217 of these patients (94%)

remaining extubated for 3 days. This experience confirms the low reintubation rates described previously. Esteban and the Spanish Lung Failure Collaborative Group have defined practical aspects of the spontaneous breathing trial. These investigators showed in a RCT of 526 patients that successful extubation was achieved equally effectively with spontaneous breathing trials lasting 30 minutes or 120 minutes (37). In a previous study, they had documented that the spontaneous breathing trial could be conducted with either a low level of PSV or a T-piece (38). In our studies, SBTs were performed with either standard T-tube circuits or flow-triggered openings of the demand valve without additional support. Incorporating flow-triggering during the spontaneous breathing trial was a convenience that minimized respiratory therapist involvement and had not been investigated by others. Taken together, these investigations support institutional variations in the specific method of conducting spontaneous breathing trials. In fact, individual physicians may wish to tailor the technique and duration of spontaneous breathing trials to individual patients.

Not only is passing a spontaneous breathing trial clinically important, but failing to pass a spontaneous breathing trial has major prognostic implications. First of all, most patients who failed a breathing trial do so fairly early (37). Vallverdu et al. (31) have studied outcomes of a 2-hour T-piece trial and found that the mean time to failure (among those who could not sustain 120 minutes of spontaneous breathing) was 39 minutes (Fig. 4). However, 36% of patients failed after the first 30 minutes of successfully breathing on their own. None of seven weaning parameters consistently predicted time to failure. Because of the

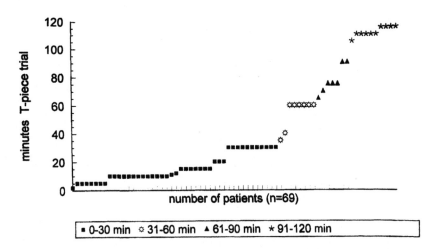

Figure 4 Time to failure of spontaneous breathing trial among 69 patients with failed attempt. Distribution of patients according to the time of spontaneous breathing in the weaning trial before reconnection to mechanical ventilation. (From Ref. 31.)

morbidity and mortality associated with reintubation, better indices need to be developed to identify patients who can sustain spontaneous breathing without distress, but who nonetheless will require reintubation after extubation (37).

V. Prediction Models

A. Prognostic Significance of a Daily Screening of Weaning Parameters

The early identification of patients who will require prolonged MV is difficult (39). The management of these chronically ventilated patients beyond their acute stay in the ICU has been addressed recently in other reports (40) and in a consensus statement by the ACCP (41). The following discussion will focus on the prognostic significance of the daily screen during the initial ventilator course. Although severity scores have some prognostic value, they are limited in value as clinical tools. During the development of the APACHE III system, an analysis was performed of data collected on 5915 mechanically ventilated patients in an attempt to predict the duration of MV. These authors, using logistic regression, determined that duration is primarily a function of the admitting diagnosis and the degree of physiological derangement as measured by the acute physiology score (42). While the predictive equation may help as a research tool, it was not meant for clinical use at the bedside. Others have concluded that a lung injury score of <1 is predictive of MV less than 15 days, but that if the lung injury score is ≥ 1, "nothing further about the expected duration of MV can be said" (43).

B. Prognosis Over Time Postintubation

The length of time on the ventilator has now been shown to be an independent contributor to hospital mortality, which supports the need for liberation from mechanical ventilation at the earliest possible time in hepatitis recovery and the need for protocols to aid this process. The relationship of patient status (discharged, deceased, and still hospitalized) to time after intubation (44) is presented in Table 1. In addition, daily screening (pass vs. fail) and extubation (successfully extubated vs. on ventilator) results are presented each day for those patients still hospitalized, along with the percentage of patients in each category who survived until discharge. The percentage of patients who survived until discharge was higher both for those who had passed the daily screening compared to those who had not yet passed (78% vs. 50%, $p = 0.001$) and for those who had been successfully extubated compared to those who still required MV (84% vs. 60%, $p = 0.001$). In addition, the difference in survival between patients who were extubated successfully and those who required continued MV remained relatively constant over time and was statistically significant for each of the seven time periods examined. By contrast, while the difference in survival between patients who had passed the daily screening and those who had not passed it was signifi-

Table 1 The Temporal Relationship of Passing the Daily Screen and Successful Extubation to Hospital Survival ($n = 300$)

Status	Days postintubation						
	3	6	9	12	15	18	21
No. discharged	2	18	34	61	86	104	115
No. deceased	18	37	56	70	82	89	96
No. remaining in hospital[a]	280	245	210	169	132	107	89
Daily screen							
No. passed (at any time)	104	133	137	114	93	78	66
Surviving until discharge, %	78	80	77	75	76	76	77
No. failed (not yet passed)	176	112	73	55	39	29	23
Surviving until discharge, %	50	47	60	65	67	69	74
p-value[b]	0.001	0.001	0.013	0.18	0.25	0.48	0.74
Extubation							
No. successful extubation	51	95	110	102	82	66	53
Surviving until discharge, %	84	89	89	88	88	89	88
No. still on ventilator	229	150	100	67	50	41	33
Surviving until discharge, %	60	47	49	48	50	49	59
p-value[c]	0.001	0.001	0.001	0.001	0.001	0.001	0.001

[a] The number of patients remaining at any given time (i.e., not discharged or deceased) will be used to determine relationships between hospital survival and passing/failing the DS or successful extubation.

[b] p-Value for null hypothesis that % surviving until discharge is same for those passing vs. failing DS. Passing the DS is associated with a higher hospital survival for the first 9–10 days, while successful extubation is associated with a higher hospital survival through day 21.

[c] p-Value for null hypothesis that % surviving is same for those successfully extubated vs. still on ventilator. (From Ref. 44.)

cant ($p = 0.001$) at 3 days postintubation, this difference decreased over time and was no longer statistically significant by 12 days postintubation ($p = 0.18$). Proportional hazards analysis of time until in-hospital death confirmed the beneficial effect of passing the daily screening during the first 10 days ($p = 0.01$) after adjustment for differences in severity of illness, age, race, gender, diagnosis, and treatment assignment.

The relationship between duration of MV and survival was significant (Fig. 5, $p = 0.02$), with the mortality rate increasing steadily throughout the first 3 weeks: the mortality rate was 33% (95% confidence interval of 26–40%) for those on MV for 1–7 days, 48% for those on MV for 8–14 days (35–59%), and 62% for those on MV 15–21 days (39–78%). Patients on MV for more than 21 days had a lower mortality of 41% (24–57%) (44). Proportional hazards analysis of time until in-hospital death confirmed this relationship between survival and duration of MV even after adjustment for differences in severity of illness, age, race, gender, diagnosis, and treatment assignment ($p = 0.001$). This observation supports longstanding anecdotal impressions and findings of a previous report of a multicenter registry of acute respiratory distress syndrome patients in which

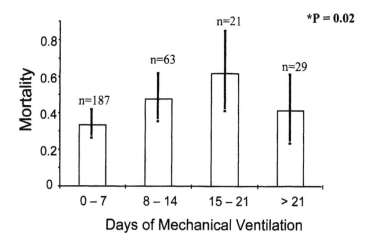

Figure 5 Duration of mechanical ventilation and survival. There was a significant relationship between the number of days of mechanical ventilation and survival ($p = 0.02$). The mortality rate increased steadily from 1 to 3 weeks of ventilator usage, and then dropped for those requiring more than 21 days of mechanical ventilation. Proportional hazards analysis of time until in-hospital death confirmed the relationship between survival and duration of mechanical ventilation even after adjustment for differences in severity of illness, age, race, gender, diagnosis, and treatment assignment ($p = 0.001$). (Adapted from data presented in Ref. 44.)

85% of the nonsurvivors had died by the fourth week, and the subsequent mortality rate was much lower than that of the population as a whole (45). At least one other investigation has found an association between mortality and the duration of MV (46).

Although reducing the length of time that patients spend on MV is essential, neither the predictors of liberation from the ventilator (i.e., use of weaning parameters) nor the number of days on MV have previously been associated independently with survival. Our data provide new information regarding the prognostic value of the daily screening of ventilated patients by RCPs and/or physicians. The daily screening predicted the likelihood of successful extubation with an accuracy of 82%, and its sensitivity and positive predictive values both approached 90%. While liberation from MV was predictive of survival at any time during the hospital stay ($p = 0.001$), the prognostic significance of the daily screening for hospital survival was related to how early after intubation it was passed. The difference in survival between patients who had passed and those who had not passed the daily screening was significant for 10 days postintubation, but progressively decreased over time.

These data provide several other important insights. Because passing the daily screening was associated with a reduced incidence of prolonged MV (3% vs. 30%, $p = 0.0001$), this monitoring technique may have useful triage implications for patients being considered for referral to regional weaning centers or for timing of tracheostomy in anticipation of a need for chronic airway support (47). For example, if the patient eventually passes the daily screen, a physician may delay tracheostomy and/or triage to a chronic ventilator facility. Although a negative screen identifies the majority of those who will require prolonged MV, the information is of little clinical use because the majority of those failing the daily screen in the first 10 days may still be extubated prior to the fourth week.

In conclusion, successfully removing the mechanical ventilator at any time is associated with higher survival rates, which may be independent of severity of illness. During the first 10 days of MV, passing the daily screen is a predictor of survival and supports attempts at optimizing liberation from MV. Failure to pass the screen of weaning parameters is of less value prognostically, since up to 29% of such patients will survive their hospital stay. While physicians should always be motivated to remove ventilators as early as possible, the time that elapses after the patient passes the daily screen but remains on MV presents a special opportunity to improve the efficiency of care.

VI. Large-Scale Implementation of a Protocol

The protocol offered here is a guide and is not meant as a rigid stand-alone device to implement directly. These tools (see Appendixes 1–3, which are daily screen and spontaneous breathing trial definitions, the Protocol Flow Sheet, and the Data Collection Sheet) may need to be modified according to institutional needs and preferences. The implementation process itself is challenging and discussed below.

The ultimate success of any patient management protocol depends upon the level of institutional commitment to improving outcomes as well as the team's leadership, persistence, and consistency in implementation. Protocolized care has been advocated in many facets of medicine, but relinquishing control of the patient's management often creates resentment and frustration on the part of physicians. Even when the evidence clearly supports change, it is very difficult to get physicians to alter their management styles (48), and what is really required is a *change of culture*. In certain circles of physicians within some institutions, there may be a low "readiness to change," and these professionals may require either motivational interventions or consultation with respected opinion leaders (48,49). Important considerations that may increase the chances of successfully changing the behavior of health care professionals include education, timely feedback, participation by physicians in the effort to change, administrative interventions, and even financial incentives and penalties (48). Each of these factors has relevance to implementation of new approaches toward MV.

While our original protocol documented the vital contributions of nonphysician health care professionals in the management of ventilated medical patients, it was conducted as a therapist-focused, rather than a therapist-driven protocol. Other groups have stressed the importance of "weaning teams" (17) and therapist-driver protocol (50,51), but there are few data documenting the feasibility and/or steps necessary to implement such protocols on a large scale with effective monitoring of protocol compliance. We sought to prospectively monitor and describe the institution-wide implementation of our previously validated approach. Importantly, we made slight modifications and reintroduced the protocol *without* the daily supervision of a weaning team, physician, or respiratory care practitioner supervisor in order to test its feasibility as a therapy-driven protocol (see Appendix 2) (34). Lastly, we wished to explore the challenges of modifying respiratory care practitioners and physicians' practice styles in the "out-of-study" setting over a one-year period.

A total of 1167 patients were enrolled in the protocol, and 9048 patient days of MV were appraised (34). The mean age was 60.1 $\pm$ 16.9 (S.D.), and there were 605 men (56.7%) and 462 women (43.3%). The principal causes of their respiratory failure were acute respiratory distress syndrome (14%), trauma (13%), chronic obstructive pulmonary disease (11%), complications related to general or cardiothoracic surgery (21%), congestive heart failure or myocardial infarction (12%), or other causes (29%). Compliance with the protocol was monitored closely using a daily data collection tool (see Appendix 3). Respiratory

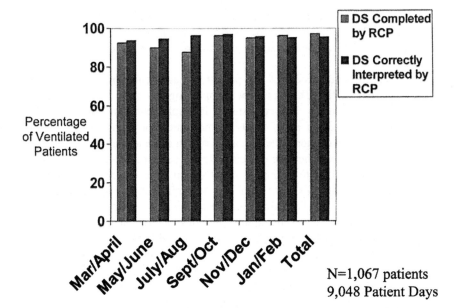

N=1,067 patients
9,048 Patient Days

Figure 6 Histogram showing completion and correct interpretation of daily screen. This shows the percent of mechanically ventilated patients ($n = 1067$ patients; 9048 patient-ventilator days) who had completion of their daily screen and correct interpretation of the daily screen data by the respiratory care practitioners during each period of implementation. Total daily screen completion rate was 97% across the year of implementation with a 95% correct interpretation rate of the data within the daily screen ($p > 0.35$). (From Ref. 34.)

care practitioners completion of the daily screen varied little on average throughout the year, with an overall completion of >95% (Fig. 6) ($p = 0.35$). Correct interpretation of the daily screen was also high (95% overall correct) ($p = 0.42$). Once the daily screening was completed and passed, the next step of the protocol was to assess the patient's ability to pass an spontaneous breathing trial. Overall compliance rates in obtaining a spontaneous breathing trial were initially low, but they increased in the fifth and sixth months and remained fairly stable thereafter. To determine whether the frequency of ordering spontaneous breathing trials differed in relation to physician specialty, we compared medical and surgical performance (Fig. 7). Across the year of implementation, spontaneous breathing trials were more often ordered on the medicine services (81% vs. 63%, $p = 0.001$).

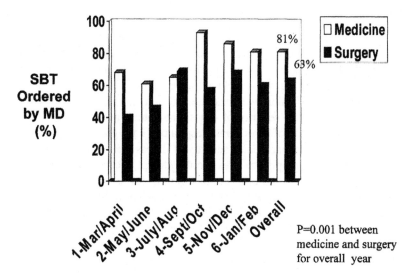

Figure 7 Histogram showing the percent of time that physicians ordered spontaneous breathing trials. Once approached by respiratory care practitioners with data that their patients had passed the daily screen, the compliance rates with spontaneous breathing trials were 81% for medicine vs. 63% for surgery ($p = 0.001$). (From Ref. 34.)

VII. Outcomes of Mechanically Ventilated Patients

We noted a fairly consistent duration of MV for our patients (between 5 and 7 days). While the duration of the spontaneous breathing trial was 2 hours unless the attending physician specifically requested an abbreviated trial, we did not monitor the frequency of 30-minute vs. 2-hour spontaneous breathing trials or their relative accuracy in predicting successful extubation (37). Throughout the year, 75% of patients who were assessed with spontaneous breathing trials (after having passed a daily screen) successfully passed their spontaneous breathing trials. While one patient had temporally associated hypotension and desaturation, no other complications were noted from spontaneous breathing trials. However, a potentially important, but unmeasured, complication of failed spontaneous breathing trial is the possibility that respiratory muscle fatigue resulting from the initial spontaneous breathing trial would adversely impact the results of the next trial.

Mechanical ventilator–associated outcomes included a reintubation rate of 14%, tracheostomy rate of 18%, and prolonged duration of MV (>21 days) of 13%. The study did not compare management with this therapist-driven protocol to a control group, nor was it our purpose to restudy the efficacy and cost savings of the protocol. Rather, we appraised the complicated interplay of program implementation and the challenges of altering physician and nonphysician behavior. Important differences from the original investigation that precluded a direct comparison of outcome measures included a major shift in the patient population, more than a third of whom were trauma and other surgical patients, the lack of prospectively recorded severity of illness indicators, and marked expansion in the participating staff of physicians, respiratory care practitioners, and nurses. Future investigations that include severity of illness measurements, complication rates, and protocol compliance rates should attempt to determine whether a varying impact on outcomes is achieved at different levels of protocol compliance. That the protocol was successful and safe in surgical ICU patients and accepted 63% of the time by surgeons overall during the first year is important new information, extending the relevance of this approach beyond medical and coronary ICUs.

VIII. Further Discussion of Implementation of Therapist-Driven Protocol

Experience has demonstrated the feasibility and challenges of implementing a previously validated protocol for discontinuation of MV. While therapist-driven protocols (TDPs) were used relatively infrequently in respiratory care departments as recently as a decade ago, surveys conducted by the American Association of Respiratory Care (52,53) showed that 60% of participating hospitals were currently using therapist-driven protocols and that one third had begun using therapist-driven protocols during the previous year. Several editorials and overviews address the scope of therapist-driven protocols, but few data have detailed the frequency of therapist-driven protocol use, implementation steps, or their impact upon ventilator weaning or management (50,51,54,55). We reintroduced a two-step process of daily screen and spontaneous breathing trial assessments (5) in our institution as a therapist-driven protocol. The lack of an overseeing "study physician," use of additional "readiness-to-wean" screen, and freedom of respiratory care practitioners to make these adjustments represented other important differences from our original protocol. Respiratory care practitioners competently performed and interpreted the daily screen, and both respiratory care practitioners and physicians improved their compliance rates in using spontaneous breathing trials in their patients who have recovered from respiratory failure. This experience demonstrated that successful implementation of the therapist-driven protocol required a commitment on the part of the hospital and its administration. The initial outlay of resources by the institution, including dedicated monitoring staff, computer support, and the time of respiratory care practitioners to attend in-

Table 2 Suggestions for Implementation of Protocols* in the ICU

To maximize the likelihood of success in achieving *both* a change in behavior and
     long-term protocol implementation:
  Identify the patient-care issue as a high-priority item within your institution (e.g.,
     ventilator weaning and timely extubation)
  Obtain baseline data (e.g., lengths of stay and complication rates)
  Base the program on medical evidence as well as reviews of other programs, and at-
     tain local expert opinion
  Acknowledge the need for a ''change in culture'' on the part of *both* physicians and
     nonphysician health care professionals
  Work hard to attain ''buy-in'' and participation of key opinion leaders/physicians
  Establish a team including the hospital administration, respiratory care practitioners,
     nurses/nurse practitioners, potentially ethicists, and physicians
  As a team, establish goals and set objective definitions of success and failure.
  Structure a graded, staged implementation process that provides the following:
    Education
    Timely feedback
    Compliance monitoring (particularly important, yet most often overlooked)
    Tracking of appropriate outcomes (including cost) via daily data collection
    Avoid complicated plans aimed at perfection; rather remain practical and useful
    Consider the entire process to be dynamic, not fixed; incorporate innovative
     changes over time to respond to lessons learned
  Avoid changing personnel too often
  Avoid overly rigid interpretation of the ''rules'' of the protocol
  Do not remove clinical judgment on part of any team members
  Acknowledge the need for and plan to have periodic refresher in-services and avoid
     the otherwise inevitable ''regression to baseline.''

---

* These general concepts may be broadly applied to numerous other patient-care protocols in critical
care.

services, was key. Several practical barriers to protocol implementation also became apparent. Although some aspects of this experience are unique to our medical center, many observations have important implications for institutions currently dealing with the need for a more systematic approach to MV and numerous
other aspects of care of the critically ill that are amenable to protocolization
(Table 2).

IX. Compliance with the Protocol

Other investigators have reported use of various weaning algorithms (56–58),
but little published information about the details of compliance with such proto-

cols exists. The first step of our approach involved the respiratory care practitioners' morning assessment using the daily screen of weaning parameters. While the >95% compliance rates in collection of the daily screen data and correct interpretation are impressive (Fig. 6), they were achieved in a setting in which many respiratory care practitioners had been involved in our original investigation. Therefore, they were familiar with how to conduct and calculate the measurements involved in the daily screening. Achieving such high compliance in a group of 117 respiratory care practitioners is reassuring, although institutions in their initial phases of implementation should not underestimate the amount of work necessary to attain such success, especially with a large group of RCPs. Others have reported compliance rates of less than 40% during weaning protocol introduction (59). Importantly, during a follow-up period in which regular reinforcements of all caregivers was discontinued, daily screen and spontaneous breathing trial compliance rates reverted to the baseline levels obtained prior to our educational interventions (unpublished observations). Thus, as with other behavioral modifications, continuous reinforcement is necessary to effect lasting change.

The second step of the protocol involved performing spontaneous breathing trials in patients who had recovered from respiratory failure, as manifested by passing the daily screening. At this point it became apparent that barriers to compliance with the protocol existed. Initially only 10% of patients who had passed their daily screening received a spontaneous breathing trial, but significant improvement occurred over the initial year of implementation. Both respiratory care practitioners and physicians contributed to this initial low compliance rate, and each group showed significant improvement in spontaneous breathing trial compliance rates over time following educational interventions. However, there appeared to be a "ceiling effect" in that there was not an increase in compliance at the end of the year of implementation despite increased familiarity with the protocol. One limitation of our report is that we did not institute direct, daily supervision of the respiratory care practitioners in their patient assessments prior to or during performance of spontaneous breathing trials. Thus, we have appraised the frequency, but not the accuracy, of respiratory care practitioner behaviors. In the absence of an independent, prospective review of all patients, the frequencies of protocol violations on the part of respiratory care practitioners or physicians are unknown. Among physician specialties, we detected variations in their frequencies of ordering spontaneous breathing trials, with higher rates on the medicine than on the surgical services. While these differences might reflect varying patient populations, management philosophies, or other undefined factors, they also reflect a higher baseline level of familiarity of the medicine staff through their exposure to the protocol during the prior study. The spontaneous breathing trial rate in surgical patients is especially remarkable when it is considered that the current implementation represented the first extension of spontaneous breathing trials to this population.

The increments in protocol compliance for both respiratory care practitioners and physicians after the fourth month of implementation coincided with the period during which in-services to all members of these groups had been completed and underscores the importance of interventions directed toward all protocol participants. The relative plateau in compliance following this "surge" probably reflects reinforcement of instruction to these groups. Alternatively, this finding might suggest that a maximum impact of our intervention is achievable by 6 months and that other approaches would be needed to effect higher compliance rates. Interestingly, it appears that in-servicing physicians and nurses contributed to respiratory care practitioners' compliance with spontaneous breathing trials. Increased general awareness of the protocol and support of its use by nurses and physicians might be expected to increase the likelihood of having respiratory care practitioners being comfortable with and feeling compelled to adhere to the protocol maneuvers. Physician compliance with the spontaneous breathing trials is a slightly different matter. There were times when the physician made an appropriate clinical decision *not* to perform a spontaneous breathing trial in a patient who passed a daily screening. For example, if the physician knew that the patient's chest x-ray had dramatically worsened or that the patient would be undergoing a surgical procedure later that day, it would be appropriate to forgo an SBT. Therefore, lack of 100% compliance in Figure 7 could be referred to as "appropriate noncompliance."

X. Other Barriers to Protocol Compliance

With a respiratory care practitioner questionnaire, we identified six commonly cited barriers that warrant consideration. The first involved house officer insecurity in advancing patients through the protocol without immediate input from their attending physicians. Even after obtaining the support of all of the participating attending physicians and in-servicing attendings and house officers, some unfamiliarity with and reservations about the protocol persisted. Some physicians among all specialties remained unaware of the importance and/or safety of weaning parameters and spontaneous breathing trials (5,33), and their approaches to patients varied. It is also noteworthy that while no attending physician order was necessary for the respiratory care practitioners to proceed with the daily screen, such an order was required for performance of an SBT because of a lack of consensus on the part of attending physicians about making this step automatic. This probably represented a major barrier to improved compliance with this phase of the protocol and was a variation from the original investigation. At some centers in which respiratory care practitioners are devoted to one unit, physicians might feel sufficiently comfortable to allow an automatic order for the spontaneous breathing trial upon the patient's passing the daily screening, greatly facilitating timely progression through the protocol.

Respiratory care practitioners also acknowledged their own inconsistency in seeking an order for a spontaneous breathing trial from physicians. While many respiratory care practitioners expressed a desire for more autonomy and decision-making responsibilities, others reported reluctance to approach certain physician groups even when respiratory care practitioners were confident that patients were successfully passing the daily screening. As with many institutional changes, protocol compliance improved over time and was probably the cumulative result of a strategy including serial reinforcement of the goals of the program during its implementation, increased "team awareness" of the protocol, experience accrued from daily patient management, and communication at the bedside. Our investigation was not designed to determine whether any single element of implementation was key to its success.

XI. Additional Caveats

Implementation proved to be a dynamic process in which an initial plan was modified based upon the prospective monitoring of compliance and feedback from all participating groups of caregivers. Alternative approaches might have more effectively promoted use of spontaneous breathing trials; the components and sequencing of our program were designed specifically for unique aspects of our ICU structure and staffing and would be expected to vary among institutions. Varying sizes and administrative structures of academic and community medical centers might be expected to pose different challenges in the implementation of this and other protocols. Differences in the number and experience of respiratory care practitioners could also have dramatic effects on protocol implementation. Protocol acceptance might be considerably easier in smaller, self-contained units with fewer staff and more direct communication channels. As in other circumstances where new care modalities are introduced, getting key physicians, respiratory care practitioners, and nurses (i.e., the opinion leaders) to "buy in" is a major element of successful protocol implementation (48,60) and was a factor in our experience.

Avoiding personnel changes as much as possible is also desirable: devoting the same therapists to a unit who are knowledgeable of the protocol and who interact with the physicians and nurses in a comfortable and consistent manner appears helpful (17). Also, overly rigid interpretation of the "rules" of the protocol seems counterproductive (see Appendixes 1 and 2). For example, determining on consecutive days that a patient failed the daily screening because the Pao_2/Fio_2 ratio was 198 (rather than >200) or their f/V_T was 107 (rather than <105) is felt to be inappropriate because some patients do not fit within the confines of specified "cut-offs" or thresholds (26,33,35,36). Continuing to advance patients through the protocol at this point and proceeding to a spontaneous breathing trial may be successful in many of these circumstances. We believe that active dialogue among caregivers can effectively identify these situations and that the protocol should not be implemented in ways that compromise clinical judgment. Lastly, future randomized investigations might compare outcomes and cost-effectiveness of patient-management strategies that are therapist-driven with those of a dedicated weaning team.

The availability of a protocol that has been validated and shown to result in better patient outcomes, increased safety, and cost savings does not assure its immediate acceptance, even within the institution where it was designed. In addition, despite implementation, suboptimal compliance with this protocol may not improve outcome. Through large-scale implementation of our program, we found that it was essential to have an awareness of not only specific elements of MV and weaning, but also general barriers to modifying health professionals' behaviors. Through graded steps every 2 months during the year of implementation, we observed improvements in protocol compliance and remarkable consistency (>95%) on the part of respiratory care practitioners in obtaining and interpreting the daily screening of weaning parameters. Important barriers to obtaining spontaneous breathing trials were identified and addressed and respiratory care practitioners and physician performance in proceeding to spontaneous breathing trials improved. Through diligence and the passage of time, an ongoing change of culture can be achieved that allows protocol implementation and appropriate modification of bedside behavior for both physicians and respiratory care practitioners. However, when this vigorous reinforcement through educational interventions is discontinued, compliance rates return to their previous baseline level.

XII. Patient Subgroups

Nuances in patient management are inevitable, and special approaches should be determined at the bedside on a case-by-case basis, but little is known about the ways approaches to MV discontinuation should be modified when patients have reduced physiological reserve or increased risks. Many physicians believe that different patient groups deserve different management approaches. Some patient groups who might require modified strategies include persons with COPD, ischemic heart disease, CHF, general surgery, trauma, neurosurgery, and, perhaps, the elderly. In our investigation of primarily medical patients (5), neither increased complication rates nor prolonged MV was found among those within any of these diagnostic groups (including persons with acute myocardial infarction or COPD). The following discussion will outline the literature concerning these subgroups and consider whether weaning protocols should be modified for these groups.

A. Chronic Obstructive Pulmonary Disease Patients

COPD affects approximately 15 million people in the United States and is the fourth most common cause of death after heart disease, cancer, and stroke (61,62). Its prevalence and mortality rates are increasing (63–65). Episodes of acute respiratory failure requiring MV in patients with COPD are associated with ICU and hospital mortality rates ranging from 1 to 16% and 11 to 46%, respectively (63,66–69). While numerous investigations have been performed to help predict the need for MV in patients with COPD (69–71), to estimate the likelihood of survival (63,66,72,73), we suspect that many physicians are unaware that the majority of COPD patients who require MV actually survive and that their mortality is not necessarily increased over that of other medical patients requiring such support. Our COPD patients' survival (Fig. 8) (75) was comparable to that in the published literature (63,66,68,69) and to that of patients with other causes of respiratory failure. In a recent multivariate analysis (63), the need for MV in

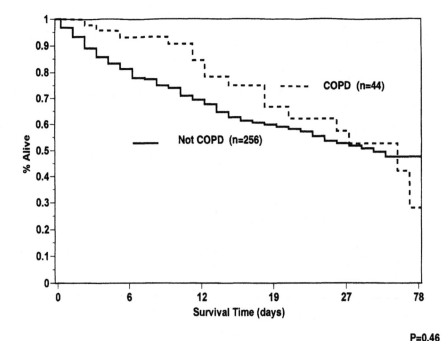

Figure 8   Kaplan-Meier analysis of in-hospital survival time between COPD and other patients. Censoring of patients at time of death and hospital discharge was performed for this analysis. There was no difference in survival between the two groups ($p = 0.46$) by Cox proportional hazards analysis. (From Ref. 75.)

COPD patients did not influence short-term or long-term outcome after adjusting for severity of illness. Rather, development of nonrespiratory organ dysfunction was the largest determinant of survival and accounted for 60% of the power of this prediction.

In our ICUs, the predictive characteristics of the daily screening worked as well for COPD patients as for persons with other diagnoses (75). Others have reported that conventional weaning criteria may be inadequate in COPD patients (76). While airway occlusion pressure at 0.1 second (i.e., $P_{0.1}$) has been shown repeatedly to be especially worthwhile in COPD patients (24,31,76,77), it has been neither widely accepted nor applied generally due to technical demands and high interindividual and intraindividual variability of this measure. As newer mechanical ventilators will begin including the $P_{0.1}$ into their software, more clinicians may examine the incorporation of this parameter into weaning protocols for COPD patients.

With the advent of noninvasive positive pressure ventilation (68,78), many have considered using PSV or bilevel positive airway pressure (BIPAP) as an aid in weaning from MV or as a means of avoiding MV altogether. Spontaneous breathing trials may have important roles in this strategy. A recent multicenter RCT by Nava et al. (79) investigated the use of a weaning protocol incorporating noninvasive PSV after extubation in patients with respiratory failure due to COPD. At 48 hours after intubation, a T-piece weaning trial (i.e., SBT) was attempted in 50 patients. If this failed, two methods of weaning were compared: (1) extubation and application of noninvasive PSV (i.e., BIPAP) by a facemask vs. (2) further invasive PSV by endotracheal tube. The average PSV in the noninvasive group was 19 ± 2 cm H_2O, while the invasive group received 17.6 ± 2.1 cm H_2O. Importantly, both groups of COPD patients received at least two spontaneous breathing trial attempts per day. The criteria to pass the spontaneous breathing trials were similar to those in our investigations (see Appendix 1) (5,34), except that the duration of successful spontaneous breathing was 3 hours and a pH of ≥7.35 was required. Outcomes of this important investigation included reduced weaning time and ICU stay, fewer instances of nosocomial pneumonia, and improved 60-day survival rates (Table 3) (79).

B. Congestive Heart Failure and Myocardial Infarction Patients

Our original investigation included 73 medical and nonsurgical cardiac patients with significant co-morbidities (5), unlike other studies that included a surgical or mixed population or excluded patients with acute coronary disease. We subsequently enrolled 123 coronary patients with myocardial infarction and congestive heart failure and 95 patients in the cardiothoracic surgical ICU (34). The latter were only enrolled if they remained on MV for over 24 hours, as they are routinely managed during the first day with a rapid "wean-to-extubation" protocol

Table 3 Noninvasive Ventilation in Weaning COPD Patients

Outcome	Invasive ($n = 25$)	BIPAP ($n = 25$)	p-value
Ventilator days	17 ± 12	10 ± 7	0.02
ICU days	24 ± 14	15 ± 5	0.005
Pneumonia	7	0	0.02
Success at 2 months	68%	88%	NS
Survival at 2 months	72%	92%	0.009

BIPAP = Bilevel positive airway pressure; COPD = Chronic obstructive airway disease; ICU = intensive care unit.
Source: Ref. 79.

and thus represented a select group. Cardiac surgical patients often have many aspects of their care (especially weaning from MV) directed by nonphysicians under protocol guidance (55,80). Importantly, none of these nearly 300 patients with cardiac diseases had a higher rate of detectable complications, suggesting that broad application of this strategy to cardiac patients is safe and effective. While others have shown that some patients have electrocardiographic changes consistent with ischemia during weaning trials (81), there have been no prospective studies documenting clinically important ischemic events resulting from management by a weaning protocol. Until such investigations are performed, bedside clinical judgment must remain an important component in individual patients. Using the above experience of safety, however, intensivists and surgeons must take care to avoid delaying extubation unnecessarily and realize that even cardiothoracic surgical patients (when not able to wean rapidly the first day) may benefit from enrollment in standard weaning protocols.

C. Neurosurgery Patients

Recognizing that neurosurgical patients receiving MV have vastly different neuromuscular and cardiopulmonary statuses than medical patients receiving MV, we have begun a series of investigations on neurosurgical patients (82,83). In our initial attempts at protocolizing the care of these patients, compliance of neurosurgeons with extubation protocols after a patient had passed a spontaneous breathing trial presented a particularly interesting dilemma. The most common reason cited for not extubating a spontaneously breathing patient was a depressed mental status. Moreover, an association was found between Glasgow coma scale (GCS) and the need for reintubation ($p = 0.0001$) (83), a finding that others have seen as well (84). Of 109 extubation attempts, only 53% occurred without any complications or reintubations. Multivariate analysis demonstrated that GCS ($p < 0.0001$) and P/F ratio ($p < 0.0001$) were independent predictors of successful extubation. GCS $\geq$ 8 was associated with success in 67% of patients, while only 21% with a GCS of <8 had successful extubation ($p < 0.0001$) (83). This observation supports the concerns of neurosurgeons regarding early liberation of patients from the ventilator. Future investigations of neurosurgical patients should ask whether the coupling of mental status measures and the GCS with result of the daily screening and spontaneous breathing trial–based strategies can improve the extubation outcomes.

Vallverdu et al. (31) studied weaning indices and MV liberation in 46 neurological patients, including ischemic stroke, intracerebral hemorrhage, subarachnoid hemorrhage, head trauma, encephalitis, metabolic encephalopathy, and brain tumor. While their average reintubation rate was 15%, 15 (33%) neurological patients needed reinstitution of invasive MV, while only 6% of the 171 other patients with acute respiratory failure or COPD required reintubation. The authors found that most predictors of weaning success lacked discriminatory ability in these patients. Interestingly, f/V_T and $P_{0.1}$ had their lowest accuracies in neurological patients (65% and 63%, respectively) and did not discriminate between weaning failure and success in these patients (31). Only maximal inspiratory pressure (MIP, $p = 0.05$) and expiratory pressure (MEP, $p = 0.001$) were different among successfully extubated neurological patients. In this group, the ability to cough and clear secretions, objectively reflected by the MEP, may help in clinical decision making. Since the need for reintubation was neither clinically nor physiologically suspected, the authors concluded that other tools need to be developed and prospectively validated to determine the optimum time to liberate patients with mental status changes and neurological impairment.

D. Elderly Patients

The present number of adults 85 years and older, estimated to be about 4 million, is expected to double by the year 2030 (85). U.S. Health Care expenditures for persons >65 years old are currently $1,740 billion (38% of total expenditures). By 2030, this amount is estimated to become $15,970 billion (74% of total). One approach to decreasing health care costs might be to limit or ration the intensive care provided to the aged in order to conserve resources (86–89). Indeed, recent data have demonstrated that elderly do receive less aggressive management for some medical illnesses (90), and data from the SUPPORT investigators have shown that age (especially >70–75 years) has great importance in the intensity of care given to patients (91–94) (Figs. 9 and 10). There are surprisingly few "expert consensus" reports regarding the decision to treat seniors with MV. One publication from the Office of Technology Assessment (95) discussed very reasonable perspectives, but few data were presented and opinions were divided as to whether or not age should be a major determinant in the use of MV.

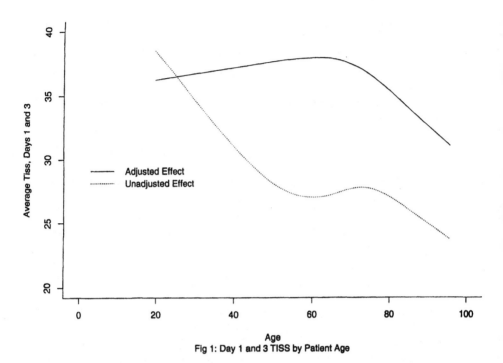

Fig 1: Day 1 and 3 TISS by Patient Age

Figure 9   The relationship between patient age and the average therapeutic intervention scoring system scores of patients enrolled in SUPPORT. The figure demonstrates that the intensity of care is lower for older patients, even after adjustment for the nature and severity of their illnesses ($p < 0.001$). An accompanying figure in the same manuscript indicated lower hospital costs also associated with age, especially above 70 years. (From Ref. 91.)

Age has been considered an important prognostic indicator of hospital outcome (88,96), but many prior investigations of MV have been limited by their retrospective design and the absence of adjustment for confounding factors such as severity of illness (97–99). Among 21 previously published reports (97–117), which included age-specific data on mechanically ventilated elderly patients, authors' conclusions were divided regarding whether age influences outcome. Seventeen of these studies were restricted to mechanically ventilated patients (97–100,104,105,107,110,112–117), and only 5 of them were prospective (100,103, 104,116,117). Of the latter, 4 concluded that age had an important effect on the outcome (100,103,116,117), while one concluded that age did not matter in outcome (104). The diversity of the designs and conclusions of these investigations

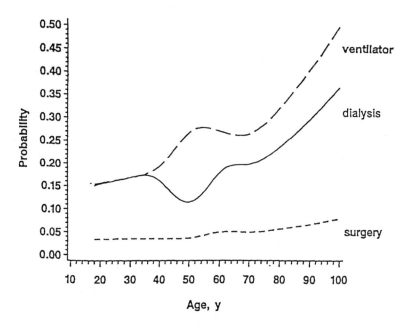

Figure 10 Relationship between patient age and the adjusted probability of a decision to withhold each life-sustaining treatment by study day 30. Results are calculated on the basis of Cox proportional hazards models adjusted for sex, income, education, insurance, prognosis, comorbid conditions, baseline function, study site, and preference for cardiopulmonary resuscitation and life-extending care. At the age of 70, the relative risk for a decision to withhold mechanical ventilation was 1.5 (95% CI 1.2–1.9), and ≥80 years the relative risk was 2.1 (1.6–2.7). (From Ref. 93.)

has only served to fuel the controversy over whether age has an independent impact on the outcomes of patients treated with MV.

In our prospectively followed cohort of 300 mechanically ventilated patients, we found that patients ≥75 years of age remained on MV a median of 4 days (interquartile ranges, 2–9) vs. 6 days (3–11) for patients <75 years ($p = 0.14$) (118). Using the time it took to pass a daily screen of weaning parameters as a marker of recovery from respiratory failure (Fig. 11). The ICU cost of care was lower [$12,822 ($9,821–$26,313) vs. $19,316 ($9,699–$39,950)] in older patients ($p = 0.03$). Median hospital costs tended to be lower in the older group, though not significantly so ($21,292 vs. 29,049, $p = 0.17$). Using multivariate logistic regression analysis to adjust for race, gender, and severity of illness, patient age of ≥75 was predictive of approximately 1 day less on the ventilator,

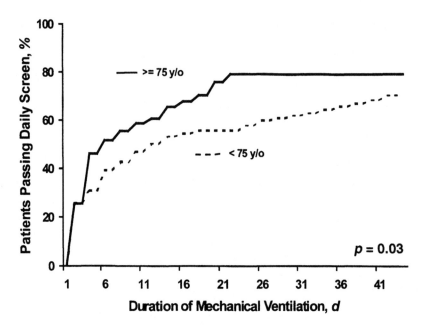

Figure 11 Kaplan-Meier analysis of the rate of recovery of respiratory failure by age. This analysis used the percent of patients passing a daily screen of weaning parameters as a surrogate marker of ''recovery'' and adjustments were made for sex, race, and severity of illness at baseline using a modified APACHE II score excluding age. Using Cox proportional hazards analysis to compare the proportions of patients who passed the daily screen in each group, elderly patients passed the daily screen earlier than younger patients [risk ratio 1.58 (95% confidence interval, 1.13–2.22), $p = 0.03$]. (From Ref. 118.)

but this was not statistically significant (95% confidence interval, -2.8 to 1.2). Multivariate analyses also confirmed that ICU and hospital LOS were not different after adjustment ($p > 0.1$), but ICU and hospital costs were lower in the elderly ($p = 0.02$). In-hospital mortality among the elderly was 38% versus 39% among younger patients ($p = 0.98$), and Cox proportional hazards analysis confirmed there was no difference in survival between the two groups (Fig. 12) (relative risk for older patients $= 0.82$, 95% confidence interval 0.52–1.29). Thus, these outcomes were not explained by differences in mortality.

Data were recently reported from 1638 patients in the MV International Study Group prevalence investigation (78). In this observational cohort, it was noted that despite a higher severity of illness, the 254 patients over the age of 75 spent significantly less time on MV than the 1355 patients under 75 years old

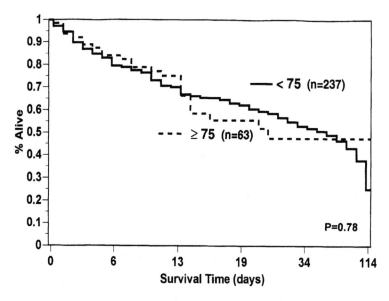

Figure 12 Kaplan-Meier analysis show the survival time of patients. After adjustment for the severity of illness at baseline as measured by the modified APACHE II score, sex, and race, Cox proportional hazards analysis showed that there was no difference in survival between those greater than or equal to 75 years old and those less than 75 years old (relative risk for older patients = 0.82, 95% CI 0.52–1.29, $p = 0.78$). (From Ref. 118.)

$(14 = 23$ vs. $21 \pm 110, p = 0.02)$. This initial analysis did not address mortality data, but further investigations will assess the relationships of age to outcomes from MV.

Women were more numerous than men among the elderly patients in our study MV (118), a finding consistent with the well-established demographics of aging. Kollef and colleagues (119) reported that women patients had a longer duration of MV ($p = 0.056$), but we detected no gender differences in the rate of recovery from respiratory failure or the duration of MV. Because of differences in access to health care for women (120) and differences among physicians in their practice styles (including the vigor of their approaches to liberation from the ventilator), further prospective analyses of gender differences in outcomes from MV are needed. We believe that the care of elderly women will represent a major future priority of critical care medicine. Gender, associated body dimensions, and age are appropriate considerations that may affect not only outcome from MV, but also objective measures of readiness to discontinue MV. Female gender, smaller endotracheal tube size (≤ 7 mm), and older age have been associ-

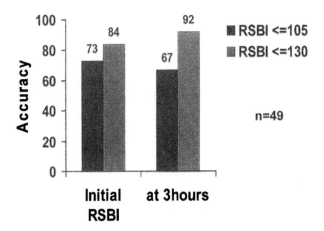

Figure 13 Accuracy of rapid shallow breathing index in elderly. Histogram demonstrating that in this group of elderly patients (>70 years old), the threshold for the rapid shallow breathing index (i.e., f/V^T) of 130 yielded a higher accuracy in predicting successful extubation than the conventional threshold of 105. Furthermore, measuring the index at 3 hours enhanced the accuracy beyond that of measurements taken at the onset of spontaneous breathing. (Adapted from Ref. 36.)

ated with an elevated f/V_T ratio (35,36), and it may be appropriate to adjust the "passing" threshold for this measurement in these instances to avoid erroneously regarding a patient as still requiring MV (Fig. 13). However, this approach will require further study.

In view of current uncertainties of physician decision making regarding the use of MV in the elderly, major pitfalls should be recognized and avoided. These include the premature application of predictive equations (113) or overreliance on anecdotal experiences. Further prospective investigations are needed in order to define "physiological age" and to determine whether or not it is truly more important than chronological age (95,121). In the absence of validated measures of "physiological age," the current observations suggest that an overreliance on chronological age is inappropriate. By using multivariate analysis to adjust for severity of illness and other variables, we found that the elderly (>75 years) spent an amount of time on the mechanical ventilator comparable to that of younger patients. They also had a lower cost of ICU and in-hospital care. Accordingly, the decision to use MV should not be based on age alone, and the appropriate use of ventilatory support in the elderly requires further prospective evaluation.

XIII. Reintubations: Distinguishing Causes

Despite the rigor with which a team of health care professionals evaluates their patients and applies an amalgam of scientific evidence and clinical experience in deciding about liberation from MV, some patients will fail requiring reintubation and going on to develop complications. Reintubation may simply be a marker of the severity of illness (31,122), but this event is associated with an 8-fold higher odds ratio for nosocomial pneumonia (12) and a 6- to 12-fold increase in mortality (37,38,84,123). During the past few years it has become clear that the most important determinants of the morbidity associated with reintubation are the proximate cause (i.e., extubation failure due to airway compromise vs. true weaning or "pump" failure) and the time to reintubation (122). Aspects of failed liberation from MV that are inherently related to the weaning approach include the following: reintubation rates, unplanned extubation, failed extubation due to airway etiologies, and weaning failure implying cardiopulmonary limitations. Each of these is relevant to implementing and monitoring the outcomes of weaning protocols.

A. Reintubation Rates

Reported reintubation rates range from 4% to 20% for different ICU populations (4,5,8,34,38,122–124), and may be as high as 33% in patients with mental status changes and neurological impairment (31). The marked variability in reintubation rates probably reflects protean factors, including differences in both patient populations and physician decision making. While hospitals often track reintubation as a quality assurance measurement, the optimal rate is not known. A reintubation rate of 0% would indicate that the managing physicians were not "pushing" vigorously to liberate patients at the earliest possible time. Alternatively, an excessively high reintubation rate might suggest reckless decision making or a very high-risk population (e.g., neurosurgical patients). While we hypothesized that an aggressive weaning protocol might increase reintubations, we found the opposite. Our protocol was the first respiratory care therapist to our knowledge that documented a lower reintubation rate than in controls (4% vs. 10%, $p = 0.04$) (5). While this may have been perceived initially as "too low," another investigation of over 500 patients reported a 6% reintubation rate when incorporating the same two-step protocol (13). Interestingly, when patients with neurological disease were excluded from the analysis of the investigation by Vallverdu et al. (31), only 8 of 125 patients (6%) required reintubation after successfully passing a similar two-step process. Two important points must be made: (1) we initially investigated only medical and coronary ICU patients, not those in postsurgical ICUs, and (2) the protocol allowed clinical decision making rather than having extubation be an automatic step, and this may have allowed a slightly lower reintubation rate. When the protocol was implemented hospital-wide in the "out-of-study setting" and changed to a TDP (without direct supervision by a managing physician), compliance decreased and reintubation rates increased to 14% (34).

B. Unplanned Extubation

This category of events in the liberation from MV may occur accidentally or as the result of the patient's deliberate self-extubation (125,126). It has been known for some time that when self-extubation occurs, patients require reintubation only about 50% of the time (9,10), a fact that should further motivate physicians to adopt proactive protocols directed toward earlier extubation (interestingly, we noted self-extubations in only 1% of intervention patients) (5). Three prospective investigations of unplanned extubation encompassing 1584 patients in over a dozen European ICUs have recently been published (84,127,128). The overall unplanned extubation rate among this entire experience was 10.8%, and 47% of the 171 self-extubated individuals were reintubated. Chevron et al. (84) prospectively studied their unplanned extubations and found a total of 66 out of 414 (16%) mechanically ventilated patients over a 15-month period. Eighty-seven percent of self-extubations were deliberate. Multivariate analysis showed inadequate sedation and oral intubation to be risk factors for unplanned extubation. Risk factors for reintubation in 37% were depressed mental status (GCS < 11), accidental nature of extubation rather than deliberate, and a Pao_2/Fio_2 ratio of <200 torr (84). Betbese et al. (128) recently reported a 7% unplanned endotracheal extubation rate (59 of 750 patients). Twenty-seven of these 59 patients (46%) required reintubation, and in this investigation the need for reintubation was not associated with survival. The two most striking factors associated with the need for reintubation were accidental rather than deliberate unplanned extubation ($p = 0.01$) and the event occurring in patients who had not yet begun weaning ($p = 0.001$) (128). Lastly, Boulain and colleagues (127) completed a multicenter prospective investigation that followed 420 patients over 2 months and found 46 unplanned extubations, of whom 28 (60.8%) were reintubated. Multivariate analysis allowed the authors to determine the following four factors associated with unplanned extubation: chronic respiratory failure, poor endotracheal tube fixation, orotracheal intubation, and inadequate intravenous sedation. These important observational studies have allowed us to summarize important features and formulate provisional recommendations for reducing the occurrence of unplanned extubations (Table 4).

C. Extubation Versus Weaning Failure

There is an important distinction between reintubation required because of *airway* compromise vs. *nonairway* precipitants. Epstein and Ciubotaru performed an analysis of prospectively collected data in 74 medical ICU patients who required

Table 4 Unplanned Extubation: Important Features and Preventive Measures

1. Unplanned extubation occurs in approximately 11% of patients receiving MV (84,127,128), although some institutions have experienced rates less than 5% (5,10)
2. Important features associated with unplanned extubation are as follows (84,127):
   Chronic respiratory failure
   Poor endotracheal tube fixation
   Orotracheal intubation
   Inadequate intravenous sedation
   Hypoactive or hyperactive delirium
   Inadequate nursing staff and occurrence during procedures, although neither has been statistically associated with unplanned extubation
3. Complications reported in patients following unplanned extubation (125–127)
   Reintubation
   Nosocomial pneumonia
   Vocal cord trauma
   Death has been reported, but, most authors have not found a higher mortality among those with unplanned vs. planned extubation
4. Reintubation is required in 50% of patients after unplanned extubation (9,10,84,127,128)
5. Important features associated with need for reintubation after unplanned extubation are as follows (84,122,127,128):
   Accidental rather than deliberate extubation
   Occurrence before active weaning has begun
   Depressed mental status
   Pao_2/Fio_2 ratio below 200 torr
6. Evidence-based suggestions for reducing the likelihood of unplanned extubation and reintubation (5,84,122,127):
   Vigilance during procedures at the patient's bedside
   Adequate sedation of agitated patients and possible use of sedation protocol
   Particular attention to orally intubated patients
   Strong fixation of the endotracheal tube
   Daily screening and assessment of patients readiness for liberation from MV

reintubation within 72 hours of extubation (122). They classified the causes for reintubation as airway-related (upper airway obstruction, aspiration, or excess pulmonary secretions) or nonairway-related (respiratory failure, congestive heart failure, encephalopathy, or other). The mortality was 42% (31 of 74) and was highest in patients who failed because of nonairway factors (53% vs. 17%, $p <$ 0.01). This group tended to be reintubated earlier by about 10 hours (mean 21 vs. 31 hours), and their mortality increased with longer interval between extubation and reintubation ($p < 0.05$). Using logistic regression, both the cause of extubation failure and increased length of time to reintubation were associated with hospital mortality (122). The authors concluded that identification of patients having nonairway problems ought to occur as early after extubation as possible, with timely reinitiation of ventilatory support. These are the patients who have a true "weaning failure," while the other patients ought to be considered "airway failure." The optimum strategies of renewed liberation efforts are likely to differ in these groups, and require clarification.

As demonstrated by numerous investigators, most patients will come off of MV without special techniques or interventions. We are in need of reliable indices that identify patients who are able to sustain spontaneous breathing but who are at risk for reintubation. These patients are likely to have long stays on the ventilator and consume an inordinate amount of resources. If an airway problem is suspected prior to extubation, one might conduct a "leak test" to help determine the likelihood of postextubation stridor. When the cuff was deflated in one investigation of the leak test (129), patients who developed postextubation stridor (i.e., airway failures) had a smaller difference between the inspiratory and expiratory tidal volumes. The authors used ROC curve analysis to determine that 105 mL was the best predictive cut-off for development of postextubation stridor.

Special considerations in weaning failure patients include reactive airways disease or COPD, cardiac diseases such as ischemic disease, congestive heart failure, uncontrolled systemic hypertension contributing to pulmonary edema, metabolic disturbances such as electrolyte disturbances or metabolic alkalosis, uncontrolled anxiety or pain, ongoing aspiration and secretion problems, neuromuscular disorders including prior use of neuromuscular blockers or diaphragm dysfunction, ongoing sepsis or other infections such as pneumonia, malnutrition or overfeeding, sedation imbalance with overutilization of narcotics or sedative/hypnotics, obesity and the need to position the patient upright or sitting in the bed to utilize gravity to maintain tidal volume, and hypothyroidism. While this list is long, it is imperative that any clinician caring for mechanically ventilated patients be aware of these commonly found reasons for failure to wean.

XIV. Conclusions

It is imperative that protocols not be put in place to supplant clinical judgment. Protocols are meant as guides for patient management, not as sets of rules engraved in stone. Likewise, protocols should not be viewed as static constructs, but rather as dynamic tools, which evolve and are molded to accommodate new data and/or health care professionals' preferences. Espousing these attitudes and incorporating new information as it becomes available will increase protocol acceptance by otherwise skeptical physicians, nurses, and respiratory care practitioners. Perhaps, soon, we will rarely hear the familiar refrain "slowly wean the ventilator as tolerated," but, rather, "the patient looks clinically stable and, according to our protocol, is ready for extubation."

Appendix 1: Definitions of Daily Screen and SBT

The Daily Screen:

Takes only about 2 minutes, patient should pass all 5 criteria:

1. Patient coughs when suction catheter passed, intact gag reflex.
2. Patient not receiving any vasopressor or sedative infusions drips
   Dopamine allowed if dose ≤ 5 µg/kg/min, and Intermittent dosing of sedatives allowed
3. $PaO_2 / FiO_2 ≥ 200$, e.g., PaO_2 of 100 / FiO_2 of 0.5 (not in %) = 200, **higher is better**
4. PEEP set ≤ 5
5. Respiratory rate / tidal volume Ratio $(f / V_t) ≤ 105$
   This is also known as the Rapid Shallow Breathing Index (RSBI), **lower is better**
   Measured after 1 minute of spontaneous breathing with ventilator rate set to 0 and pressure support set to 0.
   Average Vt calculated by dividing f into Ve (Vt = Ve / f), alternatively: $f / Vt = f^2 / Ve$
   e.g., rate (f) of 20, Ve of 10 l/min : (20x20) divided by 10 = f / Vt of 40

The Spontaneous Breathing Trial (SBT)

What is a spontaneous breathing trial and who gets one?

- A trial of spontaneous breathing for 120 minutes with "flow-by" mode, ventilator rate set to 0 and pressure support set to 0
- A patient who passes the daily screening is a candidate for a spontaneous breathing trial

Who performs the spontaneous trial? It's a TEAM EFFORT...

- Respiratory therapist performs daily screening and prompts physician to order an spontaneous breathing trial
- Respiratory therapist initiates a trial, monitors the patient during the trial in conjunction with the nurse, and re-initiates MV if criteria for trial termination are met
- ICU Nurse monitors the patient for criteria for trial termination and notifies the respiratory therapist if they are met

When is a spontaneous trial terminated?

- If the patient successfully tolerates it for two hours
- When one of the following conditions is met:
  - **Resp rate > 35 for > 5 minutes**
  - **SaO_2 < 90% during > 30 seconds of good quality measurement**
  - **20% increase or decrease in heart rate for > 5 minutes**
  - **SBP > 180 or SBP < 90 during at least one minute of continuous recording or repeated measurements**
  - **Agitation, anxiety, or diaphoresis confirmed as a change from baseline and present for > 5 minutes**

What does it mean if a patient passes a spontaneous breathing trial?

Successful completion of a 2 hour SBT indicates a 90% chance of successfully of staying off of MV for 48 hours (Ely et al, *NEJM* 1996;335:1864-69).

Appendix 2: Protocol Flow Sheet Ventilator Weaning Protocol

START

Reassess Daily

Does patient meet Daily Screen (DS)- "Readiness for SBT"?

NO → Request orders to wean ventilator settings as able

YES

Verbally notify MD that criteria are met & request order for SBT from MD.

Does MD give order for SBT?

NO → Document reason and reassess in 24 hours

YES

Explain weaning to patient & begin SBT via Flow-by or T-bar

Does patient tolerate SBT for 30 minutes to 2 hours with stable respiratory & hemodynamic parameters?

NO → Return to prior settings → Document specific termination criteria → Notify MD

YES

Notify MD with SBT results.

Does MD give order for Extubation or Trach Collar?

NO

YES

Extubate or place on Trach Collar

If patient is extubated, obtain ABG in 30 minutes

Wean FiO2 maintaining Sats > 90%

Abbreviations: ABG = arterial blood gas, DS = daily screen, RTW = readiness to wean, SBT = spontaneous breathing trial

Appendix 3: Daily Data Collection Form

The North Carolina Baptist Hospitals, Incorporated
Department of Respiratory Care
Ventilator Weaning Protocol Documentation

Please press firmly when charting, this is a two copy form.

Complete this section, when protocol is initiated.

Date enrolled in protocol: ___/___/___ Intubation date: ___/___/___ Hospital Admission date: ___/___/___ Medical record #: _____

DATE/TIME:									
Screen #1 (Enter values) Readiness to wean:									
VE									
FiO2									
PEEP									
Passes Screen? (yes, no): (Note: Must pass all 3)									
Screen #2 (Enter values) Readiness for SBT:									
Cough/Gag reflex present? (yes, no)									
Off Sedative drip / Pressors (yes, no)									
PaO2 / FiO2 ratio									
f / Vt ratio									
PEEP									
Passes Screen? (yes, no): (Note: Must pass all 5)									
If yes, obtain MD order for SBT*. ➡									
MD orders SBT*? (yes, no): If no, explain why in comments.									
SBT passed? (yes, no): If no, explain why in comments.									
Date Passes SBT: (Place sticker in chart, + call MD for orders)									
Date Extubated or to T-collar:									
Signature:									

DATE/TIME	COMMENTS	Initials	DATE/TIME	COMMENTS	Initials

*SBT = Spontaneous breathing trial   **Screen #1** Passing Criteria = VE < 15   FiO2 < .60   PEEP < 10   **Screen #2** Passing Criteria = PEEP ≤ 5   f/Vt ratio ≤ 105   PaO2 / FiO2 ratio ≥ 200

White copy to Medical Records   Yellow copy to Department

(MR2/97)

References

1. Weinberger SE, Weiss JW. Weaning from ventilatory support. N Engl J Med 1995; 332:388–389.
2. Manthous CA, Schmidt GA, Hall JB. Liberation from mechanical ventilation: a decade of progress. Chest 1998; 114:886–901.
3. Hall JB, Wood LD. Liberation of the patient from MV. JAMA 1987; 257:1621–1628.
4. Esteban A, Frutos F, Tobin MJ, Alia I, Solsona JF, Valverdu I, Fernandez R, de la Cal MA, Benito S, Tomas R. A comparison of four methods of weaning patients from MV. N Engl J Med 1995; 332:345–350.
5. Ely EW, Baker AM, Dunagan DP, Burke HL, Smith AC, Kelly PT, Johnson MM, Browder RW, Bowton DL, Haponik EF. Effect on the duration of MV of identifying patients capable of breathing spontaneously. N Engl J Med 1996; 335:1864–1869.
6. Sahn SA, Lakshminarayan S. Bedside criteria for discontinuation of mechanical ventilation. Chest 1973; 63:1002–1005.
7. Esteban A, Alia I, Ibanez J, Benito S, Tobin MJ, The Spanish Lung Failure Collaborative Group. Modes of mechanical ventilation and weaning. Chest 1994; 106: 1188–1193.
8. Brochard L, Rauss A, Benito S, Conti G, Mancebo J, Rekik N, Gasparetto A, Lemaire F. Comparison of three methods of gradual withdrawal from ventilatory support during weaning from mechanical ventilation. Am J Respir Crit Care Med 1994; 150:896–903.
9. Listello D, Sessler C. Unplanned extubation: clinical predictors for reintubation. Chest 1994; 105:1496–1503.
10. Tindol GA, Jr., DiBenedetto RJ, Kosciuk L. Uplanned extubations. Chest 1994; 105:1804–1807.
11. Stroetz RW, Hubmayr RD. Tidal volume maintenance during weaning with pressure support. Am J Respir Crit Care Med 1995; 152:1034–1040.
12. Torres A, Gatell JM, Aznar E. Re-intubation increases the risk of nosocomial pneumonia in patients needing mechanical ventilation. Am J Respir Crit Care Med 1995; 152:137–141.
13. Wood KE, Flaten AL, Reedy JS, Coursin DB. Use of a daily wean screen and weaning protocol for mechanically ventilated patients in a multidisciplinary tertiary critical care unit. Crit Care Med 1999; 27:A94–A94.
14. Luce JM. Reducing the use of Mechanical Ventilation. N Engl J Med 1996; 25: 1916–1917.
15. Kollef MH, Shapiro SD, Silver P, St.John RE, Prentice D, Sauer S, Ahrens TS, Shannon W, Baker-Clinkscale D. A randomized, controlled trial of protocol-directed versus physician-directed weaning from mechanical ventilation. Crit Care Med 1997; 25:567–574.
16. Cohen IL, Booth FV. Cost containment and mechanical ventilation in the United States. New Horizons 1994; 2:283–290.
17. Cohen IL. Weaning from mechanical ventilation—the team approach and beyond. Intensive Care Med 1994; 20:317–318.

18. Strickland JH, Jr., Hasson JH. A computer-controlled ventilator weaning system: a clinical trial. Chest 1993; 103:1220–1226.
19. Yang KL, Tobin MJ. A prospective study of indexes predicting the outcome of trials of weaning from mechanical ventilation. N Engl J Med 1991; 324:1445–1450.
20. Mohsenifar Z, Hay A, Hay J, Lewis JI, Loerner SK. Gastric intramural pH as a predictor of success or failure in weaning patients from mechanical ventilation. Ann Intern Med 1993; 119:794–798.
21. Gluck EH, Barkoviak MJ, Balk RA, Casey LC, Silver MR, Bone RC. Medical effectiveness of esophageal balloon pressure manometry in weaning patients from mechanical ventilation. Crit Care Med 1995; 23:504–509.
22. Shikora SA, Benotti PN, Johannigman JA. The oxygen cost of breathing may predict weaning from mechanical ventilation better than the respiratory rate to tidal volume ratio. Arch Surg 1994; 129:269–274.
23. Sassoon CS, Mahutte CK. Airway occlusion pressure and breathing pattern as predictors of weaning outcome. Am Rev Respir Dis 1993; 148:860–866.
24. Sassoon CSH, Te TT, Mahutte CK, Light RW. Airway occlusion pressure: an important indicator for successful weaning in patients with chronic obstructive pulmonary disease. Am Rev Respir Dis 1987; 135:107–113.
25. Gandia F, Blanco J. Evaluation of indexes predicting the outcome of ventilator weaning and value of adding supplemental inspiratory load. Intensive Care Med 1992; 18:327–333.
26. Epstein SK. Etiology of extubation failure and the predictive value of the rapid shallow breathing index. Am J Respir Crit Care Med 1995; 152:545–549.
27. Capdevila XJ, Perrigault PF, Percy PJ, Roustan JP, d'Athis F. Occlusion pressure and its ratio to maximum inspiratory pressure are useful predictors for successful extubation following T-piece weaning trial. Chest 1995; 108:482–489.
28. Yang KL. Inspiratory pressure/maximal inspiratory pressure ratio: a predictive index of weaning outcome. Intensive Care Med 1993; 9:204–208.
29. Dojat M, Harf A, Touchard D, Laforest M, Lemaire F, Brochard L. Evaluation of a knowledge-based system providing ventilatory management and decision for extubation. Am J Respir Crit Care Med 1996; 153:997–1004.
30. Vassilakopoulos T, Zakynthinos S, Roussos C. The tension-time index and the frequency/tidal volume ratio are the major pathophysiologic determinants of weaning failure and success. Am J Respir Crit Care Med 1998; 158:378–385.
31. Vallverdu I, Calaf N, Subirana M, Net A, Benito S, Mancebo J. Clinical characteristics, respiratory functional parameters, and outcome of a two-hour T-piece trial of patients weaning from mechanical ventilation. Am J Respir Crit Care Med 1999; 158:1855–1862.
32. Bellemare F, Grassino A. Effect of pressure and timing of contraction on human diaphragm fatigue. J Appl Physiol 1982; 53:1190–1195.
33. Jaeschke RZ, Meade MO, Guyatt GH, Keenan SP, Cook DJ. How to use diagnostic test articles in the intensive care unit: Diagnosing weanability using f/Vt. Crit Care Med 1997; 25:1514–1521.
34. Ely EW, Bennett PA, Bowton DL, Murphy SM, Haponik EF. Large scale implementation of a respiratory therapist-driven protocol for ventilator weaning. Am J Respir Crit Care Med 1998; 159:439–446.

35. Epstein SK, Ciubotaru RL. Influence of gender and endotracheal tube size on preextubation breathing pattern. Am J Respir Crit Care Med 1997; 154:1647–1652.

36. Krieger BP, Isber J, Breitenbucher A, Throop G, Ershowsky P. Serial measurements of the rapid-shallow-breathing index as a predictor of weaning outcome in elderly medical patients. Chest 1997; 112:1029–1034.

37. Esteban A, Alia I, Tobin M, Gil A, Gordo F, Vallverdu I, Blanch L, Bonet A, Vazquez A, dePablo R, Torres A, de la Cal MA, Macias S, for the Spanish Lung Failure Collaborative Group. Effect of spontaneous breathing trial duration on outcome of attempts to discontinue mechanical ventilation. Am J Respir Crit Care Med 1999; 159:512–518.

38. Esteban A, Alia I, Gordo F, Fernandez R, Solsona JF, Vallverdu I, Macias S, Allegue JM, Blanco J, Carriedo D, Palazon E, Carrizosa F, Tomas R, Suarez J, Goldwasser RS, The Spanish Lung Failure Collaborative Group. Extubation outcome after spontaneous breathing trials with T-tube or pressure support ventilation. Am J Respir Crit Care Med 1997; 156:459–465.

39. Scheinhorn DJ, Chao DC, Stearn-Hassenpglug M, LaBree LD, Heltsley DJ. Post-ICU mechanical ventilation. Treatment of 1,123 patients at a regional weaning center. Chest 1997; 111:1654–1659.

40. Scheinhorn DJ, Hassenpflug M, Artinian BM, LaBree L, Catlin JL. Predictors of weaning after 6 weeks of mechanical ventilation. Chest 1995; 107:500–505.

41. Make BJ, Hill NS, Goldberg AI, Bach JR, Criner G, Dunne PE, Heffner JE, Keens TG, O'Donohue WJ, Oppenheimer EA, Robert D. Mechanical ventilation beyond the intensive care unit: report of a consensus conference of the American College of Chest Physicians. Chest 1998; 113:289S–344S.

42. Seneff MG, Zimmerman JE, Knaus WA, Wagner DP, Draper EA. Predicting the duration of mechanical ventilation. The importance of disease and patient characteristics. Chest 1996; 110:469–479.

43. Troche G, Moine P. Is the duration of mechanical ventilation predictable? Chest 1997; 112:745–751.

44. Ely EW, Baker AM, Evans GW, Haponik EF. The prognostic significance of passing a DS of weaning parameters. Intensive Care Med 1998; 25:581–587.

45. Sloane PJ, Gee MH, Gottlieb JE, Albertine KH, Peters SP, Burns JR, Machiedo G, Fish JE. A multicenter registry of patients with acute respiratory distress syndrome. Physiology and outcome. Am Rev Respir Dis 1992; 146:419–426.

46. Marik P, Kaufman D. Teaching medical students in the intensive care unit: building houses with no foundation. Crit Care Med 1995; 23:1933–1934.

47. The Spanish Lung Failure Collaborative Group. Timing and clinical outcomes of ventilated patients requiring tracheostomy. Am J Respir Crit Care Med 1997; 155(4):A404.

48. Greco PJ, Eisenberg JM. Changing physicians' practices. N Engl J Med 1993; 329: 1271–1273.

49. Main DS, Cohen SJ, DiClemente CC. Measuring physician readiness to change cancer screening: preliminary results. Am J Prev Med 1995; 11:54–58.

50. Stoller JK. Why therapist-driven protocols? Respir Care 1994; 39:706–708.

51. Weber K, Milligan S. Therapist-driven protocols: the state of the art. Respir Care 1994; 39:746–755.

52. Jacobs J. How are we doing with operational restructuring and therapist-driven protocols? Am Assoc Respir Care Times 1994; 18:66–69.

53. Tietsort J. Benchmarking report on use of TDPs. Respir Care Manager 1998; 7: 1–12.

54. Shrake KL, Scaggs JE, England KR, Henkle JQ, Eagleton LE. Benefits associated with a respiratory care assessment-treatment program: results of a pilot study. Respir Care 1994; 39:715–724.

55. Wood G, MacLeod B, Moffatt S. Weaning from mechanical ventilation: physician-directed vs a respiratory-therapist-directed protocol. Respir Care 1995; 40:219–224.

56. Saura P, Blanch L, Mestre J, Valles J, Artigas A, Fernandez R. Clinical consequences of the implementation of a weaning protocol. Intensive Care Med 1996; 22:1052–1056.

57. Burn SM, Marshall M, Burns JE, Ryan B, Wilmoth D, Carpenter R, Aloi A, Wood M, Truwit JD. Desing, testing, and results of an outcomes-managed approach to patients requiring prolonged mechanical ventilation. Am J Crit Care 1998; 7:45–57.

58. Djunaedi H, Cardinal P, Greffe-Laliberte G, Jones G, MMath B, Snell CC. Does a ventilatory management protocol improve the care of ventilated patients? Respir Care 1987; 42:604–610.

59. Schriefer J. Reducing the length of stay for post-operative open heart surgical patients. Qual Connection 1993; 2:8–9.

60. Soumerai SB, McLaughlin TJ, Gurwitz JH, Guadagnoli E, Hauptman PJ, Borbas C, Morris N, McLaughlin B, Gao X, Willison DJ, Asinger R, Gobel F. Effect of local medical opinion leaders on quality of care for acute myocradial infarction. A randomized controlled trial. JAMA 1998; 279:1358–1363.

61. Higgins MW. Chronic airways disease in the United States. trends and determinants. Chest 1998; 96:328S–334S.

62. Statistical Abstract of the United States. 3. Washington, DC: U.S. Bureau of the Census, 1991.

63. Seneff MG, Wagner DP, Wagner RP'JE, Knaus WA. Hospital and 1-year survival of patients admitted to intensive care units with acute exacerbation of chronic obstructive pulmonary disease. JAMA 1995; 274:1852–1857.

64. Higgins MW, Thom T. Clinical Epidemiology of Chronic Obstructive Pulmonary Disease. New York: Marcel Dekker, 1990:23–43.

65. Niederman MS. Mechanisms and management of COPD. Chest 1998; 113:233S–287S.

66. Hudson LD. Survival data in patients with acute and chronic lung disease requiring mechanical ventilation. Am Rev Respir Dis 1989; 140:S19–S24.

67. Spicher JE, White DP. Outcome and function following prolonged mechanical ventilation. Arch Intern Med 1987; 147:421–425.

68. Brochard L, Mancebo J, Wysocki M, Lofaso F, Conti g, Rauss A, Simonneau G, Benito S, Gasparetto A, Lemaire F, Isabey D, Harf A. Noninvasive ventilation for acute exacerbations of chronic obstructive pulmonary disease. N Engl J Med 1995; 333:817–822.

69. Moran JL, Green JM, Homan SD, Leeson RJ, Leppard PI. Acute exacerbations of

chronic obstructive pulmonary disease and mechanical ventilation: a reevaluation. Crit Care Med 1998; 26:71–78.

70. Vitacca M, Clini E, Porta R, Foglio K, Ambrosino N. Acute exacerbations in patients with COPD: predictors of need for mechanical ventilation. Eur Respir J 1996; 9:1487–1493.

71. Jeffrey AA, Warren PM, Flenley DC. Acute hypercapnic respiratory failure in patients with chronic obstructive lung disease: risk factors and use of guidelines for management. Thorax 1992; 47:34–40.

72. Menzies R, Gibbons W, Goldberg P. Determinants of weaning and survival among patients with COPD who require mechanical ventilation for acute respiratory failure. Chest 1989; 95:398–405.

73. Anthonisen NR. Prognosis in chronic obstructive pulmonary disease: Results from multicenter clinical trials. Am Rev Respir Dis 1989; 140:S95–S99.

74. Ferrer M, Alonso J, Moirera J, Marraes RM, Khalaf A, Aguar MC, Plaza V, Prieto L, Anto JM, Quality of Life of Chronic Obstructive Pulmonary Disease Study Group. Chronic obstructive pulmonary disease stage and health-related quality of life. Ann Intern Med 1997; 127:1072–1079.

75. Ely EW, Baker AM, Evans GW, Haponik EF. The cost of respiratory care in mechanically ventilated patients with chronic obstructive pulmonary disease. Crit Care Med 1999.

76. Conti G, DeBlasi R, Pelaia P, Benito S, Rocco M, Antonelli M, Bufi M, Mattia C, Gasparetto A. Early prediction of successful weaning during pressure support ventilation in chronic obstructive pulmonary disease patients. Crit Care Med 1992; 29:366–371.

77. Sassoon CSH, Light RW, Lodia R, Sieck GC, Mahutte CK. Pressure-time product during continuous positive airway pressure, pressure support ventilation, and T-piece during weaning from mechanical ventilation. Am Rev Respir Dis 1991; 143: 469–475.

78. Antonelli M, Conti g, Rocco M, Bufi M, DeBlasi RA, Vivino G, Gasparetto A, Meduri GU. A comparison of noninvasive positive-pressure ventilation and conventional mechanical ventilation in patients with acute respiratory failure. N Engl J Med 1998; 339:429–435.

79. Nava S, Ambrosino N, Clini E, Prato M, Orlando GVM, Brigada P, Fracchia C, Rubini F. Noninvasive mechanical ventilation in the weaning of patients with respiratory failure due to chronic obstructive pulmonary disease: a randomized controlled trial. Ann Intern Med 1998; 128:721–728.

80. Kollef MH, Horst HM, Prang L, Brock WA. Reducing the duration of mechanical ventilation: three examples of change in the intensive care unit. New Horizons 1998; 6:52–60.

81. Chatila W, Ani S, Guaglianone D, Jacob B, Amoateng-Adjepong Y, Manthous CA. Cardiac ischemia during weaning from mechanical ventilation. Chest 1996; 109: 1577–1583.

82. Ely EW, Namen AM, Tatter S, Lucia MA, Smith AC, Landry S, Case D, Haponik EF. Impact of a ventilator weaning protocol in neurosurgical patients: a randomized, controlled trial. Am J Respir Crit Care Med 1999; 159:A370.

83. Namen AM, Ely EW, Lucia MA, Case D, Tatter S, Haponik EF. Predictors of

successful extubation in neurosurgical patients. Am J Respir Crit Care Med 2000.

84. Chevron V, Menard J, Richard J, Girault C, Leroy J, Bonomarchand G. Unplanned extubation: risk factors of development and predictive criteria for reintubation. Crit Care Med 1998; 26:1049–1053.

85. U.S. Bureau of the Census. Current Population Reports, Special Studies, P23-190. Sixty-Five Plus in the United States. Washington, DC: U.S. Printing Office, 1996.

86. Shaw AB. Age as a basis for healthcare rationing. Support for agist policies. Drugs Aging 1996; 9:403–405.

87. Baltussen R, Leidl R, Ament A. The impact of age on cost-effectiveness ratios and its control in decision making. Health Econ 1996; 5:227–239.

88. Sage WM, Hurst CR, Silverman JF, Bortz WM. Intensive care for the elderly: outcome of elective and nonelective admissions. J Am Geriatr Soc 1987; 35:312–318.

89. Singer PA. Rationing, patient preferences, and cost of care at the end of life. Arch Intern Med 1992; 152:478–480.

90. Giugliano RP, Camargo CA, Lloyd-Jones DM, Zagrodsky JD, Alexis JD, Eagle KA, Fuster V, O'Donnell CJ. Elderly patients receive less aggressive medical and invasive management of unstable angina. Arch Intern Med 1998; 158:1113–1120.

91. Hamel MB, Philips RS, Teno JM, Lynn J, Galanos AN, Davis RB, Connors AF, Desbiens N, Reding D, Goldman L. Seriously ill hospitalized adults: do we spend less on older patients? J Am Geriatr Soc 1996; 44:1043–1048.

92. Hakim RB, Teno JM, Harrell FE, Knaus WA, Wenger NS, Phillips RS, Layde PM, Califf RM, Connors AF, Lynn J. Factors associated with do-not-resuscitate orders: patients' preferences, prognoses, and physicians' judgments. SUPPORT Investigators. The Study to Understand Prognoses and Preferences for Outcome and Risks of Treatments. Ann Intern Med 1996; 125:284–293.

93. Hamel MB, Teno JM, Goldman L, Lynn J, Davis RB, Galanos AN, Desbiens N, Connors AF, Wenger NS, Phillips RS, for the SUPPORT investigators. Patient age and decisions to withhold life-sustaining treatments from seriously ill, hospitalized adults. Ann Intern Med 1999; 130:116–125.

94. Teno JM, Hakim RB, Knaus WA, Wenger NS, Phillips RS, Wu AW, Layde PM, Connors AF, Dawson NV, Lynn JA. Preferences for cardiopulmonary resuscitation: physician-patient agreement and hospital resource use. SUPPORT Investigators. J Gen Intern Med 1995; 10:179–186.

95. Goldberg AI. Life-sustaining technology and the elderly. Prolonged mechanical ventilation factors influencing the treatment decision. Chest 1988; 94:1277–1282.

96. Knaus WA, Draper EA, Wagner DP, Zimmerman JE. An evaluation of outcome from intensive care in major medical centers. Ann Intern Med 1986; 104:410–418.

97. Cohen IL, Lambrinos J. Investigating the impact of age on outcome of mechanical ventilation using a population of 41,848 patients from a statewide database. Chest 1995; 107:1673–1680.

98. Kurek CJ, Cohen IL, Lambrinos J, Minatoya K, Booth FV, Chalfin DB. Clinical and economic outcome of patients undergoing tracheostomy for prolonged mechanical ventilation in New York State during 1993: analysis of 6,353 cases under diagnosis-related group 483. Crit Care Med 1997; 25:983–988.

99. Kurek CJ, Dewar D, Lambrinos J, McLBooth FV, Cohen IL. Clinical and economic outcome of mechanically ventilated patients in New York State during 1993. Chest 1998; 114:214–222.

100. Nunn JF, Milledge JS, Singaraya J. Survival of patients ventilated in an intensive therapy unit. Br Med J 1979; 1:1525–1527.

101. Campion EW, Mulley AG, Goldstein RL, Barnett GO, Thibault GE. Medical intensive care for the elderly. A study of current use, costs, and outcomes. JAMA 1981; 246:2052–2056.

102. Fedullo AJ, Swinburne AJ. Relationship of patient age to cost and survival in a medical ICU. Crit Care Med 1983; 11:155–159.

103. Witek TJ, Schachter EN, Dean NL, Beck GJ. Mechanically assisted ventilation in a community hospital: immediate outcome, hospital charges, and follow-up of patients. Arch Intern Med 1985; 145:235–239.

104. McLean RF, McIntosh JD, Kung GY, Leung DM, Byrick RJ. Outcome of respiratory intensive care for the elderly. Crit Care Med 1985; 13:625–629.

105. Elpern EH, Larson R, Douglass P, Rosen RL, Bone RC. Long-term outcomes for elderly survivors of prolonged ventilator assistance. Chest 1989; 96:1120–1124.

106. Tran DD, Groeneveld AB, van DM, Nauta JJ, Strack van Schijndel RJ, Thijs LG. Age, chronic disease, sepsis, organ system failure, and mortality in a medical intensive care unit. Crit Care Med 1990; 18:474–479.

107. O'Donnell, A. and Bohner, B. Outcome in patients requiring prolonged mechanical ventilation: three year experience. Chest 1991; 100(2):295.

108. Pesau B, Falger S, Berger E, Weimann J, Schuster E, Leithner C, Frass M. Influence of age on outcome of mechanically ventilated patients in an intensive care unit. Crit Care Med 1992; 20:489–492.

109. Gracey DR, Naessens JM, Krishan I, Marshall M. Hospital and posthospital survival in patients mechanically ventilated for more than 29 days. Chest 1992; 101: 211–214.

110. Chelluri L, Pinsky MR, Grenvik AN. Outcome of intensive care of the "oldest-old" critically ill patients. Crit Care Med 1992; 20:757–761.

111. Stauffer JL, Fayter NA, Graves B, Cromb M, Lynch JC, Goeble P. Survival following mechanical ventilation for acute respiratory failure in adult men. Chest 1993; 104:1222–1229.

112. Swinburne AJ, Fedullo AJ, Bixby K, Lee DK, Wahl GW. Respiratory failure in the elderly. Analysis of outcome after treatment with mechanical ventilation. Arch Intern Med 1993; 153:1657–1662.

113. Cohen IL, Lambrinos J, Fein IA. Mechanical ventilation for the elderly patient in intensive care. Incremental charges and benefits. JAMA 1993; 269:1025–1029.

114. Papadakis MA, Lee KK, Browner WS, Kent DL, Matchar DB, Kagawa MK, Hallenbeck J, Lee D, Onishi R, Charles G. Prognosis of mechanically ventilated patients. West J Med 1993; 159:659–664.

115. Dardaine V, Constans T, Lasfargues G, Perrotin D, Ginies. Outcome of elderly patients requiring ventilatory support in intensive care. Aging 1995; 7:221–227.

116. Steiner T, Mendoza G, De GM, Schellinger P, Holle R, Hacke W. Prognosis of stroke patients requiring mechanical ventilation in a neurological critical care unit. Stroke 1997; 28:711–715.

117. Zilberberg MD, Epstein SK. Acute lung injury in the medical ICU. Comorbid conditions, age, etiology, and hospital outcome. Am J Respir Crit Care Med 1998; 157:1159–1164.

118. Ely EW, Evans GW, Haponik EF. Mechanical ventilation in a cohort of elderly patients admitted to an intensive care unit. Ann Intern Med 1998; 131:96–104.

119. Kollef MH, O'Brien JD, Silver P. The impact of gender on outcome from mechanical ventilation. Chest 1997; 111:434–441.

120. Yuen EJ, Gonnella JS, Louis DZ, Epstein KR, Howell SL, Markson LE. Severity-adjusted differences in hospital utilization by gender. Am J Med Qual 1995; 10: 76–80.

121. Boult C, Dowd B, McCaffrey D, Boult L, Hernandez R, Krulewitch H. Screening elders for risk of hospital admission. J Am Geriatr Soc 1993; 41:811–817.

122. Epstein SK, Ciubotaru RL. Independent effects of etiology of failure and time to reintubation on outcome for patients failing extubation. Am J Respir Crit Care Med 1998; 158:489–493.

123. Epstein SK, Ciubotaru RL, Wong JB. Effect of failed extubation on the outcome of mechanical ventilation. Chest 1997; 112:186–192.

124. Burrowes P, Wallace C, Davies JM, Campbell L. Pulmonary edema as a radiologic manifestation of venous air embolism secondary to dental implant surgery. Chest 1992; 101:561–562.

125. Coppola DP, May JJ. Self-extubation: a 12-month experience. Chest 1990; 98:165–169.

126. Vassal TN, Anh GD, Gabillet JM, Guidet B, Staikowsky F, Offenstadt G. Prospective evaluation of self-extubations in a medical intensive care unit. Intensive Care Med 1993; 19:340–342.

127. Boulain T, and the Association des Reanimateurs du Centre-Ouest. Unplanned extubations in the adult invensive care unit: a prospective multicenter study. Am J Respir Crit Care Med 1998; 157:1131–1137.

128. Betbese AJ, Perez M, Rialp G, Mancebo J. A prospective study of unplanned endotracheal extubation in intensive care unit patients. Crit Care Med 1998; 26:1180–1186.

129. Miller RL, Cole RP. Association between reduced cuff leak volume and postextubation stridor. Chest 1996; 110:1035–1040.

17

Noninvasive Ventilation to Facilitate Weaning from Mechanical Ventilation

STEFANO NAVA

S. Maugeri Foundation
Istituto di Pavia
Pavia, Italy

FIORENZO RUBINI

S. Maugeri Foundation
Istituto di Montescano
Montescano, Italy

I. A Word Lesson

"Weaning," as defined by *Stedman's Illustrated Medical Dictionary* (1), is "the act of taking from the breast and nourishing by other means." In the era of technology, it seems odd to apply this delicate and even romantic term that coincides with the beginning of life to the act of suspending mechanical ventilation, an event often associated with difficulty, pain, and disease. On the other hand, the choice of the term "weaning" seems appropriate to express all the care, dedication, and emotional support required by patients who have to abandon the security of the ventilator and the endotracheal tube and start breathing again by themselves. The person who first coined the usage of "weaning" in this context made a perceptive choice to remind us that the disconnection from mechanical ventilation is not only a matter of numbers, ventilator modes, strategies, length of hospital stay, costs and reimbursement. The lesson to be gained from the word, therefore, is that weaning should be as "natural," gradual, and atraumatic as possible.

II. Weaning Failure and Prolonged Ventilation

If we consider weaning from mechanical ventilation as only a matter of pure numbers, we could easily conclude that it is not a major clinical problem, since about 75–80% of patients mechanically ventilated for acute respiratory failure (ARF) resume spontaneous breathing quite easily (2,3).

However, in a prospective cohort of 289 consecutive intubated patients who underwent a trial of extubation, Epstein et al. (4) showed that patients who cannot be easily weaned have a poor prognosis. They found that, after adjusting for severity of illness and comorbid conditions, extubation failure had a significant independent association with increased risk for death, prolonged ICU stay, and transfer to a long-term care or rehabilitation facility.

Table 1 illustrates the rate of weaning success in published series (4–39). The weaning success rate is dramatically different between the studies depending on the case mix and referrals of any individual intensive care unit (ICU). In these studies, patients affected by primary pulmonary disorders like chronic obstructive pulmonary disease (COPD) or adult respiratory distress syndrome (ARDS) have the highest rates of failure. In particular, Brochard et al. (24) stated that "the length of weaning is first explained by etiology of the diseases, with patients with COPD being the most difficult to separate from the ventilator."

A 13-month observational cohort study was undertaken in a French ICU by Troche and Moine (40) to seek predictive criteria for the duration of mechanical ventilation. The presence of an underlying respiratory disorder was the strongest factor in predicting mechanical ventilation lasting longer than 15 days.

Among patients with respiratory disorders, the subset of COPD patients is particularly difficult to wean. This may be related to the fact that these patients are in the terminal phase of their chronic disease and their respiratory function (41) and mechanics (27) are usually severely and irreversibly compromised. Age (42,43), respiratory muscle weakness (44), hypercapnia (45), hypoxia, malnutrition (46), treatment with corticosteroids (47,48) or other agents (49,50), hemodynamic instability (51), and activity limits due to respiratory disorders (41,52) may also contribute to difficult weaning. Once these chronically ill patients have recovered from the most acute phase of their critical illness, they are still likely to require intensive nursing and/or physiotherapy for several weeks (53) before they can be weaned. In one study, these "chronically critically ill" patients, representing only 3% of the total number of patients admitted to the ICUs, used almost 40% of the total patient days of care (54). The manner in which this relatively small population cuts into hospital costs has drawn the attention from experts in the field, so that Wagner (55) has stated that "there is some level of costs of acute care that is beyond our society's economic capacity."

Weaning these patients is not only a matter of costs, just as their outcome cannot simply be considered in terms of intrahospital survival vs. death or wean-

Table 1 Rate of Weaning Failure in Published Series

Author (Ref.)	Year	Failure/total	Failure (%)	Patient type
Sahn and Lakshminarayan (5)	1973	17/100	17	COPD, ARDS, postsurgical
Tahvainen et al. (6)	1983	9/47	19	ARDS, CHF
Pourriat et al. (7)	1986	19/37	51	COPD
Gillepsie et al. (8)	1986	20/74	27	COPD
Kemper et al. (9)	1987	17/35	48	Postsurgical
Montgomery et al. (10)	1987	5/11	45	ARDS, COPD
Sassoon et al. (11)	1987	4/16	25	COPD
Tobin et al. (12)	1987	7/17	41	COPD, CHF, flail chest
Fiastro et al. (13)	1988	6/17	35	Postsurgical
Murciano et al. (14)	1988	5/16	31	COPD
Tomlinson et al. (15)	1989	10/165	6	Miscellaneous
Menzies et al. (16)	1989	26/55	47	Difficult-to-wean COPD
Shikora et al. (17)	1990	15/20	75	Postsurgical
Jabour et al. (18)	1991	22/38	42	Miscellaneous
Yang and Tobin (19)	1991	40/100	40	Miscellaneous
Conti et al. (20)	1992	7/13	53	COPD
Strickland and Hasson (21)	1993	6/15	40	Mainly COPD
Lee et al. (22)	1994	9/52	17	Miscellaneous
Nava et al. (23)	1994	19/42	45	Difficult-to-wean COPD
Brochard et al. (24)	1994	109/456	24	Miscellaneous
Levy et al. (25)	1995	1/24	4	COPD, ARDS
Stroetz and Hubmayr (26)	1995	14/31	45	Miscellaneous
Zanotti et al. (27)	1995	8/23	35	COPD
Epstein (28)	1995	18/94	19	Miscellaneous
Esteban et al. (29)	1995	130/546	24	Miscellaneous
Scheinhorn et al. (30)	1995	190/359	48	Miscellaneous difficult to wean
Epstein and Ciubataru (31)	1996	34/218	16	Miscellaneous
Amoateng-Adjepong et al. (32)	1997	23/64	36	Miscellaneous, half with sepsis
Epstein et al. (4)	1997	42/289	15	Miscellaneous
Krieger et al. (33)	1997	11/49	22	Miscellaneous older patients
Esteban et al. (34)	1997	161/484	33	Miscellaneous
Chao et al. (35)	1997	82/174	47	Mainly difficult-to-wean COPD
Jubran and Tobin (36)	1997	12/24	50	COPD
Capdevilla et al. (37)	1998	6/17	35	Miscellaneous
Jubran et al. (38)	1998	8/19	42	Miscellaneous
Vallverdu et al. (39)	1998	125/217	58	Miscellaneous

ing success vs. failure. Very few studies have looked at the "after-hospital" outcome of these patients, most of whom leave the hospital tracheotomized (56). At least two published studies, one carried out in North America (16) and the other in Europe (23), were specifically aimed at assessing the survival rates of patients with COPD who require mechanical ventilation, according to their success in the weaning process.

Menzies and coworkers (16) found that out of a total of 95 patients, 55 required mechanical ventilation for more than 15 days, 72 were weaned successfully, and 59 died within one year. Interestingly they found that the mortality rate at 1 year in the group successfully weaned was 54% vs. 87% in the group who could not reach respiratory autonomy. They also demonstrated that this latter group was characterized by a very low physical autonomy, since most of the patients were housebound.

The study carried out in Europe (23) recorded the long-term survival of 42 consecutive COPD patients requiring prolonged mechanical ventilation. The results confirmed the trend reported by Menzies et al. (16) with a mortality rate at 1 and 2 years of 23% and 32%, respectively, in the group successfully weaned vs. 62% and 78% in the group of patients who left the hospital ventilator dependent. The most logical explanation for this different outcome would be the different baseline severity of the patients' disease when they were admitted to the ICUs. Analysis of some physiological parameters recorded in the two studies confirmed that a worse premorbid level of activity, pulmonary function, maximal inspiratory pressure, $Paco_2$ level, neuromuscular drive ($P_{0.1}$), and breathing pattern during the T-piece trial were associated with weaning failure. Only in Menzie's study, however, did some of these parameters correlate with survival, but without a very strong statistical significance. In the European study, no variables were significantly associated with survival. The lack of a clear difference in premorbid parameters between survivors and nonsurvivors highlights the importance of other factors that are not strictly linked to the preadmission conditions.

Endotracheal intubation and invasive mechanical ventilation are often accompanied by complications that carry their own morbidity and mortality. Long-term sequelae may develop after complications directly related to intubation (57), such as laryngeal or tracheal injury (58), with the development of false airways, stenosis, and granulomatosis (57). The possible need for heavy sedation or paralysis during the first few days of ventilation may lead to the occurrence of generalized myopathy (59). Indeed, Kollef et al. (60) showed that the use of continuous intravenous sedation was associated with prolonged mechanical ventilation. The "abuse" of controlled mechanical ventilation may also lead to the development of selective diaphragmatic atrophy after only 48 hours, as shown in a laboratory study performed on rats (61).

Infective complications are also important. Torres and coworkers (62) considered the correlation between several risk factors and the development of nosocomial pneumonia; chronic airway obstruction and the presence of an endotracheal tube in situ for more than 3 days were significantly associated with an increased risk of nosocomial pneumonia. These findings have been confirmed by other investigators (63–65), in particular by Fagon et al. (66), who showed how this risk increased by 1% per day of invasive mechanical ventilation. Nosocomial pneumonia is responsible for a longer hospital stay as well as an increase in mortality. An endotracheal tube can predispose to the development of pneumonia by impairing cough and mucociliary clearance. Contaminated secretions can accumulate above and leak around the cuff and bacterial binding to the surface of bronchial epithelium is increased. Invasive ventilatory support also increases the risk of feeding aspiration. Elpern et al. (67) showed that about 50% of tracheotomized patients receiving prolonged ventilation had feeding aspiration. Indeed, protracted ventilation leads to the well-known side effects and complications caused by prolonged bed rest and deconditioning such as changes in skeletal muscle composition (68), altered cardiovascular responses to mild stress, bone demineralization, protein wastage, and decreased total body water (69). The central nervous system, endocrine functions, and blood composition may also be altered.

The frequent occurrence of these complications directly or indirectly attributable to invasive mechanical ventilation may explain why the so-called difficult-to-wean patients have such a poor prognosis. It is mandatory, therefore, to try to reach one of these goals: (1) to avoid intubation and, if it is needed, (2) to minimize the duration of invasive ventilation, and (3) to make weaning as "delicate" as possible, especially in "sensitive" populations like COPD patients.

III. Avoiding Intubation

Meduri et al. (70) opined that "noninvasive ventilation is the first line intervention in patients with acute hypercapnic or hypoxemic respiratory failure." The use of noninvasive ventilation clearly reduces or minimizes intubation-related short- and long-term complications.

In a prospective epidemiological survey performed on 320 consecutive patients in a French ICU, Guerin and colleagues (71) concluded that there was a significantly lower incidence of ventilator-associated pneumonia with facial mask noninvasive ventilation than with tracheal intubation.

Infectious complications are not the only side effects minimized by the use of noninvasive ventilation. For example, mechanical complications of translaryngeal intubation that cause long-term problems such as vocal cord paresis and paralysis (72–75), laryngeal granulomas, and stenosis (76,77) may also be avoided. Indeed, since almost all of the studies on noninvasive ventilation have employed assisted rather than controlled modes, avoiding the need for heavy sedation or paralysis, respiratory muscle atrophy, or drug-induced neuropathy and myopathy are seldom observed.

Noninvasive ventilation has also been shown to provide ventilatory support in patients who have declined intubation, such as those with a poor short-term prognosis due to the severity of underlying diseases (78) or advanced age (79).

Only a few studies have been performed in patients with acute hypoxemic respiratory failure. Wysocki at al. (80) designed a randomized comparison of noninvasive ventilation against conventional therapy in non-COPD patients with acute respiratory failure. A post hoc analysis in the subgroup of patients with normal or low values of $Paco_2$ (<45 mmHg) showed that the rate of endotracheal intubation in patients receiving noninvasive ventilation was 90% vs. 57% in the group treated with conventional therapy.

Contrariwise, in a randomized trial of noninvasive ventilation compared with endotracheal intubation, Antonelli and coworkers (81) more recently found that the two techniques were equally effective in improving gas exchange but that the former technique was associated with fewer complications and a shorter stay in the ICU. The rate of intubation in the noninvasive group was 31%. Overall, though, the rate of success of noninvasive ventilation in the treatment of acute hypercapnic respiratory failure is higher than in hypoxemic failure.

Recent meta-analyses or reviews (82–87) conluded that improvement of gas exchange and avoidance of intubation was obtained in 60–80% of patients with COPD, restrictive thoracic disease or postoperative extubation failure. Most of the studies dealing with the use of noninvasive ventilation in acute respiratory failure were, however, nonrandomized, and some of them did not provide enough data about inclusion and exclusion criteria. Indeed, the majority of these investigations were performed outside of the ICU, in medical wards, noninvasive respiratory units, or respiratory intensive care units, and, therefore, the populations were probably not homogeneously selected.

In fact, in their multicenter, randomized controlled study, performed in 5 different ICUs, Brochard and coworkers (88) found that the failure rate of noninvasive ventilation was higher than previously reported. This study's exclusion criteria are listed in Table 2. Despite the fact that only 11 of the 43 patients (26%)

Table 2 Causes of Exclusion from Noninvasive Ventilation

275 patients admitted to the ICUs
190 not included because of:
   51 patients (27%) required immediate intubation or already undergoing ventilation
   32 patients (17%) left heart failure
   17 patients (9%) pneumonia or sepsis
   15 patients (8%) perioperative period
   11 patients (6%) asthma
   64 patients (34%) various reasons including:
              1. respiratory rate <12 breath/m
              2. administration of sedative drugs
              3. central neural disorders (not related to hypercapnia)
              4. cardiac arrest (within the previous 5 days)
              5. cardiogenic pulmonary edema
              6. upper airway obstruction
              7. facial deformity
              8. excessive secretions with weak cough

Source: Ref. 88.

in the noninvasive ventilation group were intubated compared with 31 of 42 (74%) in the standard treatment group, it is striking that only 85 patients (about 30%) were randomized for the study out of a larger group of 275 patients. The authors concluded that noninvasive ventilation may be useful but only in a carefully selected group of patients.

From an analysis of the literature in which the causes of exclusion from protocols are not always clear, we can conclude that noninvasive ventilatory techniques may be useful to avoid intubation in an ICU setting in about 50% of COPD patients. The percentage of patients with hypoxemic failure who are candidates for noninvasive ventilation awaits further definition, although it could reasonably be expected to be lower.

IV. Reducing the Duration of Mechanical Ventilation

Early postoperative tracheal extubation is being increasingly used by anesthesiologists and intensive care specialists in patients undergoing surgical procedures, particularly cardiac surgery. The so-called fast track clinical pathway is becoming ever more popular, since it has been associated with earlier discharge from the ICU, shorter overall time spent in the hospital, and decreased utilization of resources (89–91).

Reducing the duration of mechanical ventilation is also the goal of physicians dealing with patients ventilated for an episode of acute respiratory failure. This is particularly true for the subset of patients affected by pulmonary disease in whom an initial attempt with noninvasive ventilation may be unsuccessful. Several studies have been performed in an attempt to assess the best ventilatory methods to discontinue ventilatory support at the earliest possible time.

The two most recent and important multicenter trials were performed in the mid-1990s by Brochard and coworkers (24) and Esteban and colleagues (29). Both studies compared the following methods: T-piece trials, pressure support ventilation (PSV), and synchronized intermittent mandatory ventilation (SIMV).

Brochard's study, performed on 456 patients affected by different pathologies, concluded that the outcome of weaning was influenced by the ventilatory strategy, and that the use of PSV resulted in a significant improvement over strictly defined weaning protocols using the other two techniques.

In contrast, the Spanish multicenter study, conducted on 546 patients, found that a once-daily trial of spontaneous breathing with T-piece led to extubation about three times more quickly than SIMV and about twice as quickly as PSV, with multiple daily trials of spontaneous breathing being equally successful. Both studies used very strict protocols and were well designed so that is difficult to explain their opposite results. Whatever the explanation, it is important to stress the point that in the weaning process, the ventilation mode is probably less important than optimal medical management.

Indeed, two recent papers have stressed the concept that use of a standardized protocol to wean patients from mechanical ventilation gives better results in terms of outcome and costs than the traditional practice of physician-directed weaning (92,93) (see Chapter 5). Milic-Emili (94) entitled his famous 1986 editorial "Is weaning an art or a science?" The answer to this question remains elusive even 15 years later, but in light of more recent studies there is strong evidence supporting the opinion that objective "scientific" methods improve outcomes in mechanically ventilated patients. Reflecting this view, Ely (95) concluded that "the new challenge is to effect the necessary changes in physicians' practice styles." We agree with this statement, since too many physicians, believing that weaning is mostly an art, still rely predominantly on subjective, intuitive clinical management. This belief may be bolstered by the fact that successful discontinuation from mechanical ventilation is usually a multifactorial process. Indices that assess single physiological functions are frequently unable to predict an individual's outcome (96–98), and multiple indices are rather complicated to measure and interpret (19,99).

The major limitation to "fast" extubation remains, in our opinion, the lack of guarantees for successful weaning. The removal of an endotracheal tube is, in fact, often seen as abandoning something that gives clinicians security with regards to medical management as well as legal concerns. Is it possible, in this scenario, to guarantee ventilatory support and further time for weaning and yet still remove the endotracheal tube? With this question in the forefront we shall now review and comment on the studies dealing with the substitution of one mode of ventilatory support (invasive) with another (noninvasive).

V. Weaning Through Noninvasive Ventilation

A. The History and Clinical Trials

Before going any further in this chapter we would like to stress that all the studies, and, therefore, all the conclusions drawn from them, are related to selected populations of patients affected mainly by acute-on-chronic, or hypercapnic, respiratory failure. We have stated before that the aim of this new weaning modality is to switch the patients from invasive to noninvasive ventilation early enough to avoid all the problems associated with endotracheal intubation. Because of the ethical and legal issues that this approach raises, it is important to provide evidence that noninvasive mechanical ventilation can, at least theoretically, fully substitute for invasive ventilation. Our group has first tried to provide physiological evidence. In a small group of patients, we recorded physiological parameters before and a few minutes after extubation. The patients were ventilated with the same mode and settings but used noninvasive ventilation after extubation. Figure 1 is a typical recording in an individual patient of inspiratory flow, airway pressure, and esophageal pressure measured with the balloon-catheter technique. Patients were ventilated using pressure support ventilation at an inspiratory pressure of 18 cm H_2O and an expiratory pressure of 4 cm H_2O. Invasive ventilation is shown in the left panel and noninvasive ventilation in the right panel. The two ventilatory modes produced the same pattern of breathing for the same inspiratory muscle effort, suggesting that noninvasive ventilation may theoretically fully substitute for endotracheal intubation.

Noninvasive mechanical ventilation has been used in the weaning process since the early 1990s, but none of the studies examining its use were controlled and/or randomized. The studies were usually performed after the patients had been tracheotomized. Table 3 summarizes the most important findings of these studies.

The technique was first used in the Royal Brompton Hospital in London, where Udwadia and coworkers (100) studied 22 consecutive patients referred to their hospital for weaning difficulties. Nine patients had chest wall defects, six had neuromuscular disorders, and seven primary cardiac disease. Most of the patients had hypercapnic respiratory insufficiency. All of them had undergone at least one conventional weaning attempt, including the use of pressure support

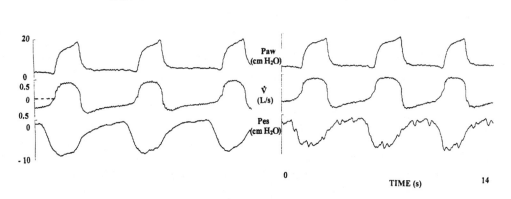

Figure 1 Typical airway pressure (Paw), flow ($\dot{V}$), and esophageal pressure (Pes) during (left) invasive pressure support ventilation and (right) noninvasive pressure support ventilation, in the same patient, minutes after he was extubated. Note that the two ventilatory modes, applied invasively or noninvasively, prodice the same pattern of breathing and inspiratory muscle effort, suggesting that noninvasive ventilation may fully substitute for endotracheal intubation when well applied.

Table 3   Weaning Through Noninvasive Ventilatory Support

Study (Ref.)	Year	Failure/ Total	%	ICU death	Patients	Study design
Udwadia (100)	1992	2/22	9	2	Miscellaneous	Prospective Uncontrolled
Goodenberger (101)	1993	0/2	0	0	Kyphoscoliosis	Retrospective Uncontrolled
Restrick (102)	1993	1/14	7	1	COPD Restrictive Dis.	Prospective Uncontrolled
Laier-Groeneveld (103)	1992	0/35	0	0	COPD Restrictive Dis.	Prospective Uncontrolled
Girault (105)	1999	4/15	27	0	COPD Restrictive Dis.	Prospective Randomized
Nava (106)	1998	3/25	12	2	COPD	Prospective Randomized
Gregoretti (107)	1998	9/22	41	6	Trauma	Prospective Uncontrolled

Most of the patients enrolled were affected by hypercapnic respiratory failure. Most were also tracheotomized.

ventilation. The decision to attempt weaning through noninvasive ventilation was taken only if the patients met the following criteria: (1) intact bulbar function with preserved cough reflex, (2) minimal airway secretion, (3) ability to breathe spontaneously for 10–15 minute, (4) low requirement of oxygen supplementation, (5) cardiac stability, and (6) functioning gastrointestinal tract.

Weaning was performed using either volume cycled ventilation or pressure support ventilation plus continuous positive airway pressure (CPAP); mechanical ventilation was continued for 16–20 hours a day in the first few days, and was then gradually decreased to nocturnal use depending on rate of progress of the individual patient. Twenty of the 22 patients were successfully supported using noninvasive ventilation, and all of these were transferred from the ICU to a step-down unit or a general ward. Only two patients failed to tolerate noninvasive ventilation; both had "pure" hypoxemic respiratory failure, one due to pulmonary fibrosis after ARDS and the other cryptogenic pulmonary fibrosis. Weaning from invasive mechanical ventilation was successful in all 20 patients, although after discharge from the hospital, two patients died of complications after having been reintubated. The duration of mechanical ventilation was not reported, but it was presumably shorter than the time spent in the hospital, which averaged 11 days. The duration of noninvasive mechanical ventilation was approximately 10% of that of invasive ventilation, as shown in Figure 2.

Follow-up at a median 21 of months showed that 16 patients were still alive and well. Although the study was not randomized or controlled, it was

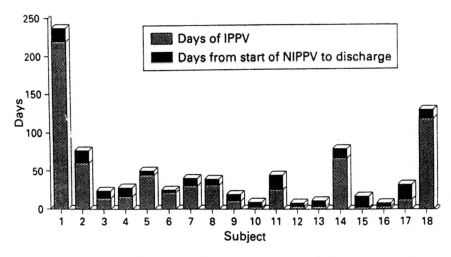

Figure 2 Number of days patients receiving invasive intermittent positive pressure ventilation (IPPV) and the number of days from the start of noninvasive ventilation (NIPPV) until hospital discharge. (From Ref. 100.)

extremely important because it was the first to demonstrate the feasibility of this method of weaning. In addition, it suggested that the technique should be used only in a selected population of patients, based not only on the disease (failure of the two patients with pulmonary fibrosis), but also on the clinical status and stability of the patients (see the exclusion criteria). Another important suggestion was that ventilators specifically designed for noninvasive ventilation should be available in units that regularly manage patients with chronic cardiorespiratory diseases or weaning problems.

During the same year, these observations were strengthened by the report of two patients affected by neuromuscular diseases in whom nocturnal invasive ventilation was replaced by nighttime noninvasive ventilation through a nasal mask allowing decannulation (101).

Restrick and coworkers (102) in the London Chest Hospital later reported on their experience of weaning patients through noninvasive ventilation. They enrolled 14 patients: 8 with COPD and 6 with restrictive disease. The patients were also at different points in the weaning process, making interpretation of the data somewhat difficult. They showed that 13 of 14 patients were successfully weaned with the new technique, while only one patient died in the ICU. The most striking result of this paper was that in 5 of 14 patients, the trials with noninvasive ventilation were started within a week of intubation, and in 3 within the first 24 hours. This experience introduced the idea that the switch from intubation to noninvasive ventilation could be carried out early, even in patients considered by the attending physician ''as individuals in whom weaning from ventilation was predicted to be difficult.''

Some other preliminary results also encouraged the use of noninvasive ventilation as a weaning technique. In Germany, Laier-Groeneveld et al. (103) showed that all but one of their 35 patients affected by chronic hypercapnic respiratory failure and considered unweanable by the attending physicians after 66 ± 44 days of mechanical ventilation had their tracheostomy removed after they were switched to noninvasive ventilation. Most of the patients continued to receive nocturnal ventilatory assistance. These studies are promising, but in this era of evidence-based medicine, randomized, controlled trials are necessary to change the attitudes of physicians towards the controversial problem of weaning.

As mentioned before, early extubation raises ethical and safety concerns. As recently stated, ''the physician should distinguish between liberation (no need for the ventilator) and extubation (no need for [the] endotracheal tube)'' (104), so that after a patient has successfully undergone a trial of unassisted breathing, or is deemed ready to be safely switched to noninvasive ventilation, one must make a second judgment as to whether the artificial airway is still needed. All of the above-mentioned studies enrolled mainly patients with tracheotomy (50/73), so that invasive ventilation could be restored quickly at any time. The technique of using noninvasive ventilation to facilitate early extubation was first developed and tested in Europe where, at the time, legal and ethical issues were perhaps less obtrusive than in the United States. It is not surprising, then, that the first randomized trials of noninvasive mechanical ventilation to expedite extubation were carried out in Europe.

The first, performed by a French group in a single ICU, was conducted on patients intubated for an episode of acute respiratory failure due to COPD or restrictive disease (105). The 33 patients were randomized to receive ''traditional'' weaning with invasive pressure support ventilation or the same modality delivered noninvasively via a face or nasal mask. The duration of mechanical ventilation and time spent in the hospital were shorter in the groups weaned noninvasively. The noninvasively weaned group also had fewer associated complications, although hospital mortality was not affected by the mode of weaning.

Similar results were obtained in a randomized, controlled trial, limited to severely ill COPD patients, that we performed in three respiratory intensive care units in Italy (106). After intubation due to emergency situations (i.e., gasping for air or respiratory arrest) or initial failure of noninvasive ventilation, 68 patients were sedated, often paralyzed and frequently suctioned during the first 6–12 hours after intubation. For the subsequent 24–36 hours, pressure support ventilation was used with a mean peak airway pressure of 21 cm H_2O. Forty-eight hours after intubation, a T-piece trial was performed, but only if the patients were hemodynamically stable, had a normal temperature, an acceptable neurological

Table 4 Definition of T-Piece Trial Failure

Respiratory rate $\geq$ 35 breaths/min
$Pao_2 \leq 50$ mmHg for $Fio_2 \geq 40\%$
Heart rate $\geq$ 145 beats/min
Sustained increase or decrease in heart rate $\geq 20\%$
Severe arrhythmia
Systolic blood pressure $\geq$ 180 mmHg or $\leq$ 70 mmHg
Agitation, anxiety, or diaphoresis

Source: Ref. 106.

status and no signs of pneumonia. Strict criteria were used to determine if the T-piece trial was a failure (see Table 4). Patients who failed the T-piece trial (a total of 50) were randomized after having been reconnected to the ventilator until previous arterial blood gas levels were reestablished. They were either extubated with immediate application of noninvasive ventilation or continued with the endotracheal tube in place and weaned conventionally.

The characteristics of the two groups of patients at the time of randomization are shown in Table 5. Both groups were weaned by daily reductions in the level of pressure support and spontaneous breathing trials at least twice a day.

Table 5 Characteristics of COPD Patients at Time of Randomization for Invasive or Noninvasive Pressure Support Ventilation

Variable	Noninvasive pressure support ventilation group	Invasive pressure support ventilation group
pH	7.31 ± 0.05	7.30 ± 0.04
$Paco_2$, mmHg	61.6 ± 11.6	63.5 ± 12.3
Pao_2:Fio_2 ratio	1.52 ± 0.3	1.64 ± 0.4
Respiratory rate, breaths/min	24.3 ± 6.1	26.2 ± 4.9
Tidal volume, mL/kg	5.82 ± 0.077	6.10 ± 0.091
Maximal inspiratory pressure, cm H_2O	−31 ± 12	−34 ± 9
Kelly and Matthay score	1.4 ± 0.2	1.3 ± 0.2
Systolic blood pressure, mmHg	125 ± 22	119 ± 16
Heart rate, beats/min	92 ± 12	89 ± 10

No major neurological alterations were observed in either group as assessed by Kelly and Matthay score, a scale specifically designed for patients affected by respiratory disorders. Data are mean + SD.
PH = hydrogen ion concentration; $Paco_2$ = arterial carbon dioxide tension; Pao_2 = arterial oxygen tension.
Source: Ref. 106.

Weaning success was defined as the absence of either reintubation or reinstitution of ventilation within the first 72 hours after suspension, while failure was defined as the inability to be weaned in 2 months, or death related to mechanical ventilation. By 60 days 22 of 25 (88%) patients ventilated noninvasively had been successfully weaned vs. 17 of 25 (68%) patients ventilated invasively. Mean duration of mechanical ventilation was significantly different (10 ± 6 vs. 16 ± 11 days, respectively). The probability of success (survival and weaning) during ventilation was found to be significantly higher in the noninvasively ventilated group, as illustrated in Figure 3. ICU stay was significantly shorter in this group (15 ± 5 vs. 24 ± 13 days). Survival rates at 60 days were also statistically different (92% for invasively ventilated group vs. 72% for the invasively ventilated group). None of the patients weaned noninvasively developed nosocomial pneumonia, whereas 7 (28%) of those treated invasively did. Overall, this study showed that use of noninvasive ventilation increased the weaning success and decreased the duration of mechanical ventilation and ICU stay.

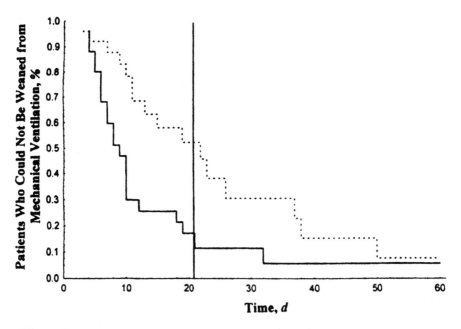

Figure 3   Kaplan-Meier curves for patients who could not be weaned from mechanical ventilation (defined as weaning failure or death linked to mechanical ventilation) in the group undergoing invasive pressure support ventilation (dashed line) and noninvasive pressure support ventilation (solid line). The vertical line represents day 21, usually considered the threshold between weanable and unweanable patients. (From Ref. 106.)

The only study thus far on hypoxemic respiratory failure was recently performed by Gregoretti and coworkers (107). The primary aim of their study was to compare blood gases, tidal volumes, and respiratory rates at equal pressures delivered invasively or noninvasively, but some important clinical data relating to facilitation of extubation were obtained from the follow-up. Twenty-two trauma patients underwent a T-piece trial of at least 15 minutes after a median period of 4 ± 2 days of invasive ventilation and were then switched to noninvasive ventilation. Nine patients (41%) were reintubated after about 2 days because of clinical deterioration, intolerance of the mask, or inability to clear the airways, and six of these died while still being ventilated. Despite the fact that this study was not controlled and not specifically aimed at assessing the feasibility of using noninvasive ventilation as a weaning technique, it demonstrates that this approach can be used in patients other than those with COPD or restrictive thoracic disease. The probability of success was, however, lower than in these latter groups, once again highlighting the possible important difference in outcome according to the underlying pathology.

B. The Rationale

Despite the promising and interesting clinical data, two physiological questions should be answered in order to understand the mechanisms of success of noninvasive ventilation as a weaning technique. The first one is why should it work, and the second is how. Theoretically, noninvasive mechanical ventilation should be reappraised as a weaning technique in COPD after an initial attempt with the same mode has failed. The four main reasons for failure of NIMV during an episode of acute respiratory failure in COPD patients are lack of cooperation, excessive secretions, severe strength-load imbalance, and hemodynamic instability.

Lack of cooperation contributes to patient-ventilator dyssynchrony and dramatically impairs the ability of the ventilator to unload the respiratory muscles (108). This may be due to hypercapnic encephalopathy, which leads on the one hand to psychomotor agitation needing sedation or on the other hand to loss of consciousness and even respiratory arrest. Despite clinical evidence that noninvasive ventilation using iron lungs is possible even in comatose patients (109), we strongly recommend endotracheal intubation in these patients.

Airway hypersecretion occurs commonly in candidates for noninvasive ventilation because many episodes of acute respiratory failure are caused by bacterial or viral agents that contribute to inflammation. Patients with a weak cough reflex, will have difficulty in cleaning the airways and are at risk for failure of noninvasive ventilation.

Strength-load imbalances are often multifactorial, related to alteration of the coupling between respiratory neuromuscular capacity and the elastic or resistive loads against which the respiratory muscle must contract (110). Infections, malnutrition (47), deconditioning, generalized weakness, sleeplessness, electrolyte disturbances (111), improper drug administration (48–51) including oxygen (112), fever, bronchospasm, endocrine abnormalities (113–115), and generalized weakness all contribute to this imbalance.

Cardiovascular instability including a systolic blood pressure of <70 mmHg and severe brady- or tachyarrhythmias are also factors that contribute to the failure of noninvasive ventilation or more often to its avoidance or discontinuation for reasons of safety.

Many of the above-mentioned problems can be swiftly (24–48 hours) corrected by protection of the airways and proper medical therapy. The institution of invasive ventilation in COPD patients is often associated with a prompt decrease in $Paco_2$, normalization of pH, and sensorial improvement. Often, patients can be instructed even while intubated, in the proper use of noninvasive ventilation, aggressive bronchial toilet, and the use of antibiotics can also quickly reduce accumulation of secretions. Ideally, the endotracheal tube should be removed as soon as possible, because it alters muciliary activity and glottic function, hindering the physiological clearance of secretions. Heavy sedation and sometimes paralysis, at least during the first 12 hours after intubation provide respiratory muscle rest and the possibility of a good sleep for these patients who have, according to relatives' reports, often passed whole nights completely awake due to severe breathlessness. This strategy should not be protracted beyond the first 12 hours in order to avoid the risk of respiratory muscle atrophy (61). Meanwhile, the pharmacological armamentarium is brought into play: bronchodilators, vasoactive agents, hydration, correction of electrolyte disturbances, and other specific drugs. Forty-eight hours is therefore often enough time to correct many of the abnormalities that cause initial failure of noninvasive ventilation. Patients may therefore be ready to be switched again to this mode even if they are not ready for complete liberation from ventilation.

The first answer to the question of how noninvasive ventilation works better than invasive ventilation is that it may avoid most of the well-known complications of prolonged intubation. The above-mentioned studies have convincingly demonstrated that infectious complications, in particular, ventilator-associated pneumonia, are avoided. With the removal of the endotracheal tube, the trachea no longer serves as a continuous reservoir for bacteria, which otherwise spread easily into the lower airways. The decrease in infectious complications may explain the diminished in the duration of hospital stay and associated costs. Another important issue linked to the removal of the endotracheal tube is that with noninvasive ventilation, adequate ventilatory support may be given through a "natural" route. Breathing through an endotracheal tube may present a considerable ventilatory challenge (116–118). For example, during pressure support ventilation, up to 10 cm H_2O may be dissipated to overcome the resistance of this tube (119,120). Recently however, Straus et al. (121) demonstrated that, compared to

T-piece breathing, the work of breathing and the pressure time product of the diaphragm (PTPdi), an index of metabolic consumption of the diaphragm, do not change much immediately after extubation. In this study, the recordings were made during mouth breathing and the nose was shut. The work of breathing dissipated in the upper airways immediately after extubation is likely to be even higher if the patient breathes through the nose. The presence of a "fluttering" or "sawtooth" inspiratory flow pattern that suggests uper airway instability and damage with tissue edema (122), commonly present in the short term after extubation, may explain why the work of breathing was not lower immediately after extubation. These findings are important because they show that spontaneous breathing through an endotracheal tube closely reflects the work of breathing after extubation. They suggested the possibility that noninvasive ventilation may reduce the increased upper airways resistance after extubation, by increasing the cross-sectional area at the level of the glottis and, therefore, providing a "bridge" to total spontaneous breathing after extubation has taken place. Table 6 shows that both invasive or noninvasive PSV (M. Vitacca and S. Nava, unpublished observations) reduce PTPdi and airway resistance compared to T-piece and to "total" spontaneous breathing, confirming that in patients not ready yet be weaned, adequate ventilation can be provided by noninvasive ventilation.

If a patients is not ready to be weaned because of incomplete recovery of respiratory muscle function, the excessive work of breathing may be a cause of T-piece trial failure after the "traditional" period of 1–2 hours. Extubation and subsequent use of noninvasive ventilation may be the ideal approach in patients not ready to be totally weaned, but fit enough to breathe spontaneously for a few hours a day of total spontaneous breathing. It is also possible that a few hours (i.e., 24–48) after extubation the airways resistance decreases due to a reduction in postextubation edema, work of breathing may fall, and, compared to a T-piece trial, endurance time may increase.

Table 6 Parameters Recorded During Invasive and Noninvasive Pressure Support Ventilation[a]

	V_T (mL)	Breathing frequency (breaths/min)	Pdi (cm H_2O)	PTPdi/m (cmH_2O × s^{-1})	$R_{,L}$ (cmH$_2$O/L/s)
Invasive PSV	515 ± 99	19.6 ± 4.5	7.6 ± 2.8	198.2 ± 84	10.7 ± 5.3
Noninvasive PSV	572 ± 179	18.0 ± 4.8	8.3 ± 4.1	202.5 ± 111.4	9.9 ± 3.7
T-piece	386 ± 57	24.5 ± 4.2	17.5 ± 3.0	389.2 ± 142.5	14.9 ± 7.1
Spontaneous breathing	431 ± 133	23.1 ± 4.2	18.2 ± 4.2	354.6 ± 158.1	12.5 ± 2.2

[a] Mean + SD recorded during a T-piece trial performed with 2 cm H_2O of CPAP and during the first 3 minutes of total spontaneous breathing immediately after extubation. Data were collected in 8 patients.

Table 7 Contraindications to the
Use of NIMV in the Weaning Process

Hemodynamic instability
Uncooperative patient
Severe hypoxia (i.e., $PaO_2/FiO_2 < 1.5$)
Fever
Sepsis or active infection
Sensorial impairment
Active cardiac ischemia or arrythmias
Weak cough reflex
Upper airway obstruction
Facial trauma
Endentolous condition
Active gastric bleeding

C. Limitations of the Techinique

Weaning through noninvasive ventilation should always be performed with caution. A recent editorial by Epstein (123) identified some of the problems linked
with this innovative technique. In response to the question "should noninvasive
mechanical ventilation be routinely used for weaning from mechanical ventilation?" he answered "clearly no." This is because the published studies pertain
only to patients affected by hypercapnic respiratory failure (pump failure) who
had been meticulously selected, since at the time of extubation they were hemodynamically stable and without fever or any sensorial impairment with a $PaO_2/$
FiO_2 ratio of ≥ 1.5, and an intact cough reflex so that clearing of the airway was
possible. Contraindications to the use of noninvasive ventilation as a weaning
technique are illustrated in Table 7.

Without large-scale studies, it is difficult to quantify how many COPD
patients admitted to ICUs and intubated may successfully undergo this technique
of weaning. In our study, noninvasive weaning was not successful in 3 of 25
patients (12%) and a further 10 of 60 (16%) patients originally enrolled in the
study (68 patients—8 with a successful T-piece weaning trial) were not even
randomized at the time of a T-piece trial due to altered neurological status or
hemodynamic instability. Thus, at least 30% of the intubated patients affected by
COPD are not likely to benefit from this technique. While this appears to be the
current situation for patients with hypercapnic respiratory failure, further studies
are clearly needed to assess the feasibility of the technique in other forms of respiratory failure, such as ARDS, postsurgical complications, or cardiac impairement.

The use of noninvasive ventilation as a weaning technique has the same
problems as those occurring with its use as a primary mode of ventilation. All

of the patients enrolled in our study developed at least one side effect, including cutaneous irritation of the nose (80%), nose abrasion (70%) that was severe in some cases, gastric distension, the need for nasotracheal tube placement (8%), and disrupted sleep and/or claustrophobia in most subjects. Nonetheless, these side effects did not prevent patients from safely undergoing the trial with noninvasive ventilation, although some patients in other studies have stopped noninvasive ventilation because of these side effects, particularly severe nose lesions (126).

Another important limitation of noninvasive ventilation to expedite weaning is personnel time, even though recent studies have shown that noninvasive mechanical ventilation is not as time-consuming (127,128) as we once thought (129). Nevertheless, successful application requires a dedicated and experienced team of physicians, nurses, and respiratory therapists. The location where noninvasive ventilation is initiated is also important. A noninvasive respiratory care unit is the most appropriate location because these units allow work in a specialized environment where medical and paramedical staff are familiar and well trained in the management of both invasive and noninvasive ventilation (128,129). Application of this weaning technique in a general or medical ICU where the personnel consider the ''monitoring of an intubated patient as a simple and classic ICU procedure, contrasting with the difficult supervision of a patient equipped with a mask'' (127). Thus, great care should be taken if weaning using noninvasive ventilation is contemplated. Frequent arterial blood gases analyses, and continuous noninvasive monitoring of Sao_2, EKG, arterial blood pressure, and ventilatory pattern are also mandatory in these patients, so they cannot be sent directly to a general medical ward.

Costs of the technique are not a major limitation since reducing the overall time spent in hospital may, at least theoretically, also reduce overall costs. This hypothesis was confirmed by controlled studies showing that the daily costs incurred by patients undergoing noninvasive ventilation are similar to those of patients receiving medical therapy or undergoing invasive mechanical ventilation (125,126). Indeed, if this technique is applied in the setting of a step-down or noninvasive respiratory care unit, it may even save resources as compared to a traditional ICU (130).

VI. Future Applications

Postextubation failure remains one of the major clinical problems in ICUs. It has been recently reported that the incidence of postextubation failure of patients ventilated in ICUs is relatively high (131), although values ranging from 3.3% to 23.5% have been reported (4). The prognosis of these patients is poor since their hospital mortality exceeds 30–40%, with the cause of extubation failure (i.e., nonairway problems) and the time to reintubation being independent pre-

dictors of outcome (132). Since clinical evidence suggests that the act of reintubation itself is an insufficient explanation for the high mortality rate, it has been
claimed that the clinical deterioration occurring during the time of unsupported
ventilation allows the development of multiple organ failure, which leads to poor
prognosis. This period of unsupported ventilation may be, in some cases, unduly
protracted because physicians avoid new intubation due to the very poor chance
of survival or because of concerns about worsening the patient's clinical status
as a result of the well-known complications associated with intubation. Bearing
in mind the importance of this time factor, early institution of a noninvasive
form of mechanical ventilation in those patients who show signs of "incipient"
respiratory failure, or even the sequential use of this technique right from the
time of extubation, may be attractive strategies that deserve future study.

The so-called "sequential use" of noninvasive ventilation is an interesting
application by Hilbert and coworkers (133). It consists of periods of noninvasive
ventilation, delivered by a home care ventilator, lasting at least 30 minutes every
3 hours. During ventilation-free intervals, patients are systematically resumed on
noninvasive ventilation if Sao_2 is <85% or respiratory rate is >30 breaths/min.
This sequential use has been successfully employed in the management of patients
with acute exacerbations of COPD and may be applied to all patients identified at
risk of postextubation failure. Noninvasive mechanical ventilation delivered in this
fashion has been shown to improve the outcome of patients with COPD and postextubation hypercapnic respiratory failure, compared to matched subjects treated conventionally (134). This study has the obvious limitation that it used historically
matched controls, but the two groups seem to have been well matched. Table 8
shows the outcome of the patients; the use of sequential noninvasive pressure sup-

Table 8 Outcome of Patients with Postextubation Hypercapnic Respiratory
Insufficiency and Treated with Noninvasive Pressure Support Ventilation or Standard
Medical Therapy (Control)[a]

	NIPSV group (*n* = 30)	*p*-value	Control group (*n* = 30)
Patients requiring intubation, %	6 (20)	<0.001	20 (67)
Deaths, %	2 (7)	NS	6 (20)
Outcome in survivor days			
Duration of ventilatory assistance	6 ± 4	<0.01	11 ± 8
Length of ICU stay	8 ± 4	<0.01	14 ± 8

[a] Latter group composed of historically matched patients.
Source: Ref. 134.

port significantly reduced the need for endotracheal intubation, the mean duration of ventilatory assistance and the length of ICU stay, while it had no statistically significant effects on mortality. Mortality was, however, three times higher in the conventionally treated group, suggesting that a study on a larger group of patients could have shown a significant difference in survival. This study also demonstrated a lower incidence of pneumonia in the group treated noninvasively (7% vs. 20%) (134). Considering these promising results, randomized controlled studies are needed to confirm the feasibility and efficacy of the application of noninvasive ventilation to avoid postextubation failure, not only in patients with postextubation hypercapnic but also in those with hypoxemic respiratory failure.

Another potentially important application for noninvasive ventilation is to treat unplanned extubation, which occurs in 3–13% of intubated patients (135–137). Chevron and coworkers (138) have demonstrated that this event occurrs particularly frequently in patients with oral intubation and insufficient sedation. After "unplanned" extubation, 63% of patients did not require reintubation, but when reintubation was mandatory, the mortality of the patients reached approximately 40%. Causes of death in this group were not specified, but in keeping with other studies, infectious complications, including bronchial aspiration, may have played an important role. These complications could be reduced by using noninvasive ventilation.

Early extubation following cardiac or other types of surgery has recently received much attention because financial constraints have encouraged the minimization of postoperative intensive care and have induced anesthesiologists to alter their practice accordingly. The decrease in the duration of intubation has, however, so far been obtained with the use of "lighter" volatile agent–based anesthesia (139), the balanced combination of anesthetics and opioids (140,141), or following strict postoperative intensive care managements protocols. Surprisingly little attention has been given to the ventilatory strategy, including the possible use of noninvasive ventilation, which could theoretically shorten the time of postoperative intubation. Table 9 is a scheme of a possible future applications of noninvasive ventilation to shorten intubation or to avoid it.

Table 9 Possible Future Applications of NIMV in the Field of Weaning

"Sequential" use immediately after extubation
Postextubation failure
Unplanned extubation
Management of extubation following cardiac surgery

VII. Conclusions

In the late 1980s, noninvasive mechanical ventilation was proposed as an alternative treatment for patients with acute respiratory failure (142,143). The technique was considered promising, but it was introduced with caution and even suspicion. At first, it was often reserved for patients who refused endotracheal intubation or who were affected by moderate respiratory failure so that invasive ventilatory treatment was not mandatory (79). Ten years later noninvasive ventilation may be considered as "first-line treatment" for acute hypercapnic respiratory failure (70), while promising results are being obtained with its use in hypoxic respiratory failure (81).

The application of noninvasive ventilation in the early weaning of intubated patients represents a new frontier in the clinical use of this ventilatory mode, but it should be carefully validated as was its use in acute respiratory failure. So far, we have fairly strong evidence that it may work in a selected population of COPD patients with hypercapnic respiratory failure under the supervision of experienced

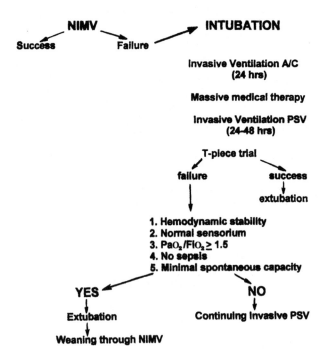

Figure 4 Proposed flow of patients with COPD and acute hypercapnic respiratory failure admitted to the hospital.

teams and in appropriate environments. However, its application in other situations, such as weaning of hypoxic patients, postextubation failure, and in the postsurgical period, remains promising but speculative. Careful selection of patients and strict guidelines must be followed before randomized, controlled studies can validate the use of noninvasive ventilation to facilitate weaning in these other populations. Figure 4 shows a proposed algorithm for the management of ventilation and extubation in patients with COPD, as well as the essential criteria that patients should meet to be switched from invasive to noninvasive ventilation.

Acknowledgment

The partial financial support of Telethon-Italy (Grant n. 1125C) is gratefully acknowledged.

References

1. Stedman's Illustrated Medical Dictionary. 24th ed. Baltimore: Williams and Wilkins, 1992:1575.
2. Goldstone J, Moxham J. Weaning from mechanical ventilation. Thorax 1991; 46: 56–62.
3. Lemaire F. Difficult weaning. Intensive Care Med 1993; 19:S69–S73.
4. Epstein SK, Ciubataru RL, Wong JB. Effect of failed extubation on the outcome of mechanical ventilation. Chest 1997; 112:186–192.
5. Sahn SA, Lakshminaraya S. Bedside criteria for discontinuation of mechanical ventilation. Chest 1973; 63:1002–1005.
6. Tahvanainen J, Salmenpera M, Nikki P. Extubation criteria after weaning from intermittent mandatory ventilation and continuous positive airway pressure. Crit Care Med 1983; 11:702–707.
7. Pourriat JL, Lamberto C, Hoang PH, Fournier JL, Vasseur B. Diaphragmatic fatigue and breathing pattern during weaning from mechanical ventilation in COPD patients. Chest 1986; 90:703–707.
8. Gillepsie DJ, Marsh HM, Divertie MB, Meadows JA. Clinical outcome of respiratory failure in patients requiring prolonged (>24 hours) mechanical ventilation. Chest 1986; 90:364–369.
9. Kemper M, Weissman C, Askanazi J, Hyman AI, Kinney JM. Metabolic and respiratory changes during weaning from mechanical ventilation. Chest 1987; 92:979–983.
10. Montgomery AB, Holle RH, Neagley SR, Pierson DJ, Schoene RB. Prediction of successful ventilator weaning using airway occlusion pressure and hypercapnic challange. Chest 1987; 91:496–499.
11. Sassoon CS, Te TT, Mahutte CK, Light RW. Airway occlusion pressure. An important indicator for successful weaning in patients with chronic obstructive pulmonary disease. Am Rev Respir Dis 1987; 135:107–113.

12. Tobin MJ, Guenther SM, Perez W, Lodato RF, Mador MJ, Allen SJ, Dantzker DR. Konno-Mead analysis of ribcage-abdominal motion during successful and unsuccessful trials of weaning from mechanical ventilation. Am Rev Respir Dis 1987; 35:1320–1328.

13. Fiastro JF, Habib MP, Shon BY, Campbell SC. Comparison of standard weaning parameters and the mechanical work of breathing in mechanically ventilated patients. Chest 1988; 94:232–238.

14. Murciano D, Boczkowski J, Legocguic Y, Milic-Emili JM, Pariente R, Aubier M. Tracheal occlusion pressure: a simple index to monitor respiratory muscle fatigue during acute respiratory failure in patients with chronic obstructive pulmonary disease. Ann Intern Med 1988; 108:800–805.

15. Tomlinson JR, Miller KS, Lorch DG, Smith L, Reines HD, Sahn SA. A prospective comparison of IMV and T-piece weaning from mechanical ventilation. Chest 1989; 96:348–352.

16. Menzies R, Gibbons W, Goldberg P. Determinants of weaning and survival among patients with COPD who require mechanical ventilation for acute respiratory failure. Chest 1989; 95:398–405.

17. Shikora SA, Bistrian BR, Borlase BC, Blackburn GL, Stone MD, Benotti PN. Work of breathing: reliable predictor of weaning and extubation. Crit Care Med 1990; 18:157–162.

18. Jabour ER, Rabil DM, Truwit JD, Rochester DF. Evaluation of a new weaning index based on ventilatory endurance and the efficiency of gas exchange. Am Rev Respir Dis 1991; 155:531–537.

19. Yang KL, Tobin MJ. A prospective study of indexes predicting the outcome of trials of weaning from mechanical ventilation. N Engl J Med 1991; 324:1445–1450.

20. Conti G, de Blasi R, Benito S, Rocco M, Antonelli M, Bufi M, Mattia C, Gasparetto A. Early prediction of successful weaning during pressure support ventilation in COPD patients. Crit Care Med 1992; 20:366–371.

21. Strickland JH, Hasson JH. A computer-controlled ventilator weaning system. A clinical trial. Chest 1993; 103:1220–1226.

22. Lee KH, Hui KP, Chan TB, Tan WC, Lim TK. Rapid shallow breathing (frequency-tidal volume ratio) did not predict extubation outcome. Chest 1994; 105:540–543.

23. Nava S, Rubini F, Zanotti E, Ambrosino N, Bruschi C, Vitacca M, Fracchia C, Rampulla C. Survival and prediction of successful ventilator weaning in COPD patients requiring mechanical ventilation for more than 21 days. Eur Respir J 1994; 7:1645–1652.

24. Brochard L, Rauss A, Benito S, Conti G, Mancebo J, Rekik N, Gasparetto A, Lemaire F. Comparison of three methods of gradual withdrawal from ventilatory support during weaning from mechanical ventilation. Am J Respir Crit Care Med 1994; 150:896–903.

25. Levy MM, Miyasaki A, Langston D. Work of breathing as a weaning parameter in mechanically ventilated patients. Chest 1995; 108:1018–1020.

26. Stroetz RW, Hubmayr RD. Tidal volume maintenance during weaning with pressure support. Am J Respir Crit Care Med 1995; 152:1034–1040.

27. Zanotti E, Rubini F, Iotti G, Braschi A, Palo A, Bruschi C, Fracchia C, Nava S.

Elevated static compliance of the total respiratory system: early predictor of weaning unsuccess in severe COPD patients mechanically ventilated. Intensive Care Med 1995; 21:399–405.

28. Epstein SK. Etiology of extubation failure and the predictive value of the rapid shallow breathing index. Am J Respir Crit Care Med 1995; 152:545–549.

29. Esteban A, Frutos F, Tobin MJ, Alia I, Solsona JF, Valverdu' I, Macias S, Allegue JM, Blanco J, Carriedo D, Leon M, de la Cal MA, Taboada F, Gonzales de Velasco J, Palazon E, Carrizosa F, Tomas R, Suarez J, Goldwasser R. A comparison of four methods of weaning from mechanical ventilation. Spanish Lung Failure Collaborative Group. N Engl J Med 1995; 332:345–350.

30. Scheinhorn DJ, Hassenpflug M, Artinian BM, LaBree L, Catlin JL. Predictors of weaning after 6 weeks of mechanical ventilation. Chest 1995; 107:500–505.

31. Epstein SK, Ciubataru RL. Influence of gender and endotracheal tube size on pre-extubation breathing pattern. Am J Respir Crit Care Med 1996; 154:1647–1652.

32. Amoateng-Adjepong Y, Jacob BK, Ahmad M, Manthous CA. The effect of sepsis on breathing pattern and weaning outcomes in patients recovering from respiratory failure. Chest 1997; 112:472–477.

33. Krieger BP, Isber J, Breitenbucher A, Throop G, Ershowsky P. Serial measurements of the rapid-shallow-breathing index as a predictor of weaning outcome in elderly medical patients. Chest 1997; 12:1029–1034.

34. Esteban A, Alia I, Gordo F, Fernandez R, Solsona JF, Vallerdu' I, et al. Extubation outcome after spontaneous breathing trials with T-tube or pressure support ventilation. Am J Respir Crit Care Med 1997; 156:459–465.

35. Chao DC, Scheinhorn DI, Stearn-Hassenpflug. Patient-ventilator trigger asynchrony in prolonged mechanical ventilation. Chest 1997; 112:1592–1599.

36. Jubran A, Tobin M. Passive mechanics of lung and chest wall in patients who failed or succeeded in trials of weaning. Am J Respir Crit Care Med 1997; 155:916–921.

37. Capdevilla X, Perrigault PF, Ramonatxo M, Roustan JP, Peray P, d'Athis F, Prefault C. Changes in breathing pattern and respiratory muscle performance parameters during difficult weaning. Crit Care Med 1998; 26:79–87.

38. Jubran A, Mathru M, Dries D, Tobin MJ. Continuous recordings of mixed venous oxygen saturation during weaning from mechanical ventilation and the ramifications thereof. Am J Respir Crit Care Med 1998; 158:1763–1769.

39. Vallerdu' I, Calaf N, Subirana M, Net A, Benito S, Mancebo J. Clinical characteristics, respiratory functional parameters, and the outcome of a two-hour T-piece trial in patients weaning from mechanical ventilation. Am J Respir Crit Care Med 1998; 158:1855–1862.

40. Troche G, Moine P. Is the duration of mechanical ventilation predictable? Chest 1997; 112:745–751.

41. Vitacca M, Clini E, Porta R, Foglio K, Ambrosino N. Acute exacerbations in patients with COPD:predictors of need for mechanical ventilation. Eur Respir J 1996; 9:1487–1493.

42. Seneff MG, Zimmerman JE, Knaus WA, Wagner DP, Draper EA. Predicting the duration of mechanical ventilation. The importance of disease and patient characteristics. Chest 1996; 110:469–479.

43. Tolep K, Higgins N, Muza S, Criner G, Kelsen SG. Comparison of diaphragm

strength between healthy adult elderly and young men. Am J Respir Crit Care Med 1995; 152:677–682.

44. Vassilakopoulos T, Zakynthinos S, Roussos C. The tension-time index and the frequency/tidal volume ratio are the major pathophysiologic determinants of weaning failure or success. Am J Respir Crit Care Med 1998; 158:378–385.

45. Juan G, Calverley P, Talamo C, Schnader J, Roussos C. Effect of carbon dioxide on diaphragmatic function in human beings. N Engl J Med 1984; 310:874–879.

46. Lewis MI and Sieck GC. Effect of acute nutritional deprivation on diaphragmatic structure and function in adolescent rats. J Appl Physiol 1992; 73:974–978.

47. Nava S, Gayan-Ramirez G, Rollier H, Bisschop A, Dom R, de Bock V, Decramer M. Effects of acute steroid administration on ventilatory and peripheral muscles in rats. Am J Respir Crit Care Med 1996; 153:1888–1896.

48. Williams TJ, O'Hehir RE, Czarny D, Horne M, Bowes G. Acute myopathy in severe acute asthma treated with intravenously administered corticosteroid. Am Rev Respir Dis 1988; 137:460–463.

49. Op de Coul A, Lambregts P, Koeman J, van Puyenbroek M, Laak H, Gabreels-Festen. Neuromuscular complications in patients given Pavulon (pancuronium bromide) during artificial ventilation. Clin Neurol Neurosurg 1985; 87:17–22.

50. Gooch J, Suchyta M, Balbierz J, Petajan J, Clemmer T. Prolonged paralysis after treatment with neuromuscular junction blocking agents. Crit Care Med 1991; 100: 1125–1130.

51. Nava S, Bellemare F. Cardio-circulatory failure and apnea in shock. J Appl Physiol 1989; 66:184–189.

52. Connors AF, Dawson NV, Thomas C, Harrell FE, Desbiens N, Fulkerson WJ, Kussin P, Bellamy P, Goldman L, Knaus WA for the SUPPORT Investigators. Outcome following acute exacerbation of severe chronic obstructive lung disease. Am J Respir Crit Care Med 1996; 154:959–967.

53. Nava S. Rehabilitation of patients admitted to a Respiratory Intensive Care Unit. Arch Phys Med Rehabil 1998; 79:849–854.

54. Daly BJ, Rudy ED, Thompson KS, Happ MB. Development of a special care unit for chronically ill patients. Heart-Lung 1991; 20:45–52.

55. Wagner DP. Economics of prolonged mechanical ventilation. Am Rev Respir Dis 1989; 140:514–518.

56. Scheinhorn DJ, Chao DC, Stearn-Hassenpflug M, LaBree LD, Heltsley DJ. Post-ICU mechanical ventilation: treatment of 1123 patients at a regional weaning center. Chest 1997; 111:1654–1659.

57. Stauffer JL. Complications of translaryngeal intubation. In: Tobin M, ed. Principles and Practice of Mechanical Ventilation. New York: McGraw-Hill, 1994:711–747.

58. Belson TP. Cuff induced tracheal injury in dogs following prolonged intubation. Laryngoscope 1983; 93:549–555.

59. Berek K, Margreiter J, Willeit J, Berek A, Schmutzard E, Mutz NJ. Polyneuropathies in critically ill patients: a prospective evaluation. Intensive Care Med 1996; 22: 849–855.

60. Kollef MH, Levy NT, Ahrens TS, Schaiff R, Prentice D, Sherman G. The use of continuous IV sedation is associated with prolongation of mechanical ventilation. Chest 1998; 114:541–548.

61. Le Bourdelles G, Vires N, Bockzowki J, Seta N, Pavlovic D, Aubier M. Effects of mechanical ventilation on diaphragmatic contractile properties in rats. Am J Respir Crit Care Med 1994; 149:1539–1544.

62. Torres A, Aznar R, Gatell JM, Jimenez P, Gonzales J, Ferrer A, Celis R, Rodriguez-Roisin R. Incidence, risk, and prognosis factors of nosocomial pneumonia in mechanically ventilated patients. Am Rev Respir Dis 1990; 142:523–528.

63. Craven DE, Kunches LM, Kilinsky V, Lichtenberg DA, Make BJ, McCrabe WR. Risk factors for pneumonia and fatality in patients receiving continuous mechanical ventilation. Am Rev Respir Dis 1986; 133:792–796.

64. Fagon JY, Chastre J, Hance AJ, Montravers P, Novara A, Gilbert C. Nosocomial pneumonia in ventilated patients: a cohort study evaluating attributable mortality and hospital stay. Am J Med 1993; 94:281–288.

65. Torres A, De La Bellacasa JP, Xaubet A, Gonzales J, Rodriguez-Roisin R, Jimenez De Anta MT, Agusti-Vidal A. Diagnostic value of quantitative cultures of bronchoalveolar lavage and telescoping plugged catheters in mechanically ventilated patients with bacterial pneumonia. Am Rev Respir Dis 1989; 140:306–310.

66. Fagon JY, Chastre J, Domart Y, Troulliet JL, Pierre J, Darne C, Gibert C. Nosocomial pneumonia in patients receiving continuous mechanical ventilation. Prospective analysis of 52 episodes with use of protected specimen brush and quantitative culture techniques. Am Rev Respir Dis 1989; 139:877–884.

67. Elpern EH, Scott MG, Petro L, Ries MH. Pulmonary aspiration in mechanically ventilated patients with tracheostomies. Chest 1994; 105:563–566.

68. Bortz WM. Disuse and aging. JAMA 1982; 248:1203–1208.

69. Haines RF. Effect of bed rest and exercise on body balance. J Appl Physiol 1974; 86:323–327.

70. Meduri GU, Turner RE, Abou-Shala N, Wunderink R, Tolley E. Noninvasive positive pressure ventilation via face mask:first-line intervention in patients with acute hypercapnic and hypoxemic respiratory failure. Chest 1996; 109:179–193.

71. Guerin C, Girard R, Chemorin C, De Varax R, Fournier G. Facial mask noninvasive mechanical ventilation reduces the incidence of nosocomial pneumonia. A prospective epidemiological survey from a single ICU. Intensive Care Med 1997; 23:1024–1032.

72. Peppard SB, Dickens JH. Laryngeal injury following short-term intubation. Ann Otol Rhinol Laryngol 1983; 92:327–330.

73. Burns HP, Dayal VS, Scott A, van Nostrand AWP, Bryce DP. Laryngotracheal trauma: observations on its pathogenesis and its prevention following prolonged orotracheal intubation in the adult. Laryngoscope 1979; 89:1316–1325.

74. Whited RE. Laryngeal dysfunction following prolonged intubation. Ann Otol Rhinol Laryngol 1979; 88:474–478.

75. Colice GL. Resolution of laryngeal injury following translaryngeal intubation. Am Rev Respir Dis 1992; 145:361–364.

76. Supance JS, Reilly JS, Doyle WJ, Bluestond CD, Hubbard J. Acquired subglottic stenosis following prolonged endotracheal intubation. Arch Otolaryngol 1982; 108:727–731.

77. Weber AL, Grillo HC. Tracheal stenosis: an analysis of 151 cases. Radiol Clin North Am 1978; 16:291–308.

78. Meduri Gu, Fox RC, Abou-Shala N, Leeper K, Wunderink RG. Noninvasive mechanical ventilation via face mask in patients with acute respiratory failure who refused endotracheal intubation. Crit Care Med 1994; 22:1584–1590.

79. Benhamou D, Girault C, Faure C, Portier F, Muir JF. Nasal mask ventilation in acute respiratory failure. Experience in elderly patients. Chest 1992; 102:912–917.

80. Wysocki M, Tric L, Wolff MA. Noninvasive pressure support ventilation in patients with acute respiratory failure: a randomized comparison with conventional therapy. Chest 1995; 107:761–768.

81. Antonelli M, Conti G, Rocco M, Bufi M, De Blasi RA, Vivino G, Gasparetto A, Meduri GU. A comparison of noninvasive positive-pressure ventilation and conventional mechanical ventilation in patients with acute respiratory failure. N Engl J Med 1998; 339:429–435.

82. Elliott M, Moxham J. Noninvasive mechanical ventilation by nasal or face mask. In: Martin Tobin, ed. Principles and Practice of Mechanical Ventilation. New York: McGraw-Hill 1994:427–453.

83. Keenan SP, Kernerman PD, Cook DJ, Martin CM, McCormack D, Sibbald WJ. Effect of noninvasive positive pressure ventilation on mortality in patients admitted with acute respiratory failure: a meta-analysis. Crit Care Med 1997; 25:1685–1692.

84. Meyer JT, Hill NS. Noninvasive positive pressure ventilation to treat respiratory failure. Ann Intern Med 1994; 120:760–770.

85. Hillberg RE, Johnson D. Noninvasive ventilation. N Engl J Med 1997; 337(24):1746–1752.

86. Elliott MW. Noninvasive ventilation in chronic obstructive pulmonary disease. N Engl J Med 1995; 333(13):870–871.

87. Ambrosino N, Nava S, Rubini F. Noninvasive mechanical ventilation in the treatment of acute respiratory failure in chronic obstructive pulmonary disease. State of the art. Monaldi Arch Chest Dis 1993; 48:144–154.

88. Brochard L, Mancebo J, Wysocki M, Lofaso F, Conti G, Rauss A, Simonneau G, Benito S, Gasparetto A, Lemaire F, Isabey D, Harf A. Noninvasive ventilation for acute exacerbations of chronic obstructive pulmonary disease. N Engl J Med 1995; 833:817–822.

89. London MJ, Shroyer AL, Coll JR, MaWhinney S, Fullerton DA, Hammermeister KE, Grover FL. Early extubation following cardiac surgery in a veterans population. Anesthesiology 1998; 88:1447–1458.

90. Engelman RM, Rousou JA, Flack JE, Deaton DW, Humphrey CB, Ellison LH, Allmendinger PD, Owen SG, Pekow PS. Fast-track recovery of the coronary bypass patient. Ann Thorac Surg 1994; 58:1742–1746.

91. Silbert BS, Santamaria JD, O'Brien JL, Blyth CM, Kelly WJ, Molnar RR, and the Fast Track Cardiac Care Team. Chest 1998; 113:1481–1488.

92. Ely WE, Baker AM, Dunagan DP, Burke HL, Smith AC, Kelly PT, Johnson MM, Browder RW, Bowton DL and Haponik E. Effect on the duration of mechanical ventilation of identifying patients capable of breathing spontaneously. N Engl J Med 1996; 335:1864–1869.

93. Kollef MH, Shapiro SD, Silver P, St. John RE, Prentice D, Sauer S, Ahrens TS, Shannon W, Baker-Clinkscale D. A randomized, controlled trial of protocol-

directed versus physician-directed weaning from mechanical ventilation. Crit Care Med 1997; 25:567–574.

94. Milic-Emili J. Is weaning an art or a science? Am Rev Respir Dis 1986; 134:1107–1108.

95. Ely EW. Challenges encountered in changing physicians' practice styles: the ventilator weaning experience. Intensive Care Med 1998; 24:539–541.

96. Tobin MJ, Perez W, Guenther SM, Semmer BJ, Mador MJ, Allen SJ, Lodato RF, Dantzker DR. The pattern of breathing during successful and unsuccesful trials of weaning from mechanical ventilation. Am Rev Respir Dis 1986; 134:1111–1118.

97. Milbern SM, Downs JB, Jumper LC Evaluation of criteria for discontinuing mechanical ventilatory support. Arch Surg 1978; 113:1441–1443.

98. Hubmayr RD, Loosbrock LM, Gillepsie DJ, Rodarte JR. Oxygen uptake during weaning from mechanical ventilation. Chest 1988; 94:1148–1155.

99. Jabour ER, Rabil DM, Truwit JD, Rochester DF. Evaluation of a new weaning index based on ventilatory endurance and the efficiency of gas exchange. Am Rev Respir Dis 1991; 144:531–537.

100. Udwadia ZF, Santis GK, Steven MH, Simonds AK. Nasal ventilation to facilitate weaning in patients with chronic respiratory insufficiency. Thorax 1992; 47:715–718.

101. Goodenberger DM, Couser J, May JJ. Successful discontinuation of ventilation via tracheostomy by substitution of nasal positive pressure ventilation. Chest 1992; 102:1277–1279.

102. Restrick LJ, Scott AD, Ward EM, Feneck RO, Cornwell WE, Wedzicha JA. Nasal intermittent positive-pressure ventilation in weaning intubated patients with chronic respiratory disease from assisted intermittent, positive-pressure ventilation. Respir Med 1993; 87:199–204.

103. Laier-Groeneveld G, Kupfer J, Huttemann U, Criee CP. Weaning from invasive mechanical ventilation. Am Rev Respir Dis 1992; 145:A518.

104. Manthous C, Schmidt GA, Hall J. Liberation from mechanical ventilation. A decade of progress. Chest 1998; 114:886–901.

105. Girault C, Daudenthun I, Chevron V, Tamoin F, Leroy J, Bonmarchand G. Noninvasive ventilation as a new weaning technique in acute on chronic respiratory failure. Intensive Care Med 1997; 23:A79.

106. Nava S, Ambrosino N, Clini E, Prato M, Orlando G, Vitacca M, Brigada P, Fracchia C, Rubini F. Noninvasive mechanical ventilation in the weaning of patients with respiratory failure due to chronic obstructive pulmonary disease. A randomized, controlled trial. Ann Intern Med 1998; 128:721–728.

107. Gregoretti C, Beltrame F, Lucangelo U, Burbi L, Conti G, Turello M, Gregori D. Physiologic evaluation of non-invasive pressure support ventilation in trauma patients with acute respiratory failure. Intensive Care Med 1998; 24:785–790.

108. Nava S, Bruschi C, Rubini F, Palo A, Iotti G, Braschi A. Respiratory response and inspiratory effort during pressure support ventilation in COPD patients. Intensive Care Med 1995; 21:871–879.

109. Corrado A, De Paola E, Gorini M, Messori A, Bruscoli G, Nutini S, Tozzi D, Ginanni R. Intermittent negative pressure ventilation in the treatment of hypoxic

hypercapnic coma in chronic respiratory insufficiency. Thorax 1996; 51:1077–1082.

110. Zakynthinos S, Vassilakopoulos T and Roussos C. The load of inspiratory muscles in patients needing mechanical ventilation. Am J Respir Crit Care Med 1995; 152: 1248–1255.

111. Aubier M, Murciano D, Lecocguic Y, Viires N, Jacquens Y, Squara P, Pariente R. Effect of hypophosphatemia on diaphragmatic contractility in patients with acute respiratory failure. N Engl J Med 1985; 13:420–424.

112. Derenne JP, Fleury B, Pariente R. Acute respiratory failure of chronic obstructive pulmonary disease. Am Rev Respir Dis 1988; 138:1006–1033.

113. Siafakas NM and Bouros D. Respiratory muscles in endocrinopathies. Respir Med 1993; 87:351–358.

114. Gipson GJ, Edmonds JP, Huges GRV. Diaphragm function and lung involvement in systemic lupus erythematosus. Am J Med 1977; 63:926–932.

115. Nava S, Rubini F. Respiratory muscle dysfunction. In: Milic-Emili J, ed. Applied Physiology in Respiratory Mechanics. Berlin: Springer-Verlag, 1998:34–38.

116. Shapiro M, Wilson RK, Casar G, Bloom K, Teague RB. Work of breathing through different sized endotracheal tubes. Crit Care Med 1986; 14:1028–1031.

117. Conti G, Rocco M, De Blasi A, Lappa A, Antonelli M, Buffi M, Gasparetto A. A new device to remove obstruction from endotracheal tubes during mechanical ventilation in critically ill patients. Intensive Care Med 1994; 20:573–576.

118. Banner PM, Kirby RR, Blanch PB. Site of pressure measurement during spontaneous breathing with continuous positive airway pressure: effect on calculating imposed work of breathing. Crit Care Med 1992; 20:528–533.

119. Brochard L, Rua F, Lorino H, Lemaire F, Harf A. Inspiratory pressure support compensates for the additional work of breathing caused by the endotracheal tube. Anesthesiology 1991; 75:739–754.

120. Fiastro FJ, Habib MP, Quan SF. Pressure support compensation for inspiratory work due to endotracheal tubes and demand continuous positive airway pressure. Chest 1988; 93:499–505.

121. Straus C, Louis B, Isabey D, Lemaire F, Harf A, Brochard L. Contribution of the endotracheal tube and the upper airway to breathing workload. Am J Respir Crit Care Med 1998; 157:23–30.

122. Neukirch F, Weitzenblum E, Liard R, Korobaeff M, Henry C, Orvoen-Frija E, Kauffmann F. Frequency and correlates of the saw-tooth pattern of flow-volume curves in an epidemiological survey. Chest 1992; 101:425–431.

123. Epstein SK. June 1998 editorial on Critical Care Journal Club, Respiratory Failure and Mechanical Ventilation section. *www.thoracic.org*.

124. Vitacca M, Rubini F, Foglio K, Scalvini S, Nava S, Ambrosino N. Non-invasive modalities of positive pressure ventilation improve the outcome of acute exacerbation in COLD patients. Intensive Care Med 1993; 19:450–455.

125. Nava S, Evangelisti I, Rampulla C, Compagnoni ML, Fracchia C, Rubini F. Human and financial costs of noninvasive mechanical ventilation in patients affected by COPD and acute respiratory failure. Chest 1997; 111:1631–1638.

126. Kramer N, Meyer TJ, Mecharg J, Cece RD, Hill NS. Randomized, prospective trial

of noninvasive positive pressure ventilation in acute respiratory failure. Am J Respir Crit Care Med 1995; 151:1799–1806.

127. Chevrolet JC, Jolliet P, Abajo B, Toussi A, Louis M. Nasal positive pressure ventilation in patients with acute respiratory failure. Difficult and time-consuming procedure for nurses. Chest 1991; 100:775–782.

128. Nava S, Confalonieri M, Rampulla C. Intermediate respiratory intensive care units in Europe: a European prospective. Thorax 1998; 53:798–802.

129. Bone RC, Balk RA. Non-invasive respiratory care unit. Chest 1988; 93:390–394.

130. Byrick RB, Mazer CD, Caskennette GM. Closure of an intermediate care unit. Impact on critical care utilization. Chest 1993; 104:876–881.

131. Torres A, Gatell JM, Aznar E, el-Ebiary M, Puig de la Bellacasa J, Gonzales J, Ferrer M, Rodriguez-Roisisn R. Re-intubation increases the risk of nosocomial pneumonia in patients needing mechanical ventilation. Am J Respir Crit Care Med 1995; 152:137–141.

132. Espstein SK, Ciubotaru RL. Independent effects of etiology of failure and time to reintubation on outcome for patients failing extubation. Am J Respir Crit Care Med 1998; 158:489–493.

133. Hilbert G, Gruson D, Gbikpi-Benissan G, Cardinaud JP. Sequential use of noninvasive pressure support ventilation for acute exacerbations of COPD. Intensive Care Med 1997; 23:955–961.

134. Hilbert G, Gruson D, Portel L, Gbikpi-Benissan G, Cardinaud JP. Noninvasive pressure support ventilation in COPD patients with postextubation hypercapnic respiratory insufficiency. Eur Respir J 1998; 11:1349–1353.

135. Whelan J, Simpson SQ, Levy H. Unplanned extubation. Predictors of successful termination of mechanical ventilatory support. Chest 1994; 105:1808–1812.

136. Tindol GA, DiBenedetto RJ, Kosciuk L. Unplanned extubations. Chest 1994; 105: 1804–1807.

137. Stauffer JL, Olson DE, Petty TL. Complications and consequences of endotracheal intubation and tracheotomy. Am J Med 1981; 70:65–76.

138. Chevron V, Menard JF, Richard JC, Girault C, Leroy J, Bonmarchand G. Unplanned extubation: risk factors of development and predictive criteria for reintubation. Crit Care Med 1998; 26:1049–1053.

139. Shapiro BA, Lichtenthal PR. Inhalation-based anesthetic techniques are the key to early extubation of the cardiac surgical patient. J Cardiothorac Vasc Anesth 1993; 7:135–136.

140. Higgins TL. Safety issues regarding early extubation after coronary artery bypass surgery. J Cardiothorac Vasc Anesth 1995; 9:24–29.

141. Sherry KM, McNamara J, Brown JS, Drummond M. An economic evaluation of propofol/fentanyl compared with midazolam/fentanyl on recovery in the ICU following cardiac surgery. Anaesthesia 1996; 51:312–317.

142. Bach JR, Alba A, Mosher R, Delaubier A. Intermittent positive pressure ventilation via nasal access in the management of respiratory insufficiency. Chest 1987; 92: 168–170.

143. Meduri GU, Conoscenti CC, Menashe P, Nair S. Noninvasive face mask ventilation in patients with acute respiratory failure. Chest 1989; 95:865–870.

18

Strategies to Avoid Ventilator-Induced Lung Injury

**JEAN-DAMIEN RICARD and
DIDIER DREYFUSS**

Hôpital Louis Mourier, Colombes
IFROZ, Faculté de Médecine Xavier
  Bichat
Paris, France

GEORGES SAUMON

IFROZ, Faculté de Médecine Xavier
  Bichat
Paris, France

I. Introduction

Mechanical ventilation has been part of basic life support for several decades. Several potential drawbacks and complications have been identified early in the use of mechanical ventilation (1). Of these, ventilator-induced lung injury (VILI) has recently received much attention in both the experimental (2) and the clinical field (3–6). The purpose of this chapter is to review the different situations in which VILI can occur based on animal studies and to detail different ventilator strategies the clinician may use in order to avoid VILI.

II. Evidence for VILI

A. Ventilation of Intact Lungs

High-Volume VILI

Webb and Tierney were the first to demonstrate that mechanical ventilation could cause pulmonary edema in intact animals (7). They were able to show in rats subjected to positive airway pressure ventilation that pulmonary edema was more severe and occurred more rapidly when the animals were ventilated with 45 cm

H_2O than with 30 cm H_2O peak airway pressure. Animals ventilated for 1 hour with 14 cm H_2O peak airway pressure did not develop edema. It was later confirmed that ventilation with high airway pressure produces capillary permeability alterations, nonhydrostatic pulmonary edema and tissue damage resembling that observed during ARDS (8) (Fig. 1). Further studies demonstrated that VILI depended mainly on lung volume and especially on the end-inspiratory volume (9). The corresponding pressure is termed "plateau" pressure, and its clinical importance has been emphasized in a Consensus Conference on mechanical ventilation (10). The respective roles of increased airway pressure and increased lung volume on the development of VILI were clarified by showing that mechanical ventilation of intact rats with large or low tidal volume (V_T), but with identical peak airway pressures (45 cm H_2O) (9) did not result in the same lung alterations. Pulmonary edema and cellular ultrastructural abnormalities were encountered only in rats subjected to high tidal volume and not in those in which lung distention was limited by thoraco-abdominal strapping (9). Furthermore, animals ventilated with large V_T but negative airway pressure (by means of an iron lung) still developed pulmonary edema thus demonstrating that airway pressure is not a determinant for pulmonary edema (9). Consequently, it was suggested that the term "volutrauma" would be more appropriate than barotrauma in this situation (11,12). Other investigators have reached the same conclusions with different protocols and species. Hernandez and coworkers compared the capillary filtration coefficient (a measure of capillary permeability) of the lungs of rabbits ventilated with 15, 30, and 45 cm H_2O peak airway pressures with that of animals ventilated with the same airway pressures but with limitation of thoraco-abdominal excursions by plaster casts placed around the chest and the abdomen (13). The capillary filtration coefficient of the lungs removed after ventilation was normal in animals ventilated at 15 cm H_2O peak pressure, increased by 31% at 30 cm H_2O peak pressure and by 430% at 45 cm H_2O peak pressure in animals without restriction of lung distention. In striking contrast, limiting lung inflation prevented the in-

Figure 1 (a) Macroscopic aspects of rat lungs after mechanical ventilation at 45 cm H_2O peak airway pressure: (left) normal lungs; (middle) after 5 minutes of high airway pressure mechanical ventilation (note the focal zones of atelectasis, in particular at the left lung apex); (right) after 20 minutes, the lungs were markedly enlarged and congestive; edema fluid fills the tracheal cannula. (From Ref. 2.) (b) Changes in the ultrastructural appearance if the blood-air barrier after mechanical ventilation of a closed-chest rat for 20 minutes at 45 cm H_2O peak airway pressure. Very severe changes in the alveolar/capillary barrier result in diffuse alveolar damage. The epithelial layer is totally destroyed leading to denudation of the basement membrane (arrows). Hyaline membranes (HM), composed of cell debris and fibrin (f), occupy the alveolar space (AS). En = endothelial cells; IE = interstitial edema; In = interstitium. (From Ref. 8.)

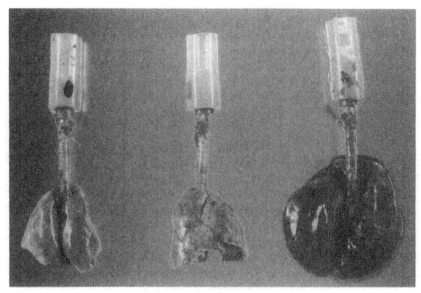

(a)

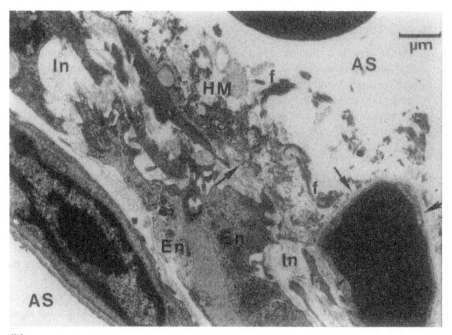

(b)

crease of the capillary filtration coefficient (13). Carlton and coworkers confirmed this observation in lambs (14). The critical role of lung overinflation was further underlined by Adkins and coworkers (15). They studied the effect of ventilation at 30–55 cm H_2O peak airway pressure in young rabbits in comparison with adult animals. They found that the lung capillary filtration coefficient increased more in the young rabbits than in the adult ones, probably because the lung and chest wall compliance of young animals were larger, allowing greater lung overdistention for the same peak airway pressure. Besides the lung distention that occurs during mechanical ventilation, the rate at which lung volume varies may also affect microvascular permeability. Peevy and coworkers (16) used isolated perfused rabbit lungs to determine the capillary filtration coefficient of lungs ventilated with various tidal volumes and inspiratory flow rates. They found that small tidal volumes with a high flow rate increased the filtration coefficient to the same extent (approximately six times baseline value) as ventilation with a markedly higher V_T but a lower inspiratory flow rate for the same peak airway pressure.

Taken together, these experimental studies have demonstrated that large volume rather than high intrathoracic pressures per se results in the ventilator-induced lung edema in intact animals.

Low Lung VILI

Unlike high-volume lung injury (which can be observed in noninjured animals), low lung volume injury is not seen in healthy lungs, which can tolerate mechanical ventilation with physiological tidal volumes and low levels of PEEP for prolonged periods of time without any apparent damage. Taskar and colleagues (17) have shown that the repetitive collapse and reopening of terminal units during 1 hour does not seem to damage healthy lungs (although it does alter gas exchange and reduces compliance).

B. Ventilation of Damaged Lungs

High-Volume Lung Injury

Several investigators have evaluated the effect of mechanical ventilation with overdistension on damaged lungs. Results from these studies consistently stress the increased susceptibility of diseased lungs to the detrimental effects of mechanical ventilation.

The first studies were performed on isolated lungs. Bowton and Kong (18) showed that isolated perfused rabbit lungs injured by oleic acid gained significantly more weight when ventilated with 18 mL/kg body weight (bw) than when ventilated with 6 ml/kg bw V_T. Hernandez and colleagues (19) compared the effects of oleic acid alone, mechanical ventilation alone, and a combination of them both on the capillary filtration coefficient and wet-to-dry weight ratio of isolated perfused lungs from young rabbits. These measurements were not significantly affected by low doses of oleic acid or mechanical ventilation with a peak inspiratory pressure of 25 cm H_2O for 15 minutes. However, the filtration coefficient increased significantly when oleic acid injury was followed by mechanical ventilation. The wet-to-dry weight ratio (a marker of edema severity) of these lungs was significantly higher than that of the lungs subjected to oleic acid injury or ventilation alone. The same workers also showed that the increased filtration coefficient produced by ventilating isolated blood-perfused rabbit lungs with 30–45 cm H_2O peak pressure was greater when surfactant was inactivated by instilling dioctyl-succinate (20). Whereas light microscope examination showed only minor abnormalities (minimal hemorrhage and vascular congestion) in the lungs of animals subjected to ventilation alone, or surfactant inactivation alone, the combination of the two caused severe damage (edema and flooding, hyaline membranes, and extensive alveolar hemorrhage).

These results on isolated lungs suggested that VILI might develop at lower airway pressure in abnormal lungs. Whether this could also be the case in intact animals was investigated by comparing the effects of different degrees of lung distention during mechanical ventilation in rats whose lungs had been injured by α-naphthylthiourea (ANTU) (21). ANTU infusion alone caused moderate interstitial pulmonary edema of the permeability type. Mechanical ventilation of intact rats for 2 minutes resulted in a permeability edema whose severity depended on the tidal volume amplitude. It was possible to calculate how much mechanical ventilation would theoretically injure lungs diseased by ANTU by summing up the separate effect of mechanical ventilation alone or ANTU alone on edema severity (Fig. 2a). The results showed that the lungs of the animals injured by ANTU ventilated at high volume (45 mL/kg bw) had more severe permeability edema than predicted (Fig. 2a), indicating synergism between the two insults rather than additivity. Even minor alterations, such as those produced by spontaneous ventilation during prolonged anesthesia [which degrades surfactant activity and promotes focal atelectasis (22,23)], are sufficient to synergistically increase the harmful effects of high-volume ventilation (Fig. 2b) (21). The extent to which lung mechanical properties have deteriorated prior to ventilation is a key factor in this synergy. The amount of edema produced by high-volume mechanical ventilation in the lungs of animals given ANTU or that had undergone prolonged anesthesia was inversely proportional to the respiratory system compliance measured at the very beginning of mechanical ventilation (21). Thus, the more severe the existing lung abnormalities before ventilation, the more severe the VILI. The reason for this synergy requires clarification. The presence of local alveolar flooding in animals given the most harmful ventilation protocol was the most evident difference from those ventilated with lower, less harmful, tidal volumes (21). It is conceivable that flooding reduced the number of alveoli that received

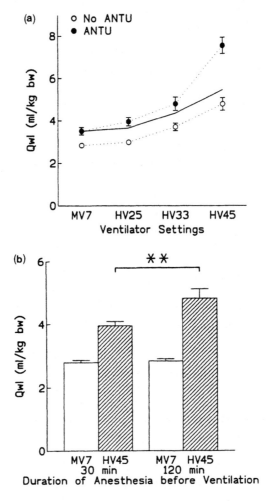

Figure 2 Interaction between previous lung alterations and mechanical ventilation on pulmonary edema. (a) Effect of previous toxic lung injury. Extravascular lung water (Qwl) after mechanical ventilation in normal rats (open circles) and in rats with mild lung injury produced by α-naphthylthiourea (ANTU) (closed circles). V_T varied from 7 to 45 mL/kg bw. The solid line represents the Qwl value expected for the aggravating effect of ANTU on ventilation edema assuming additivity. ANTU did not potentiate the effect of ventilation with V_T up to 33 mL/kg bw. In contrast, ventilation at 45 mL/kg bw V_T resulted in an increase in edema that greatly exceeded additivity, indicating synergy between the two insults. (b) Effect of lung functional alteration by prolonged anesthesia. Intact rats were anesthetized and breathed spontaneously for 30–120 minutes prior to with 7 mL/kg bw (open bars), or at 45 mL/kg bw V_T (shaded bars) V_T in intact rats. Qwl of animals ventilated with a high V_T was significantly higher than in those ventilated with a normal V_T. Qwl was not affected by the duration of anesthesia in animals ventilated with a normal V_T. In contrast, 120 minutes of anesthesia before high V_T ventilation resulted in a larger increase in Qwl than did 30 minutes of anesthesia (**$p < 0.01$). (From Ref. 21.)

the tidal volume, exposing them to overinflation and rendering them more susceptible to injury, further reducing the aerated lung volume and resulting in positive
feedback. The same reasoning applies to prolonged anesthesia, during which the
aerated lung volume was probably gradually reduced by atelectasis (21). Both
flooding and atelectasis decrease compliance, likely to an extent that is correlated
with their spreading. It is thus not surprising that the lower the lung distensibility
before ventilation (as inversely reflected by quasi-static compliance, an index of
the amount of lung that remains open), the more severe the alterations induced
by high-volume ventilation (21). Thus, uneven distribution of ventilation that
occurs during acute lung injury (24) may render lungs more prone to regional
overinflation and injury. To explore this possibility, alveolar flooding was produced by instilling 2 mL saline into the trachea. The rats were then immediately
ventilated for 10 minutes with tidal volumes of up to 33 mL/kg. Flooding with
saline did not significantly affect microvascular permeability when tidal volume
was low. As tidal volume was increased, capillary permeability alterations were
larger in flooded than in intact animals, reflecting further impairment of their
endothelial barrier (Fig. 3). There was also a correlation between end-inspiratory

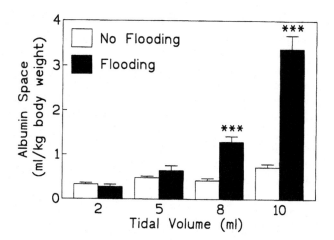

Figure 3   Effect of increasing V_T during mechanical ventilation for 10 minutes on an
indice of lung capillary permeability alteration (i.e., extravascular albumin distribution
space in lungs) of rats with intact lungs (open bars) or with alveolar flooding (closed bars)
produced by saline instillation. There was a moderate increase in albumin space in intact
rats at the larger V_T. Lung flooding did produce significant increases of albumin space
when V_T was normal or moderately increased. Albumin space was significantly increased
with V_T of 8 and 10 mL (i.e., 24 and 32 mL/kg bw). The increase in albumin space
exceeded additivity, indicating a positive interaction between the two insults (***$p <$
0.001 as compared with intact animals). (From Ref. 58.)

airway pressure, the pressure at which was found the lower inflection point on the PV curve, and capillary permeability alterations in flooded animals ventilated with a high tidal volume (25). Thus, the less compliant and recruitable the lung was after saline flooding, the more severe were the changes in permeability caused by lung distention.

Low-Volume Ventilation

There may be an increase in trapped gas volume during pulmonary edema and acute lung injury, especially when surfactant properties are altered, because of terminal units closure (26). Under such conditions, the slope of the inspiratory pressure-volume curve of the respiratory system often displays an abrupt increase at low lung volume. This change reflects the massive opening of previously closed units and has been termed the "lower inflection point." Most clinicians are aware of the importance of this phenomenon in terms of arterial oxygenation, since setting PEEP above this inflection point usually results in a very abrupt decrease in shunt and increase in Pao_2 (27–30).

Attention has focused only relatively recently on the possibility that pulmonary lesions may be aggravated if this inflection point lies within the tidal volume. Experimental evidence for this was initially provided by studies comparing conventional mechanical ventilation with high-frequency oscillatory ventilation in premature or surfactant-depleted lungs (see Sec. III.D). More recently, studies performed during conventional mechanical ventilation of surfactant-depleted lungs with various levels of PEEP also support the possibility that the repeated opening and closing of terminal units cause additional injury (31–33). Sykes and coworkers (31,32) studied this issue ventilating rabbits whose lungs were depleted of surfactant by lavage. Peak inspiratory pressure was 15 mmHg at the beginning of the experiment and 25 mmHg at the end (5 hours later), because lung compliance decreased (tidal volume was set but not stated). PEEP was adjusted so that FRC was either above or below the lower inflection point on the inspiratory limb of the pressure-volume curve. This resulted in PEEP levels of about 1–2 mmHg (below inflection) and 8–12 mmHg (above inflection). The mortality rates in the two groups were identical, but the arterial Pao_2 was better preserved and there was less hyaline membranae formation in the high PEEP group (31,32). This lessening of pathological alterations occurred even when the mean airway pressures in the low and high PEEP groups were kept at the same level by adjusting the inspiratory/expiratory time ratio (32). Muscedere and colleagues (33) recently reported similar results for isolated, unperfused, lavaged rabbit lungs ventilated with a low (5–6 mL/kg bw) tidal volume and with a PEEP set below or above the inflection point. However, Sykes and colleagues could not replicate these findings in rabbits with hydrochloric acid–injured lungs using the same ventilation settings (34). The reality of the repetitive opening and closure of terminal units and the significance of the lower inflection point on the PV curve have been recently challenged by Martynowicz and coworkers (35). They studied the regional expansion of oleic acid–injured lungs using the parenchymal marker technique. They found that the gravitational distribution of volume at the functional residual capacity was not affected by oleic acid injury and that the injury was not associated with decreased parenchymal volume of dependent regions. In addition, they found that the temporal inhomogeneity of regional tidal expansion did not increase with oleic acid injury. Their findings are therefore in contradiction with the hypothesis that a gravitational gradient in superimposed pressure during VILI produces compression atelectasis of dependent lung that in turn produces shear injury from cyclic recruitment and collapse (35). They propose a different explanation for the occurrence of a lower inflection point on the PV curve, namely the displacement of air/liquid interfaces along the tracheobronchial tree rather than alveolar recruitment and derecruitment and thus a different mechanism by which PEEP restores the regional tidal expansion of dependent regions. It therefore remains unsettled whether injury caused by the repetitive reopening of collapsed terminal units and the protective effect of PEEP is restricted to the peculiar situation of surfactant depletion. It may be that repeated opening and closing during tidal ventilation may damage unstable lung units. PEEP may prevent diffuse alveolar damage during prolonged ventilation at high lung volume by stabilizing distal units.

III. Strategies to Prevent VILI

A. Roles of V_T, PEEP, and Overall Lung Distention

The influence of positive end-expiratory pressure on acute lung injury (and more specifically on ventilator-induced pulmonary edema) must be studied with respect to the level of V_T used. Indeed, PEEP increases functional residual capacity and opens the lung but also displaces end-inspiratory volume towards total lung capacity when V_T is kept constant possibly thus favoring overinflation. PEEP may also affect hemodynamics and lung fluid balance. Therefore, close analysis of the numerous studies which have been done to clarify the relationships between PEEP, oxygenation, and the accumulation of extravascular lung water during hydrostatic or permeability type edema must take into account the experimental approach used, i.e., intact animals or isolated lungs (for which lung water content will differ) and whether or not V_T is reduced (thus increasing or not end-inspiratory lung volume).

Effects of PEEP When V_T Is Kept Constant

Application of PEEP may result in lung overinflation if it is followed by a significant change in FRC owing to the increase in end-inspiratory volume. Depending on the homogeneity of ventilation distribution, this overinflation will affect preferentially the more distensible areas, thus accounting for the usual lack of reduction or even the worsening of edema reported with PEEP during most experiments (36). In intact animals, application of PEEP does not counteract the accumulation of edema fluid during hydrostatic type edema (37) or permeability type edema (37,38), though it improves oxygenation (37) because of the re-opening of flooded alveoli. In isolated ventilated-perfused lung, PEEP aggravates edema fluid accumulation (39). Thus, for a given V_T, increasing FRC with PEEP has dissimilar effects on edema accumulation in isolated lungs and in intact animals. In the latter, the lack of effect of PEEP depends on the balance between PEEP-induced increase in end-inspiratory lung volume, which decreases interstitial pressure and favors fluid filtration in extraalveolar vessels and the hemodynamic depression due to elevated intrathoracic pressure that will decrease filtration pressure. In contrast, the preservation of perfusion rate in isolated-perfused lungs favors the increase in edema.

Effects of PEEP When V_T Is Reduced

Edema is less severe when V_T is decreased and end-inspiratory lung volume is kept constant by increasing FRC with PEEP during high-volume ventilation (2). Webb and Tierney showed that edema was lessened by 10 cm H_2O PEEP application during ventilation with 45 cm H_2O peak airway pressure (7). The authors attributed this beneficial effect of PEEP to the preservation of surfactant activity. It was shown later that although PEEP decreased the amount of edema, it did not change the severity of the permeability alterations as assessed by the increase in dry lung weight (9). However, no alveolar damage was observed in animals ventilated with PEEP in comparison with those ventilated in ZEEP. The only ultrastructural alterations observed with PEEP consisted of endothelial blebbing (9). This preservation of the epithelial layer has received no satisfactory explanation. It may be that PEEP prevented repetitive opening and closing of terminal units, thereby decreasing shear stress at this level. Similar observations have been made by other investigators either in intact animals (40,41) or in perfused canine lobes (42). The potential role of hemodynamic alterations induced by PEEP should be considered. For a given end-inspiratory airway pressure, application of PEEP produces an increase in intrathoracic pressure which adversely affects cardiac output (43,44). Indeed, rats submitted to high peak airway pressure ventilation with 10 cm H_2O PEEP had more severe edema when the hemodynamic alterations induced by PEEP were corrected with dopamine (45). The amount of edema was correlated with systemic blood pressure, suggesting that improvement in cardiac output and increased filtration were responsible for this aggravation. In conclusion, the reduction of edema and of the severity of cell damage by PEEP during ventilation-induced pulmonary edema may be linked to reduced tissue stress (by decreasing volume-pressure excursion) and capillary filtration, as well as to the preservation of surfactant activity.

Importance of Overall Lung Distention

Lung volume at the end of inspiration (i.e., the overall degree of lung distention) is probably the main determinant of VILI severity. Rats ventilated with a low V_T and 15 cm H_2O PEEP developed pulmonary edema whereas rats ventilated with the same V_T but 10 cm H_2O PEEP did not (45). Similarly, doubling V_T (which was not deleterious in animals ventilated in ZEEP) resulted in edema in the presence of 10 cm H_2O PEEP. Thus the safety of a given V_T depends on how much FRC is increased.

In conclusion, ventilation-induced lung injury and edema occurs when a certain degree of lung overinflation is reached. This situation is met when V_T is increased at a given end-inspiratory pressure. By contrast, when PEEP is added to reach the same end-inspiratory pressure, it seems to slow the development of edema and diminish the severity of tissue injury, although the occurrence of microvascular permeability alterations is not prevented (9,45). Finally, when PEEP results in additional overinflation, there is greater edema (45).

B. High-Frequency Oscillatory Ventilation

The search for a way of avoiding the large changes in pressure-volume generated by conventional mechanical ventilation, which could be responsible for additional lung damage during acute respiratory failure, has led to the development of high frequency oscillatory ventilation (HFO). Studies on prematurely delivered lambs (46), baboons (47), and adult rabbits made surfactant-deficient by repeated saline lavage (48–50) indicate that the efficiency of HFO on the lessening of lung lesions depends on the performance of a preliminary sustained static inflation (also called "lung conditioning") to recruit the greatest possible number of lung units before starting HFO (51).

Hamilton and coworkers (48) compared oxygenation and lung pathology in saline-lavaged rabbits ventilated by conventional mechanical ventilation with a 6 cm H_2O PEEP and HFO at similar mean airway pressure (15 cm H_2O). Both groups underwent static inflation at 25–30 cm H_2O for 15 seconds. HFO-treated animals had considerably higher Pao_2. More importantly, whereas conventionally ventilated rabbits had extensive hyaline membrane formation, the lungs of HFO-treated animals had few if any hyaline membranes.

Meredith and coworkers, working on premature baboons, showed that hyaline membrane disease was prevented when HFO was preceded by a recruitment maneuver (47). The importance of successful recruitment for preventing lung injury during HFO was illustrated by the severity of the changes in microvascular and alveolar permeability and histological damage, which were similar to those

caused by conventionally ventilating premature newborn lambs, when recruitment was not successful (46). Failure to achieve recruitment was ascribed to the
inability of premature lungs to secrete enough surfactant (46).

Another study (49) also indicated the pivotal role of lung recruitment. Rabbits made surfactant-deficient (by repeated lung lavage) were subjected to conventional mechanical ventilation with a PEEP (8 cm H_2O) below the inflection
point on the pressure-volume curve and a mean airway pressure of 18–19 cm
H_2O, or to HFO at two levels of mean airway pressure (9–10 and 15–16 cm
H_2O) resulting in low or high lung volumes. All animals underwent recruitment
by static lung inflation at an airway pressure of 30 cm H_2O for 15 seconds and
were then connected to the conventional or HFO ventilator. Lung mechanical
properties were better preserved in the HFO–high-lung volume animals. Indeed,
at the end of the experimental period (7 hours) lung compliance was significantly
greater in HFO–high-volume animals than in those ventilated with HFO–low-
volume or conventional mechanical ventilation. Consequently, HFO–high-
volume animals had a lung volume above FRC three times that of animals ventilated with HFO at low lung volume and five times that of animals conventionally
ventilated. These preserved mechanical properties resulted in markedly better
oxygenation. HFO–high-volume animals had also considerably less hyaline
membrane and bronchiolar epithelium necrosis. This study suggests that reopening an atelectasis-prone lung is not sufficient to prevent injury due to shear
stress when ventilation causes the repeated collapse and opening of terminal airways. It is thus important to keep most of the lung open (52) by applying sufficient mean airway pressure during HFO. Avoiding large pressure volume variations with HFO does not totally prevent lung injury if sufficient functional
residual capacity cannot be maintained.

The prevention of VILI by HFO was essentially demonstrated in the particular context of surfactant deficiency. Its efficiency during other types of lung
injury is largely unknown (51,53).

C. Partial Liquid Ventilation

Partial liquid ventilation (54) with perfluorocarbons has been developed during
the last decade as an alternative to conventional gas mechanical ventilation
for the treatment of acute respiratory failure. Several investigators using different models of acute respiratory failure (surfactant depletion, oleic acid, hydrochloric acid, prematurity) have reported improvement in gas exchange, lung
mechanics, and lung histology (55). Although some investigators have shown a
dose-dependent improvement in gas exchange with Perflubron (LiquiVent®) in
a rabbit model of surfactant depletion (56), others have highlighted the risk of
barotrauma (namely pneumothorax) with the use of large volumes of perfluorocarbon combined with high PEEP or increased tidal volume (57). Until recently,

the effect of partial liquid ventilation on VILI received little attention. Mechanical nonuniformity of diseased lungs may predispose them to VILI by overinflation of the more compliant (ventilatable), aerated zones (21). Perfluorocarbon may reduce this nonuniformity by suppressing air/liquid interfaces and allowing reopening of collapsed or liquid-filled areas. The effect of perfluorocarbon instillation on hyperinflation-induced lung injury during alveolar flooding was investigated in rats (58). Saline was instilled into the trachea to mimic alveolar edema and reduce aerated lung volume. Alveolar flooding significantly aggravated VILI, as attested by an increase in capillary permeability alterations. Tracheal instillation of a low dose (3.3 mL/kg) of Perflubron (LiquiVent®) in these flooded lungs considerably reduced VILI and decreased permeability alterations (Fig. 4). Whereas saline instillation alone raised the lower inflection point (opening pressure) of the respiratory system pressure-volume curve to values as high as 25 cm H_2O, and produced a significant increase in the end-inspiratory pressure, the administration of Perflubron significantly reduced the pressure of the lower inflection point and normalized end-inspiratory pressure (Fig. 5). Interestingly, these decreases were correlated with the lessening of capillary permeability alterations. However, in some instances, Perflubron instillation failed to reduce these alterations. Animals in which this occurred

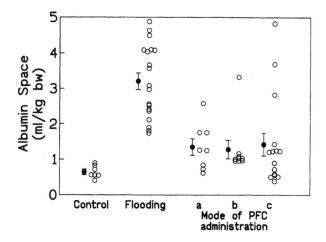

Figure 4 Effect of Perflubron (LiquiVent®) instillation on permeability pulmonary edema as assessed by the extravascular albumin distribution space in the lungs of rats ventilated with 33 mL/kg bw V_T. Flooding significantly increased albumin space ($p < 0.001$). Perflubron given as a bolus (a), by slow infusion before flooding (b), or as a bolus dose after flooding (c) resulted in a significant decrease in albumin space whose values remained higher than in controls ($p < 0.05$). Closed circles with error bar indicate means ± SEM. (From Ref. 58.)

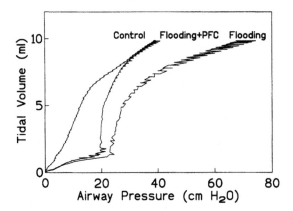

Figure 5 Representative pressure-volume curves of the respiratory system of rats ven-tilated with 33 mL/kg bw V_T. Intact animals (controls) had no discernible lower inflec-tion point. Flooding produced an inflection point; additionally, the slope of the linear part of the curve was reduced and end-inspiratory pressure increased markedly. Perflubron (LiquiVent®) reduced the pressure at which the lower inflection occurred and normalized the end-inspiratory pressure. (From Ref. 58.)

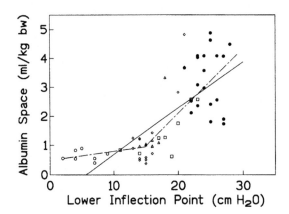

Figure 6 Correlation between the lower inflection point pressure and albumin space in controls (open circles), flooded animals (closed circles), and animals given a bolus dose of Perflubron before flooding (open squares), a slow infusion before flooding (open trian-gles), or a bolus dose after flooding (open diamonds). All animals were ventilated with 33 mL/kg bw V_T. Segmented regression analysis revealed that the best fit was obtained with two joined linear segments. The slope of the first segment is essentially zero. Animals in which Perflubron reduced the lower inflection point pressure had normal or near-normal values for albumin space. There was a threshold for pressure values of around 15 cm H_2O. (From Ref 58.)

had pressures similar to those of animals given saline alone, suggesting that Perflubron administration was unable to "reopen" flooded areas (Fig. 6). Thus in this setting, administration of small doses of Perflubron considerably reduced the harmful effects of mechanical ventilation (58). Nevertheless, the appropriate dose of perfluorocarbon during partial liquid ventilation remains to be determined. To further investigate the effect of partial liquid ventilation on VILI with respect to the dosage of perfluorocarbon, intact animals received increasing doses of Perflubron (LiquiVent®) (from 6 to 20 mL/kg) (59). Hyperinflation-induced pulmonary edema tended to decrease with doses of Perflubron lower than 10 mL/kg as compared to animals not given Perflubron. By contrast, ventilator-induced pulmonary edema was aggravated in animals given 13 and 16 mL/kg, and even more so in animals given 20 mL/kg Perflubron. End-inspiratory pressure was significantly correlated with the capillary permeability alterations. In this setting, administration of small doses of Perflubron (<10 mL/kg) tends to decrease hyperinflation edema and thus protect lungs against volutrauma (58). Larger doses (>20 mL/kg) significantly worsen volutrauma by reducing the volume of aerated lung. These observations suggest that monitoring the end-inspiratory pressure could help detect the risk of volutrauma during partial liquid ventilation.

D. Surfactant

By contrast with the numerous studies on gas exchange improvement after surfactant administration in experimental models of lung injury, few experimental studies have specifically addressed the issue of surfactant administration during VILI. Verbrugge and coworkers have studied the effect of surfactant administration on lung function and alveolar permeability during high peak inspiratory pressure mechanical ventilation of rats (60). Rats were ventilated for 20 minutes with 45 cm H_2O peak inspiratory pressure either with exogenous surfactant at increasing doses (50, 100, or 200 mL/kg) or with an equivalent volume of saline. Lung function was assessed by the Gruenwald index, the amount of active surfactant in bronchoalveolar lavage fluid and the minimal surface tension of the crude lavage fluid. Lung function was better preserved in rats that received 200 mL/kg exogenous surfactant than in all other ventilated animals. Alveolar permeability as assessed by the Evans blue dye influx was significantly reduced in animals receiving the highest doses of surfactant (60).

IV. Clinical Studies

To date, the only mechanical ventilation strategy to prevent VILI that has proved to be efficient in terms of mortality reduction in acute respiratory distress syndrome (ARDS) patients is tidal volume reduction.

A. Tidal Volume Reduction

The clinical relevance of experimental VILI (2) has very recently received a resounding illustration by a NIH randomized trial (6) that showed a 22% reduction of mortality in patients suffering from acute respiratory distress syndrome when lung mechanical stress was lessened by V_T reduction during mechanical ventilation. That excessive tissue stress may occur during mechanical ventilation of ADRS patients was brought to attention only 3 years after the description of ARDS by Jere Mead and coworkers in a visionary paper (61). These authors calculated that tissue stretch around atelectatic areas might be considerable, even at moderately high airway pressure. This led them to speculate that "mechanical ventilators, by applying high transpulmonary pressure to the nonuniformly expanded lungs of some patients who would otherwise die of respiratory insufficiency, may cause the hemorrhage and hyaline membranes found in such patients' lungs at death" (61). In the trial recently completed by the ARDS network (6), 861 patients were randomized either to a traditional ventilation strategy (12 mL/kg predicted body weight tidal volume and plateau pressure of 50 cm H_2O or less) or to a lower tidal volume strategy (6 mL/kg predicted body weight and plateau pressure of 30 cm H_2O or less). The trial was stopped prematurely because mortality was significantly lower in the group treated with lower tidal volumes than in the group treated with traditional tidal volumes (31.0% vs. 39.8%, $p = 0.007$). The wonder is that after more than 30 years of experimental and clinical research involving drugs such as glucocorticoids, alprostadil, nitric oxyde, ketoconazole, procysteine, lisofylline, and ventilatory strategies such as extracorporeal membrane oxygenation, extracorporeal carbon dioxide removal, pressure-controlled inversed i:e ratio ventilation, prone positioning, partial liquid ventilation (all reviewed in Ref. 62), the simplest intervention conceivable such as turning the tidal volume knob of any basic respirator was sufficient by its own to reduce by 22% the mortality of ARDS (6). The results of the NIH trial (6) contrast with those of two previous randomized controlled trials on tidal volume reduction (4,5). These two studies failed to show any benefit of tidal volume reduction on mortality of ARDS patients. Reasons for these negative results may be found in the difference in magnitude of V_T reduction which was greater in the NIH trial (5.6 mL/kg) than in Stewart and coworkers' trial (3.6 mL/kg) (5) or in Brochard and coworkers' trial (3.2 mL/kg) (4). A threshold may thus possibly exist.

B. Alveolar Recruitment

The potential beneficial effect of a mechanical ventilation strategy of ARDS patients that favors alveolar recruitment has been evaluated by Amato and coworkers (3). In this prospective, randomized, controlled trial, a conventional mechanical ventilation strategy based on a 12 mL/kg bw V_T, minimal PEEP, and normal carbon dioxide levels was compared to a protective ventilation strategy including PEEP set above the lower inflection point on the static PV curve, 6 mL/kg bw V_T, driving pressures of less than 20 cm H_2O above PEEP value, and permissive hypercapnia. Although 28-day mortality was significantly lower in the protective-ventilation group, the difference in survival to hospital discharge was not significant. By contrast, occurrence of barotrauma was much more frequent in the conventional-ventilation group than in the protective-ventilation group (42% vs. 7%, $p = 0.02$). According to protocol, PEEP levels differed significantly between the two groups (16.4 cm H_2O during the first 36 hours for the protective-ventilation group and 8.7 cm H_2O for the conventional-ventilation group during the same period). Therefore, it is not clear whether the trend towards an improved prognosis resulted from V_T reduction, increased PEEP, or both? Interestingly, in the NIH trial, PEEP levels were very much similar during the first 3 days of protocol (9.2 cm H_2O in the low V_T group and 8.6 cm H_2O in the conventional-ventilation group). However, and most interestingly, Pao_2/Fio_2 was significantly lower in the low V_T group despite a very slightly higher level of PEEP (i.e., greater alveolar recruitment) (6). These results clearly confirm the experimental concept of high-volume VILI, whereas they cast doubt on the clinical relevance of low lung volume lung injury. In conclusion, the potential benefit of alveolar recruitment by setting high levels of PEEP remains to be proven. The ARDS network is currently conducting a trial comparing two levels of PEEP in combination with low V_T.

C. Surfactant, Partial Liquid Ventilation, and High-Frequency Oscillatory Ventilation

Surfactant Therapy

Surfactant-replacement therapy for patients with ARDS has been less successful in adults than in neonates. To date, two clinical randomized, controlled trials have been published in extenso in adult ARDS (63,64). In the first study that included over 700 patients (63), aerosolized administration of a synthetic surfactant had no effect on oxygenation, duration of mechanical ventilation, or survival. Reasons for the negative results of this study may be found in the nature of the surfactant and its administration modality. First, the surfactant used was protein-free, which may not be the most effective surfactant preparation. Second, surfactant administration was ensured by aerosolization, which may have greatly impeded surfactant delivery to the distal air spaces. In a smaller, albeit randomized controlled pilot trial, Gregory and coworkers (64) studied the effect of several doses of a bovine modified surfactant preparation (beractant) on oxygenation parameters, lung mechanics, and occurrence of side effects in 59 adult ARDS patients. Fio_2 was significantly reduced at 120 hours and 7 days after surfactant administration in the group of patients receiving up to 100 mg $\times$ 4 surfactant. In a whole, surfactant administration was well tolerated. Finally, mortality was not significantly reduced. This study differs considerably from the first one because of the nature and the delivery mode (tracheal instillation) of the surfactant preparation, and these differences may well explain the diverging results.

Partial Liquid Ventilation

Partial liquid ventilation has been investigated in both pediatric and adult patients with ARDS. To our knowledge, no prospective randomized trial in neonates has been published in extenso, although encouraging results have been published in an open study including 13 premature infants with very severe respiratory failure (65). One adult, prospective, randomized trial has been published in abstract form (66). In this study, 90 adult patients were randomized across 18 U.S. centers with 2 partial liquid ventilation for 1 conventional gas ventilation. Sixty-five patients received a mean 22 mL/kg Perflubron (LiquiVent®) with maintenance dosing for an average of 79.6 hours. There were no differences in 28-day mortality and ventilator-free days between the two study groups. Conversely, oxygenation parameters and lung mechanics did not differ between the groups. An international, multicenter randomized controlled trial comparing two doses of Perflubron® and a conventional mechanical ventilation strategy for the treatment of adult ARDS is currently being performed. The first results are expected at the beginning of 2001.

High-Frequency Oscillatory Ventilation

By contrast with the neonatal experience in HFO, no prospective randomized controlled trial comparing HFO and a conventional mechanical ventilation strategy for the treatment of adult ARDS has been published. Recently, a pilot study showed significant improvements in gas exchange and Pao_2/Fio_2 in 13 of 17 severe ARDS patients who were failing inverse ratio mechanical ventilation (mean lung injury score 3.81 and mean Pao_2/Fio_2 68.6) (67). These beneficial effects of HFO must be confirmed by a prospective randomized controlled trial.

V. Conclusion

The results of experimental studies and of clinical trials clearly show that improvement of ARDS prognosis is the result of a more physiological approach of mechanical ventilation, which takes into account the impairment of lung mechanical properties. Questions that remain unanswered are the following:

Should we apply V_T reduction in every patient or try to tailor it according
    to the information provided by the PV curve analysis (68,69)?
Should the hypercapnia that result from the reduced V_T be tolerated? Indeed, in the recent NIH trial, hypercapnia was very mild because of

increased respiratory rate. Recent experimental data suggest that hypercapnia might be beneficial during acute lung injury (70).

What is the optimal PEEP level?

Should we try to improve lung mechanics with perfluorocarbon or surfactant administrations?

Well-conducted randomized studies should provide answers to these questions in the near future.

References

1. Pingleton SK. Complications of acute respiratory failure. Am Rev Respir Dis 1988; 137:1463–1493.
2. Dreyfuss D, Saumon G. Ventilator-induced lung injury: lessons from experimental studies. Am J Respir Crit Care Med 1998; 157:294–323.
3. Amato MB, Barbas CS, Medeiros DM, Magaldi RB, Schettino GP, Lorenzi-Filho G, Kairalla RA, Deheinzelin D, Munoz C, Oliveira R, Takagaki TY, Carvalho CR. Effect of a protective-ventilation strategy on mortality in the acute respiratory distress syndrome. N Engl J Med 1998; 338:347–354.
4. Brochard L, Roudot-Thoraval F, Roupie E, Delclaux C, Chastre J, Fernandez-Mondejar E, Clementi E, Mancebo J, Factor P, Matamis D, Ranieri M, Blanch L, Rodi G, Mentec H, Dreyfuss D, Ferrer M, Brun-Buisson C, Tobin M, Lemaire F. Tidal volume reduction for prevention of ventilator-induced lung injury in acute respiratory distress syndrome. The Multicenter Trail Group on Tidal Volume reduction in ARDS. Am J Respir Crit Care Med 1998; 158:1831–1838.
5. Stewart TE, Meade MO, Cook DJ, Granton JT, Hodder RV, Lapinsky SE, Mazer CD, McLean RF, Rogovein TS, Schouten BD, Todd TR, Slutsky AS. Evaluation of a ventilation strategy to prevent barotrauma in patients at high risk for acute respiratory distress syndrome. Pressure- and Volume-Limited Ventilation Strategy Group. N Engl J Med 1998; 338:355–361.
6. The Acute Respiratory Distress Syndrome Network. Ventilation with lower tidal volumes as compared with traditional tidal volumes for acute lung injury and the acute respiratory distress syndrome. N Engl J Med 2000; 342:1301–1308.
7. Webb HH, Tierney DF. Experimental pulmonary edema due to intermittent positive pressure ventilation with high inflation pressures. Protection by positive end-expiratory pressure. Am Rev Respir Dis 1974; 110:556–565.
8. Dreyfuss D, Basset G, Soler P, Saumon G. Intermittent positive-pressure hyperventilation with high inflation pressures produces pulmonary microvascular injury in rats. Am Rev Respir Dis 1985; 132:880–884.
9. Dreyfuss D, Soler P, Basset G, Saumon G. High inflation pressure pulmonary edema. Respective effects of high airway pressure, high tidal volume, and positive end-expiratory pressure. Am Rev Respir Dis 1988; 137:1159–1164.
10. Slutsky AS. Consensus conference on mechanical ventilation—January 28–30, 1993 at Northbrook, Illinois, USA. Intensive Care Med 1994; 20:64–79.

11. Dreyfuss D, Saumon G. Barotrauma is volutrauma, but which volume is the one responsible? [editorial]. Intensive Care Med 1992; 18:139–141.

12. Dreyfuss D, Soler P, Saumon G. Spontaneous resolution of pulmonary edema caused by short periods of cyclic overinflation. J Appl Physiol 1992; 72:2081–2089.

13. Hernandez LA, Peevy KJ, Moise AA, Parker JC. Chest wall restriction limits high airway pressure-induced lung injury in young rabbits. J Appl Physiol 1989; 66: 2364–2368.

14. Carlton DP, Cummings JJ, Scheerer RG, Poulain FR, Bland RD. Lung overexpansion increases pulmonary microvascular protein permeability in young lambs. J Appl Physiol 1990; 69:577–583.

15. Adkins WK, Hernandez LA, Coker PJ, Buchanan B, Parker JC. Age affects susceptibility to pulmonary barotrauma in rabbits. Crit Care Med 1991; 19:390–393.

16. Peevy KJ, Hernandez LA, Moise AA, Parker JC. Barotrauma and microvascular injury in lungs of nonadult rabbits: effect of ventilation pattern. Crit Care Med 1990; 18:634–637.

17. Taskar V, John J, Evander E, Robertson B, Jonson B. Healthy lungs tolerate repetitive collapse and reopening during short periods of mechanical ventilation. Acta Anaesthesiol Scand 1995; 39:370–376.

18. Bowton DL, Kong DL. High tidal volume ventilation produces increased lung water in oleic acid-injured rabbit lungs. Crit Care Med 1989; 17:908–911.

19. Hernandez LA, Coker PJ, May S, Thompson AL, Parker JC. Mechanical ventilation increases microvascular permeability in oleic acid-injured lungs. J Appl Physiol 1990; 69:2057–2061.

20. Coker PJ, Hernandez LA, Peevy KJ, Adkins K, Parker JC. Increased sensitivity to mechanical ventilation after surfactant inactivation in young rabbit lungs. Crit Care Med 1992; 20:635–640.

21. Dreyfuss D, Soler P, Saumon G. Mechanical ventilation-induced pulmonary edema. Interaction with previous lung alterations. Am J Respir Crit Care Med 1995; 151: 1568–1575.

22. Huang YC, Weinmann GG, Mitzner W. Effect of tidal volume and frequency on the temporal fall in compliance. J Appl Physiol 1988; 65:2040–2047.

23. Ward HE, Nicholas TE. Effect of artificial ventilation and anaesthesia on surfactant turnover in rats. Respir Physiol 1992; 87:115–129.

24. Tsang JY, Emery MJ, Hlastala MP. Ventilation inhomogeneity in oleic acid–induced pulmonary edema. J Appl Physiol 1997; 82:1040–1045

25. Dreyfuss D, Saumon G. Liquivent® instillation reduces ventilation-induced lung injury in flooded lungs (abstr). Am J Respir Crit Care Med 1997; 155:A391.

26. Hughes JMB, Rosenzweig DY. Factors affecting trapped gas volume in perfused dog lungs. J Appl Physiol 1970; 29:332–339.

27. Falke KJ, Pontoppidan H, Kumar A, Leith DE, Geffin B, Laver MB. Ventilation with end-expiratory pressure in acute lung disease. J Clin Invest 1972; 51:2315–2323.

28. Suter PM, Fairley B, Isenberg MD. Optimum end-expiratory airway pressure in patients with acute pulmonary failure. N Engl J Med 1975; 292:284–289.

29. Matamis D, Lemaire F, Harf A, Brun-Buisson C, Ansquer JC, Atlan G. Total respiratory pressure-volume curves in the adult respiratory distress syndrome. Chest 1984; 86:58–66.

30. Benito S, Lemaire F. Pulmonary pressure-volume relationship in acute respiratory distress syndrome in adults: role of positive end-expiratory pressure. J Crit Care 1990; 5:27–34.

31. Argiras EP, Blakeley CR, Dunnill MS, Otremski S, Sykes MK. High peep decreases hyaline membrane formation in surfactant deficient lungs. Br J Anaesth 1987; 59: 1278–1285.

32. Sandhar BK, Niblett DJ, Argiras EP, Dunnill MS, Sykes MK. Effects of positive end-expiratory pressure on hyaline membrane formation in a rabbit model of the neonatal respiratory distress syndrome. Intensive Care Med 1988; 14:538–546.

33. Muscedere JG, Mullen JB, Gan K, Slutsky AS. Tidal ventilation at low airway pressures can augment lung injury. Am J Respir Crit Care Med 1994; 149:1327–1334.

34. Sohma A, Brampton WJ, Dunnill MS, Sykes MK. Effect of ventilation with positive end-expiratory pressure on the development of lung damage in experimental acid aspiration pneumonia in the rabbit. Intensive Care Med 1992; 18:112–117.

35. Martynowicz MA, Minor TA, Walters BJ, Hubmayr RD. Regional expansion of oleic acid-injured lungs. Am J Respir Crit Care Med 1999; 160:250–258.

36. Rizk NW, Murray JF. PEEP and pulmonary edema. Am J Med 1982; 72:381–383.

37. Hopewell PC, Murray JF. Effects of continuous positive-pressure ventilation in experimental pulmonary edema. J Appl Physiol 1976; 40:568–574.

38. Luce JM, Huang TW, Robertson HT, Colley PS, Gronka R, Nessly ML, Cheney FW. The effects of prophylactic expiratory positive airway pressure on the resolution of oleic acid-induced lung injury in dogs. Ann Surg 1983; 197:327–336.

39. Toung T, Saharia P, Permutt S, Zuidema GD, Cameron JL. Aspiration pneumonia: beneficial and harmful effects of positive end-expiratory pressure. Surgery 1977; 82:279–283.

40. Corbridge TC, Wood LDH, Crawford GP, Chudoba MJ, Yanos J, Sznadjer JI. Adverse effects of large tidal volume and low PEEP in canine acid aspiration. Am Rev Respir Dis 1990; 142:311–315.

41. Colmenero Ruiz M, Fernández Mondéjar E, Fernández Sacristán MA, Rivera Fernández R, Vazquez Mata G. PEEP and low tidal volume ventilation reduce lung water in porcine pulmonary edema. Am J Respir Crit Care Med 1997; 155:964–970.

42. Bshouty Z, Ali J, Younes M. Effect of tidal volume and PEEP on rate of edema formation in in situ perfused canine lobes. J Appl Physiol 1988; 64:1900–1907.

43. Permutt S. Mechanical influences on water accumulation in the lungs. In: Pulmonary Edema. Fishman AP, Renkin EM, eds. Washington, D.C.: American Physiology Society, 1979:175–193.

44. Luce JM. The cardiovascular effects of mechanical ventilation and positive end-expiratory pressure. JAMA 1984; 252:807–811.

45. Dreyfuss D, Saumon G. Role of tidal volume, FRC, and end-inspiratory volume in the development of pulmonary edema following mechanical ventilation. Am Rev Respir Dis 1993; 148:1194–1203.

46. Solimano A, Bryan AC, Jobe A, Ikegami M, Jacobs H. Effects of high-frequency and conventional ventilation on the premature lamb lung. J Appl Physiol 1985; 59: 1571–1577.

47. Meredith KS, DeLemos RA, Coalson JJ, King RJ, Gerstmann DR, Kumar R, Kuehl

TJ, Winter DC, Taylor A, Clark RH, Null Jr DM. Role of lung injury in the pathogenesis of hyaline membrane disease in premature baboons. J Appl Physiol 1989; 66: 2150–2158.

48. Hamilton PP, Onayemi A, Smyth JA, Gillan JE, Cutz E, Froese AB, Bryan AC. Comparison of conventional and high-frequency ventilation: oxygenation and lung pathology. J Appl Physiol 1983; 55:131–138.

49. McCulloch PR, Forkert PG, Froese AB. Lung volume maintenance prevents lung injury during high frequency oscillatory ventilation in surfactant-deficient rabbits. Am Rev Respir Dis 1988; 137:1185–1192.

50. Sugiura M, McCulloch PR, Wren S, Dawson RH, Froese AB. Ventilator pattern influences neutrophil influx and activation in atelectasis-prone rabbit lung. J Appl Physiol 1994; 77:1355–1365.

51. Froese AB, Bryan AC. High frequency ventilation. Am Rev Respir Dis 1987; 135: 1363–1374.

52. Lachmann B. Open up the lung and keep the lung open. Intensive Care Med 1992; 18:319–321.

53. Slutsky AS. High frequency ventilation. Intensive Care Med 1991; 17:375–376.

54. Fuhrman BP, Paczan PR, DeFrancisis M. Perfluorocarbon-associated gas exchange. Crit Care Med 1991; 19:712–722.

55. Lachmann B, Fraterman A, Verbrugge SJC. Liquid ventilation. In: Marini JJ, Slutsky AS, eds. Physiological Basis of Mechanical Ventilation. New York: Marcel Dekker, 1998:1131–1154.

56. Tütüncü AS, Akpir K, Mulder P, Erdmann W, Lachmann B. Intratracheal perfluorocarbon administration as an aid in the ventilatory management of respiratory distress syndrome. Anesthesiology 1993; 79:1083–1093.

57. Cox PN, Frndova H, Tan PS, Nakamura T, Miyasaka K, Sakurai Y, Middleton W, Mazer D, Bryan AC. Concealed air leak associated with large tidal volumes in partial liquid ventilation. Am J Respir Crit Care Med 1997; 156:992–997.

58. Dreyfuss D, Martin-Lefevre L, Saumon G. Hyperinflation-induced lung injury during alveolar flooding in rats: effect of perfluorocarbon instillation. Am J Respir Crit Care Med 1999; 159:1752–1757.

59. Ricard J-D, Dreyfuss D, Saumon G. Bell shape dose-dependent effect of Perflubron (PFC) instillation during high volume mechanical ventilation in rats (abstr). Am J Respir Crit Care Med 2000; 161:A25.

60. Verbrugge SJC, Vazquez de Anda G, Gommers D, Neggers SJCMM, Sorm V, Böhm SH, Lachmann B. Exogenous surfactant preserves lung function and reduces alveolar Evans blue dye influx in a rat model of ventilation-induced lung injury. Anesthesiology 1998; 89:467–474.

61. Mead J, Takishima T, Leith D. Stress distribution in lungs: a model of pulmonary elasticity. J Appl Physiol 1970; 28:596–608.

62. Ware LB, Matthay MA. The acute respiratory distress syndrome. N Engl J Med 2000; 342:1334–1349.

63. Anzueto A, Baughman RP, Guntupalli KK, Weg JG, Wiedemann HP, Artigas Raventos A, Lemaire F, Long W, Zaccardelli DS, Pattishall EN. Aerosolized surfactant in adults with sepsis-induced acute respiratory distress syndrome. N Engl J Med 1996; 334:1417–1421.

64. Gregory TJ, Steinberg KP, Spragg R, Gadek JE, Hyers TM, Longmore WJ, Moxley MA, Cai G-Z, Hite RD, Smith RM, Hudson LD, Crim C, Newton P, Mitchell BR, Gold AJ. Bovine surfactant therapy for patients with acute respiratory distress syndrome. Am J Respir Crit Care Med 1997; 155:1309–1315.

65. Leach CL, Greenspan JS, Rubenstein SD, Shaffer TH, Wolfson MR, Jackson JC, DeLemos R, Fuhrman BP. Partial liquid ventilation with perflubron in premature infants with severe respiratory distress syndrome. The LiquiVent Study Group. N Engl J Med 1996; 335:761–767.

66. Bartlett R, Croce M, Hirschl R, Gore D, Wiedemann H, Davis K, Zwischenberger J. A phase II randomized, controlled trial of partial liquid ventilation (PLV) in adult patients with acute hypoxemic respiratory failure (AHRF) (abstr). Crit Care Med 1997; 25:A35.

67. Fort P, Farmer C, Westerman J, Johannigman J, Beninati W, Dolan S, Derdak S. High-frequency oscillatory ventilation for adult respiratory distress syndrome—a pilot study. Crit Care Med 1997; 25:937–947.

68. Roupie E, Dambrosio M, Servillo G, Mentec H, el Atrous S, Beydon L, Brun-Buisson C, Lemaire F, Brochard L. Titration of tidal volume and induced hypercapnia in acute respiratory distress syndrome. Am J Respir Crit Care Med 1995; 152:121–128.

69. Dambrosio M, Roupie E, Mollet JJ, Anglade MC, Vasile N, Lemaire F, Brochard L. Effects of positive end-expiratory pressure and different tidal volumes on alveolar recruitment and hyperinflation. Anesthesiology 1997; 87:495–503.

70. Laffey JG, Engelberts D, Kavanagh BP. Buffering hypercapnic acidosis worsens acute lung injury. Am J Respir Crit Care Med 2000; 161:141–146.

19

Strategies for Diagnosing, Managing, and Avoiding Ventilator-Associated Pneumonia

DANA LUSTBADER, ARUNABH, and ALAN M. FEIN

North Shore University Hospital
Manhasset, New York

Pneumonia is the leading cause of nosocomial infections resulting in death (1). The crude mortality rate for nosocomial pneumonia ranges from 20 to 50% (1,2). Critically ill patients who require mechanical ventilation are prone to developing ventilator-associated pneumonia (VAP), the incidence of which is estimated to range from 10 to 25% (1,3). VAP may increase the risk of death by up to 43% and is associated with prolonged intensive care unit and hospital length of stay (2–4). VAP that occurs during the first 3 days of hospitalization is called early-onset pneumonia and is often caused by antibiotic-sensitive bacteria such as *Haemophilus influenzae, Streptococcus pneumoniae*, and oxacillin-sensitive *Staphylococcus aureus, Moraxella catarrhalis*, and uncommonly by anerobes (5). Late-onset VAP occurring more than 3 days after admission is generally a result of infection by antibiotic-resistant pathogens such as *Pseudomonas aeruginosa, Acinetobacter* or *Enterobacter* species, oxacillin-resistant *S. aureus*, and *Legionella pneumophila* (6). This chapter reviews the epidemiology of VAP and selected controversies surrounding its diagnosis, treatment, and prevention.

I. Introduction

Despite numerous technological advances, the diagnosis of VAP remains difficult. Substantial progress has been made in our understanding of VAP during the past decade, but controversies persist regarding the use of quantitative diagnostic methods, initial treatment, and efficacy of prevention strategies (1,3,7–11). In most hospitals, the diagnosis of VAP is made clinically with the knowledge that specificity is low (8,9,12,13). The specificity may be increased with the use of quantitative bacteriology after bronchoscopy with bronchoalveolar lavage (BAL) or protected specimen brush (PSB), nondirected BAL (NBAL), and quantitative endotracheal aspirates (QEA). There have been no outcome studies comparing these methods to clinical diagnosis alone, in terms of antibiotic use, morbidity, mortality, and cost (8,9,13–20).

Aspiration of bacteria colonizing the oropharynx and stomach with leakage around the endotracheal tube cuff, or direct inoculation of some pathogens, increase bacterial entry into the lower respiratory tract (21–24). Oropharyngeal and gastric colonization, reflux, aspiration, and nosocomial sinusitis may also be contributing factors (21–27).

Despite the initiation of effective antibiotic therapy, the mortality rate for VAP remains high (11,28,29). Prevention of VAP appears to decrease patient morbidity, mortality, and hospital costs, but its importance has not generally been appreciated and introduced into clinical practice (1,3,5).

II. Epidemiology

The epidemiology and natural history of nosocomial pneumonia has changed considerably during the last few decades and even within the last 5 years. It is difficult to predict whether this is due to the introduction of various preventive strategies or to the changing patient population. In addition, the use of invasive devices and respiratory therapy equipment may also contribute to an altered history of this disease process. For example, in the early days of mechanical ventilation, nosocomial pneumonia was frequently associated with the use of mainstream reservoir nebulizers for humidification of respirator gas (30). Today, however, the mechanical ventilator is an uncommon source of microorganisms leading to VAP. Host defense impairment and aspiration are much more commonly implicated.

The bacterial pathogens associated with VAP vary with time of presentation, method of diagnosis, and patient comorbidities (Table 1) (1,13,17,19,23,31–33). Accurate accounting of the incidence of VAP is difficult to obtain because of the nonstandardized diagnostic criteria used. To facilitate standardization of data, infection rates for VAP are reported per thousand ventilator days (34). According to 1996 National Nosocomial Surveillance System (NNIS), the mean rate of VAP in the United States ranges from 6.4 to 20.9 cases per thousand ventilator days (35). Rates of nosocomial pneumonia are increased 6- to 21-fold for intubated patients (25,36–38). It has been estimated that crude rates of VAP are in

Table 1 Pathogens Associated with
Nosocomial Pneumonia

Early-onset pneumonia (<3 days)
  Streptococcus pneumoniae
  Haemophilus influenzae
  Moraxella catarrhalis
  Methicillin-sensitive *Staphylococcus aureus* (MSSA)
Late-onset pneumonia (>3 days)
  Methicillin-resistant *Staphylococcus aureus* (MRSA)
  Pseudomonas aeruginosa
  Enterobacter species
  Acinetobacter species
  Klebsiella pneumoniae
  Serratia marcescens
  Escherichia coli
  Legionella pneumophila

---

the range of 1–3% per day of intubation and mechanical ventilation, but this rate declines after the first week (1,2,39,40,41).

Patients in the ICU with nosocomial pneumonia appear to have a 2- to 10-fold increased risk of mortality compared with ICU patients without pneumonia (4,25,42,43). Recently several studies concluded that one third to one half of all deaths occurring in those with nosocomial pneumonia are directly attributable to the presence of infection (3,4,44). If one accepts this concept of attributable mortality from VAP, then efforts at better understanding strategies for diagnosing, managing, and avoiding VAP could yield benefits in terms of reduced mortality and medical costs (1,45,46).

III. Pathogenesis

The pathogenesis of VAP usually requires two distinct processes to take place: first, the bacterial colonization of the aerodigestive tract and, second, aspiration of these contaminated secretions into the patient's lower airways (6). These pathogens may be a part of the host's endogenous flora or may be acquired from other patients, staff, devices, or the hospital environment. The risk factors for VAP can be broadly classified into factors that alter host defenses and factors that increase adherence to bacteria. Introduction of highly beneficial but complex medical technology, the emergence of antimicrobial resistance among hospital microorganisms, and at times inadequate surveillance for infections, accompanied by a low intensity of infection control by many hospitals have contributed to emergence of VAP as a major health hazard (33,47). Although VAP may result from bacteremia, translocation of bacteria from the gastrointestinal tract, or direct inoculation of the lower airway, aspiration of bacteria from the oropharynx appears to be the most common route of infection. The stomach and lower gastrointestinal tract have not been demonstrated to be a significant source of organisms causing VAP (21–26).

The endotracheal tube facilitates aspiration of contaminated secretions and bacterial colonization of the tracheobronchial tree via mucosal injury, pooling of contaminated secretions above the endotracheal tube cuff, and elimination of the cough reflex (23,24,26). Bacteria may also be directly inoculated from the hands of medical personnel or from contaminated respiratory therapy equipment. In contrast to healthy persons, patients with VAP have high rates of oropharyngeal colonization with bacterial pathogens (21,48). Host factors, endogenous host flora, and the use of antibiotics appear to alter oropharyngeal colonization and bacterial adherence to epithelial cells (49,50). Although the stomach is normally sterile because of the potent bactericidal activity of hydrochloric acid, gastric colonization may result from advanced age, achlorhydria, various gastrointestinal diseases, malnutrition, or use of antacids and H_2 receptor antagonists (51,52). Another risk factor for VAP is enteral feedings, as contamination of tube fed material has been identified as a source of colonization resulting in VAP. Similarly, supine positioning of these patients has been identified as a risk factor (26).

In summary, bacteria causing VAP may originate from the patient's endogenous flora, other patients, hospital personnel, or other environmental sources. Aspiration or direct in-oculation are the major routes of bacterial entry into the lower respiratory tract. The bacterial load and host's lung response are important factors for pathogenesis. Oropharyngeal and gastric colonization with bacteria, cross-infection, as well as the indiscriminate use of antibiotics or invasive devices substantially increase the risk of VAP.

IV. Diagnosis

Understanding the pathogenesis and treatment of bacterial nosocomial pneumonia is limited by the lack of a gold standard for diagnosing lower respiratory tract infection. This makes the accurate diagnosis of VAP particularly challenging.

A. Clinical Diagnostic Criteria

Clinical diagnosis of VAP is often difficult in critically ill patients. Clinical signs of pneumonia such as fever, pulmonary infiltrates on chest radiographs, purulent sputum production, and blood leukocytosis lack specificity in differentiating VAP from other causes of pulmonary infiltrates (13). Fagon et al. (53) showed that in 84 ventilated patients suspected of having VAP, only 27 in fact had pneumonia, and the presence of pneumonia was accurately diagnosed by clinical criteria in only 62% of those predicted. The mean value of blood leukocytes, temperature, Pao_2/Fio_2, and radiological findings were the same in patients who had pneumonia and in those who did not. Wunderink et al. (54) reviewed 69 mechanically ventilated patients who died, 24 of whom had autopsy-proven pneumonia. They showed that no single radiographic sign had a diagnostic accuracy of greater than 68%. Radiographically, air bronchograms were the only sign that correlated well with pneumonia but correctly predicted only 64% of VAP.

Because tracheobronchitis alone does not appear to be associated with poor prognosis, antimicrobial therapy may not be justified. In contrast, Fagon et al. (3) showed that VAP increased mortality by 25% and is associated with a 54% crude mortality rate compared to only 27% mortality in matched controls without pneumonia confirming prior results (4,44).

B. Protected Specimen Brush Technique

The use of the bronchoscopic PSB technique to obtain uncontaminated lower airway secretions for culture was first used in 1979 by Wimberley (55). A special double-catheter system that houses a sterile brush is inserted through the bronchoscope, generally in the region of maximal radiographic infiltrate. The inner brush is extended beyond the distal end of the outer catheter to obtain a specimen and is considered to be free of upper airway contamination. A quantitative bacterial count of at least 10^3 colony-forming units (cfu)/mL is the standard threshold for the diagnosis of pneumonia (56). Cook et al. (57) showed in a meta-analysis of 18 studies using the PSB technique in a total of 524 critically ill patients a sensitivity of 89% and a specificity of 94.3% for diagnosing nosocomial pneumonia. Although the cutoff point of 10^3 cfu/mL to diagnose pneumonia is well established in patients not receiving antibiotics, the culture results of PSB in patients receiving prior antibiotics may be difficult to interpret (58). The PSB technique is of limited value in patients with recent pulmonary infiltrates who have received new antibiotics because a negative finding indicates either that the patient has been successfully treated for pneumonia and the bacteria are eradicated or that pneumonia was never there to begin with. Therefore, a negative PSB result does not rule out the presence of lung infection for patients receiving antibiotics. Concentrations of $<10^3$ cfu/mL may be associated with incipient pneumonia or pulmonary microabscesses.

C. Quantitative Cultures of Bronchoalveolar Lavage

Bronchoscopy with BAL involves wedging the bronchoscope under visual control into a midsize bronchus and lavaging with aliquots of saline. The disadvantage of this technique is the possibility of sampling secretions from the bronchial tree of patients with bronchitis or heavy airway colonization. Immediate examination of the specimen with Gram stain showing more than 5% BAL cells with intracellular bacteria is highly predictive of pneumonia. Used in this manner, Gram stain on the BAL has a sensitivity of 55–100% and a specificity of 66–100% (10,17,19). The technique used to identify intracellular bacteria in BAL cells is easy and available in most laboratories. Since the lavage fluid samples a greater area of lung tissue than does the PSB technique, BAL can also have a lower false-negative rate than the PSB technique. BAL may identify other causes of pulmonary infiltrates such as pulmonary hemorrhage or malignancy (9). Combining these two techniques may improve overall accuracy in diagnosing VAP.

D. Nondirected BAL

Because bronchoscopy is an invasive technique that is costly and not always available, nondirected BAL has been suggested as an effective alternative that can be performed by nonphysicians (15,16,59,60). This method relies on quantitative cultures but is simpler, less expensive, and appears to provide results similar to those obtained by bronchoscopy (18,19).

Some investigators have been concerned about the lack of reliability of quantitative bacteriology in the absence of standardized clinical criteria for the diagnosis of VAP. Pugin et al. reported a good correlation between bronchoscopic diagnosis and NBAL using the clinical pulmonary infection score (CPIS) and quantitative bacteriology (bacterial index) (61). The CPIS incorporates a standardized quantitative assessment of the patient's temperature, leukocyte count and differential, oxygenation, presence of infiltrates or ARDS on chest radiograph, and results of semi-quantitative Gram stain and culture of tracheal aspirates. A modified CPIS scoring system used with a mean colony count from NBAL of $>10^4$ organisms/mL was associated with the development of VAP (15,16). Serial microbiological surveillance culture and the CPIS are valuable methods for the diagnosis of VAP, but further studies are needed to improve our understanding of the risk and cost benefits.

E. Quantitative Endotracheal Aspirates

Invasive diagnostic testing is not without problems. Currently, there is no randomized clinical trial comparing the use of invasive diagnostic methods to clinical judgment alone in the outcome of patients with VAP, especially mortality (58). Although quantitative QEA may be a simple way to diagnose VAP, its use may be limited by its poor specificity (18,19,62,63). Sanchez-Nieto et al. (64) compared quantitative bronchoscopic cultures of BAL and/or PSB versus QEA in 51 ventilated patients in a prospective randomized study. To distinguish colonization from true infection in the QEA group, a threshold of 10^5 cfu/mL was used. They found no significant difference in crude mortality rate or adjusted mortality rates, ICU length of stay, or ventilator days when management was directed by bronchoscopic data, which led to more frequent antibiotic changes. In summary, the operating characteristics of various invasive and semi-invasive strategies lack sufficient sensitivity and specificity to recommend them as definitive alternatives to clinical diagnosis.

V. Treatment

The use of effective antibiotics may improve survival for patients with VAP. Initial use of antibiotics ineffective against isolated organisms is associated with increased mortality with an odds ratio of 5.8 (31). Pathogens most commonly associated with inadequate initial empiric antibiotic treatment of culture-positive VAP include *Pseudomonas aeruginosa, Acinetobacter* species, *Klebsiella pneumoniae*, and *Enterobacter* species (28,29,65,66). Often these organisms are associated with antibiotic resistance (Table 2) and increased mortality. Methicillin-resistant *S. aureus* (MRSA) was the next most common pathogen associated with inadequate antibiotic therapy. Although they are important oropharyngeal organisms, anaerobes are uncommonly recovered pathogens in patients with VAP, perhaps obviating the need for anaerobic coverage (67).

Initial antimicrobial therapy should be aimed against antibiotic resistant gram-negative bacteria and MRSA (Table 3). Broad-spectrum treatment should not be prolonged, however, unless supported by appropriate culture data in order to minimize the emergence of antibiotic-resistant strains of bacteria (5). Routine prophylactic antibiotic therapy for patients with neutropenic fever and respiratory failure is beneficial, at least until white blood cell counts recover. The use of empiric broad-spectrum antibiotics in other patients without infection is harmful and facilitates colonization and superinfection with resistant organisms (5). Previous exposure to antibiotics is a significant risk factor for ventilator-associated pneumonia. Colonization of the upper respiratory tract by resistant organisms such as MRSA and *P. aeruginosa* correlates with the development of pneumonia

Table 2 Risk Factors for
Antibiotic Resistance

Immunosuppression
Advanced age
High-acuity illness
Multiple comorbidities
Devices and procedures
Resistance in the hospital and ICU
Ineffective infection control and compliance
Increased prophylactic and empiric antibiotic use

Table 3 Treatment of Ventilator-Associated Pneumonia

Risk factors[a]	Usual pathogens	Antibiotics
None	*S. pneumoniae* *H. influenzae* Non-*Pseudomonas* gram-negative bacilli *S. aureus*	Second or nonpseudomonal third- generation cephalosporin or beta-lactam + beta lactamase in- hibitor or fluoroquinolone or clindamycin + aztreonam
Present	*P. aeruginosa* Methicillin-resistant *S. aureus* (MRSA) Non-*Pseudomonas* gram-negative bacilli	Consider two antibiotics: antipseudomonal lactam agent and/or fluoroquinolone and/or aminoglycoside Also consider vancomycin

[a] Risk factors include late-onset VAP, prior antibiotic use, ICU stay, high-dose steroids, shock, advanced age, immunosuppression, coma.

(68). Eliminating the unnecessary use of antibiotics could help prevent these antibiotic-resistant nosocomial infections.

VI. Risk Factors and Prevention

Risk factors for VAP may be grouped into host factors, conditions that favor colonization, aspiration, and cross-contamination, and complications from antibiotic therapy or invasive devices (3,5,7). Host factors such as advanced age and comorbidities significantly increase the risk of pneumonia and colonization of the upper airway but are not practical targets for prevention. However, infection-control programs that implement nosocomial pneumonia-prevention policies (Table 4) to minimize colonization, cross-contamination, and inappropriate use of antibodies are associated with a reduction in the incidence of VAP (1,69,70).

A. Nonpharmacological Strategies

Bacterial colonization of the trachea with potential pathogens occurs in up to 75% of patients admitted to an intensive care unit (71). Education of unit personnel, proper use of infection-control measures, and surveillance programs reduce the risk of patient colonization and infection. Frequent hand washing is an effec-

Table 4   Strategies for the Prevention of VAP

Recommended strategies
  Remove endotracheal and nasogastric tubes as soon as possible
  Prevent unnecessary reintubation
  Noninvasive positive pressure ventilation
  Oral intubation (avoid nasal route)
  Infection-control programs
  Hand washing
  Semirecumbent position of patient
  Nutrition
  Avoid gastric overdistention
  Maintenance of endotracheal tube cuff pressure
  Continuous subglottic suctioning
  Antibiotics for neutropenic fever
Strategies with undetermined effectiveness
  Humidification with heat and moisture exchanger
  Gowns and gloves
  Prophylactic antibiotics for comatose patients
  Prophylactic immune globulin
  Granulocyte colony-stimulating factor (G-CSF)
  Limit stress-ulcer prophylaxis
  Aerosolized antibiotic prophylaxis
  Selective digestive decontamination
Ineffective strategies
  Routine changes of ventilator circuit
  Routine changes of in-line suction catheters
  Chest physiotherapy

tive means of removing contaminating bacteria and preventing cross-contamination (72). The use of gloves and gowns for contact with all patients has been shown to decrease the rates of nosocomial infections in pediatric ICUs (73). Their use, however, appears to be much more effective when directed at specific antibiotic-resistant pathogens, such as vancomycin-resistant enterococi (5).

Reducing pulmonary aspiration (26), atelectasis, maintaining patients in the semi-upright position, and reducing unplanned extubations (74) are simple prevention measures that have risk and cost-benefit ratios that strongly favor implementation. Similarly, prolonged nasal intubation should be avoided because it predisposes to nosocomial sinusitis and in turn VAP (27). The routine use of chest physiotherapy has not been shown to be effective and may be associated with other risks in this patient population like arterial oxygen desaturation (75).

Endotracheal tubes may facilitate the entry of bacteria into the lungs leading to VAP (22–24,27,76). Transmigration of bacteria and aspiration of pooled subglottic secretions around the endotracheal tube cuff into the trachea can occur. Special endotracheal tubes with a separate dorsal lumen above the cuff to suction these secretions may reduce this risk (23,24). The pressure in the cuff should also be adequate to reduce the leakage of subglottic secretions into the airway.

Accurate assessment of the patient's nutritional status is thought to be important, and early initiation of enteral feeding could help prevent VAP (50). Nearly all patients receiving mechanical ventilation have a tube inserted to manage gastric secretions, prevent gastric distention, or provide nutritional support. Such interventions may be a source of contamination and actually promote oropharyngeal colonization, aspiration, and VAP (1,27,36,69,77,78). Gastric overdistension can be reduced by limiting the use of narcotics and anticholinergic drugs and by monitoring the residual gastric volumes.

Changing mechanical ventilator breathing circuits frequently or on a scheduled basis increases the risk of developing VAP (1,79,80). Condensate in the tubing circuit may inadvertently be transmitted to the respiratory tract (1,81) and should be cleared. Heat and moisture exchangers reduce the incidence of VAP by minimizing the development of condensate within the ventilator circuits (82). Recent improvements in these designs obviate the need for daily changes of these devices (83). Medication nebulizers, resuscitation bags, spirometers, and oxygen analyzers are also potential sources of cross-contamination. These devices should be properly disinfected and not transferred between patients (1,6,84).

The last decade has seen an increasing use of noninvasive ventilation in critically ill patients who previously would have been placed on conventional mechanical ventilation. Patients able to tolerate noninvasive ventilation have a lower incidence of nosocomial pneumonia than those who are intubated (85,86). Reintubation is associated with an even higher rate of VAP (74). Management of respiratory failure without tracheal intubation may hold great promise as a primary preventive strategy in this disease.

There have been both sporadic and endemic occurrences of nosocomial pneumonia resulting from *L. pneumophila* (1,87). These outbreaks are usually associated with contaminated water sources. Intervention strategies should include treatment of the hospital water with heat or hyperchlorination to decrease or eliminate the organism. Recommendations for providing bottled water to high-risk, immunocompromised patients or cleaning the contaminated cooling tower are outlined in the Centers for Disease Control/Hospital Infection Control Practices Advisory Committee guidelines (1).

B. Pharmacological Strategies

Critically ill patients at highest risk for clinically important gastrointestinal bleeding are those requiring mechanical ventilation for more than 48 hours and those with coagulopathy (88). It is hypothesized, however, that the use of antacids, H_2

receptor antagonists, and possibly sucralfate may be associated with an increased risk of VAP (42,49,88–90). Pooled data from randomized trials in a meta-analysis showed no significant difference in the incidence of pneumonia between patients receiving an H_2 receptor antagonist and those receiving sucralfate (90). A prospective randomized controlled trial comparing ranitidine to sucralfate in ventilated patients showed no significant difference in the rate of VAP, ICU length of stay, or mortality between the two groups, but there was a trend toward a lower incidence of VAP in the sucralfate group (89).

Previous exposure to antibiotics is a risk factor for VAP, particularly that caused by resistant organisms (5). Restricting antibiotic use or offering guidelines for their use may help to reduce the incidence of resistant VAP caused by resistant organisms (91,92). The use of broad-spectrum antibiotics for the primary prevention of VAP cannot be recommended as it may lead to increased antibiotic resistance among subsequent hospital acquired infections. Changing or rotating the antibiotic classes used for the treatment of suspected bacterial infections and avoiding the use of a single class of antimicrobial agents may reduce the rate of nosocomial pneumonia caused by antibiotic-resistant pathogens (93).

Selective decontamination of the digestive tract (SDD) with nonabsorbable enteral antibiotics or antifungals, sometimes in combination with parenteral antibiotics, remains controversial as a way to prevent infection in the ICU (94,95). This technique attempts to prevent the development of nosocomial pneumonia by preventing colonization with potentially pathogenic aerobic Gram-negative bacilli and possibly *Candida albicans* while permitting growth of normal anaerobic bacteria that appear to be protective. SDD has been frequently implemented as a protective strategy in Europe, but unresolved issues persist regarding its use in the United States. Several meta-analyses have failed to identify a survival benefit, although a reduction in nosocomial pneumonia rate has been shown (96,97). The differential impact of SDD on pneumonia incidence versus mortality may be attributed to the wide variability in definition of pneumonia used in these studies, the way mortality is attributed to VAP, or the high risk of differences in the patient population for death due to other causes. In a prospective randomized trial of more than 1500 ICU patients, most requiring mechanical ventilation, mortality rates were not affected by SDD. The frequency of ICU-acquired infections was higher after SDD was discontinued, however, mainly from *Acinetobacter* species and Enterobacteriaceae (98). Although antimicrobial resistance among these organisms was not increased during the first year after the study, longer follow-up may be required. In addition, low-level resistance is difficult to detect and often precedes high-level resistance. Since antibiotic resistance has become a major concern and ICUs appear to be the primary location of pathogens that are multiply resistant, limiting antibiotic use is important (99). Other concerns with the use of SDD include associated costs and, ultimately, lack of a clearly demonstrated mortality benefit.

Efforts have been made to boost patient immunity. One study conducted in critically ill surgical patients found that the use of immunoglobulin compared with placebo reduced the overall incidence of nosocomial infection and pneumonia, particularly in postoperative surgical patients (100). Similarly, granulocyte colony-stimulating factor (G-CSF), a hematopoietic growth factor that increases both neutrophil number and function, has been shown to improve survival in nonneutropenic animal models of bacterial pneumonia (101). However, prophylactic G-CSF in an animal pneumonia model had detrimental effects on survival with *E. coli* pneumonia despite beneficial effects with *S. aureus* pneumonia, perhaps related to increased inflammatory tissue injury or augmented host defenses (102–104). The host defense system is in a delicate balance between the pro-inflammatory and the anti-inflammatory state. As new areas surrounding host-pathogen interactions are discovered, newer therapeutic modalities to alter the immune system in a beneficial way may be identified.

VII. Summary

The definitive diagnosis of VAP remains elusive today. Empiric antibiotic therapy should be considered for patients with suspected pneumonia based on clinical criteria. Invasive diagnostic studies of the lower respiratory tract in this patient population has led to a better understanding of the pathogenic events leading to VAP but has not altered the mortality associated with the disease. Outcome studies comparing different diagnostic strategies are critical to assess both the risk and cost benefit of invasive versus noninvasive diagnostic approaches. Accurate diagnosis of VAP is important to reduce the use of unnecessary antibiotics, particularly in this era of increased antibiotic resistance. Preventive strategies such as semi-upright positioning, oral intubation rather than nasal intubation, controlled antibiotic use, and aspiration of subglottic secretions need to be carefully evaluated in randomized controlled trials.

References

1. Tablan OC, Anderson LJ, Arden NH, et al. Guideline for prevention of nosocomial pneumonia: Part I. Issues on prevention of nosocomial pneumonia, 1994. Infect Control Hosp Epidemiol 1994; 15:588–625.
2. Kollef MH. Ventilator-associated pneumonia: a multivariate analysis. JAMA 1993; 270:1965–1970.
3. Craven DE, Steger KA. Nosocomial pneumonia in mechanically ventilated adult patients: Epidemiology and prevention in 1995. Semin Respir Infect 1996; 11:32–53.
4. Heyland DK, Cook DJ, Griffith L, Keenan SP, Brun-Buisson C, Canadian Care Trials Group. The attributable morbidity and mortality of ventilator-associated

pneumonia in the critically ill patient. Am J Respir Crit Care Med 1999; 159:1249–1256.

5. Kollef MH. The prevention of ventilator associated pneumonia. N Engl J Med 1999; 340:627–634.
6. Niederman MS, Craven DE, Fein AM, Schultz DE. Pneumonia in the critically ill hospitalized patient. Chest 1990; 97:170–281.
7. Craven DE, Steger KA. Epidemiology of nosocomial pneumonia: new concepts on an old disease. Chest 1995; 108:1S–16S.
8. Niederman MS, Torres A, Sunner W. Invasive diagnostic testing is not needed routinely to manage suspect ventilator-associated pneumonia. Am J Respir Crit Care Med 1994; 150:565–569.
9. Chastre J, Fagon JY. Invasive diagnostic testing should be routinely used to manage ventilated patients with suspected pneumonia. Am J Respir Crit Care Med 1994; 150:570–574.
10. Cook DJ, Brun-Buisson C, Guyatt GH, et al. Evaluation of new diagnostic technologies: Bronchoalveolar ravage and the diagnosis of ventilator-associated pneumonia. Crit Care Med 1994; 22:1314–1322.
11. Niederman MS. An approach to empiric therapy of nosocomial pneumonia. Med Clin North Am 1993; 78:1123–1141.
12. Bryant LR, Mobin-Uddin K, Dillon ML, et al. Misdiagnosis of pneumonia in patients needing mechanical respiration. Arch Surg 1973; 106:286–288.
13. Fagon JY, Chastre J, Hance AJ, et al. Detection of nosocomial lung infection in ventilated patients: use of a protected specimen brush and quantitative culture techniques in 147 patients. Am Rev Respir Dis 1988; 138:110–116.
14. Chastre J, Fagon JY, Soler P, et al. Diagnosis of nosocomial bacterial pneumonia in intubated patients undergoing ventilation: comparison of the usefulness of bronchoalveolar lavage and the protected specimen brush. Am J Med 1988; 85:499–506.
15. A'Court CHD, Garrard CS, Crook D, et al. Microbiological lung surveillance in mechanically ventilated patients, using nondirected lavage and quantitative culture. QJ Med 1993; 86:635–648.
16. Garrard CS, Court CD. The diagnosis of pneumonia in the critically ill. Chest 1995; 108:17S–25S.
17. Pugin J, Auckenthaler R, Mili N, et al. Diagnosis of ventilator-associated pneumonia by bacteriologic analysis of bronchoalveolar lavage fluid. Am Rev Respir Dis 1991; 143:1121–1129.
18. El-ebiary M, Torres A, Gonzalez J, et al. Quantitative cultures of endotracheal aspirates for the diagnosis of ventilator-associated pneumonia. Am Rev Respir Dis 1993; 148:1552–1557.
19. Torres A, De La Bellacasa JP, Xaubet A, et al. Diagnostic value of quantitative cultures of bronchoalveolar lavage and telescoping plugged catheters in mechanically ventilated patients with bacterial pneumonia. Am Rev Respir Dis 1989; 140:306–310.
20. Marquette CH, Georges H, Wallet F, et al. Diagnostic efficiency of endotracheal aspirates with quantitative bacterial cultures in intubated patients with suspected pneumonia. Am Rev Respir Dis 1993; 148:138–144.

21. Johnson WGJ, Pierce AK Sanford J, et al. Nosocomial respiratory infections with Gram-negative bacilli: The significance of colonization of the respiratory tract. Ann Intern Med 1972; 77:701–706.
22. Craven DE, Driks MR. Pneumonia in the intubated patient. Semin Respir Infect 1987; 2:20–33.
23. Valles J, Artigas A, Rello J, et al. Continuous aspiration of subglottic secretions in the prevention of ventilator-associated pneumonia. Ann Intern Med 1995; 122: 179–186.
24. Rello J, Sonora R, Jubert P, Artigas A, Rue M, Valles J. Pneumonia in intubated patients: role of respiratory airway care. Am J Respir Crit Care Med 1996; 154: 111–115.
25. Cross AS, Roupe B. Role of respiratory assistance devices in endemic nosocomial pneumonia. Am J Med 1981; 70:681–685.
26. Torres A, Serra-Battles J, Ros E, et al. Pulmonary aspiration of gastric contents in patients receiving mechanical ventilation: the effect of body position. Ann Intern Med 1992; 116:540–542.
27. Rouby J, Laurent P, Gosnach M, et al. Risk factors and clinical relevance of nosocomial maxillary sinusitis in the critically ill. Am J Respir Crit Care Med 1994; 150: 776–783.
28. Luna CM, Vujacich P, Niederman MS, et al. Impact of BAL data on the therapy and outcome of ventilator-associated pneumonia. Chest 1997; 111:676–685.
29. Rello J, Gallego M, Mariscal D, et al. The value of routine microbial investigation in ventilator-associated pneumonia. Am J Respir Crit Care Med 1997; 156:196–200.
30. Reinarz JA, Pierce AK, Mays BB, et al. The potential role of inhalational therapy equipment in nosocomial pulmonary infection. J Clin Invest 1965; 44:831–839.
31. Fagon JY, Chastre J, Domart Y, et al. Nosocomial pneumonia in patients receiving continuous mechanical ventilation: prospective analysis of 52 episodes with use of a protected specimen brush and quantitative culture techniques. Am Rev Respir Dis 1989; 139:877–884.
32. Torres A, Aznar R, Gatell JM, et al. Incidence, risk, and prognosis factors of nosocomial pneumonia in mechanically ventilated patients. Am Rev Respir Dis 1990; 142:523–528.
33. Rello J, Quintana E, Ausina V, et al. Incidence, etiology, and outcome of nosocomial pneumonia in mechanically ventilated patients. Chest 1991; 100:439–444.
34. Wunderink RG, Mayhall G, Gilbert C. Methodology for clinical investigation of ventilator associated pneumonia: epidemiology and therapeutic intervention. Chest 1992; 102:580S–588S.
35. Centers for Disease Control. National Nosocomial Infections Surveillance Report. Data from April 1986-October 1986. CDC Internet site. (http:www.cdc.gov/ncidod/disease/hip/nnis).
36. Celis R, Torres A, Gatell JM, et al. Nosocomial pneumonia: a multivariate analysis of risk and prognosis. Chest 1988; 93:318–324.
37. Haley RW, Hooton TM, Culver DH, et al. Nosocomial infections in US hospitals, 1975–1976: estimated frequency by selected characteristics of patients. Am J Med 1981; 70:947–959.

38. Langer M, Mosconi P, Cigada M, et al. The Intensive Care Unit Group of Infection Control. Long-term respiratory support and risk of pneumonia in critically ill patients. Am Rev Respir Dis 1989; 140:302–305.

39. Vincent J, Bihari DJ, Suter PM, et al. The prevalence of nosocomial infection in intensive care units in Europe: results of the European Prevalence of Infection in Intensive Care (EPIC) study. JAMA 1995; 274:639–644.

40. Jarvis WR, Edwards JR, Culver DH, et al. Nosocomial infection rates in adult and pediatric intensive care units in the United States. Am J Med 1991; 91(suppl 3B): 185S–190S.

41. George DL. Epidemiology of nosocomial ventilator-associated pneumonia. Infect Control Hosp Epidemiol 1993; 14:163–169.

42. Craven DE, Kunches LM, Mlinsky V, et al. Risk factors for pneumonia and fatality in patients receiving continuous mechanical ventilation. Am Rev Respir Dis 1986; 133:792–796.

43. Torres A, Aznar R, Gatell JM, et al. Incidence, risk, and prognosis factors of nosocomial pneumonia in mechanically ventilated patients. Am Rev Respir Dis 1990; 142:523–528.

44. Leu HS, Kaiser DL, Mori M, et al. Hospital-acquired pneumonia: attributable mortality and morbidity. Am J Epidemiol 1989; 129:1258–1267.

45. Craven DE, Steger KA. Ventilator-associated bacterial pneumonia: challenges in diagnosis, treatment and prevention. New Horizons 1998; 6(2):S30–S45.

46. Craig CP, Connelly S. Effect of intensive care unit nosocomial pneumonia on duration of stay and mortality. Am J Infect Control 1984; 12:233–238.

47. Rello J, Quintana E, Ausina V, et al. Risk factors for *Staphylococcus aureus* pneumonia in critically ill patients. Am Rev Respir Dis 1990; 142:1320–1324.

48. Torres A, El-Ebiary M, Gonzalez J, et al. Gastric and pharyngeal flora in nosocomial pneumonia acquired during mechanical ventilation. Am Rev Respir Dis 1993; 148:352–357.

49. Niederman MS. Gram-negative colonization of the respiratory tract: pathogenesis and clinical consequences. Semin Respir Infect 1990; 5:173–184.

50. Niederman MS, Mantovani R, Schoch P, et al. Patterns and routes of tracheobronchial colonization in mechanically ventilated patients: the role of nutritional status in colonization of the lower airway by Pseudomonas species. Chest 1989; 95:155–161.

51. Daschner F, Kappstein I, Engels I, et al. Stress ulcer prophylaxis and ventilation pneumonia: Prevention by antibacterial cytoprotective agents. Infect Control 1988; 9:59–65.

52. Donowitz LG, Page MC, Mileur GL, Guenthner SH. Alteration of normal gastric flora in critical care patients receiving antacid and cimetidine therapy. Infect Control 1986; 7:23–26.

53. Fagon JY, Chastre J, Hance AJ, Domart Y, Trouillet JL, Gilbert C. Evaluation of clinical judgment in the identification and treatment of nosocomial pneumonia in ventilated patients. Chest 1993; 103:547–553.

54. Wunderink RG, Woldenderg LS, Zeiss J, et al. The radiologic diagnosis of autopsy proven ventilator associated pneumonia. Chest 1992; 101:458–463.

55. Wimberley N, Faling LJ, Bartlett JG. A fiberoptic bronchospcopy technique to ob-

tain uncontaminated lower airway secretions for bacterial culture. Am Rev Respir Dis 1979; 119:337–343.

56. Chastre J, Viau F, Brun P, et al. Prospective evaluation of the protected specimen brush for the diagnosis of pulmonary infection in ventilated patients. Am Rev Respir Dis 1984; 130:924–929.

57. Cook DJ, Fitzgerald JM, Guyatt GH, Walter S. Evaluation of the protected brush catheter and bronchoalveolar lavage in the diagnosis of nosocomial pneumonia. J Intensive Care Med 1991; 6:196–205.

58. Niederman MS, Torres A, Summer W. Invasive diagnostic testing is not needed routinely to manage suspected ventilator-associated pneumonia. Am J Resp Crit Car Med 1994; 150:565–569.

59. Pipemo D, Gaussorgues P, Bachmann P, et al. Diagnostic value of nonbronchoscopic bronchoalveolar lavage during mechanical ventilation. Chest 1988; 93:223–227.

60. Kollef MH, Bock KR, Richards RD, et al. The safety and diagnostic accuracy of minibronchoalveolar lavage in patients with suspected ventilator-associated pneumonia. Ann Intern Med 1995; 122:743–748.

61. Pugin J, Auckenthaler R, Mili N, et al. Diagnosis of ventilator-associated pneumonia by bacteriologic analysis of bronchoscopic and nonbronchoscopic blind bronchoalveolar lavage fluid. Am Rev Respir Dis 1988; 138:117–120.

62. Torres A, Martos A, Puig de la Bellacasa J, et al. Specificity of endotracheal aspiration, protected specimen brush and bronchoalveolar lavage in mechanically ventilated patients. Am Rev Respir Dis 1993; 147(4):952–957.

63. Jourdain B, Novara A, Joly-Guillou ML, et al. Role of quantitative cultures of endotracheal aspirates in the diagnosis of nosocomial pneumonia. Am J Respir Crit Care Med 1995; 152(1):241–246.

64. Sanchez-Nieto JM, Torres A, Garcia-Cordoba F, El-Ebiary M, Carrillo A, Ruiz J, Nunez ML, Niederman M. Impact of invasive and noninvasive quantitative culture sampling on outcome of ventilator-associated pneumonia. Am J Respir Crit Care Med 1998; 157:371–376.

65. Alvarez-Lerma F. Modification of empiric antibiotic treatment in patients with pneumonia acquired in the intensive care unit: ICU-Acquired Pneumonia Study Group. Intensive Care Med 1996; 22:387–394.

66. Kollef MH, Ward S. The influence of mini-BAL cultures on patient outcomes: implications for the antibiotic management of ventilator associated pneumonia. Chest 1998; 113:412–420.

67. Marik PE, Careau P. The role of anaerobes in patients with ventilator-associated pneumonia and aspiration pneumonia. Chest 1999; 115:178–183.

68. Garrouste-Orgeas M, Chevret S, Arlet G, et al. Oropharyngeal or gastric colonization and nosocomial pneumonia in adult intensive care unit patients: a prospective study based on genomic DNA analysis. Am J Respir Crit Care Med 1997; 156:1647–1655.

69. Joiner GA, Salisbury D, Bollin GE. Utilizing quality assurance as a tool for reducing the risk of nosocomial ventilator pneumonia. Am J Med Qual 1996; 11:228–230.

70. Kelleghan SI, Salemi C, Padilla S, et al. An effective continuous quality improve-

ment approach to prevention of ventilator associated nosocomial pneumonia. Am J Infect Control 1993; 21:322–330.

71. Pingleton SK, Hinthorn DR, Liu C. Enteral nutrition in patients receiving mechanical ventilation: Multiple sources of tracheal colonization include the stomach. Am J Med 1986; 80:827–832.

72. Debbeling BN, Stanley GL, Sheetz CT et al. Comparative efficacy of alternative hand washing agents in reducing nosocomial infections in intensive care units. N Engl J Med 1992; 327:88–93.

73. Klein BS, Perloff WH, Maki DG, et al. Reduction of nosocomial infection during pediatric intensive care by protective isolation. N Engl J Med 1989; 320:1714–1721.

74. Torres A, Gatell JM, Aznar E, et al. Re-intubation increases the risk of nosocomial pneumonia in patients needing mechanical ventilation. Am J Respir Crit Care Med 1995; 152:137–141.

75. Hall JC, Tarala RA, Tapper J, Hall JL. Prevention of respiratory complications after abdominal surgery: a randomized clinical trial. Br Med J 1996; 312:148–152.

76. Craven DE, Barber TW, Steger KA, et al. Nosocomial pneumonia in the 90's: update of epidemiology and risk factors. Semin Respir Infect 1990; 5:157–172.

77. Holzapfel L, Chevret S, Madinier G, et al. Influence of long term oro- or nasotracheal intubation on nosocomial maxillary sinusitis and pneumonia: results of a prospective, randomized, clinical trial. Crit Care Med 1993; 21:1132–1138.

78. Pingleton SK. Enteral nutrition as a risk factor for nosocomial pneumonia. Eur J Clin Microbiol Infect Dis 1989; 8:51–55.

79. Kollef M, Shapiro S, Fraser V, et al. Mechanical ventilation with or without 7-day circuit changes: a randomized controlled trial. Ann Intern Med 1995; 123:168–174.

80. Kollef MH. Prolonged use of ventilator circuits and ventilator associated pneumonias: a model for identifying the optimal clinical practice Chest 1998; 113:267–269.

81. Craven DE, Goularte TA, Make B. Contaminated condensate in mechanical ventilator circuits: a risk factor for nosocomial pneumonia. Am Rev Respir Dis 1984; 129:625–628.

82. Djedaini K, Billiard M, Mier L, et al. Changing heat and moisture exchangers every 48 hours rather than 24 hours does not affect their efficacy and the incidence of nosocomial pneumonia. Am J Resp Crit Care Med 1995; 152:1562–1569.

83. Kirton OC, FeHaven B, Morgan J, Morejon O, Civetta J. A prospective randomized comparison of an in-line heat moisture exchange filter and heated wire humidifiers: rates of ventilator early onset (community acquired) pneumonia or late onset (hospital acquired) pneumonia and incidence of endotracheal tube occlusion. Chest 1997; 112:1055–1059.

84. Craven DE, Lichtenberg DA, Goularte TA, et al. Contaminated medication nebulizers in mechanical ventilator circuits: a source of bacterial aerosols. Am J Med 1984; 77:834–838.

85. Antonelli M, Conti G, Rocco M, et al. A comparison of non-invasive positive pressure ventilation and conventional ventilation in patients with acute respiratory failure. N Engl J Med 1998; 339:429–435.

86. Guerin C, Girard R, Chemorin C, De Varax R, Fournier G. Facial mask non-invasive mechanical ventilation reduces the incidence of nosocomial pneumonia. A prospective epidemiological survey from a single ICU. Intensive Care Med 1997; 23: 1024–1032.
87. Marrie TJ, MacDonald S, Clarke K, et al. Nosocomial Legionnaires' disease: lessons from a four-year prospective study. Am J Infect Control 1991; 19:79–85.
88. Cook DJ, Fuller HD, Guyatte GH, et al. Risk factors for gastrointestinal bleeding in critically ill patients. N Engl J Med 1994; 330:377–381.
89. Cook DJ, Guyatt GH, Marshall J, et al. Comparison of sucralfate and ranitidine for the prevention of upper gastrointestinal bleeding in patients requiring mechanical ventilation. N Engl J Med 1998; 338:791–797.
90. Cook DJ, Reeve BK, Guyatt GH, et al. Stress ulcer prophylaxis in critically ill patients: resolving discordant meta-analysis. J Am Med Assoc 1996; 275:308–314.
91. Goldman DA, Weinstein RA, Wenzel RP, et al. Strategies to prevent and control the emergence and spread of antimicrobial resistant microorganisms in hospitals: a challenge to hospital leadership. J Am Med Assoc 1996; 275:234–240.
92. Evans RS, Pestotnik SL, Classen DC, et al. A computer assisted management program for antibiotics and other anti-infective agents. N Engl J Med 1998; 338:232–238.
93. Kollef MH, Vlasnik J, Sharpless L, Pasque C, Murphy D, Fraser V. Scheduled change of antibiotic classes: a strategy to decrease the incidence of ventilator associated pneumonia. Am J Respir Crit Care Med 1997; 156:1040–1048.
94. Sanchez Garcia M, Cambronero GJA, Lopez Diaz J, et al. Effectiveness and cost of selective decontamination of the digestive tract in critically ill, intubated patients. A randomised double blind, multicenter trial. Am J Respir Crit Care Med 1998; 158:908–916.
95. Gastinne H, Wolff M, Delatour F, Faurisson F, Chevrett S. A controlled trial in intensive care units of selective decontamination of the digestive tract with nonabsorbable antibiotics. N Engl J Med 1992; 326:594–599.
96. Heyland D, Cook DJ, Jaeschke R, Griffith L, Lee HN, Guyatt GH. Selective decontamination of the digestive tract: an overview. Chest 1995; 105:1221–1229.
97. Kollef MH. The role of selective digestive tract decontamination on mortality and respiratory tract infections. A meta-analysis. Chest 1994; 105:1101–1108.
98. Hammond JMJ, Potgieter PD. Long-term effects of selective decontamination on antimicrobial resistance. Crit Care Med 1995; 23(1):637–645.
99. Bartlett JG. Selective decontamination of the digestive tract and its effect on antimicrobial resistance. Crit Care Med 1995; 23(1):613–615.
100. The intravenous immunoglobulin collaborative study group. Prophylactic intravenous administration of standard immune globulin as compared with core-lipopolysaccharide immune globulin in patients at high risk of post surgical infections. N Engl J Med 1992; 327:234–240.
101. Lundlad R, Nesland JM, Giercksky. Granulocyte colony-stimulating factor improves rurvival rates and reduces concentrations of bacteria, endotoxin, tumor necrosis factor and endothelin-1 in fulminant intra-abdominal sepsis in rats. Crit Care Med 1996; 24:820–826.
102. Mitchell PL, Mooreland B, Stevens MC, et al. Granulocyte stimulating factor in

established febrile neutropenia. Randomized study of pediatric patients. J Clin Oncology 1997; 15:1163–1170.

103. Nelson S. A question of balance. Am J Respir Crit Care Med 1999; 159:1365–1367.

104. Karzai W, Specht U, Parent C, Haberstroh J, Wollersen K, Natanson C, Banks SM, Eichacker PQ. G-CSF during *E. coli* versus *S. aureus* pneumonia in rats has fundamentally different and opposite effects. Am J Respir Crit Care Med 1999; 159:1377–1382.

20

Effects of Mechanical Ventilation on Heart–Lung Interactions

MICHAEL R. PINSKY

University of Pittsburgh Medical Center
Pittsburgh, Pennsylvania

I. Introduction

Ventilation can have profound cardiovascular effects that can be either beneficial or detrimental to the host (1). Directionally opposite hemodynamic responses to seemingly similar ventilatory maneuvers can occur between patients. The reasons for such hemodynamic responses may not appear logical on the surface, but when dissected free of clinical bias, the reasoning not only is often clear but leads to a deeper understanding of the patient's cardiopulmonary reserve. It is the goal of this chapter to develop that deeper understanding on a general level so that individual patient responses can be appreciated.

Heart–lung interactions can be assessed by the effects of ventilation on the circulation or the effects of the circulation on ventilation. This review will focus on the effects of ventilation on the circulatory system. Four primary interactions can be identified that comprise most heart-lung interactions: Ventilation is exercise; inspiration increases lung volume; spontaneous inspiration decreases intrathoracic pressure (ITP); and positive-pressure ventilation increases ITP. To simplify the discussion the term intrathoracic pressure will be used to refer to a nonspecific intrathoracic surface pressure. When specific surface pressures are identified, they will be referred to as the lateral chest wall, diaphragm and juxta-cardiac pleural pressures, or pericardial pressure, where appropriate.

Clearly, acute left ventricular (LV) failure can impair gas exchange by inducing pulmonary edema. Similarly, profound hypotension in a patient with air trapping can increase dead space ventilation. However, the circulation can also impair gas exchange by limiting the energy delivery to the respiratory muscles, first inducing hypopnea and then apnea. This effect can be grouped under the heading of "ventilation is exercise." This category will be discussed in the next section, and the remainder of this chapter will deal with the other three primary categories.

II. Spontaneous Ventilation Is Exercise

Spontaneous ventilatory efforts require contraction of the respiratory muscles. The diaphragm and intercostal muscles comprise the bulk of the musculature, although secondary muscles of respiration can also add to the metabolic load of ventilation. With marked hyperpnea, abdominal wall muscles and muscles of the shoulder girdle can markedly increase total O_2 demand of the respiratory apparatus. The vascular supply to the respiratory muscles comes from a number of arterial feeding branches, and the ability of these vessels to dilate exceeds the theoretical maximal O_2 extraction of these muscles (2). Thus, respiratory muscle blood flow is not the limiting factor determining maximal ventilatory effort under normal conditions.

Although ventilation normally requires less than 5% of total O_2 delivery to meet its demand (2), in lung disease states, the work of breathing can increase metabolic demand for O_2 up to 30% of total O_2 delivery (2–5). If the supply-demand balance of O_2 delivery is disrupted, then blood flow to other organs as well as to the respiratory muscles may be compromised. In profound circulatory shock, the increased metabolic demand of spontaneous ventilation can induce both tissue hypoperfusion and lactic acidosis (6,7).

The institution of mechanical ventilatory support eliminates spontaneous ventilatory efforts and reduces this metabolic demand. Total body O_2 consumption will therefore decrease, and Svo_2 must increase if cardiac output and Cao_2 remains constant. Accordingly, in the setting of right-to-left shunts, initiating mechanical ventilatory support may have the effect of increasing arterial oxygenation without actually altering gas exchange in the lungs.

Finally, if cardiac output is severely limited, as is often the case with end-stage cardiac disease, the hypoperfusion of the respiratory muscles leads to a terminal chain of events that starts with hypopnea and progresses through to apnea and then cardiac arrest (8). In this scenario, one would hypothesize that the primary cause of death in patients with severe cardiomyopathies would be apneic cardiac arrest. Although not validated, these data fit the epidemiological data demonstrating that the majority of cardiac deaths occur in the early morning hours when respiratory drive is least.

In fact, numerous clinical studies have documented that weaning places increased metabolic demand on the heart and can precipitate ischemia in patients with limited cardiovascular reserve. Thus, one can consider weaning to be a cardiac stress test. Lemaire et al. (9) demonstrated that the institution of spontaneous ventilation in patients with chronic obstructive lung disease induced an immediate and profound LV failure state characterized by markedly increased LV filling pressures, pulmonary edema, and, if not rapidly reversed by reinstitution of mechanical ventilation, acute cardiovascular collapse (9). Similar data with evidence of LV dysfunction was seen by Richard et al. (10), who attempted to wean patients with chronic airflow obstruction (10). Focusing on coronary ischemia using thallium-201 myocardial perfusion imaging demonstrated that myocardial ischemia rapidly develops during weaning in patients with coronary artery disease (1,121).

III. Inspiration Increases Lung Volume

When tissue volume changes, so does the vascular resistance of that organ. For the lung, changes in volume alter both global autonomic tone and local pulmonary vascular resistance. Furthermore, with hyperinflation the expanded lungs compress the heart within the cardiac fossa in a fashion analogous to tamponade. These concepts will be elaborated on in the following sections.

A. Autonomic Tone

The lungs have a rich neuronal network of integrated somatic and autonomic fibers that originate, traverse through, and end in the thorax. They mediate multiple homeostatic processes. For example, respiratory sinus arrhythmia and antidiuretic hormone (ADH)–induced fluid retention are both autonomic-controlled processes. Inflation induces immediate changes in autonomic output that cause phase-specific changes in heart rate and non–phase-specific changes in arterial tone and contractility. Lung inflation to normal tidal volumes (<10 mL/kg) increases heart rate via parasympathetic tone withdrawal (13,14), referred to as respiratory sinus arrhythmia (15). The presence of respiratory sinus arrhythmia denotes normal autonomic tone (16). Similarly, loss of respiratory sinus arrhythmia has been used clinically to identify dysautonomia.

The reappearance of respiratory sinus arrhythmia precedes the return of peripheral autonomic control in diabetics with peripheral neuropathy (17) and can thus be used as a sensitive marker of effective diabetic control. Some minimal amount of respiratory-associated heart rate change reflects local right atrial volume changes because they persist even in the dennervated human heart following cardiac transplantation (18). Lung inflation to larger tidal volumes (>15 mL/kg) decreases heart rate and causes reflex vasodilation (19,20–24). Blocking sympathetic afferent fibers also blocks this reflex (22,25). Although this effect usually occurs only with very large tidal volumes, in the setting of acute lung injury with loss of ventilated lung units, ventilation with what would otherwise be normal tidal volumes will induce a local overdistention and stimulate this response. However, this concern is probably of little clinical consequence because unilateral lung hyperinflation (unilateral PEEP) does not appear to influence systemic hemodynamics (26).

On the other hand, high-frequency ventilation tends to be better tolerated hemodynamically than conventional ventilation, probably because of the smaller tidal volumes and lack of sympathetic withdrawal. On the opposite end of this spectrum, high-frequency ventilation with hyperinflation in the neonate can cause hypotension (19,22), probably by the above-described sympathetic blockade.

Independent of these phasic reflex arcs, ventilation also alters control of intravascular fluid balance via hormonal release. Both positive-pressure ventilation and sustained hyperinflation induced by positive end-expiratory pressure (PEEP) stimulate a variety of endocrinological responses that induce fluid retention via right atrial stretch receptors. In essence, lung distention compresses the right atrium, eliciting a sympathetic response to fluid retained by the kidneys. Plasma norepinepherine, plasma rennin activity (27,28), and atrial natriuretic peptide (29) increase during positive-pressure ventilation with or without PEEP. Reciprocally, when patients with congestive heart failure are given sustained nasal continuous positive airway pressure (CPAP), plasma atrial natriuretic peptide activity decreases in parallel with improvements in blood flow (30,31), suggesting that when hemodynamics are improved, the body responds by reducing this stress response.

B. Determinants of Pulmonary Vascular Resistance

Tissue pressure is a major determinant of microcirculatory vascular resistance in every organ. In the lung, tissue pressure relative to vascular pressure varies throughout every breath, reflecting changes in lung volume. Lung inflation, independent of changes in ITP, primarily affects cardiac function and cardiac output by altering right ventricular (RV) afterload and both RV and LV preload (32,33–38). Increasing pulmonary vascular resistance is important because the RV has a minimal ability to eject blood into a pressurized circuit. When either venous return is augmented or RV outflow resistance increased, RV volumes increase rapidly. Just as for the left ventricle, RV afterload reflects RV systolic wall stress (39), which, by the law of LaPlace, is proportional to the radius of curvature of the right ventricle (a function of end-diastolic volume) and transmural pressure (a function of systolic RV pressure) (40).

In the absence of pulmonic obstruction, transmural systolic RV pressure is also transmural systolic pulmonary artery pressure (Ppa), which is Ppa relative to ITP. Transmural Ppa can increase by either of two mechanisms: (1) an increase in pulmonary arterial pressure without an increase in pulmonary vasomotor tone as may occur with either a marked increase in blood flow (exercise) or passive increases in outflow pressure (LV failure), or (2) an increase in pulmonary vascular resistance by either active changes in vasomotor tone or passive lung hyperinflation. If transmural Ppa increases during positive-pressure ventilation it is usually due to an increase in pulmonary vascular resistance, because neither blood flow (41) nor LV filling (42) usually increases. If transmural Ppa increases by any mechanism, RV ejection will be impeded (43). This will result in an immediate decrease in RV stroke volume (44), RV dilation, and a secondary reduction in venous return (39,41) that usually takes a few beats to become manifest. This process of decreasing RV ejection, increasing RV wall stress and falling venous return rapidly induces acute cor pulmonale and obstructive circulatory shock. If RV dilation continues, RV free wall ischemia and infarction can develop, because RV coronary perfusion cannot be sustained across such high wall stresses (45). Accordingly, acute cor pulmonale is characterized by profound decreases in cardiac output that are resistant to fluid loading therapies. Furthermore, rapid intravascular fluid loading in acute cor pulmonale can precipitate profound cardiovascular collapse due to excessive RV dilation, LV compression and RV ischemia.

Hypoxic Pulmonary Vasoconstriction

Alveolar hypoxia also increases transmural Ppa by increasing pulmonary vasomotor tone. The mechanism by which pulmonary vasomotor tone actually increases is complex and not fully understood. If regional alveolar Po_2 (PAO_2) decreases below approximately 60 mmHg, pulmonary vasomotor tone in that region increases, reducing local blood flow (46). This process is called hypoxic pulmonary vasoconstriction and is mediated, in part, by variations in the synthesis and release of nitric oxide by pulmonary vascular endothelial cells. The pulmonary vascular endothelium normally synthesizes nitric oxide, a potent vasodilator, at a continual but low level, maintaining a generalized and active state of pulmonary vasodilation. Nitric oxide production is highly regulated, and acidosis, alveolar hypoxia, or hypoxemia can all inhibit nitric oxide production.

Hypoxic pulmonary vasoconstriction presumably evolved as a mechanism for matching ventilation to perfusion when regional impairments in ventilation exist. However, if global alveolar hypoxia occurs, as is the case with sleep apnea or high-altitude or severe obstructive lung disease, then overall pulmonary vasomotor tone increases, increasing pulmonary vascular resistance and impeding RV ejection (39). This is part of the rationale for giving low-flow O_2 to all patients with chronic obstructive lung disease. The supplemental O_2 minimizes both hypoxic pulmonary vasoconstriction, improving hemodynamics and exercise tolerance, and also limits the hypoxia-induced pulmonary vascular remodeling. Importantly, at low lung volumes, as may be seen in patients with acute lung injury, alveoli spontaneously collapse as a result of loss of interstitial traction and surfactant deactivation and become hypoxic (47,48). Accordingly, some of the increased pulmonary vascular resistance seen in patients with acute respiratory distress syndrome (ARDS) is due to hypoxic pulmonary vasoconstriction. Thus, (PEEP) therapy, if it also recruits collapsed lung units, should also reduce pulmonary vasomotor tone.

Lung Volume–Induced Changes in Pulmonary Vascular Resistance

Changes in lung volume may either reduce or increase pulmonary vascular resistance (Fig. 1). Increasing lung volume may reduce active pulmonary vasomotor

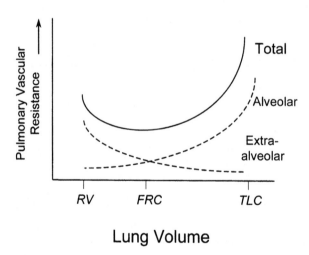

Lung Volume

Figure 1 Schematic diagram of the relation between changes in lung volume and pulmonary vascular resistance, where the extra-alveolar and alveolar vascular components are separated. Note that pulmonary vascular resistance is minimal at resting lung volume or functional residual capacity (FRC). As lung volume increases toward total lung capacity (TLC) or decreases toward residual volume (RV), pulmonary vascular resistance also increases. However, the increase in resistance with hyperinflation is due to increased alveolar vascular resistance, whereas the increase in resistance with lung collapse is due to increased extra-alveolar vessel tone.

tone if the basal state of the lung has increased vascular tone due to hypoxic pulmonary vasoconstriction. The ventilatory maneuver increases global alveolar Po_2 (Pao_2) (49–52), increases alveolar ventilation, and thus reverses acute respiratory acidosis (53), and decreases central sympathetic output by minimizing respiratory distress (54,55). Importantly, these effects do not require positive-pressure breaths as much as expansion of collapsed alveoli and reduced work of breathing (56). Accordingly, lung recruitment maneuvers, such as bag-sigh-suctioning, the application of CPAP to spontaneously breathing patients, or application of PEEP during positive-pressure ventilation may all reverse increased pulmonary vasomotor tone.

Changes in lung volume can also profoundly alter pulmonary vascular resistance by passively compressing the alveolar vessels (46,47,51). Conceptually, the pulmonary circulation can be separated into two groups of blood vessels, depending on what pressure surrounds them (51). The large pulmonary arteries and veins, as well as the heart and intrathoracic great vessels of the systemic circulation, sense interstitial pressure or ITP as their surrounding pressure and can be called extra-alveolar vessels. The small pulmonary arterioles, venules, and alveolar capillaries sense alveolar pressure as their surrounding pressure and are referred to as alveolar vessels. Since alveolar pressure minus ITP is the transpulmonary pressure, changes in lung volume must alter transpulmonary pressure, thus altering the transmural vascular pressure gradient in extra-alveolar compared to intra-alveolar vessels. The radial interstitial forces of the lung that keep airways patent (50,57,58) also act upon the extra-alveolar vessels. As lung volume increases, the radial interstitial forces increase, increasing the diameter of both extra-alveolar vessels and the conducting airways. The extra-alveolar vessel diameter increases as lung volume increases, dilating these vessels, whereas intra-alveolar vessels are compressed by alveolar pressures at high lung volumes (59). At low lung volumes, on the other hand, the radial interstitial traction decreases, decreasing the cross-sectional diameter and increasing the resistance of extra-alveolar vessels (50,60). This effect is primarily due to the obligatory collapse of the terminal airways and results in alveolar hypoxia. Thus, at small lung volumes pulmonary vascular resistance is increased owing to the combined effect of hypoxic pulmonary vasoconstriction and extra-alveolar vessel collapse.

Increases in lung volume above resting lung volume can increase pulmonary vascular resistance (60,61). With preexisting hyperinflation and loss of pulmonary vasculature, as occurs with either chronic bronchitis or emphysema, this increase in pulmonary vascular resistance can rapidly lead to RV dilation and failure (acute cor pulmonale) (62) and RV ischemia (45). This is related to the fact that if pulmonary pressure increases enough to exceed intralumenal vascular pressure, the pulmonary vasculature will collapse at the vascular loci where extra-alveolar vessels pass into the alveoli. The vascular effect of this collapse will be to reduce the pulmonary vascular cross-sectional area, increasing pulmonary vascular resistance. Similarly, increasing lung volume by stretching and distending the alveolar septa may also compress alveolar capillaries, although this mechanism is less well substantiated. Thus, if lung volumes are reduced, increasing lung volume back to baseline levels should decrease pulmonary vascular resistance. However, excessive increases in lung volume, as occurs with dynamic hyperinflation, will raise pulmonary vascular resistance (63).

C. Ventricular Interdependence

The heart functions as two pumps in series that beat (fill and eject) in parallel, while sharing a common intraventricular septum and housed in a common pericardial sac. Changes in RV output must invariably alter LV filling because the two ventricles are linked in series through the pulmonary vasculature. However, LV preload can also be altered by changes in RV end-diastolic volume through ventricular interdependence (64). Because there is a fixed total cardiac volume, increasing RV end-diastolic volume must limit the LV end-diastolic volume. Functionally, this will make the LV appear to become stiffer, in that for the same filling pressure LV end-diastolic volume will decrease. Increasing RV end-diastolic volume will also induce a shift of the intraventricular septum into the LV, thereby decreasing LV diastolic compliance (65). Thus, for the same LV filling pressure, RV dilation will decrease LV end-diastolic volume and, therefore, cardiac output. This interaction is believed to be the major determinant of the phasic changes in arterial pressure and cardiac output seen in cardiac tamponade. Since spontaneous inspiration increases systemic venous return to the RV (see above), this will result in an inspiratory decrease in LV preload, LV stroke volume, and arterial pulse pressure, referred to as pulsus paradoxus. Although common in subjects during spontaneous ventilation, this mechanism is probably not important during positive-pressure ventilation, wherein RV volumes usually decrease with inspiration. Maintaining a relatively constant rate of venous return, either by volume resuscitation (66) or vasopressor infusion (67), will minimize the tamponade effect. Thus, phasic changes in arterial pressure have been used as a marker of functional hypovolemia (68).

D. Mechanical Heart–Lung Interactions

If lung volumes greatly increase, then the heart can be compressed by the two lungs expanding in the cardiac fossa (69). It has been long known that with hyperinflation juxtacardiac ITP increases more than either lateral chest wall or diaphragmatic ITP (70,72). This compressive effect of the inflated lung can be seen with either spontaneous hyperinflation (73) or positive pressure–induced hyperinflation (57,58). This would lead a clinician at the bedside to conclude that LV contractility was reduced because LV stroke work and cardiac output would decrease with the application of PEEP, despite the same LV filling pressure, when

LV filling pressure is estimated as intralumenal LV pressure alone (without reference to either pericardial or pleural pressure) (66,73,74). However, since LV filling pressure is actually intralumenal pressure minus extramural pressure and LV preload is more accurately defined as LV end-diastolic volume, numerous studies have shown that when patients are fluid resuscitated to return LV end-diastolic volume to its original level, both LV stroke work and cardiac output also return to their original levels (35,66) despite the continued application of PEEP (76). Thus, PEEP has no primary hemodynamic effects unrelated to changes in lung volume and the compressive effects on the heart.

IV. Relationship Between Airway Pressure, Intrathoracic Pressure, and Lung Volume

Positive-pressure ventilation has profound hemodynamic consequences that are often proportional to the increase in airway pressure (Paw) (67,77). However, for the same increase in peak, mean, or end-expiratory Paw, patients often have markedly different hemodynamic responses that cannot be explained by their baseline hemodynamic state. A major source of this apparent inconsistency rests in equating changes in airway pressure (Paw) with changes in both pleural pressure (Ppl) and lung volume. Is it reasonable to equate Paw with predicted hemodynamic effects? Practically, yes, because Paw can be measured easily at the bedside in patients receiving mechanical ventilation, mean Paw reflects mean alveolar pressure, and increases in Paw qualitatively reflect increases in both lung volume and ITP. However, the association between Paw and lung volume and ITP is highly variable among subjects because of individual differences in ventilatory patterns, airway resistance, and lung and chest wall compliance. Since many of the hemodynamic effects of ventilation are due to changes in lung volume, measures of Paw or its change will not accurately reflect changes in lung volume if airway resistance or chest and lung compliance vary. Furthermore, even if lung volume and ITP could be discerned from changes in Paw, they may not accurately reflect changes in pericardial pressure (Ppc), which is a primary determinant of transmural LV pressure. Since the primary determinants of the hemodynamic responses to ventilation are due to changes in intrathoracic pressure and lung volume (49), not Paw, using Paw to predict hemodynamic consequences of mechanical ventilation is fraught with both bias and error.

Lung expansion pushes the chest wall outward, the diaphragm downward, and the cardiac fossa in upon itself. This induces an increase in lateral wall, diaphragmatic, and juxtacardiac Ppl, as well as Ppc. The degree of increase in each of these surface pressures in response to dynamic lung expansion is a function of the compliance and inertness of the chest wall, diaphragm-abdominal contents, and heart. Novak et al. (70) demonstrated that the changes in Ppl induced by positive-pressure ventilation are not similar in all regions of the thorax and increase differently as inspiratory flow rate and frequency increase. Pleural pressure at the diaphragm increases least during positive-pressure inspiration, and juxtacardiac Ppl increases most.

This result seems intuitively obvious because the diaphragm is very compliant, whereas the rib cage has to overcome both resistance to bony distortion and intercostal muscle inertia. However, with a marked reduction in diaphragmatic compliance, experimentally induced by abdominal binding or clinically seen with bowel wall swelling and lumenal distention, diaphragmatic ITP increases by a similar amount as lateral chest wall Ppl. Further, both increase more for the same increase in lung volume than would have been the case in the absence of abdominal stiffness. Thus, in the setting of acute abdominal distention, one may incorrectly assume that the lung is injured and is becoming stiffer, when in fact the lung compliance may be normal but chest wall compliance (here referred to as the entire chest wall-diaphragm apparatus) is restricting expansion (70). This distinction is important because increasing Paw to overcome chest wall stiffness should do so only to the extent that ITP also increases, thus inducing greater hemodynamic consequences. Instead, if lung compliance is reduced, as occurs in acute lung injury states, then similar increases in Paw should not increase ITP as much but should also recruit collapsed and injured alveolar units, improving gas exchange while having fewer hemodynamic effects.

Furthermore, a hydrostatic pressure gradient exists in the pleural space, increasing from nondependent to dependent regions. Dependent regions have a higher baseline pressure than nondependent regions. In the supine subject, steady-state apneic Ppl along the horizontal plane from apex to diaphragm is similar, whereas anterior Ppl is less and posterior gutter Ppl is greater (Fig. 2).

Similarly, if pericardial constriction limits cardiac dilation, then measures of Ppc will underestimate actual Ppc. Thus, estimates of LV filling pressure made from intracavitary LV pressure relative to Ppl will overestimate actual LV filling pressure even if Ppl is measured from a juxtacardiac location. Pinsky and Guimond (71) demonstrated in a canine model of acute ventricular failure that the induction of heart failure was associated with a greater increase in Ppc than juxtacardiac Ppl. Furthermore, with progressive increases in PEEP, juxtacardiac Ppl increased while Ppc remained constant until they equalized, and then both increased equally (72,78).

The interaction of Paw, lung volume, and ITP in the setting of lung disease is complex and can be different for the same pathological condition depending on the tidal volume, inspiratory flow rate, and respiratory frequency. The presence of parenchymal disease, airflow obstruction, and extrapulmonary processes that directly alter chest wall-diaphragmatic contraction also profoundly alters these interactions. If lung injury induces alveolar flooding or increased pulmonary parenchymal stiffness, then greater increases in Paw will be required to distend the

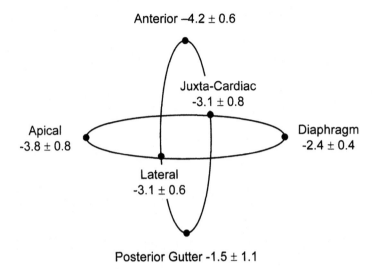

Figure 2 Apneic pleural pressure (Ppl) (mean ± SE) in torr for six pleural regions of the right hemithorax of an intact supine canine model: ANT, anterior; AP, apical; PG, posterior gutter; DI, diaphragmatic; JC, juxtacardiac; and LAT, lateral. Ellipses, regional measurements defining three orthogonal planes. (Adapted from Ref. 70.)

lungs to a constant end-inspiratory volume. However, if tidal volume is kept constant, then both lateral wall Ppl and Ppc increase equally during both normal and acute lung injury conditions (79). Thus, the primary determinant of the increase in Ppl and Ppc during positive-pressure ventilation is lung volume change (80). Also, if the increase in lung volume is sustained, then the increase in ITP is greater than the increase in Ppc. Presumably, Ppc does not increase as much as ITP because increasing lung volume reduces filling of the ventricles, reducing their size within the cardiac fossa (Fig. 3).

Because the distribution of alveolar collapse and lung compliance in ARDS is nonhomogeneous, lung distention during positive-pressure ventilation must overdistend some regions of the lung at the expense of noncompliant or poorly compliant regions (81). Accordingly, Paw will reflect lung distention of lung units that were aerated prior to inspiration, but may not reflect the degree of lung inflation of initially nonaerated lung units. However, Romand et al. (79) and Scharf and Ingram (82) demonstrated that despite this nonhomogeneous alveolar distention, if tidal volume is kept constant, then Ppl will increase equally, independent of the mechanical properties of the lung. In support of this concept, Pinsky et al. (83) demonstrated in postoperative patients that the percentage of Paw increase that is transmitted to the pericardial surface is not constant from

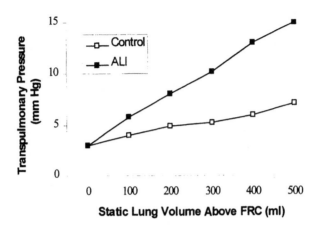

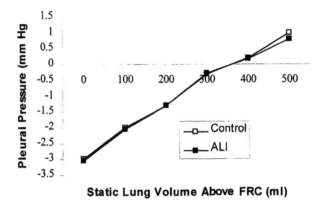

Figure 3 Relation between airway pressure (Paw) and tidal volume (Vt) and between pleural pressure (Ppl) and Vt in control and oleic acid–induced acute lung injury (ALI) conditions in a canine model. Note that despite greater increases in Paw for the same Vt during ALI as compared to control conditions, Ppl and Ppc increase similarly during both control and ALI conditions for the same increase in Vt. (Adapted from Ref. 79.)

one subject to the next as PEEP is increased (Fig. 4). Unfortunately, these workers could not use compliance changes to correct for all of the pressure transmission differences among patients. Thus, one cannot accurately predict the amount of increase in Ppc or Ppl that will occur in patients as PEEP is increased. Accordingly, assuming some constant fraction of Paw transmission to the pleural surface as a means of calculating the effect of increasing Paw on Ppl is misleading and potentially dangerous to patient management.

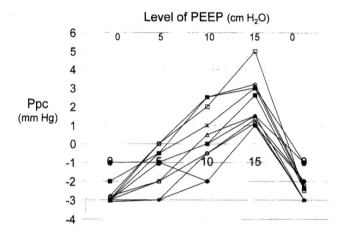

Figure 4 Relation between pericardial pressure (Ppc) and airway pressure as apneic levels of positive end-expiratory pressure (PEEP) were progressively increased from zero to 15 cm H_2O and then back to zero in 5 cm H_2O increments in patients immediately following open heart surgery. Note that although Ppc increases in all subjects as PEEP is increased from 0 to 15 cm H_2O, the initial Ppc value and the proportional change in Ppc among incremental increases in PEEP are quite different among subjects, such that no specific proportion of airway pressure transmission to the pericardial surface can be assumed to occur in all patients. (Adapted from Ref. 83.)

Although it may be difficult to know the actual Ppl, it is possible to determine the change in Ppl induced by ventilation and ventilatory maneuvers. The two methods by which one can vary ITP by an exact amount are by either inspiratory or expiratory maneuvers against an occluded airway, referred to as Mueller and Valsalva maneuvers, respectively. Since lung volume does not change, transpulmonary pressure is constant so that the change in ITP is equal to the change in Paw (84). Normal spontaneous or positive-pressure ventilatory efforts can be used to assess the relative change in ITP in the absence of airway obstruction. Since intrathoracic vascular structures sense ITP as their surrounding pressure, dynamic and rapid swings in ITP, as may occur during ventilation, will be reflected in intrathoracic vascular pressure swings. Both right atrial pressure and pulmonary artery diastolic pressure swings tend to closely follow Ppl swings during ventilation. Regrettably, the only way to obtain these data is by invasive hemodynamic monitoring.

Measures of esophageal pressure using balloon-tipped catheters have been used for many years to monitor changes in ITP. Although esophageal pressure is accurate at reflecting negative swings in Ppl during spontaneous inspiration in upright-seated individuals (77) and in recumbent dogs in the left lateral position

(85), it underestimates both the positive swings in Ppl and the mean increase in Ppl seen with increases in lung volume during positive-pressure ventilation. During Mueller and Valsalva maneuvers, however, because lung volume does not change, swings in esophageal pressure accurately reflect swings in Ppl (78). In fact, the validity of esophageal balloon pressure recordings is documented by demonstrating that both Paw and esophageal pressures increase by similar amounts during a Valsalva maneuver.

V. Hemodynamic Effects of Changes in Intrathoracic Pressure

The heart is housed within the thorax, a pressure chamber within a pressure chamber. Therefore, changes in ITP will affect the pressure gradients for both systemic venous return to the RV and systemic outflow from the LV, independent of the heart itself. Increases in ITP, by increasing right atrial pressure and decreasing transmural LV systolic pressure, will reduce these pressure gradients and thereby decrease intrathoracic blood volume. Continual decreases in ITP will augment venous return and impede LV ejection, thereby increasing intrathoracic blood volume. Although both venous return and LV ejection are simultaneously altered by these changes in ITP, it is helpful to analyze the effects of ITP on venous return and LV ejection separately because their resultant hemodynamic effects can be different.

A. Systemic Venous Return

Blood passively flows back to the heart from the periphery through low pressure–low resistance venous conduits. Once the high pressure arterial flow reaches the capillaries, most of the vascular pressure has been spent on overcoming the high resistance of arterioles and precapillary sphincters. Approximately 4/7 of the circulating blood volume resides in venous reservoirs, and the rate of return of blood to the heart is a major determinant of cardiac output. Systemic venous return to the heart from these venous reservoirs is directly influenced by right atrial pressure (Pra) (86). Since Pra is the downstream pressure for venous return, changes in Pra constitute a primary determinant in the instantaneous rate of venous blood flow back to the right ventricle. Since the right atrium is highly compliant, changes in ITP are directly transmitted to Pra. Increases in ITP, as may occur with positive-pressure ventilation, will decrease the pressure gradient for venous return. If Pra increases enough to equal or exceed the upstream pressure in the venous reservoirs, venous blood flow will cease. This is a presumed cause of circulatory collapse for massive pulmonary embolism as well as the cause of circulatory arrest from constriction.

The relation between Pra and venous return describes a curve with a negative slope and a positive pressure intercept, referred to as the venous return curve (Fig. 5). The zero flow Pra intercept is the upstream pressure in the venous reservoirs, referred to variously as mean circulatory pressure or mean systemic pressure. Mean systemic pressure can be measured with accuracy only during acute circulatory arrest with a patent arterio-venous connection (86). When so measured in normal anesthetized humans, values have ranged between 7 and 11 mmHg. Mean systemic pressure is a function of blood volume, peripheral vasomotor tone, and the distribution of blood within the vasculature (87). Assuming a Pra of near zero, this translates into a driving pressure for venous return of only 10 mmHg or less. Such a low driving pressure is adequate under most circumstances, but underscores the profound effect that slight changes in Pra may have on this flow.

Pra changes rapidly during the ventilatory cycle in phase with the changes in ITP, whereas mean systemic pressure usually does not. Accordingly, variation in right atrial pressure is the major determinant of fluctuations in the pressure gradient for systemic venous return during ventilation (41,88) and explains most of the observed changes in pulmonary blood flow seen during the ventilatory

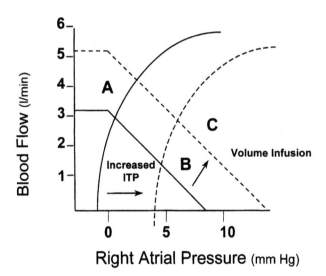

Figure 5 Schematic representation of the effects of increasing or decreasing intrathoracic pressure (ITP) on steady-state venous return. Note that decreases in ITP that decrease right atrial pressure to below zero relative to atmospheric pressure will only increase venous return by a limited amount, whereas increases in ITP will progressively decrease venous return to a complete circulatory standstill.

cycle. Both positive-pressure ventilation and hyperinflation during spontaneous ventilation increase ITP, raising right atrial pressure relative to atmospheric pressure. Thus, venous return decreases (44), RV filling first and then RV stroke volume (44,41,89–96). During normal spontaneous inspiration with decreases in ITP, the converse fall occurs, namely, Pra decreases, accelerating venous blood flow and increasing RV filling and stroke volume (44,67,91,94,97,98).

This simple relation has been challenged by studies showing that positive-pressure inspiration-associated diaphragmatic descent increases intra-abdominal pressure (99,100). Since intra-abdominal pressure is the surrounding pressure of the abdominal vasculature, this increase in pressure also induces a proportional increase in mean systemic pressure. Thus, the pressure gradient for venous return may not be reduced by PEEP, especially in patients with hypervolemia or tense ascites. Potentially, abdominal pressurization by diaphragmatic descent may be the major mechanism by which the decrease in venous return is minimized during positive-pressure ventilation (100–104). Thus, ventilation may have less of an effect on venous return than originally postulated.

Finally, with exaggerated swings in ITP, as occur with obstructed inspiratory efforts, venous return behaves as if abdominal pressure is additive to mean systemic pressure in defining total venous blood flow (105–107). This is analogous to the increase in systemic venous pressure induced by skeletal muscle contraction in exercise. Recent interest in inverse ratio ventilation has raised questions about its hemodynamic effects because its application includes a large component of hyperinflation. However, Mang et al. (109) demonstrated in an animal model of acute lung injury that if total PEEP (intrinsic PEEP plus excess extrinsic PEEP) was similar, no hemodynamic differences between conventional ventilation and inverse ratio ventilation were seen.

B. Right Ventricular Filling

The normal right ventricle is highly compliant. In fact, under normal conditions, it is extremely difficult to document that RV filling pressure increases at all as diastolic RV filling occurs. When RV filling pressure, defined as right atrial pressure minus Ppc, was directly measured in patients undergoing open chest operations, it was insignificantly altered as RV volume was varied by acute volume loading (110). Although right atrial pressure increases with volume loading, Ppc also increases, such that RV filling pressure, defined as right atrial pressure minus pericardial pressure, remains unchanged.

Similar patterns are seen when RV volume is reduced by the application of PEEP in postoperative cardiac patients (111). This suggests that under normal conditions, most of the increase in right atrial pressure seen during volume loading reflects pericardial compliance and cardiac fossa stiffness rather than changes in RV distending pressure. These observations collectively imply that RV wall stretch is unaltered during RV filling. Presumably conformational changes in RV geometry rather than actual RV distention are the primary mechanisms that allow for RV enlargement (78). Thus, changes in right atrial pressure do not follow changes in RV end-diastolic volume and are a poor marker of RV filling. When cardiac contractility is reduced and intravascular volume is expanded, the relation is still not linear. RV filling pressure may increase as a result of decreased RV diastolic compliance, increased pericardial compliance, increased end-diastolic volume, or a combination of all three. Thus, measures of Pra are of limited value in assessing RV filling, although increased Pra does indicate an expanded intravascular blood volume.

Taylor et al. (64) documented in an isolated asystolic canine heart preparation that there is a curvilinear relation between RV filling pressure and volume, such that as RV end-diastolic volume increased above a threshold level, RV filling pressure increased greatly. Furthermore, Pinsky and Guimond (71) demonstrated that in dogs with acute ventricular failure, volume loading increased Ppc more than ITP, consistent with pericardial rather than cardiac fossal restraint. In further support of this view, as PEEP is increased in the setting of volume overload heart failure, ITP but not Ppc selectively increases until it equals Ppc, then both ITP and Ppc increase equally if PEEP is increased further. Pinsky et al. (83) subsequently demonstrated similar phenomena in postoperative cardiac surgery patients. We can conclude from these studies that PEEP, and by extension, lung expansion, compresses the heart within the cardiac fossa in a fashion analogous to pericardial tamponade, but it is the expansion of the lungs and not pericardial restraint that increases ITP and limits ventricular filling (4,112).

Under normal conditions at rest, venous return to the heart is maintained at near maximal levels (22,96,97) because RV filling occurs with minimal changes in Pra (112). This hemodynamically favorable condition occurs because of two complementary processes. First, spontaneous inspiration decreases ITP, so even if RV filling pressure were to increase as venous return accelerated, the increase would be minimal or nonexistent if seen from the perspective of Pra relative to atmosphere. Second, under most conditions the RV fills with minimal or no increase in transmural pressure. Thus, Pra usually decreases during spontaneous inspiration even though RV filling is augmented. The more Pra remains near zero relative to atmospheric pressure, the closer to maximal is the pressure gradient for systemic venous blood flow (86,92). This mechanism can only work if instantaneous RV output equals venous return to the RV from the prior beat. Otherwise the RV would overdistend, increasing Pra and decreasing venous return.

Normal physiology and vascular architecture work to keep venous return near maximal. First, significant conformational changes in RV shape can occur that result in significant increases in RV volume without requiring any increase in RV distending pressure. Second, for the same RV wall stretch at end-diastole

(RV preload), the pulmonary arterial inflow circuit is highly compliant, such that marked changes in RV stroke volume do not result in significant changes in pulmonary outflow pressure (44,113). Finally, normal spontaneous inspiration is followed by passive expiration, with a slight increase in ITP and drop in venous return, such that RV volume returns to apneic values (41).

Since spontaneous inspiratory efforts decrease ITP and lower Pra, one sees an increase in venous return with spontaneous inspiration (33,92–95). However, this augmentation of venous return is limited (107,108) because decreases in ITP below atmospheric pressure causes large systemic veins to collapse as they enter the thorax (86). This flow limitation functions as a safety valve for the heart because ITP can decrease greatly during inspiratory efforts in patients with airway obstruction (23). If venous return was not flow-limited, the RV might become overdistended and either fail or impede LV filling (interdependence) with each vigorous inspiratory effort (114).

This beautifully adaptive coupling between venous return and RV function during spontaneous ventilation will rapidly become dysfunctional if either RV diastolic compliance decreases or if right atrial pressure increases independent of changes in RV end-diastolic volume. Regrettably, both these conditions commonly occur in critically ill patients and explain much of the observed hemodynamic dysfunction they display. RV diastolic compliance rapidly decreases if pulmonary hypertension develops as may occur with a massive pulmonary embolism, bronchospasm, hyperinflation, or ARDS. Dissociation between Pra and RV end-diastolic volume occurs during both tamponade and positive-pressure inspiration. This is an important concept to remember. During positive-pressure inspiration, Pra and RV filling pressure become dissociated because Pra is artificially increased by the increasing ITP, decreasing the rate of venous return and reducing RV end-diastolic volume. This is the primary process by which positive-pressure ventilation impairs normal circulatory adaptive processes. With weaning from mechanical ventilatory support, if pulmonary hypertension develops (increased sympathetic tone or hyperinflation) or a poorly contracting RV is given an increased load, then acute RV failure may develop. Thus, during weaning from mechanical ventilation, occult RV failure may become manifest as a rapid rise in Pra associated with a decrease in cardiac output.

Since the primary effect of any form of ventilation on cardiovascular function in normal subjects is to alter RV preload via altering venous blood flow, the detrimental effect of positive-pressure ventilation on cardiac output can be minimized by either fluid resuscitation to increase mean systemic pressure (Fig. 5) (67,89,105,106) or by keeping both mean ITP and swings in lung volume as low as possible. This can be accomplished by prolonging expiratory time, decreasing tidal volume, and avoiding excessive amounts of PEEP (1,3,40,91–95,115).

C. Left Ventricular Preload and Ventricular Interdependence

Changes in venous return must eventually result in directionally similar changes in LV preload, because the two ventricles are in series. If systemic venous return were selectively reduced by a Valsalva maneuver, for example, RV end-diastolic volume would decrease but LV end-diastolic volume would remain constant (84). In actuality, RV filling declines after about three heartbeats, lowering RV stroke volume and causing a progressive decline in LV end-diastolic volume and, thus, stroke volume. As the Valsalva maneuver is sustained, LV filling and cardiac output both begin to decrease (69,116). This phase delay in changes in output from the RV to the LV is exaggerated if tidal volume or respiratory rate is increased in the setting of hypovolemia (3,36,37,66,74,75,96,115,117–121) and can be used to identify hypovolemia and preload responsiveness in ventilator-dependent patients (68).

Changes in RV volumes can also alter LV end-diastolic volumes directly, through the process of ventricular interdependence. The ventricles share a common intraventricular septum, are housed in a common pericardial sac that limits absolute cardiac volume, and are collectively influenced by changes in lung volume via compression or expansion of the cardiac fossa, so changes in RV end-diastolic volume directly affect LV diastolic compliance (Fig. 6). Increasing RV

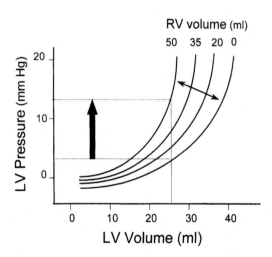

Figure 6 Schematic diagram of the effect of increasing right ventricular (RV) volumes on the left ventricular (LV) diastolic pressure-volume (filling) relationship. Note that increasing RV volumes decrease LV diastolic compliance, such that a higher filling pressure is required to generate a constant end-diastolic volume. (Adapted from Ref. 64.)

volume decreases LV diastolic compliance by shifting the intraventricular septum into the LV. However, positive-pressure ventilation usually decreases RV volumes, minimizing ventricular interdependence (64,119–122). Jardin et al. demonstrated this in humans using echocardiography (36). They showed that although PEEP resulted in some degree of right-to-left intraventricular septal shift, the shift was small. Furthermore, although increases in lung volume during positive-pressure ventilation cause some septal shift, the primary effect of PEEP is to compress both ventricles into each other, decreasing bi-ventricular volume (123). Thus, it should come as no surprise that the decrease in cardiac output during PEEP, if present, is simply due to a decrease in LV end-diastolic volume. Furthermore, if LV end-diastolic volume is restored to its original value, cardiac output will also be restored (124,125) without a change in LV diastolic compliance (66).

During spontaneous inspiration, on the other hand, marked increases in RV volume transiently shift the intraventricular septum into the LV (65), decreasing LV diastolic compliance and LV end-diastolic volume (64,122,126). This transient RV dilation-induced septal shift is the primary cause of inspiration-associated decreases in arterial pulse pressure in otherwise normal subjects. With hyperinflation, however, the pericardium is stretched downward by the descending diaphragm reducing maximal pericardial volume (127). Thus, in the setting of acute cardiac enlargement or pericardial effusion, and/or with vigorous and large tidal volumes, the swings in arterial pulse pressure (which reflect swings in LV stroke volume) during one respiratory cycle can be exaggerated. If such swings in arterial pulse pressure are greater than 10 mmHg, this phenomenon is referred to as pulsus paradoxus (97). Since spontaneous inspiratory efforts can also occur during positive-pressure ventilation and especially during partial ventilatory assist, pulsus paradoxus can be seen in mechanically ventilated patients.

D. Left Ventricular Afterload

Although LV preload is usually equated with maximal LV wall stretch prior to systole and is proportional to LV end-diastolic volume, LV afterload is more difficult to define. LV afterload reflects the strain of myocardial ejection during systole and can be equated to systolic wall tension. Systolic wall tension, by the law of LaPlace, is proportional to the product of transmural LV pressure and the radius of curvature of the LV, which itself is proportional to LV volume. Maximal LV wall tension normally occurs at the end of isometric contraction, reflecting both a maximal LV radius of curvature (end-diastolic volume) and aortic pressure (diastolic pressure) product. During ejection, LV pressure increases to peak systolic pressure, but LV volume decreases much more. Thus, under normal conditions, the LV unloads itself during systole.

However, when LV dilation exists, as in congestive heart failure, maximal LV wall stress occurs during LV ejection because the maximal product of the radius and pressure occurs at this time, and end-ejection does not offer the straining ventricle any reprieve from the increased wall stress. Accordingly, LV afterload varies depending on the baseline level of cardiac contractility and intravascular volume. Based on the above discussion, if LV volume or ejection pressure increases, then LV afterload will also increase, increasing myocardial O_2 demand. Similarly, if either LV volume or ejection pressure decreases, LV afterload will also decrease.

Both LV volume and ejection pressure are affected by ventilation and ventilatory maneuvers. Thus, although the primary effect of ventilation on cardiovascular function is to vary LV preload, changes in LV afterload also occur and can be the dominant hemodynamic effect. Although the above discussion illustrated how ventilation could alter LV end-diastolic volume by a variety of mechanisms, ventilation alters LV ejection pressure by only one simple process.

LV ejection pressure is the transmural LV systolic pressure, which can be measured as intralumenal LV pressure minus pericardial pressure, which can be further approximated as arterial pressure relative to ITP. Normal homeostatic processes functioning through baroreceptors located in the carotid body maintain arterial pressure constant with respect to atmosphere. Increases in arterial pressure induced by increasing ITP will induce a reflex peripheral vasodilation so as to maintain arterial pressure constant but also causing transmural LV pressure to decrease. Recall that LV afterload is the product of LV transmural pressure and volume. Accordingly, if transmural arterial pressure were to remain constant as ITP increased but LV end-diastolic volume were to decrease because of the associated decrease in systemic venous return, then LV wall tension would also decrease (128). Thus, by either mechanism, increases in ITP decrease LV afterload.

Using the same logic, decreases in ITP at a constant arterial pressure will increase LV transmural pressure increasing LV afterload (84,129). Since marked decreases in ITP commonly occur during vigorous spontaneous inspiratory efforts, especially in the setting of upper airway obstruction or bronchospasm, spontaneous ventilation can increase afterload in patients being weaned from mechanical ventilation, inducing heart failure, myocardial ischemia, and infarction (129–131). Similarly, removing spontaneous inspiratory efforts by initiating mechanical ventilation is often associated with an improvement in LV systolic function in patients with severe LV failure (132). Similar "auto-EPAP" effects of expiratory grunting have been reported in infants during crying (37) and in an adult with severe LV failure (133).

Pulsus paradoxus is the primary cardiovascular sign of heart-lung interactions. Originally, it was used as a means to identify subjects with constrictive pericarditits secondary to tuberculosis, but it occurs during spontaneous inspiration under all conditions characterized by marked pericardial restraint. For example, tamponade and constrictive pericarditis, hyperinflation as well as loaded spontaneous ventilatory efforts and acute cor pulmonale are all associated with pulsus paradoxus. In all of these examples, inspiration is associated with a decrease in LV stroke volume relative to apnea (127,134–137). Perhaps the most common mechanism creating an inspiratory decrease in both LV stroke volume and systolic arterial pressure is the increased venous return–induced transient shift of the intraventricular septum into the LV lumen owing to pericardial volume restraint. Since negative swings in ITP increase LV ejection pressure (LV pressure minus ITP) as well as LV end-systolic volume (84), the increase in LV afterload and reduction of LV stroke volumes are of a greater magnitude than would be the case if only end-diastolic volume increased.

Ventilation can also alter LV systolic function independent of the effects on LV end-diastolic volume and ejection pressure. For example, obstructive sleep apnea induces a marked increase in peripheral vasomotor tone that increases atrial impedance (138). Similarly, increasing ejection pressure causes greater reductions and delays in shortening in those regions of the myocardium less able to increase their force of contraction in response to the increased load. This results in load-dependent regional wall motion abnormalities that reduce the synchrony of contraction of the global myocardium (139) and can produce ischemia-induced decreases in contractility if coronary blood flow is fixed and compromised (140). Ischemia has the added detriment of directly reducing LV diastolic compliance (141). These two hemodynamic effects have received little attention in the literature but may prove to be very important once methods of assessing regional asynchrony and myocardial O_2 demand are made available at the bedside.

If ITP increases rapidly, then arterial pressure increases as well and by a similar amount. Thus, both arterial pressure relative to ITP (transmural arterial pressure or LV ejection pressure) (84) and aortic blood flow (68) remain constant. However, sustained increases in ITP decrease venous return and eventually decrease aortic blood flow and arterial pressure (84). Since baroreceptor mechanisms maintain arterial pressure constant (23), if ITP increased arterial pressure without changing transmural arterial pressure, then the periphery would reflexively vasodilate to maintain a constant extrathoracic arterial pressure-flow relation (118). Unfortunately, the coronary circulation is housed in the thorax, so coronary perfusion pressure will decrease despite no change in arterial pressure. Furthermore, compression of the coronaries by the expanding lungs may obstruct coronary blood flow further. Thus, these combined effects can decrease coronary blood flow and induce myocardial ischemia (142–144).

E. Myocardial Energetics and Ventilation

Myocardial oxygen demand (Mvo_2) is determined by numerous factors including primarily myocardial wall stress and heart rate. As we saw above, under normal conditions LV wall stress is greatest at the point of aortic valve opening. The associated LV end-diastolic volume and diastolic pressure product is usually maximal at that time. Because the heart is in the chest but receives its venous return and ejects its stroke volume from and into extrathoracic compartments, respectively, changes in ITP will directly alter Mvo_2 independent of any increased metabolic stress that spontaneous breathing may require. Increasing ITP will decrease venous return reducing LV end-diastolic volume and LV ejection pressure. The combined effect of these two actions is to reduce both myocardial wall stress and Mvo_2.

The work performed by the contracting LV increases by a similar amount whether ITP increases above atmospheric pressure or increases from a negative value to atmospheric, as long as the absolute change in ITP is similar. In both cases, the LV ejection pressure will decrease in proportion to the relative increase in ITP. However, the effect on venous return of removing large negative levels of ITP differs from that of adding positive ITP. Importantly, although an increase in ITP is limited in its ability to reduce Mvo_2, owing to the obligatory decrease in venous return, removing large negative swings in ITP acts in a similar fashion to reduce LV ejection pressure but does not reduce venous return. Venous return does not increase further as right atrial pressure becomes negative, owing to the venous collapse inducing flow limitation so large negative swings in ITP selectively increase LV ejection pressure.

Large negative swings in ITP, as seen during vigorous inspiratory efforts in the setting of airway obstruction (asthma, upper airway obstruction, vocal cord paralysis) or stiff lungs (interstitial lung disease, pulmonary edema and acute lung injury) selectively increase LV afterload. This mechanism has been postulated as the cause of the often observed LV failure and pulmonary edema seen in these conditions (23,32), especially if LV systolic function is already compromised (9,145). Furthermore, removing large negative swings in ITP by either bypassing upper airway obstruction (endotracheal intubation) or by instituting mechanical ventilation or PEEP should selectively reduce LV afterload without significantly decreasing either venous return or cardiac output (67,86,117,146–148). This concept has significant clinical implications. The institution of endotracheal intubation and positive-pressure breathing may markedly improve hemodynamics and reduce LV ischemia if it selectively reduces LV afterload while maintaining venous return.

Reversing this argument, weaning from mechanical ventilation is associated with increases in both metabolic demand and LV afterload. Thus, weaning is a form of cardiac stress testing. Numerous studies have documented that weaning induces ischemia in patients with coronary artery disease (149–152) and its termination (reinstitution of mechanical ventilation) reverses ischemic ECG changes (147,148).

VI. Patient-Specific Heart–Lung Interactions

Based on the above discussion, it should be clear that spontaneous and positive-pressure ventilation have profound hemodynamic consequences. However, given different cardiac, vascular, and ventilatory states, the same maneuver might have opposite effects on cardiovascular stability. Furthermore, different modes of mechanical ventilatory support require varying degrees of patient effort, alter lung volumes differently, and induce different patterns of ITP during the ventilatory cycle. Thus, almost any hemodynamic effect can be explained by heart–lung interactions. This, in and of itself, is a profound limitation of the general concepts listed above, because it can be seen that almost any hemodynamic effect can occur during ventilation given the right circumstances. Yet this is also the primary strength of heart–lung physiology, because common interventions that induce different hemodynamic effects can be explained rationally and specific treatments that can alleviate almost any dysfunction can be implemented. Furthermore, it can be predicted that all forms of ventilation that induce similar changes in ITP, lung volume, and work of breathing will have identical hemodynamic effects regardless of the type of ventilation or settings used. In fact, equalizing hemodynamic effects when switching from one mode of ventilation to another is an excellent method of ensuring that similar levels of ITP, lung volume, and work of breathing were achieved with the two modes.

Thus, the following generalities hold across most modes of mechanical ventilation. In patients with markedly increased work of breathing, hypervolemia, or impaired LV pump function, adding mechanical ventilatory support usually improves cardiovascular function by decreasing global O_2 demand and Mvo_2, independent of any effects on intrapulmonary gas exchange. At the other end of the spectrum, patients likely to develop hyperinflation (e.g., patients with chronic airflow obstruction of acute bronchospasm) or who are hypovolemic (either absolute or apparent) are apt to become hemodynamically unstable if mechanical ventilation is initiated, despite improving arterial oxygenation. Similarly, since withdrawal of ventilatory support is an exercise stress test, patients with limited cardiovascular reserve may not wean from mechanical ventilatory support even if their weaning parameter values are acceptable (10,145).

When different modes of mechanical ventilation with similar airway pressures and PEEP induce different hemodynamic responses, these differences are explainable by different effects on lung volume and ITP (153). Importantly, when two different modes of ventilation induce similar changes in ITP and ventilatory effort, their hemodynamic effects will be similar, even if airway waveforms differ markedly. This is best illustrated for partial ventilatory support modalities such as pressure support ventilation and intermittent mandatory ventilation. Both result in similar hemodynamic responses when matched for similar tidal volumes (154). Similarly, tissue oxygenation was similar in 12 stable ventilator-dependent patients when switched between assist-control, intermittent mandatory ventilation, and pressure-support ventilation at matched tidal volumes (155). To take this validation to its limits, even when high-frequency jet ventilation is compared to other modes of mechanical ventilatory support, hemodynamics are similar to large tidal volume ventilation (156). Three common clinical scenarios demonstrate this phenomenon.

A. Chronic Obstructive Pulmonary Disease

Patients with COPD who develop respiratory failure and/or require mechanical ventilatory support often develop dynamic hyperinflation. The net result of this hyperinflation is compression of the heart within the cardiac fossa, increasing right atrial pressure, decreasing LV diastolic compliance, and increasing pulmonary vascular resistance. Dynamic hyperinflation is also referred to as intrinsic PEEP. Intrinsic PEEP alters hemodynamic function in a fashion similar to extrinsic PEEP (157–159). Although matching intrinsic PEEP with externally applied PEEP decreases the work cost of spontaneous breathing, it has no measurable detrimental hemodynamic effect. Similarly, CPAP has no measurable hemodynamic effect when delivered below the level of intrinsic PEEP (160). Finally, there is little hemodynamic difference between increasing airway pressure to generate a breath and decreasing extrathoracic pressure (iron lung-negative pressure ventilation) (161). Both alter heart–lung interactions similarly, with the exception of the potential effect of negative pressure breathing devices on intra-abdominal pressure.

Patients with severe COPD receiving mechanical ventilation may go into cardiogenic pulmonary edema during weaning despite having adequate weaning parameters (9). This probably reflects a complex hemodynamic effect consisting of adverse responses of the LV, as described earlier, as well as altered pulmonary vascular resistance that impairs RV ejection independent of any effects of weaning on Mvo_2 and LV ejection (10). The difficulty that clinicians have in predicting weaning success at the bedside using measures of ventilatory reserve, airflow, and gas exchange parameters may reflect an ignorance of the patient's cardiovascular reserve and the exercise load that spontaneous breathing places on the circulation (68). Occult cardiovascular insufficiency may play a major role in the development of failure to wean in critically ill patients (58).

B. Acute Lung Injury

Patients with acute lung injury usually benefit significantly from positive-pressure ventilation. Since increases in ITP reduce intrathoracic blood volume (92), pulmonary edema often is minimized. The addition of PEEP decreases intrathoracic blood volume even more (111,112) without altering LV contractile function (163). Although lung water may increase slightly during PEEP therapy, the distribution does not affect gas-exchanging regions of the lung and is of questionable significance. However, the increase in airway pressure does not mean that ITP also increases by some fixed proportion. In fact, the primary determinant of the increase in ITP during positive-pressure ventilation is the associated increase in lung volume (79). In 18 ventilator-dependent but hemodynamically stable patients, Singer et al. (164) found that the degree of hyperinflation, not the increase in airway pressure, correlated with the decrease in cardiac output. Thus, to the extent that increases in lung volume are matched between different modes of mechanical ventilation, cardiac output will also decrease to a similar extent (104,165). That these effects reflect primarily a preload phenomenon is validated by numerous studies showing that if LV end-diastolic volume is held constant, PEEP has minimal hemodynamic effects (163,165,167,168). The PEEP-induced reduction in cardiac output is due to a decreased pressure gradient for venous return, as was elegantly shown by Gunter et al. (169), who minimized the decrease in cardiac output in ventilator-dependent septic patients by lower body compression. Unfortunately, PEEP may have other detrimental effects in patients with acute lung injury, such as increased leukocyte retention in human lungs (151).

A few clinical reports serve to underscore these statements. Lessard et al. (170) compared volume-controlled conventional ventilation with pressure-controlled and pressure-controlled inverse ratio ventilation in nine patients with ARDS. Total PEEP and tidal volume were consistent between treatment arms, so the changes in ITP were similar among the three therapies and no significant hemodynamic effects were seen. Chan and Abraham (171) saw similar results in 10 ARDS patients matched for tidal volumes and total PEEP. However, when pressure-controlled ventilation with a smaller tidal volume was compared to volume-controlled, not surprisingly, pressure-controlled ventilation was associated with a higher cardiac output (172,173).

C. Congestive Heart Failure

Increases in cardiac output with increases in airway pressure suggest the presence of congestive heart failure (148,174). Calvin et al. (150) noted that patients with cardiogenic pulmonary edema had no decrease in cardiac output when given PEEP. Grace and Greenbaum (146) demonstrated that adding PEEP to patients with heart failure increased cardiac output if pulmonary artery occlusion pressure initially exceeded 18 mmHg. Rasanen et al. documented that decreasing levels of ventilatory support in patients with myocardial ischemia and acute LV failure worsened ischemia (148,149) and could be minimized by preventing spontaneous inspiratory effort-induced negative swings in ITP (147). Since weaning from mechanical ventilatory support is a form of exercise stress test, withdrawal of ventilatory support can unmask cardiac failure in otherwise stable patients with acute respiratory failure (9). Such patients may require cardiovascular pharmacological support to be weaned from mechanical ventilation (145).

The cardiovascular benefits of positive airway pressure in patients with heart failure can also be seen by withdrawing negative swings in ITP. Examples include the use of low levels of CPAP in patients with heart failure and/or obstructive sleep apnea (150,151). Levels of CPAP as low as 5 cm H_2O can increase cardiac output in congestive heart failure patients. On the other hand, cardiac output decreases in normal subjects and heart failure patients without volume overload treated with similar levels of CPAP. Nasal CPAP can also accomplish the same results in patients with obstructive sleep apnea and heart failure (152,175). Prolonged nighttime nasal CPAP can selectively improve respiratory muscle strength as well as LV contractile function in the setting of preexistent heart failure (174). That these effects reflect real hemodynamic improvement is supported by the associated reductions in serum catecholamine levels (177).

If positive airway pressure augments LV ejection in heart failure states, then systolic arterial pressure should not decrease and may actually increase as compared to spontaneous ventilation. This is referred to as reverse pulsus paradoxus and was seen in 10 post–cardiac surgery patients (174). Furthermore, the relation between ventilatory efforts and systolic arterial pressure may be used to rapidly identify which patients may benefit from cardiac assist by increases in ITP and which patients may not (178–180). Patients who increase their systolic arterial pressure during ventilation relative to an apneic baseline tend to have a greater degree of volume overload (179) and heart failure (176), whereas those subjects in whom systolic arterial pressure decreases tend to be volume responsive. Although the mechanism by which this systolic pulse pressure varies appears not to be due to a change in stroke volume (181), monitoring the ventilation-associated changes in pulse pressure appears to accurately predict preload responsiveness and cardiac output changes in ventilator-dependent patients with acute lung injury (68).

VII. Summary and Conclusions

Mechanical ventilation influences the cardiovascular system in numerous ways, both beneficial and detrimental. Heart–lung interactions in patients receiving mechanical ventilation are complex, and seemingly similar ventilatory maneuvers can yield diametrically opposite responses, depending on patient factors. Fortunately, hemodynamic responses to different ventilator settings can usually be explained by a consideration of effects on the important factors that determine the cardiovascular responses. Most of these factors are taken into consideration if one recognizes that spontaneous ventilation may be viewed as a form of exercise, that lung volume is a more important determinant of cardiovascular responses than airway or intrathoracic pressure, and that positive-pressure mechanical ventilation exerts many of its effects via increases in intrathoracic pressure.

While considering these factors, it is well to keep in mind that depending on initial lung volume, increases can augment or diminish cardiac output, that intrathoracic pressure as measured by esophageal pressure does not necessarily reflect pericardial pressure, and that the influence of intrathoracic pressure varies depending on changes in lung volume as determined by lung compliance. The heart can be thought of as a pump within a pump, and depending on pressure changes within the thoracic pump, major alterations may occur in the function of the cardiac pump. For example, the phenomenon of ventricular interdependence, in which the filling of one ventricle affects filling of the other, is heavily influenced by changes in lung volume and differences in mean systemic versus intrathoracic pressure.

By taking into consideration the specific factors that determine cardiovascular effects of mechanical ventilation, one can anticipate patterns of response in particular patient subsets. For example, in patients with severe airway obstruction, the increased lung compliance and airway resistance give rise to dynamic hyperinflation that compresses the heart within the cardiac fossa, increases right atrial pressure, decreases LV diastolic compliance, increases pulmonary vascular resistance, and, in the end, can have profound deleterious hemodynamic effects. In addition, weaning of COPD patients from mechanical ventilation may bring out LV dysfunction and induce cardiogenic pulmonary edema, particularly if there are large negative intrathoracic pressure swings. Patients with acute lung injury usually benefit from positive-pressure ventilation because increased intrathoracic pressure decreases intrathoracic blood volume and reduces pulmonary vascular resistance. Patients with congestive heart failure also usually benefit from positive-pressure ventilation, particularly if there is volume overload and impaired ventricular systolic function. In this situation, increased intrathoracic pressure serves to reduce myocardial tension and left ventricular afterload. By taking into consideration the numerous heart-lung interactions that occur during mechanical ventilation, clinicians can select ventilator settings that optimize cardiovascular function.

References

1. Cournaud A, Motley HL, Werko L, et al. Physiologic studies of the effect of intermittent positive pressure breathing on cardiac output in man. Am J Physiol 1948; 152:162–174.
2. Roussos C, Macklem PT. The respiratory muscles. N Engl J Med 1982; 307:786–797.
3. Grenvik A. Respiratory, circulatory and metabolic effects of respiratory treatment. Acta Anaesth Scand (suppl) 1966.

4. Shuey CB, Pierce AK, Johnson RL. An evaluation of exercise tests in chronic obstructive lung disease. J Appl Physiol 1969; 27:256–261.

5. Stock MC, David DW, Manning JW, Ryan ML. Lung mechanics and oxygen consumption during spontaneous ventilation and severe heart failure. Chest 1992; 102: 279–283.

6. Kawagoe Y, Permutt S, Fessler HE. Hyperinflation with intrinsic PEEP and respiratory muscle blood flow. J Appl Physiol 1994; 77:2440–2448.

7. Aubier M, Vires N, Sillye G, Mozes R, Roussos C. Respiratory muscle contribution to lactic acidosis in low cardiac output. Am Rev Respir Dis 1982; 126:648–652.

8. Vires N, Sillye G, Rassidakis A, et al. Effect of mechanical ventilation on respiratory muscle blood flow during shock. Physiologist 1980; 23:1–8.

9. Lemaire F, Teboul JL, Cinoti L, Giotto G, Abrouk F, Steg G, Macquin-Mavier I, Zapol WM. Acute left ventricular dysfunction during unsuccessful weaning from mechanical ventilation. Anesthesiology 1988; 69:171–179.

10. Richard C, Teboul J-L, Archambaud F, Hebert J-L, Michaut P, Auzepy P. Left ventricular function during weaning of patients with chronic obstructive pulmonary disease. Intensive Care Med 1994; 20:181–186.

11. (a) Hurford et al. Thallium-201 myocardial perfusion impaired during weaning from MV in ventilator-dependent patients. Anesthesiology 1991; 74:1007–1016. (b) Hurford et al. Association of myocardial ischemia with failure to wean. Crit Care Med 1995; 23:1475–1480.

12. Chatila et al. Cardiac ischemia during weaning from MV. Chest 1995; 109:1421–1422.

13. Glick G, Wechsler AS, Epstein DE. Reflex cardiovascular depression produced by stimulation of pulmonary stretch receptors in the dog. J Clin Invest 1969; 48:467–472.

14. Painal AS. Vagal sensory receptors and their reflex effects. Physiol Rev 1973; 53: 59–88.

15. Anrep GV, Pascual W, Rossler R. Respiratory variations in the heart rate. I. The reflex mechanism of the respiratory arrhythmia. Proc R Soc Lond B Biol Sci 1936; 119:191–217.

16. Taha BH, Simon PM, Dempsey JA, Skatrud JB, Iber C. Respiratory sinus arrhythmia in humans: an obligatory role for vagal feedback from the lungs. J Appl Physiol 1995; 78:638–645.

17. Bernardi L, Calciati A, Gratarola A, Battistin I, Fratino P, Finardi G. Heart rate-respiration relationship: computerized method for early detection of cardiac autonomic damage in diabetic patients. Acta Cardiol 1986; 41:197–206.

18. Bernardi L, Keller F, Sanders M, Reddy PS, Griffith B, Meno F, Pinsky MR. Respiratory sinus arrhythmia in the totally denervated human heart. J Appl Physiol 1989; 67:1447–1455.

19. Glick G, Wechsler AS, Epstein DE. Reflex cardiovascular depression produced by stimulation of pulmonary stretch receptors in the dog. J Clin Invest 1969; 48:467–472.

20. Cassidy SS, Eschenbacher WI, Johnson Jr RL. Reflex cardiovascular depression during unilateral lung hyperinflation in the dog. J Clin Invest 1979; 64:620–626.

21. Daly MB, Hazzledine JL, Ungar A. The reflex effects of alterations in lung vol-

ume on systemic vascular resistance in the dog. J Physiol (London) 1967; 188: 331–351.

22. Shepherd JT. The lungs as receptor sites for cardiovascular regulation. Circulation 1981; 63:1–10.

23. Stalcup SA, Mellins RB. Mechanical forces producing pulmonary edema in acute asthma. N Engl J Med 1977; 297:592–596.

24. Vatner SF, Rutherford JD. Control of the myocardial contractile state by carotid chemo- and baroreceptor and pulmonary inflation reflexes in conscious dogs. J Clin Invest 1978; 63:1593–1601.

25. Pick RA, Handler JB, Murata GH, Friedman AS. The cardiovascular effects of positive end-expiratory pressure. Chest 1982; 82:345–350.

26. Fuhrman BP, Everitt J, Lock JE. Cardiopulmonary effects of unilateral airway pressure changes in intact infant lambs. J Appl Physiol 1984; 56:1439–1448.

27. Payen, DM, Brun-Buisson CJL, Carli PA, Huet Y, Leviel F, Cinotti L, Chiron B. Hemodynamic, gas exchange, and hormonal consequences of LBPP during PEEP ventilation. J Appl Physiol 1987; 62:61–70.

28. Frage D, de la Coussaye JE, Beloucif S, Fratacci MD, Payen DM. Interactions between hormonal modifications during PEEP-induced antidiuresis and antinatriuresis. Chest 1995; 107:1095–1100.

29. Frass M, Watschinger B, Traindl O, Popovic R, Podolsky A, Gisslinger H, Flager S, Golden M, Schuster E, Leithner C. Atrial natriuretic peptide release in response to different positive end-expiratory pressure levels. Crit Care Med 1993; 21:343–347.

30. Wilkins MA, Su XL, Palayew MD, Yamashiro Y, Bolli P, McKenzie JK, Kryger MH. The effects of posture change and continuous positive airway pressure on cardiac natriuretic peptides in congestive heart failure. Chest 1995; 107:909–915.

31. Shirakami G, Magaribuchi T, Shingu K, Suga S, Tamai S, Nakao K, Mori K. Positive end-expiratory pressure ventilation decreases plasma atrial and brain natriuretic peptide levels in humans. Anesth Analg 1993; 77:1116–1121.

32. Bromberger-Barnea B. Mechanical effects of inspiration on heart functions: a review. Fed Proc 1981; 40:2172–2177.

33. Brecher GA, Hubay CA. Pulmonary blood flow and venous return during spontaneous respiration. Circ Res 1955; 3:40–214.

34. Goldstein JA, Vlahakes GJ, Verrier ED. The role of right ventricular systolic dysfunction and elevated intrapericardial pressures in the genesis of low output in experimental right ventricular infarction. Circulation 1982; 65:513–520.

35. Jardin F, Farcot JC, Boisante L. Influence of positive end-expiratory pressure on left ventricular performance. N Engl J Med 1981; 304:387–392.

36. Jardin FF, Farcot JC, Gueret P, Prost JF, Ozier Y, Bourdarias JP. Echocardiographic evaluation of ventricles during continuous positive pressure breathing. J Appl Physiol 1984; 56:619–627.

37. Prec KJ, Cassels DE. Oximeter studies in newborn infants during crying. Pediatr 1952; 9:756–761.

38. Luce JM. The cardiovascular effects of mechanical ventilation and positive end-expiratory pressure. J Am Med Assoc 1984; 252:807–811.

39. Maughan WL, Shoukas AA, Sagawa K, Weisfeldt ML. Instantaneous pressure-volume relationships of the canine right ventricle. Circ Res 1979; 44:309–315.

40. Sibbald WJ, Driedger AA. Right ventricular function in disease states: pathophysiologic considerations. Crit Care Med 1983; 11:339.

41. Pinsky MR. Instantaneous venous return curves in an intact canine preparation. J Appl Physiol 1984; 56:765–771.

42. Buda, AJ, Pinsky, MR, Ingels NB, et al. Effect of intrathoracic pressure on left ventricular performance. N Engl J Med 1979; 301:453–459.

43. Piene H, Sund T. Does pulmonary impedance constitute the optimal load for the right ventricle? Am J Physiol 1982; 242:H154–H160.

44. Pinsky MR. Determinants of pulmonary arterial flow variation during respiration. J Appl Physiol 1984; 56:1237–1245.

45. Johnston WE, Vinten-Johansen J, Shugart HE, Santamore WP. Positive end-expiratory pressure potentiates the severity of canine right ventricular ischemia-reperfusion injury. Am J Physiol 1992; 262:H168–H176.

46. Madden JA, Dawson CA, Harder DR. Hypoxia-induced activation in small isolated pulmonary arteries from the cat. J Appl Physiol 1985; 59:113–118.

47. Hakim TS, Michel RP, Chang HK. Effect of lung inflation on pulmonary vascular resistance by arterial and venous occlusion. J Appl Physiol 1982; 53:1110–1115.

48. Quebbeman EJ, Dawson CA. Influence of inflation and atelectasis on the hypoxic pressure response in isolated dog lung lobes. Cardiovasc Res 1976; 10:672–677.

49. Whittenberger JL, McGregor M, Berglund E, et al. Influence of state of inflation of the lung on pulmonary vascular resistance. J Appl Physiol 1960; 15:878–882.

50. Dawson CA, Grimm DJ, Linehan JH. Lung inflation and longitudinal distribution of pulmonary vascular resistance during hypoxia. J Appl Physiol 1979; 47:532–536.

51. Howell JBL, Permutt S, Proctor DF, et al. Effect of inflation of the lung on different parts of the pulmonary vascular bed. J Appl Physiol 1961; 16:71–76.

52. West JB, Dollery CT, Naimark A. Distribution of blood flow in isolated lung; relation to vascular and alveolar pressures. J Appl Physiol 1964; 19:713–724.

53. Marshall BE, Marshall C. Continuity of response to hypoxic pulmonary vasoconstriction. J Appl Physiol 1980; 49:189–196.

54. Fuhrman BP, Everitt J, Lock JE. Cardiopulmonary effects of unilateral airway pressure changes in intact infant lambs. J Appl Physiol 1984; 56:1439–1448.

55. Fuhrman BP, Smith-Wright DL, Kulik TJ, Lock JE. Effects of static and fluctuating airway pressure on the intact, immature pulmonary circulation. J Appl Physiol 1986; 60:114–122.

56. Thorvalson J, Ilebekk A, Kiil F. Determinants of pulmonary blood volume. Effects of acute changes in airway pressure. Acta Physiol Scand 1985; 125:471–479.

57. Hoffman EA, Ritman EL. Heart-lung interaction: effect on regional lung air content and total heart volume. Ann Biomed Eng 1987; 15:241–257.

58. Olson LE, Hoffman EA. Heart-lung interactions determined by electron beam x-ray CT in laterally recumbent rabbits. J Appl Physiol 1995; 78:417–427.

59. Grant BJB, Lieber BB. Compliance of the main pulmonary artery during the ventilatory cycle. J Appl Physiol 1992; 72:535–542.

60. Hakim TS, Michel RP, Minami H, Chang K. Site of pulmonary hypoxic vasocon-

striction studied with arterial and venous occlusion. J Appl Physiol 1983; 54:1298–1302.

61. Lopez-Muniz R, Stephens NL, Bromberger-Barnea B, Permutt S, Riley RL. Critical closure of pulmonary vessels analyzed in terms of Starling resistor model. J Appl Physiol 1968; 24:625–635.

62. Block AJ, Boyson PG, Wynne JW. The origins of cor pulmonale, a hypothesis. Chest 1979; 75:109–114.

63. Canada E, Benumnof JL, Tousdale FR. Pulmonary vascular resistance correlated in intact normal and abnormal canine lungs. Crit Care Med 1982; 10:719–723.

64. Taylor RR, Corell JW, Sonnenblick EH, Ross Jr, J. Dependence of ventricular distensibility on filling the opposite ventricle. Am J Physiol 1967; 213:711–718.

65. Brinker JA, Weiss I, Lappe DL, et al. Leftward septal displacement during right ventricular loading in man. Circulation 1980; 61:626–633.

66. Marini JJ, Culver BN, Butler J. Mechanical effect of lung distention with positive pressure on cardiac function. Am Rev Respir Dis 1980; 124:382–386.

67. Braunwald E, Binion JT, Morgan WL, Sarnoff SJ. Alterations in central blood volume and cardiac output induced by positive pressure breathing and counteracted by metraminol (Aramine). Circ Res 1957; 5:670–675.

68. Michard F, Chemla D, Richard C, Wysocki M, Pinsky MR, Lecarpentier Y, Teboul JL. Clinical use of respiratory changes in arterial pulse pressure to monitor the hemodynamic effects of PEEP. Am J Respir Crit Care Med 1999; 159(3):935–939.

69. Butler J. The heart is in good hands. Circulation 1983; 67:1163–1168.

70. Novak RA, Matuschak GM, Pinsky MR. Effect of ventilatory frequency on regional pleural pressure. J Appl Physiol 1988; 65:1314–1323.

71. Pinsky, MR, JG Guimond. The effects of positive end-expiratory pressure on heart-lung interactions. J Crit Care 1991; 6:1–11.

72. Tsitlik JE, Halperin HR, Guerci AD, Dvorine LS, Popel AS, Siu CO, Yin FCP, Weisfeldt ML. Augmentation of pressure in a vessel indenting the surface of the lung. Ann Biomed Eng 1987; 15:259–284.

73. Cassidy SS, Wead WB, Seibert GB, Ramanathan M. Changes in left ventricular geometry during spontaneous breathing. J Appl Physiol 1987; 63:803–811.

74. Cassidy SS, Robertson CH, Pierce AK, et al. Cardiovascular effects of positive end-expiratory pressure in dogs. J Appl Physiol 1978; 4:743–749.

75. Conway CM. Hemodynamic effects of pulmonary ventilation. Br J Anaesth 1975; 47:761–766.

76. Berglund JE, Halden E, Jakobson S, Landelius J. Echocardiographic analysis of cardiac function during high PEEP ventilation. Intensive Care Med 1994; 20:174–180.

77. Milic-Emili J, Mead J, Turner JM. Improved method for assessing the validity of the esophageal balloon technique. J Appl Physiol 1964; 19:207–211.

78. Kingma I, Smiseth OA, Frais MA, Smith ER, Tyberg JV. Left ventricular external constraint: relationship between pericardial, pleural and esophageal pressures during positive end-expiratory pressure and volume loading in dogs. Ann Biomed Eng 1987; 15:331–346.

79. Romand JA, Shi W, Pinsky MR. Cardiopulmonary effects of positive pressure ventilation during acute lung injury. Chest 1995; 108:1041–1048.

80. O'Quinn RJ, Marini JJ, Culver BH, et al. Transmission of airway pressure to pleural pressure during lung edema and chest wall restriction. J Appl Physiol 1985; 59: 1171–1177.

81. Gattinoni L, Mascheroni D, Torresin A, Fumagalli R, Vesconi S, Rossi GP, Rossi F, Baglioni S, Bassi F, Nastri G, Persenti A. Morphological response to positive end-expiratory pressure in acute respiratory failure. Intensive Care Med 1986; 12: 137–142.

82. Scharf SM, Ingram RH Jr. Effects of decreasing lung compliance with oleic acid on the cardiovascular response to PEEP. Am J Physiol 1977; 233:H635–H641.

83. Pinsky MR, Vincent JL, DeSmet JM. Estimating left ventricular filling pressure during positive end-expiratory pressure in humans. Am Rev Respir Dis 1991; 143: 25–31.

84. Buda AJ, Pinsky MR, Ingels NB, et al. Effect of intrathoracic pressure on left ventricular performance. N Engl J Med 1979; 301:453–459.

85. Marini JJ, Rodriguez RM, Lamb V. The inspiratory workload of patient-initiated mechanical ventilation. Am Rev Respir Dis 1986; 134:902–909.

86. Guyton AC, Lindsey AW, Abernathy B, et al. Venous return at various right atrial pressures and the normal venous return curve. Am J Physiol 1957; 189:609–615.

87. Goldberg HS, Rabson J. Control of cardiac output by systemic vessels: circulatory adjustments of acute and chronic respiratory failure and the effects of therapeutic interventions. Am J Cardiol 1981; 47:696.

88. Kilburn KH. Cardiorespiratory effects of large pneumothorax in conscious and anesthetized dogs. J Appl Physiol 1963; 18:279–283.

89. Chevalier PA, Weber KC, Engle JC, et al. Direct measurement of right and left heart outputs in Valsalva-like maneuver in dogs. Proc Soc Exp Biol Med 1972; 139:1429–1437.

90. Guntheroth WC, Gould R, Butler J, et al. Pulsatile flow in pulmonary artery, capillary and vein in the dog. Cardiovasc Res 1974; 8:330–337.

91. Guntheroth WG, Morgan BC, Mullins GL. Effect of respiration on venous return and stroke volume in cardiac tamponade. Mechanism of pulsus paradoxus. Circ Res 1967; 20:381–390.

92. Guyton AC. Effect of cardiac output by respiration, opening the chest, and cardiac tamponade. In: Guyton AC, Circulatory Physiology: Cardiac Output and Its Regulation. Philadelphia: Saunders, 1963:378–386.

93. Holt JP. The effect of positive and negative intrathoracic pressure on cardiac output and venous return in the dog. Am J Physiol 1944; 142:594–603.

94. Morgan BC, Abel FL, Mullins GL, et al. Flow patterns in cavae, pulmonary artery, pulmonary vein and aorta in intact dogs. Am J Physiol 1966; 210:903–909.

95. Morgan BC, Martin WE, Hornbein TF, et al. Hemodynamic effects of intermittent positive pressure respiration. Anesthesiology 1960; 27:584–590.

96. Scharf SM, Brown R, Saunders N, Green LH. Hemodynamic effects of positive pressure inflation. J Appl Physiol 1980; 49:124–131.

97. Wise RA, Robotham JL, Summer WR. Effects of spontaneous ventilation on the circulation. Lung 1981; 159:175–192.

98. Scharf SM, Brown R, Saunders N, et al. Effects of normal and loaded spontaneous inspiration on cardiovascular function. J Appl Physiol 1979; 47:582–590.

99. Fessler HE, Brower RG, Wise RA, Permutt S. Effects of positive end-expiratory pressure on the canine venous return curve. Am Rev Respir Dis 1992; 146: 4–10.

100. Takata M, Robotham JL. Effects of inspiratory diaphragmatic descent on inferior vena caval venous return. J Appl Physiol 1992; 72:597–607.

101. Chihara E, Hasimoto S, Kinoshita T, Hirpose M, Tanaka Y, Morimoto T. Elevated mean systemic filling pressure due to intermittent positive-pressure ventilation. Am J Physiol 1992; 262:H1116–H1121.

102. Takata M, Wise RA, Robotham JL. Effects of abdominal pressure on venous return: abdominal vascular zone conditions. J Appl Physiol 1990; 69:1961–1972.

103. Barnes GE, Laine GA, Giam PY, Smith EE, Granger HJ. Cardiovascular responses to elevation of intra-abdominal hydrostatic pressure. Am J Physiol 1985; 248: R208–R213.

104. Lichtwarck-Aschoff M, Zeravik J, Pfeiffer UJ. Intrathoracic blood volume accurately reflects circulatory volume status in critically ill patients with mechanical ventilation. Intensive Care Med 1992; 18:142–145.

105. Magder S, Georgiadis G, Cheong T. Respiratory variations in right atrial pressure predict the response to fluid challenge. J Crit Care 1992; 7:76–85.

106. Terada N, Takeuchi T. Postural changes in venous pressure gradients in anesthetized monkeys. Am J Physiol 1993; 264:H21–H25.

107. Scharf S, Tow DE, Miller MJ, Brown R, McIntyre K, Dilts C. Influence of posture and abdominal pressure on the hemodynamic effects of Mueller's maneuver. J Crit Care 1989; 4:26–34.

108. Tarasiuk A, Scharf SM. Effects of periodic obstructive apneas on venous return in closed-chest dogs. Am Rev Respir Dis 1993; 148:323–329.

109. Mang H, Kacmarek RM, Ritz R, Wilson RS, Kimball WP. Cardiorespiratory effects of volume- and pressure-controlled ventilation at various I/E ratios in an acute lung injury model. Am J Respir Crit Care Med 1995; 151:731–736.

110. Tyberg JV, Taichman GC, Smith ER, Douglas NWS, Smiseth OA, Keon WJ. The relationship between pericardial pressure and right atrial pressure: an intraoperative study. Circulation 1986; 73:428–432.

111. Pinsky MR, Vincent JL, DeSmet JM. Effect of positive end-expiratory pressure on right ventricular function in man. Am Rev Respir Dis 1992; 146:681–687.

112. Jayaweera AR, Ehrlich W. Changes of phasic pleural pressure in awake dogs during exercise: potential effects on cardiac output. Ann Biomed Eng 1987; 15:311–318.

113. Sibbald WH, Calvin J, Driedger AA. Right and left ventricular preload, and diastolic ventricular compliance: implications of therapy in critically ill patients. Critical Care State of the Art. Fullerton, CA: Society of Critical Care, 1982.

114. Lores ME, Keagy BA, Vassiliades T, Henry GW, Lucas CL, Wilcox BR. Cardiovascular effects of positive end-expiratory pressure (PEEP) after pneumonectomy in dogs. Ann Thorac Surg 1985; 40:464–473.

115. Harken AH, Brennan MF, Smith N, Barsamian EM. The hemodynamic response to positive end-expiratory ventilation in hypovolemic patients. Surgery 1974; 76: 786–793.

116. Sharpey-Schaffer EP. Effects of Valsalva maneuver on the normal and failing circulation. Br Med J 1955; 1:693–699.

117. Peters J, Kindred MK, Robotham JL. Transient analysis of cardiopulmonary interactions II. Systolic events. J Appl Physiol 1988; 64:1518–1526.
118. Pinsky MR, Matuschak GM, Klain M. Determinants of cardiac augmentation by increases in intrathoracic pressure. J Appl Physiol 1985; 58:1189–1198.
119. Rankin JS, Olsen CO, Arentzen CE, et al. The effects of airway pressure on cardiac function in intact dogs and man. Circulation 1982; 66:108–120.
120. Robotham JL, Rabson J, Permutt S, Bromberger-Barnea B. Left ventricular hemodynamics during respiration. J Appl Physiol 1979; 47:1295–1303.
121. Ruskin J, Bache RJ, Rembert JC, Greenfield JR. Pressure-flow studies in man: effect of respiration on left ventricular stroke volume. Circulation 1973; 48:79–85.
122. Olsen CO, Tyson GS, Maier GW, et al. Dynamic ventricular interaction in the conscious dog. Circ Res 1983; 52:85–104.
123. Bell RC, Robotham JL, Badke FR, Little WC, Kindred MK. Left ventricular geometry during intermittent positive pressure ventilation in dogs. J Crit Care 1987; 2: 230–244.
124. Qvist J, Pontoppidan H, Wilson RS, Lowenstein E, Laver MB. Hemodynamic responses to mechanical ventilation with PEEP: the effects of hypovolemia. Anesthesiology 1975; 42:45–53.
125. Denault AY, Gorcsan III J, Deneault LG, Pinsky MR. Effect of positive pressure ventilation on left ventricular pressure-volume relationship. Anesthesiology 1993; 79:A315.
126. Janicki JS, Weber KT. The pericardium and ventricular interaction, distensibility and function. Am J Physiol 1980; 238:H494–H503.
127. Blaustein AS, Risser TA, Weiss JW, Parker JA, Holman L, McFadden ER. Mechanisms of pulsus paradoxus during resistive respiratory loading and asthma. J Am Coll Cardiol 1986; 8:529–536.
128. Beyar R, Goldstein Y. Model studies of the effects of the thoracic pressure on the circulation. Ann Biomed Eng 1987; 15:373–383.
129. Pinsky MR, Summer WR, Wise RA, Permutt S, Bromberger-Barnea B. Augmentation of cardiac function by elevation of intrathoracic pressure. J Appl Physiol 1983; 54:950–955.
130. Cassidy SA, Wead WB, Seibert GB, Ramanathan M. Geometric left-ventricular responses to interactions between the lung and left ventricle: positive pressure breathing. Ann Biomed Eng 1987; 15:285–295.
131. Scharf SM, Brown R, Warner KG, Khuri S. Intrathoracic pressure and left ventricular configuration with respiratory maneuvers. J Appl Physiol 1989; 66:481–491.
132. Pinsky MR, Summer WR. Cardiac augmentation by phasic high intrathoracic support (PHIPS) in man. Chest 1983; 84:370–375.
133. Pinsky MR, Matuschak GM, Itzkoff JM. Respiratory augmentation of left ventricular function during spontaneous ventilation in severe left ventricular failure by grunting: an auto-EPAP effect. Chest 1984; 86:267–269.
134. Strohl KP, Scharf SM, Brown R, Ingram RH Jr. Cardiovascular performance during bronchospasm in dogs. Respiration 1987; 51:39–48.
135. Scharf SM, Graver LM, Balaban K. Cardiovascular effects of periodic occlusions of the upper airways in dogs. Am Rev Respir Dis 1992; 146:321–329.

136. Viola AR, Puy RJM, Goldman E. Mechanisms of pulsus paradoxus in airway obstruction. J Appl Physiol 1990; 68:1927–1931.

137. Scharf SM, Graver LM, Khilnani S, Balaban K. Respiratory phasic effects of inspiratory loading on left ventricular hemodynamics in vagotomized dogs. J Appl Physiol 1992; 73:995–1003.

138. Latham RD, Sipkema P, Westerhof N, Rubal BJ. Aortic input impedance during Mueller maneuver: an evaluation of "effective strength." J Appl Physiol 1988; 65:1604–1610.

139. Virolainen J, Ventila M, Turto H, Kupari M. Effect of negative intrathoracic pressure on left ventricular pressure dynamics and relaxation. J Appl Physiol 1995; 79: 455–460.

140. Garpestad E, Parker JA, Katayama H, et al. Decrease in ventricular stroke volume at apnea termination is independent of oxygen desaturation. J Appl Physiol 1994; 77:1602–1608.

141. Gomez A, Mink S. Interaction between effects of hypoxia and hypercapnia on altering left ventricular relaxation and chamber stiffness in dogs. Am Rev Respir Dis 1992; 146:313–320.

142. Abel FL, Mihailescu LS, Lader AS, Starr RG. Effects of pericardial pressure on systemic and coronary hemodynamics in dogs. Am J Physiol 1995; 268:H1593–H1605.

143. Khilnani S, Graver LM, Balaban K, Scharf SM. Effects of inspiratory loading on left ventricular myocardial blood flow and metabolism. J Appl Physiol 1992; 72: 1488–1492.

144. Satoh S, Watanabe J, Keitoku M, Itoh N, Maruyama Y, Takishima T. Influences of pressure surrounding the heart and intracardiac pressure on the diastolic coronary pressure-flow relation in excised canine heart. Circ Res 1988; 63:788–797.

145. Beach T, Millen E, Grenvik A. Hemodynamic response to discontinuance of mechanical ventilation. Crit Care Med 1973; 1:85–90.

146. Grace MP, Greenbaum DM. Cardiac performance in response to PEEP in patients with cardiac dysfunction. Crit Care Med 1982; 20:358–360.

147. Rasanen J, Nikki P, Heikkila J. Acute myocardial infarction complicated by respiratory failure. The effects of mechanical ventilation. Chest 1984; 85:21–28.

148. Rasanen J, Vaisanen IT, Heikkila J, et al. Acute myocardial infarction complicated by left ventricular dysfunction and respiratory failure. The effects of continuous positive airway pressure. Chest 1985; 87:156–162.

149. Rasanen J. Respiratory failure in acute myocardial infarction. Appl Cardiopulm Pathophysiol 1988; 2:271–279.

150. DeHoyos A, Liu PP, Benard DC, Bradley TD. Haemodynamic effects of continuous positive airway pressure in humans with normal and impaired left ventricular function. Clin Sci Colch 1995; 88:173–178.

151. Naughton MT, Rahman MA, Hara K, Flora JS, Bradley TD. Effect of continuous positive airway pressure on intrathoracic and left ventricular transmural pressures in patients with congestive heart failure. Circulation 1995; 91:1725–1731.

152. Lin M, Yang Y-F, Chiang H-T, Chang M-S, Chiang BN, Cheitlin MD. Reappraisal of continuous positive airway pressure therapy in acute cardiogenic pulmonary edema. Chest 1995; 107:1379–1386.

153. Pinsky MR, Matuschak GM, Bernardi L, Klain M. Hemodynamic effects of cardiac cycle-specific increases in intrathoracic pressure. J Appl Physiol 1986; 60:604–612.

154. Drics DJ, Kumar P, Mathru M, Mayer R, Zecca A, Rao TL, Freeark RJ. Hemodynamic effects of pressure support ventilation in cardiac surgery patients. Am Surg 1991; 57:122–125.

155. Sternberg R, Sahebjami H. Hemodynamic and oxygen transport characteristics of common ventilatory modes. Chest 1994; 105:1798–1803.

156. Bayly R, Sladen A, Guntapalli K, Klain M. Synchronous versus nonsynchronous high frequency jet ventilation: effects on cardiorespiratory variables and airway pressures in postoperative patients. Crit Care Med 1987; 15:915–923.

157. Ranieri VM, Giuliani R, Cinnella G, et al. Physiologic effects of positive end-expiratory pressure in patients with chronic obstructive lung disease during acute ventilatory failure and controlled mechanical ventilation. Am Rev Respir Dis 1993; 147:5–13.

158. Baigorri F, De Monte A, Blanch L, et al. Hemodynamic response to external counterbalancing of auto-positive end-expiratory pressure in mechanically ventilated patients with chronic obstructive lung disease. Crit Care Med 1994; 22:1782–1791.

159. Pinsky MR. Through the past darkly: Ventilatory management of patients with chronic obstructive pulmonary disease. Crit Care Med 1994; 22:1714–1717.

160. Ambrosino N, Nava S, Torbicki A, Riccardi G, Fracchia C, Opasich C, Rampulla C. Hemodynamic effects of pressure support and PEEP ventilation by nasal route in patients with stable chronic obstructive pulmonary disease. Thorax 1993; 48:523–528.

161. Ambrosino N, Cobelli F, Torbicki A, Opasich C, Pozzoli M, Fracchia C, Rampulla C. Hemodynamic effects of negative-pressure ventilation in patients with COPD. Chest 1990; 97:850–856.

162. Brochard L, Isabey D, Piquet J, et al. Reversal of acute exacerbations of chronic obstructive lung disease by inspiratory assistance with a face mask. N Engl J Med 1990; 323:1523–1530.

163. Dhainaut JF, Devaux JY, Monsallier JF, Brunet F, Villemant D, Huyghebaert MF. Mechanisms of decreased left ventricular preload during continuous positive pressure ventilation in ARDS. Chest 1986; 90:74–80.

164. Singer M, Vermaat J, Hall G, Latter G, Patel M. Hemodynamic effects of manual hyperinflation in critically ill mechanically ventilated patients. Chest 1994; 106:1182–1187.

165. Hartmann M, Rosberg B, Jonsson K. The influence of different levels of PEEP on peripheral tissue perfusion measured by subcutaneous and transcutaneous oxygen tension. Intensive Care Med 1992; 18:474–478.

166. Huemer G, Kolev N, Kurz A, Zimpfer M. Influence of positive end-expiratory pressure on right and left ventricular performance assessed by Doppler two-dimensional echocardiography. Chest 1994; 106:67–73.

167. Jardin F. PEEP and ventricular function. Intensive Care Med 1994; 20:169–170.

168. Goertz A, Heinrich H, Winter H, Deller A. Hemodynamic effects of different ventilatory patterns. A prospective clinical trial. Chest 1991; 99:1166–1171.

169. Gunter JP, deBoisblanc BP, Rust BS, Johnson WD, Summer WR. Effect of syn-

chronized, systolic, lower body, positive pressure on hemodynamics in human septic shock: a pilot study. Am J Respir Crit Care Med 1995; 151:719–723.

170. Lessard MR, Guerot E, Lorini H, Lemaire F, Brochard L. Effects of pressure-controlled with different I : E ratios versus volume-controlled ventilation on respiratory mechanics, gas exchange and hemodynamics in patients with adult respiratory distress syndrome. Anesthesiology 1994; 80:983–991.

171. Chan K, Abraham E. Effects of inverse ratio ventilation on cardiorespiratory parameters in severe respiratory failure. Chest 1992; 102:1556–1561.

172. Abraham E, Yoshihara G. Cardiorespiratory effects of pressure controlled ventilation in severe respiratory failure. Chest 1990; 98:1445–1449.

173. Poelaert JI, Visser CA, Everaert JA, Koolen JJ, Colardyn FA. Acute hemodynamic changes of pressure-controlled inverse ratio ventilation in the adult respiratory distress syndrome. A transesophageal echocardiographic and Doppler study. Chest 1993; 104:214–219.

174. Abel JG, Salerno TA, Panos A, et al. Cardiovascular effects of positive pressure ventilation in humans. Ann Thorac Surg 1987; 43:36–43.

175. Buckle P, Millar T, Kryger M. The effect of short-term nasal CPAP on Cheyne-Stokes respiration in congestive heart failure. Chest 1992; 102:31–35.

176. Granton JT, Naughton MT, Benard DC, Liu PP, Goldstein RS, Bradley TD. CPAP improves inspiratory muscle strength in patients with heart failure and central sleep apnea. Am J Respir Crit Care Med 1996; 153:277–282.

177. Naughton MT, Benard DC, Liu PP, Rutherford R, Rankin F, Bradley TD. Effects of nasal CPAP on sympathetic activity in patients with heart failure and central sleep apnea. Am J Respir Crit Care Med 1995; 152:473–479.

178. Baeaussier M, Coriat P, Perel A, Lebret F, Kalfon P, Chemla D, Lienhart A, Viars P. Determinants of systolic pressure variation in patients ventilated after vascular surgery. J Cardiothorac Vasc Anesth 1995; 9:547–551.

179. Coriat P, Vrillon M, Perel A, Baron JF, LeBret F, Saada M, Viars P. A comparison of systolic blood pressure variations and echocardiographic estimates of end-diastolic left ventricular size in patients after aortic surgery. Anesth Analg 1994; 78:46–53.

180. Szold A, Pizov R, Segal E, Perel A. The effect of tidal volume and intravascular volume state on systolic pressure variation in ventilated dogs. Intensive Care Med 1989; 15:368–371.

181. Denault A, Gasior TA, Gorcsan J, Mandarino WA, Deneault LG, Pinsky MR. Determinants of aortic pressure variation during positive-pressure ventilation in man. Chest 1999; 116:176–186.

21

Extubation Failure

Predictions and Consequences

SCOTT K. EPSTEIN

Tufts University School of Medicine
New England Medical Center
Boston, Massachusetts

I. Introduction

The process of liberating patients from mechanical ventilation has been under active investigation for more than a quarter of a century (1). Liberation has two components: the first, traditionally termed weaning, consists of two elements, readiness testing and progressive withdrawal (2). The former element refers to the initial brief period of minimal support (e.g., a spontaneous breathing trial), typically carried out with a T-tube (T-piece) circuit, continuous positive airway pressure (CPAP) circuit, or low levels of pressure support ventilation (PSV). The latter element refers to a slower process, in which the work of breathing is more gradually transferred from machine to patient, until the level of support is minimal. Extensive investigation has focused on determining when readiness testing can be commenced (3,4) and on which modes of ventilator support best advance the process of progressive withdrawal (5–8).

In either case, the culmination of these efforts is the removal of a translaryngeal endotracheal tube, or extubation. In the past, this second component of liberation received little emphasis, being perceived as a simple and automatic step at the end of the weaning process. Yet, for weaning and liberation to be successful, the patient must be successfully extubated. Perhaps this common definition of success led many investigators to also lump together weaning and extubation failure. The latter is defined by the need for reinstitution of ventilatory support, typically reinsertion of an endotracheal tube (reintubation). In the unique case of patients with a tracheostomy tube in place, the removal of the tube has been termed decannulation. Extubation also differs from weaning in that it can be planned or unplanned. More recently, the distinction between weaning and extubation failure has become evident as investigators have identified the particular pathophysiological causes and unique outcomes for each.

II. Prevalence of Extubation Failure

A. Overview

There is no consensus on what constitutes an acceptable extubation failure rate. Higher failure rates may reflect inadequate assessment prior to or during weaning trials, i.e., premature extubation. Conversely, a very low extubation failure rate may be a consequence of overly stringent extubation criteria and result in a needlessly prolonged duration of mechanical ventilation. The prevalence of extubation failure may be represented as failures per total number of patients ventilated, failures per total number of patients undergoing weaning trials, or failures per total number of patients extubated. For example, Vallverdu et al. noted a 48-hour reintubation rate of 10.6% when all patients were included and 15.5% when the analysis was restricted to extubated patients (9). The time frame for extubation failure has also been defined variably as the need for reintubation within 24, 48, or 72 hours of extubation. Table 1 shows that the prevalence of extubation failure ranges from 2 to 20%. The wide range is likely explained by the time frame studied, differences in patient severity of illness, and the variable criteria employed for deciding when to reintubate. Planned extubation is typically the result of several decisions (10). First, screening criteria must be satisfied prior to subjecting the patient to a weaning trial. These criteria have not been uniform but often contain some combination of the following: temperature $\leq 38°C$; hemoglobin ≥ 8 g/dL; respiratory rate ≤ 35 breaths/min; tidal volume $\geq 4-5$ mL/kg; negative inspiratory force (NIF) more negative than -20 to -30 cm H_2O; hemodynamic stability (not on vasopressors agents other than dopamine or dobutamine < 5 μg/kg/min); no sedation or sedative infusions; adequate cough; minimal respiratory secretions; $Pao_2 = 60$ mmHg or $Sao_2 = 90\%$ on 40–50% Fio_2 or $Pao_2/Fio_2 = 150-200$ and an adequate neurological status (e.g., Glasgow Coma Scale > 11). Studies of weaning typically employ stringent criteria for determining the tolerance for a weaning trial. For example, intolerance is characterized by the development of hypoxemia, hypercapnia, hemodynamic instability, signs of increased work of breathing, agitation, or diaphoresis during a weaning trial lasting 30–120 minutes (5–7,9,11). In contrast, few studies have employed such rigorous criteria for determining tolerance for extubation. Rather the decision to reintubate is typically left to interns, residents, fellows, or attending physicians. Clearly, the lack of objective reintubation criteria is a major limitation of nearly all studies of extubation failure. Other factors may also impact on the prevalence of extubation failure (Table 2).

B. Patient Populations

The prevalence of extubation failure varies with the patient population studied. In general, failure rates are lowest for postoperative cardiac surgical patients. For example, Reyes et al. found a reintubation rate of just 3.3% in patients after cardiac surgery (12). The rate was higher for patients randomized to an early extubation strategy (extubation at 6 hours after admission to the ICU, 5.8%) compared to a conventional strategy (extubation at 8 a.m. the day following surgery, 1.3%). In contrast, London and coworkers found comparable failure rates among 304 "fast track" and 255 convention extubations in cardiac surgery patients (5.0% vs. 6.3%) (13). In a large retrospective study, Rady and Ryan found an extubation failure rate of 6.6% in over 11,000 cardiac surgical patients (14). Similar rates of extubation failure have been observed in studies of general surgical and specialized surgical populations (15,16). The prevalence of extubation failure in trauma units has generally been below 5%, using all intubated patient as the denominator (17,18). In contrast to these surgical/trauma series, with few exceptions, the prevalence of extubation failure among medical intensive care unit patients or mixed MICU/SICU patients has been substantially higher, up to 20% (Table 1).

C. Age

A number of investigators have noted that extubation failure patients tend to be older than those successfully liberated from mechanical ventilation (7,10,14, 19,20). Capdevila et al. noted that reintubated patients averaged two decades older than those successfully extubated (69 vs. 48 years, $p < 0.001$) (19). Esteban et al. and Del Rosario and colleagues found much smaller but still significant differences between successfully extubated and reintubated patients (7,20). In univariate analysis, Epstein and coworkers noted that extubation failure patients were approximately a decade older (64.2 vs. 55.1 years, $p < 0.01$) (10). In multivariate analysis, older age was an independent predictor for discharge to a long-term care or rehabilitation unit but not for hospital mortality or prolonged ICU stay. Using multivariate analysis, Rady and Ryan noted that age ≥ 65 years was an independent risk factor for extubation failure after cardiac surgery (14).

Table 1 Incidence of Extubation Failure

Study (Ref.)	Type of ICU	Number of patients studied	Preextubation mode of ventilation	Time to EF	%EF	Mortality for EF (mortality for ES)
Zwillich (97)	Mixed	354	NR	24	5.9	NR
Schachter (158)	Mixed	251	IMV	NR	10.8	NR
Tahvanainen (77)	Medical	47[a]	T-piece CPAP	48	19.0	22.2[b] (5.3)
DeHaven (27)	Surgical trauma	48[a]	CPAP	NR	6.3	NR
Demling (17)	Surgical	400	T-piece CPAP	168	5.5	40.0
	Burn/trauma	300	T-piece CPAP	168	3.3	10.0
Krieger (111)	Medical/surgical	269[a]	T piece	48	10.4	NR
Jones (36)	Medical/surgical	106[a]	T piece CPAP	NR	4.7	NR
Sassoon (139)	Medical	40[a]	CPAP	48	12.5	NR
Stauffer (159)	Medical/surgical	255[a]	NR	NR	17.3	NR
Mohsenifar (160)	Respiratory	21[a]	PSV	24	14.3	NR
Lee (28)	Medical	52[a]	CPAP PSV	24	17.0	33.3
Brochard (5)	Medical/surgical (first weaning trial)	122[a]	T-piece	48	17.2	NR
	(>1 weaning trial)	109	T-piece PSV IMV	48	11.0	NR
Esteban (6)	Medical/surgical (first weaning trial)	372[a]	T piece	48	15.6	NR
	(>1 weaning trial)	115	T piece PSV IMV	48	20	NR

Capdevila (19)	Multidisciplinary	67[a]	T piece	48	18	NR
Epstein (22)	Medical	218[a]	PSV + IMV	72	15.6	NR
Khan (112)	Pediatric	208[a]	NR	48	16.3	NR
Miller (57)	Medical	100[a]	CPAP	NR	17.0	NR
DeHaven (51)	Trauma	589[a]	CPAP	72	7.8	NR
Leitch (161)	Multidisciplinary	163[a]	PSV	24	1.8	NR
Daley (18)	Trauma	405	NR	72	4.7	8.3
Ely (3)	MICU/CCU	300	T piece CPAP	48	5.7	NR
Epstein (10)	Medical	289[a]	PSV+IMV	72	14.5	42.5 (11.7)
Esteban (7)	Medical/surgical	397[a]	T piece PSV	48	18.6	27.0[b] (2.6)
Jacob (15)	Surgical (general and cardiac)	176[a]	NR	24	4.5	NE
Reyes (12)	Cardiothoracic	272	T-piece	168	3.3	NR
Kollef (4)	Medical/surgical	357	T piece PSV IMV	NR	11.5	NR
Vallverdu (9)	Medical/surgical	148[a]	T piece	48	15.5	34.8[b]
Esteban (11)	Medical/surgical	453	T piece	48	13.5	41.0 (12.5)
Esteban (103)	Multidisciplinary	1,692[a]	T-piece PSV IMV + PSV	48	15.0	37.0 (15.0)
Rady (14)	Cardiothoracic	11,330[a]	CPAP + PSV	168	6.6	21.0 (2.0)
Ely (39)	Multidisciplinary	1,067	T-piece CPAP	48	14.0	NR

EF, Extubation failure; ES, extubation success; NR, not reported.

[a] Number of extubated patients (all others also include mechanically ventilated patients not extubated).

[b] ICU mortality (all others are hospital mortality).

Table 2 Factors That May Influence Extubation
Failure Rate

Patient population (medical, general surgical, cardiac surgical, postoperative, trauma)
Age
Gender
Severity of illness
Indication for mechanical ventilation
Duration of mechanical ventilation
Individual weaning trial duration prior to extubation
Number of weaning trials prior to extubation
Preextubation mode of ventilatory support
Use of protocol-directed weaning approach
Use of sedation
Temporal definition of extubation failure (e.g., 24 vs. 48 vs. 72 hours)

D. Gender

Independent of hormonal status, physiological differences have been noted in spontaneously breathing and mechanically ventilated women and men (21–23), but whether gender impacts on outcome for mechanically ventilated patients remains controversial. The best evidence suggests that, in surgical but *not* medical intensive care units, the mortality for mechanically ventilated women may be higher than that seen for men (24,25). In a study of 580 mechanically ventilated MICU patients, women tended toward a lower likelihood of extubation failure, but this was not statistically significant (women 13.4% vs. men 18.3%, $p = 0.19$) (24). Kollef and co-investigators noted reintubation rates of 10.6% in women and 12.5% in men, though the breakdown of planned versus unplanned extubations was not specified (25).

E. Severity of Illness

The impact of severity of illness on extubation failure has been recently investigated. Separate studies by Capdevila and Esteban found no difference in SAPS and SAPS II, respectively, comparing reintubated to successfully extubated patients (7,19). A study of MICU patients found no difference in APACHE II score at the onset of mechanical ventilation but noted a slightly higher score at weaning onset in patients destined to fail extubation (12 vs. 10, $p < 0.05$) (10). Taken together these studies indicate no definite association between severity of illness and extubation failure. In contrast, patients with extubation failure after cardiac surgery were more likely to have single or multiple organ failure (14).

F. Indication for Mechanical Ventilation

A lengthy list of processes can precipitate respiratory failure and the need for mechanical ventilation. Given the differences in pathophysiology, the cause for respiratory failure may also affect the likelihood of extubation failure. For example, the presence of underlying lung disease influences the likelihood of extubation failure. In a study looking at first trial extubation failure, reintubation occurred in 35.7% (15/42) of neurological and 8.6% (8/93) of acute respiratory failure patients, while no (0/13) patient with COPD failed (9). In contrast, Esteban and coworkers found no difference in the prevalence of extubation failure for patients with coma (22%), COPD (24%), and acute lung injury (17%) (7). In the study of Del Rosario et al., 5 of 12 patients with CHF experienced extubation failure compared to just 2 of 22 with COPD (20). Similarly, a study of MICU patients found that patients with a cardiac etiology of respiratory failure were more likely to experience extubation failure (10). In a study of mechanically ventilated COPD patients, 18.5% manifested extubation failure and were reintubated within 72 hours of extubation (26).

G. Duration of Mechanical Ventilation Prior to Extubation

The impact of duration of mechanical ventilation on outcome remains controversial. In general, the prevalence of extubation failure has been lower in studies with a shorter mean duration of mechanical ventilation (e.g., less than 72 hours) (15,27). In contrast, similar extubation failure rates have been reported in studies with preextubation duration of ventilation ranging from 5 to 14 days (5,28). Several studies with mean duration of mechanical ventilation of less than one week found no difference in duration of mechanical ventilation prior to extubation when directly comparing patients requiring reintubation to those successfully extubated (7,10). In contrast, Rady and Ryan noted a longer preextubation duration of ventilation among cardiac surgery patients requiring reintubation (14). Del Rosario and colleagues observed that extubation failure patients tended to be ventilated longer prior to extubation (14 vs. 7 days) (20). Studies examining translaryngeal extubation failure after markedly prolonged mechanical ventilation (e.g., greater than 21 days) are generally not available because such patients uniformly have a tracheostomy tube in place (29).

H. Time After Extubation

The prevalence of extubation failure depends upon the time frame studied. Investigators have characterized reintubation occurring with 24, 48, or 72 hours as consistent with extubation failure. In general, the majority of patients with extubation failure fail within the first 24 hours of extubation. For example, in one study of MICU patients, the reintubation rate was 8% at 24, 11% at 48, and 14%

at 72 hours (10). Using a 48-hour threshold, Esteban et al. noted that 59% of patients with extubation failure were reintubated within 12 hours and 75% within 24 hours (30). Although occasional patients may fail extubation after 72 hours, most reintubations after that point occur after transfer out of the ICU when the patient has demonstrated substantial recovery. These "late" reintubations, which appear to result from distinctly new events or processes, have been associated with a very high mortality rate (53%) (10).

I. Individual Weaning Trial Duration

The optimal duration of individual weaning trials remains controversial. Too brief a trial may result in premature extubation and increase the likelihood of extubation failure. Too prolonged a trial may lead to "iatrogenic" weaning failure, especially when the imposed work of breathing through the endotracheal tube and ventilatory circuit is elevated (31). Nevertheless, tolerance for a prolonged weaning trial may identify patients with a low likelihood of extubation failure (32). The majority of investigators have employed a 1- to 2-hour spontaneous (T-piece) breathing trial (3,5–7,9,19,33). In a physiological study, Vassilakopoulos and colleagues noted no cases of extubation failure among 30 patients who were able to tolerate a 6-hour spontaneous breathing trial (32). Pressure support ventilation and intermittent mandatory ventilation (IMV) weaning trials have varied from 2 (6,7) to 24 hours (5) in duration. Unfortunately, these studies do not provide head-to-head comparisons of different duration for weaning trial duration. Recently, 526 medical and surgical ICU patients were randomized to either a 30-minute or a 120-minute T-piece breathing trial (11). Among the approximately 80% of patients successfully completing the weaning trial and extubated, the reintubation rates were similar (30 minute, 13.5% vs. 120 minute, 13.4%). In contrast, a trend toward a higher reintubation rate after 48 hours was observed among patients in the 120 minute group (1.3% vs. 7.3%, $p = 0.13$). It is important to note that this study looked only at the patient's first weaning trial and not subsequent attempts. Further investigation is necessary to define the impact of weaning trial duration on extubation failure, especially for modes other than T-piece.

J. Preextubation Mode of Ventilation

Although controversial, some recent studies indicate that work of breathing may increase after extubation compared to spontaneous breathing through the endotracheal tube (34,35). If true, then preextubation modes of ventilation providing partial support, such as CPAP, IMV, or PSV, may result in higher extubation failure rates compared to T-piece trials. In general, the reported prevalence of extubation failure appears similar for T-piece, PSV, IMV, combined PSV and IMV, and CPAP (Table 1). Several studies provide direct head-to-head comparison of reintubation rates for different preextubation modes. Jones et al. compared a one-hour trial of CPAP of 5 cm H_2O to T-piece in 106 patients and found no difference in reintubation rate (36). Esteban and colleagues compared a single initial 2-hour T-piece trial with a 2-hour trial of PSV 7 cm H_2O in 484 medical and surgical ICU patients (7). Although weaning trial failure was more likely in the T-piece group, the 48-hour reintubation rate was similar among extubated patients (18.5 vs. 18.8%). Two randomized trials have compared different preextubation modes of ventilation among patients failing an initial T-piece trial. Brochard et al. observed extubation failure in 3/35 (8.6%) with T-piece, 6/43 (13.9%) with IMV, and 3/31 (9.7%) with PSV (5) Esteban and coinvestigators, noted that reintubation occurred in 5/32 (15.6%) with intermittent T-piece trials, 7/29 (24.1%) with once daily T-piece trials, 4/24 (16.7%) with IMV, and 7/30 (23.3%) with PSV (6). Although the total number of patients studied was limited, these studies do not indicate an effect of preextubation mode of ventilation on extubation outcome.

K. Number of Weaning Trials Prior to Extubation

The prevalence of extubation failure is often reported without stratifying for number of weaning trials before weaning success is achieved and extubation attempted. Thus, the rate of extubation failure after initial or multiple subsequent weaning trials varies substantially between studies, and no clear conclusion can be drawn. The studies of Esteban and Brochard have reported first trial reintubation rates of 15–19% (5–7,11). In contrast, Brochard and colleagues found a reintubation rate of 11% among patients who failed an initial 2-hour T-piece trial but passed a weaning trial one or more days later (5). Esteban et al. noted an extubation failure rate of 20% among the 115 patients who required more than one weaning trial (6). In a subsequent study the same investigators noted extubation failure in 6/64 (9.4%) patients requiring more than one weaning trial before success was achieved (7).

L. Protocol-Directed Weaning

Nearly all the studies listed in Table 1 required that patients pass a screen of weaning parameters (see above) before allowing them to embark on a weaning trial. Use of a more formalized, protocol-directed weaning approach leads to reduced duration of mechanical ventilation and reduced duration of weaning (3,4,37,38). Furthermore, at least one study suggested that a protocol-directed approach may reduce the need for reintubation. Ely and coworkers noted a trend toward a reduction in 48-hour extubation failure rate (3% vs. 8%, $p = 0.08$) among patients who underwent daily screening and spontaneous breathing trials (3). In contrast, in a subsequent study examining large-scale implementation of a therapist-directed protocol, the same authors noted a substantially higher

48-hour extubation failure rate of 14.0% (39). Saura and colleagues, comparing a weaning protocol to retrospective controls, found no difference in reintubation rate (17% vs. 14% in the control group) (37). Similarly, Kollef et al. found no difference in reintubation rate when weaning was protocol-directed compared to when it was physician-directed (12.8% vs. 10.1%) (4). Taken together these studies suggest that although protocol-directed weaning has important benefits in duration of ventilation and length of stay, the incidence of extubation failure is not diminished.

M. Sedation

Bolus dose or continuous intravenous sedation is commonly administered to patients on mechanical ventilation. These medications may predispose to extubation failure by adversely affecting ventilatory drive and the mechanisms of airway protection. Kollef et al. in a prospective observational study noted that patients who had received continuous intravenous sedation, principally lorazepam and/or fentanyl, had a greater incidence of reintubation compared to those on bolus or no sedation (15.1% vs. 4.7%, $p = 0.005$) (40). Similarly, the frequency of extubation failure is higher for post–cardiac surgery patients undergoing "fast track" weaning and extubation (12). Such patients are less likely to have recovered from the sedative effects of anesthesia, which could contribute to the higher reintubation rate.

III. Pathophysiology of Extubation Failure

A. Overview

Recent investigations have helped identify the pathophysiologic basis for weaning failure (32,41,42). The most common mechanism is likely an imbalance between respiratory load and the capacity of the respiratory muscle pump. Less commonly abnormal gas exchange is responsible for failure. There is also increasing appreciation that cardiac disease and psychological factors can contribute to ventilator dependence (43–46). Although these factors can also contribute to extubation failure, their prevalence is likely to differ from that observed with weaning failure. Extubation failure is also characterized by a unique set of circumstances that can manifest when the translaryngeal endotracheal tube is removed, such as upper airway obstruction, aspiration, and an inability to manage pulmonary secretions. A number of recent studies have examined the causes of extubation failure (Table 3).

B. Upper Airway Obstruction

Controversy exists about how work of breathing after extubation compares to that present prior to removal of the endotracheal tube (47). A number of studies

Table 3 Studies Reporting the Causes of Extubation Failure

Study (n = total number of patients with extubation failure)	Causes for extubation failure, number of patients (% of all patients with extubation failure)	Ref.
Tahvanainen (n = 9)	Acute pulmonary edema, 3 (33) CO2 retention, 3 (33) Hypoxia, 4 (44) Inability to clear airways, 1 (11) Unconsciousness, 1 (11)	77
Demling (n = 10)	Airway protection, 2 (20) Pulmonary toilet, 3 (30) Airway and pulmonary toilet, 3 (30) Positive pressure ventilation, 2 (20)	17
Demling (n = 22)	Cardiovascular compromise, 4 (18) Pulmonary edema, 7 (32) Hypoventilation, 7 (32) Pulmonary toilet, 5 (23) Inadequate ventilation, 6 (27)	17
Capdevila (n = 12)	Respiratory distress, 8 (67) Deterioration of blood gases, 3 (25) Pulmonary edema, 1 (8)	19
Epstein (n = 18)	Original respiratory process, 6 (33) Congestive heart failure, 6 (33) Upper airway obstruction, 3 (17) Aspiration/secretions, 4 (22) Encephalopathy, 2 (11) New process (pneumonia/PE), 1 (6)	75
Miller (n = 17)	Respiratory fatigue, 6 (35) Atelectasis, 5 (29) Stridor, 3 (18) Pulmonary edema, 2 (12) Apnea (6)	57
Daley (n = 24)	Respiratory distress/secretions, 11 (46) Stridor, 9 (38) Mental status change, 3 (13) Surgery, 1 (4)	18
DeHaven (n = 46)	Secretions, 11 (24) Stridor, 9 (20) Hypoxemia/secretions, 11 (24) Hypoxemia, 12 (26) Hypercapnia, 2 (4) Seizure/CPR, 1 (2)	51
Khan (n = 34)	Poor effort, 8 (24) Excessive effort, 14 (42) Altered mental status/absent airway reflexes, 2 (6)	112

Table 3   Continued

Study (n = total number of patients with extubation failure)	Causes for extubation failure, number of patients (% of all patients with extubation failure)	Ref.
	Cardiovascular instability, 3 (9)	
	Inadequate oxygenation, 3 (9)	
	Respiratory acidosis, 3 (9)	
	Unknown, 1 (3)	
Esteban (n = 74)	Respiratory failure, 60 (81)	7
	(hypoxemia, hypercapnia, increased WOB)	
	Upper airway obstruction, 14 (19)	
Vallverdu (n = 23)	Secretions/aspiration, 7 (30)	9
	Upper airway obstruction, 2 (9)	
	Encephalopathy, 3 (13)	
	Atelectasis, 4 (17)	
	Sepsis, 1 (4)	
	Bronchopulmonary infection, 1 (4)	
	Cardiorespiratory arrest, 1 (4)	
	Hypoxemia, 2 (9)	
	Bronchospasm, 1 (4)	
	Angina, 1 (4)	
Epstein (n = 74)	Respiratory failure, 21 (33)	76
	Congestive heart failure, 17 (23)	
	Aspiration/secretions, 12 (16)	
	Upper airway obstruction, 11 (15)	
	Encephalopathy, 7 (9)	
	Other (sepsis, GI bleeding), 6 (8)	
Esteban (n = 61)	Upper airway obstruction, 9 (15)	11
	Hypoxemia, 20 (33)	
	Respiratory acidosis, 7 (11)	
	Signs of increased respiratory work, 23 (38)	
	Impaired clearance of secretions, 17 (28)	
	Cardiac failure, 4 (7)	
	Decreased consciousness, 11 (18)	
	Other, 5 (8)	
	Unknown, 3 (5)	
Rady (n = 748)	Acute respiratory failure, 406 (54)	14
	Acute hemodynamic deterioration, 153 (20)	
	Respiratory distress, 122 (16)	
	Airway protection, 60 (8)	
	Acute neurological event, 7 (1)	
Davis (n = 20)	Hypoxemia, 9 (45)	162
	Hypercarbia, 3 (15)	
	Excessive secretions, 3 (15)	
	All mechanisms combined, 5 (25)	

have indicated that work of breathing through the endotracheal tube and the ventilator apparatus may be considerable (48–52). It has been suggested that because of adherence of secretions to the inner lumen of the tube, tube kinking and head/neck position that in situ endotracheal tubes may manifest a significantly reduced diameter leading to increased airflow resistance (53). In contrast, several recent studies suggest that postextubation work of breathing is greater than preextubation work though the anatomic sites of narrowing remain ill-defined (34,35). Although the difference is significant statistically, the clinical relevance has not been elucidated. Alternatively, others have noted that postextubation work is similar to that found when measured through the endotracheal tube as the patient breaths on a T-tube circuit (54). One limitation of these studies is that analysis has been limited primarily to successfully extubated patients. Few data are available on the work of breathing experienced by patients failing extubation.

There is little doubt that intubation can cause laryngotracheal injury and lead to glottic or subglottic narrowing of the airway because of inflammation, granuloma formation, ulceration, or edema (53,55,56). By increasing airway resistance, these processes can increase the resistive work of breathing after extubation and precipitate extubation failure. The prevalence is variable and depends on whether an anatomical (direct visualization) or clinical (stridor) definition is used (55–59). In a prospective study of 700 adults, Darmon et al. noted that laryngeal edema occurred in 4.2% of extubated patients (60). Laryngeal edema was more common in women and those requiring more than 36 hours of intubation. Other authors have found that laryngotracheal complications increase with longer duration of intubation or with female gender (56,60–62). Miller and Cole observed stridor in 6% (5% excluding self-extubation) of 100 episodes of mechanical ventilation in a medical ICU (57). Comparing those with and without postextubation stridor, no difference was found in age, duration of mechanical ventilation prior to extubation, number of times intubated, endotracheal tube adjustments, cuff pressure, or use of steroids. Only half of these patients with stridor required reintubation. Others have noted that the majority who develop postextubation upper airways obstruction can be managed without reintubation (60,62). Overall, the reported incidence of upper airway obstruction among patients with extubation failure ranges from 9 to 38%, with the highest values reported in trauma patients (Table 3).

C. Excess Respiratory Secretions (Inability to Protect Airway)

The prevalence of excess respiratory secretions or aspiration among patients with extubation failure ranges from 11 to 46% (Table 3). Effective swallowing and adequate cough are crucial defense mechanisms for reducing aspiration into and clearing secretions from the tracheobronchial tree. After extubation, defective swallowing can result from the presence of a nasogastric tube, depressed mental status, or the effects of sedation. Structural and functional laryngeal incompetence and consequent aspiration are potentially important problems after extubation. Unfortunately, traditional assessment of respiratory muscle function does not accurately reflect the function of the muscles of airway protection (63). One third of patients intubated for 18 hours will aspirate radiopaque dye when it is administered immediately after extubation (64). In a study of 34 patients (mean duration of mechanical ventilation 11 days), de Larminat et al. demonstrated alterations in the swallowing reflex using installation of small volumes of normal saline into the posterior pharynx after extubation (65). Immediately after extubation the electromyographically determined swallowing latency was significantly increased compared to controls. These alterations in the swallowing reflex had substantially resolved by 2 days after extubation. Among trauma patients, 45% were found to have endoscopic evidence of aspiration 24 hours after extubation (66). The incidence of swallowing dysfunction is even higher after more prolonged mechanical ventilation (67).

Effective cough requires adequate expiratory muscle function. Recent studies suggest that inadequate expiratory muscle function, measured either by maximal expiratory pressure or by reduced peak expiratory flow, can contribute to extubation failure (9,68). Inspiratory muscle function, by ensuring adequate lung volume from which to initiate a cough, may also be important. For example, it has been demonstrated that tracheobronchial clearance is abnormal in subjects with bilateral diaphragmatic weakness (69).

D. Cardiac Failure or Ischemia

Lemaire and coworkers have elegantly demonstrated that patients with both COPD and cardiovascular disease can develop acute left ventricular dysfunction during unsuccessful weaning trials (43). With the development of pulmonary edema, gas exchange deteriorates and elastic work of breathing increases. Myocardial ischemia can result both from increased myocardial oxygen demand and decreased supply. Cardiac dysfunction can also lead to decreased respiratory muscle function (70–72). In the study of Lemaire and colleagues, an increase in transmural pulmonary artery occlusion pressure during weaning occurred 5–10 minutes after the assumption of spontaneous breathing through a T-tube circuit (43). Few studies have examined the incidence of cardiac ischemia during weaning. In a prospective MICU/CCU study, using an ST segment monitoring system, electrocardiographic evidence of ischemia was found in 6/93 (6%) patients during weaning trials, contributing to weaning failure in 4 (73).

The change from positive pressure to negative pressure (spontaneous) respiration may also contribute to myocardial dysfunction by increasing left ventricular preload and afterload. Given that many patients are weaned with some form of positive pressure (74), the change to negative swings in intrathoracic pressure may occur only *after* extubation. This may explain why the incidence of cardiac failure among patients with extubation failure may be as high as 33% (Table 3). The incidence is lowest when T-piece trials are used (9,11,19) and highest when partial support modes are used (75–77).

E. Encephalopathy

Encephalopathy or an abnormal mental status, resulting from either underlying neurological disease or from sedative medications, can contribute to extubation failure through several mechanisms. Among patients with extubation failure, encephalopathy is deemed to be the cause in 6–18% of cases (Table 3). Importantly, encephalopathy may interact with other causes, such as upper airway obstruction or excess secretions, to contribute to extubation failure. For example, in pediatric patients a poor correlation was found between airway anatomic abnormalities and the need for reintubation. Rather, these authors found that extubation failure better correlated with neurological impairment (78).

F. Respiratory Failure

Because of the various definitions used, the true incidence of respiratory failure as a cause for extubation failure is not known (Table 3). Definitions have included hypoxemia, hypercapnia, signs of increased respiratory work, use of accessory respiratory muscles, presence of thoracoabdominal paradox, or tachypnea. As noted earlier, weaning failure most commonly results from an imbalance between respiratory load and capacity (32,41,42). The rationale of a weaning trial is to detect the presence or absence of imbalance to ensure the patient has adequately recovered and that "premature extubation" will not occur. Though a weaning trial may appear to be successful, load/capacity imbalance can still occur and lead to extubation failure. One explanation is the weaning trial may be of insufficient duration to adequately assess the interaction between load and capacity. It has also been difficult to predict, in individual patients, the level of partial support that just overcomes the imposed work of breathing (79). Higher levels of support may assist an insufficiently recovered patient to "pass" a weaning trial, only to fail extubation when ventilatory support is removed. Additionally, weaning trials may lead to respiratory muscle fatigue that only becomes clinically detectable after extubation (80). Similarly, routinely used methods for assessing the presence of load/capacity imbalance during a weaning trial may not be sufficiently sensitive. For example, Murciano et al. noted diaphragmatic electromyographic evidence of fatigue *prior* to extubation among five patients who required reintubation within 48 hours (80). These patients had shown no signs of weaning trial intolerance during a one-hour spontaneous breathing trial. Lastly, a new process can occur after extubation (e.g., pneumonia, pulmonary embolism, exacerbation of airways disease) that can lead to a new load/capacity imbalance.

G. Other Processes

A small number of extubations (probably <10%) are attributable to the development of gastrointestinal bleeding, sepsis, seizures, or the need for surgery (Table 3).

IV. Extubation Outcome

A. Overview

Numerous studies have examined the outcome for patients who require mechanical ventilation. Many of these have examined specific categories of acute respiratory failure, such as COPD (81–84), or acute lung injury (85–87), or have focused on patients with particular underlying comorbid conditions such as bone marrow transplantation (88,89), HIV (90,91), cirrhosis (92,93), malignancy (94,95), or congestive heart failure (96). Only recently have investigators directed their attention to the issue of how extubation outcome impacts on ICU and hospital survival.

B. Extubation Success

Relatively few studies have specifically analyzed the in-hospital mortality for patients who are successfully extubated. Although extubation success is viewed as a positive outcome, the mortality and morbidity for these patients is still considerable. Epstein et al., studying MICU patients in an academic tertiary care center, found that 29/241 (12%) successfully extubated patients still died during their hospitalization (10). Eight (28%) of these died after requiring late reintubation, usually from a new or unrelated process, more than 72 hours after extubation. On average patients spent another 4.5 days in the ICU and 16.3 days in the hospital after successful extubation. Among hospital survivors, 24% required transfer to a rehabilitation or long-term care unit. Esteban and coworkers found an in-hospital mortality of 12.5% (49/392) among successfully extubated patients, with 60% of deaths occurring after the patient had been transferred out of the ICU (11). In contrast, among cardiac surgical patients, a mortality of just 2% was noted among those successfully extubated (14).

C. Extubation Failure

Older studies suggested that "premature extubation" was not associated with increased mortality (97). Over the last decade investigators have focused on defining the outcome of patients who fail extubation and require reintubation. These studies indicate that mortality depends on the patient population under investigation. Hospital mortality for reintubated patients is below 10% for patients in trauma units (17,18). In contrast, mortality has ranged from 21 to 43% for patients in general surgical or medical ICUs and after cardiac surgery (Table 2).

Recent investigators have further demonstrated that, in univariate analyses, that mortality for extubation failure ranges from 2.5 to 10 times greater than that of successfully extubated patients (7,9–11,77). It is also clear that other secondary outcomes are dramatically affected by extubation failure. Among MICU patients, extubation failure resulted in a substantially longer length of ICU and hospital stay (Fig. 1). On average, reintubated patients spent 12 additional days on mechanical ventilation, 21 additional days in the ICU, and 30 additional days in the hospital. Among hospital survivors, two thirds required transfer to a long-term care facility or rehabilitation unit.

Extubation failure increases the likelihood of tracheostomy, especially among trauma and surgical patients. For example, Daley and coworkers found that 62% of reintubated trauma patients required tracheostomy (18). Combining two consecutive studies of MICU/SICU patients, Esteban and colleagues noted that 50 of 135 (37%) reintubated patients required tracheostomy (7,11). In contrast, 15 of 74 (20%) medical patients with extubation failure eventually received a tracheostomy (76).

The above studies have focused principally on heterogeneous populations. Although data are limited, poor outcome is also seen for homogeneous groups of patients. For example, Nevins and Epstein noted that COPD patients failing extubation were more likely to die than those successfully extubated (36% vs. 6%, $p < 0.0001$) (26). Among survivors, 78% of extubation failure patients

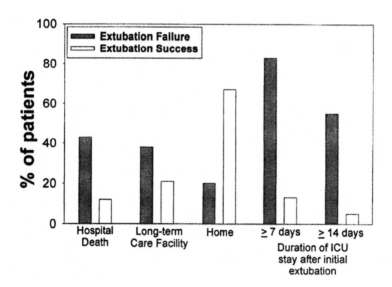

Figure 1   Effect of failed extubation on outcome of medical intensive care unit patients. (Adapted from Ref. 10.)

needed transfer to a chronic care facility compared to 32% of successfully extubated patients ($p < 0.001$). Extubation failure significantly prolonged the duration of mechanical ventilation and intensive care unit and hospital stay.

Several investigators have demonstrated that the cause of extubation failure is an important determinant of outcome. For example, mortality is highest for patients reintubated because of respiratory failure, cardiac failure, encephalopathy, or other causes (gastrointestinal bleeding and sepsis) and lowest when extubation failure results from upper airway obstruction, aspiration, or excess pulmonary secretions (Fig. 2) (7,11,18,76).

These investigations have raised several important questions. First, why is mortality so high for extubation failure? Second, why is mortality variable for different patient populations? The increased mortality associated with extubation failure could reflect patients with greater underlying severity of illness or the presence of significant comorbid conditions. Alternatively, failed extubation may not directly cause a poor outcome but rather serve as an additional independent marker of severity of illness. The act of reintubation may result in life-threatening complications. Lastly, significant clinical deterioration may occur

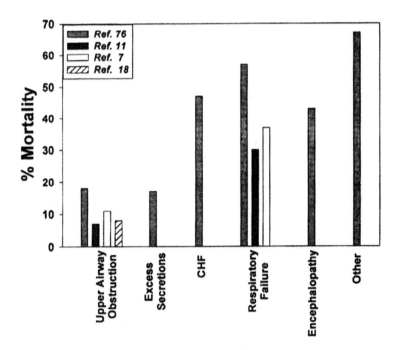

Figure 2   Effect of cause of extubation failure on hospital mortality.

between the time of extubation and eventual reinstitution of adequate ventilatory support.

Severity of Illness

Sicker patients may be prone to extubation failure. If true, poor outcome may relate to the severity of illness and be independent of extubation failure. In a study of MICU patients, no differences were found in APACHE II score (measured 6 hours after onset of first mechanical ventilation) or the presence of significant comorbid conditions (cirrhosis, active malignancy, HIV, transplantation) when extubation success and extubation failure patients were compared (10). The APACHE II score was slightly higher at the onset of weaning among those destined to develop extubation failure. Using a multiple logistic regression model controlling for APACHE II, comorbid conditions, age, and acute renal failure, extubation failure was found to be an independent predictor of hospital mortality, prolonged ICU stay (greater than 7 or 14 days of ICU care) and need for transfer to rehabilitation or chronic care. Esteban et al. also controlled for severity of illness (using SAPS II), days of mechanical ventilation prior to weaning and reason for initiation of ventilation and similarly found extubation failure to be a powerful independent predictor of poor outcome (relative risk 11.2, 95% CI 4.6–26.9) (7). In contrast, Rady and Ryan, using a multivariate model in cardiac surgical patients, found that extubation failure increased the duration of mechanical ventilation, length of ICU and hospital stay, but not mortality (14). These authors controlled for single and multiple organ dysfunction which may have resulted *from* extubation failure, thereby confounding their analysis.

Complications of Reintubation

Emergent tracheal intubation is frequently associated with significant complications, but direct immediate attributable mortality is low. Schwartz and coworkers, studying 297 emergent adult intubations, noted 7 deaths (3%) within 30 minutes of the procedure (98). Nearly all were hypotensive or receiving vasopressor agents prior to reintubation. Reintubation for extubation failure can be performed electively or may be required emergently and has been associated with numerous complications (Table 4). In a study of 61 MICU patients, Rashkin and Davis noted that those requiring reintubation had a higher rate of complications than those not reintubated (63% vs. 31%, $p < 0.05$) (99). Similarly, Daley et al. recorded complications in 50% of reintubated trauma patients including pneumonia (50%), atelectasis (43%) or pleural effusion (7%) (18).

In an observational study, Torres and coinvestigators found that 38% of patients with ventilator associated pneumonia had previously undergone reintubation (61% of reintubated patients developed pneumonia) (100). The authors postulated that changing the endotracheal tube may lead to aspiration of oropharyn-

Table 4 Complications of Reintubation

Esophageal intubation
Barotrauma (pneumothorax, pneumomediasti- num, subcutaneous emphysema)
Aspiration of gastric or oropharyngeal contents
Pneumonia
Arrhythmia
Lobar collapse/atelectasis
Myocardial ischemia
Airway injury
Right mainstem intubation

geal secretions pooled in the posterior pharynx. In a subsequent case-control study, these investigators found that reintubation increased the risk of nosocomial pneumonia sixfold (101). Forty-seven percent of reintubated patients developed pneumonia after reintubation compare to just 10% of controls. Reintubation increased the duration of ICU stay and increased the crude mortality from 20% to 35%, with one half of the deaths being attributable to nosocomial pneumonia. Semi-recumbent position (perhaps fostering gravitational movement of oropharyngeal secretions to the lower airways) during the interval between extubation and reintubation, was significantly associated with the development of pneumonia. The frequency of nosocomial pneumonia also seems to increase when cardiac surgical patients experience extubation failure (14).

In contrast, recent investigators have been unable to demonstrate an increased mortality attributable to complications resulting from reintubation after extubation failure. Esteban and coworkers noted that 15% of reintubated patients suffered a complication but this was not associated with increased mortality (7). In a subsequent study, the investigators observed that 11/61 reintubated patients (18%) suffered a complication, including 6 with pneumonia and 3 with cardiovascular complications (11). Mortality was similar between those with complications (45.4%) and those without complications (30.0%). Epstein and Ciubotaru observed a total of 21 (28%) complications in 74 reintubated MICU patients, including pneumonia (13), arrhythmia (3), atelectasis/lobar collapse (3), myocardial infarction (2), and cerebrovascular accident (2) (76). Mortality for patients with complications (38%) was similar to those without complications (43%). Pneumonia resulting from reintubation was not associated with increased mortality (with pneumonia, 46% vs. without pneumonia, 41%). Taken together, these studies indicate that although complications of reintubation are frequent, mortality may not increase as a consequence. This conclusion is also supported by the observation that mortality is very much dependent upon why and when extubation failure occurs.

Time to Reintubation

Increased mortality of extubation failure may be related to deterioration that occurs during the interval between extubation and reintubation. For example, Torres and coworkers noted a lower incidence of pneumonia in patients who were immediately reintubated compared to those with delayed reintubation (101). Therefore, elapsed time from extubation to reintubation may be a crucial determinant of outcome. The adverse consequence of delayed reestablishment of adequate ventilatory support was recently suggested by a randomized controlled trial of noninvasive positive pressure ventilation (NPPV) for acute respiratory failure in an emergency department. A trend toward increased mortality was found for patients randomized to NPPV. Among patients eventually requiring invasive mechanical ventilation, the NPPV group experienced a longer delay from emergency department arrival to the time of intubation (26 hours vs. 5 hours). Delaying intubation and mechanical ventilation may have allowed physiological deterioration and organ dysfunction to occur (102).

A number of studies have indirectly examined the impact of time to reintubation on outcome of extubation failure. Tahvanainen and colleagues observed a 22% mortality among reintubated patients with a mean time to reintubation of 9.3 ± 5.6 hours (77). In Demling's series, general surgical patients were reintubated a mean of 2.2 days after extubation and suffered a 40% mortality rate (17). Only 1 of 7 reintubated within 24 hours died. The same authors observed only a 10% mortality among reintubated trauma patients, all of whom had ventilatory support reestablished in less than 24 hours (mean 15.5 hours). Similarly, in another series of trauma patients, an 8% mortality was seen among 24 patients reintubated after a mean of 11.6 hours after extubation (18). These studies suggest that mortality is lowest when ventilatory support is more rapidly reestablished.

One weakness of these reports is the failure to control for severity of illness, comorbid conditions, and the cause of extubation failure. The latter factor is particularly important because it is anticipated that upper airway obstruction or difficulty handling excess pulmonary secretions may lead to earlier reintubation. To address this issue, Epstein and Ciubotaru studied 74 medical patients reintubated within 72 hours of extubation (76). Mortality was lowest for those reintubated within 12 hours and increased with duration of time to reestablishment of ventilator support (Fig. 3). After controlling for severity of illness, presence of significant comorbid conditions, organ failure, and cause of reintubation, time to reintubation was found to be an independent predictor of outcome. In a preliminary report, Esteban et al. found mortality rates of 28, 54, and 48% among patients

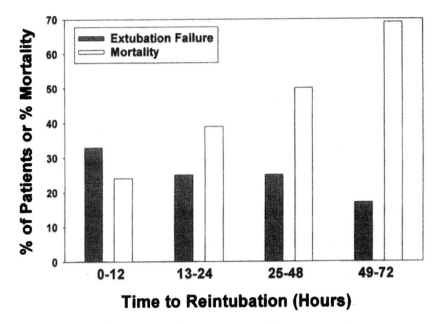

Figure 3   Effect of time to reintubation on hospital mortality. Filled bars represent %
of patients with extubation failure at 0–12, 13–24, 25–48, and 49–72 hours. Open bars
represent % mortality for each time period. (Adapted from Ref. 76.)

reintubated within 0–12, 12–24, and 24–48 hours (103), respectively. These studies support the hypothesis that clinical deterioration after extubation may contribute to the elevated mortality of extubation failure. An important clinical implication is that very early reestablishment of ventilatory support has the potential to
improve outcome.

V. Prediction of Extubation Outcome

A. Why Predict Outcome?

Given the association of extubation failure and increased mortality, the ability
to accurately foretell extubation outcome is of substantial importance. Increasing
duration of mechanical ventilation is associated with increasing risk for numerous
complications (104) including ventilator-associated pneumonia (105), thrombo-
embolism, gastrointestinal bleeding (106), oxygen toxicity, and airway injury
(55,56,61,97). Although data are conflicting, some complications, such as ventilator-associated pneumonia, may increase mortality (105). Therefore, an additional

important goal of prediction is to identify the earliest time at which a patient can be liberated from mechanical ventilation in order to reduce the likelihood of these complications. Lastly, intensive care unit costs rise with increasing duration of stay. Patients with a high probability of extubation success may be appropriate for early transfer out of the ICU, once extubated. Timely liberation of a patient from mechanical ventilation also opens up an ICU bed, a valuable and increasingly scarce resource. In contrast, patients at increased risk for extubation failure warrant a longer duration of observation in the intensive care unit after extubation to allow for early recognition of deterioration and rapid reinstitution of ventilatory support. Although it can be argued that expert clinicians can foretell extubation outcome based on clinical assessment, the level of expertise of those making these crucial decisions may vary widely. Thus, extubation predictors may serve to guide decision making with the potential for broad applicability in diverse settings.

B. Rules of Test Interpretation

A critical evaluation of extubation predictors requires an understanding of the basic tools of clinical decision analysis (107). The terms most commonly used are sensitivity, specificity, positive predictive value, and negative predictive value. These terms can be most easily explained with a 2-by-2 table, designed to allow the systematic comparison of the results of the test (e.g., the extubation predictor) under evaluation and a "gold standard" (Fig. 4). When applied to

Gold Standard

		Extubation Success	Extubation Failure
Test Result	Positive ($f/V_T \leq 105$)	True Positive (TP)	False Positive (FP)
	Negative ($f/V_T > 105$)	False Negative (FN)	True Negative (TN)

Sensitivity = TP / (TP + FN)   PPV = TP / (TP + FP)
Specificity = TN / (TN + FP)   NPV = TN / (TN + FN)

Figure 4 Two-by-two table comparing the "gold standard" (extubation outcome) to the results of a predictor test (f/V_T).

extubation, the test (e.g., the f/V_T or rapid shallow breathing index) is used to detect whether the patient can be successfully extubated and is then compared to the actual outcome of extubation (e.g., the gold standard).

The term *sensitivity* refers to the ratio of true positives (e.g., $f/V_T \leq 105$ breaths/min/L and successful extubation) to the sum of true positives plus false negatives (e.g., all patients successfully extubated). The term *specificity* is the ratio of all patients who have both a negative test ($f/V_T > 105$ breaths/min/L) and fail extubation (true negatives) to all patients who fail extubation (true negatives plus false positives). Though important characteristics of a clinical test, sensitivity and specificity are of less value to the clinician than the positive predictive value (PPV) and negative predictive value (NPV). It is crucial to realize that while sensitivity and specificity are properties of a test itself, independent of the particular patient sample in whom the test is used, the PPV and NPV depend not only on the sensitivity and specificity of the test, but also on the prevalence of the condition being measured.

A common error in the application of diagnostic information to decision making is the failure to consider the prevalence (e.g., the prior or pretest probability) of the condition under investigation. Numerous studies have emphasized the importance of this in the interpretation of ventilation-perfusion scans for pulmonary embolism, PPD skin testing for tuberculous infection and solitary lung nodules for malignancy. Unfortunately, the importance of the pretest probability of weaning or extubation success in interpreting and applying predictors has been infrequently considered (107). By combining the pretest probability of extubation success with the true-positive rate (TPR or sensitivity) and false-positive rate (FPR, 1-specificity) of the extubation predictor a posttest probability can be generated using Bayes' theorem (107).

Careful analysis of these principles demonstrates that extubation predictors are most useful when the range of pretest probability of extubation success is approximately 0.50–0.80. Conversely, when the pretest probability of successful extubation is very high, a positive test (e.g., $f/V_T \leq 105$ breaths/min/L) has marginal impact on the posttest probability. In contrast, when the pretest probability is very low, although a positive test will increase the likelihood of success, extubation failure may still remain the most likely outcome.

Similar observations are made when examining patients with negative tests (e.g., $f/V_T > 105$ breaths/min/L). When the pretest probability of extubation success is very high, the likelihood of successful extubation may remain significant even when the $f/V_T > 105$. In distinction, a negative test minimally affects the posttest probability when the pretest probability of success is very low. Thus, even for a very accurate extubation predictor (assuming that a perfect test with a sensitivity and specificity of unity is unlikely to exist), at the extremes of probability, the posttest probability may differ little from the pretest value. It is also clear that identical test results (e.g., two patients with a positive test, $f/V_T \leq 105$

breaths/min/L) can translate into very different posttest probabilities of success because of the crucial influence of the pretest probability. Analogously, patients with very different f/V_T values may actually have the same posttest probability of extubation success when the pretest probabilities are very different.

C. Differences in Predicting Weaning and Extubation Outcome

Numerous weaning and extubation predictors have been examined over the last quarter of a century. The ideal predictor should be easy to measure, highly reproducible, and accurate in foretelling outcome. Predictors will function best when they reflect the pathophysiology of failure. In general, predictors have proven to be far less accurate in predicting extubation outcome than weaning outcome. Several explanations for this difference in accuracy have been offered (107).

One reason is that many predictors are designed to detect or reflect the pathophysiology of weaning failure rather than the distinct pathophysiology of extubation failure. For example, parameters such as negative inspiratory force, vital capacity, minute ventilation, maximal voluntary ventilation, and the breathing pattern are measurements related to load/capacity considerations. Another explanation is that although the definitions of weaning and extubation success are identical (e.g., successful removal of the endotracheal tube without need for reinsertion in the following 24–72 hours), the definitions for failure are distinct. Weaning failure is defined as an inability to tolerate a weaning trial, necessitating reinstitution of ventilatory support (with the endotracheal tube still in place), characterized by either objective (e.g., hypercapnia, hypoxemia, acidosis, tachypnea, hyper- or hypotension, tachy- or bradycardia) or subjective (e.g., agitation, diaphoresis, distress) criteria for failure. In contrast, extubation failure refers specifically to the need for reintubation within 24–72 hours of extubation. Furthermore, investigators have demonstrated that a percentage of patients with "weaning" failure have no detectable pathophysiological cause for failure (41,51,52). In some cases, this occurs because "signs" of weaning failure (e.g., tachypnea, tachycardia, agitation, or diaphoresis) may reflect anxiety of the patient rather than true weaning intolerance. In other instances, true load/capacity imbalance exists but can be primarily attributed to either the endotracheal tube or other ventilatory circuitry. In either case, the result is that some patients who appear to fail weaning trials can be successfully extubated, that is, weaning failure does not equal extubation failure (51,52). Once a patient passes a weaning trial, the probability of successful extubation ranges from 80 to 95%. Given the principles of Bayes theorem, this high pretest probability of success means that the false-positive rate will be fairly low (e.g., most positives are true positives leading to a high PPV) and the false-negative rate high (e.g., low NPV). The above factors explain, in part, why the PPVs are similar and the NPVs divergent when comparing studies examining weaning failure and those examining extubation failure.

D. Predictors

Traditional Predictors

Numerous investigators have measured maximal inspiratory pressure (MIP, or negative inspiratory force, NIF), vital capacity, minute ventilation, maximal voluntary ventilation, and indices of oxygenation or gas exchange in an effort to predict outcome. The overwhelming majority of studies have focused on weaning alone or have combined weaning and extubation into a single outcome (1,9,15,33,108–110). Few investigators have specifically examined the value and accuracy of predictors of extubation outcome alone (Table 5). Many studies compare mean values, without analysis based on threshold cutoffs (e.g., a definition of what constitutes a positive versus a negative test). In general, accuracy of traditional predictors, measured prior to a weaning trial, has been lower when applied to extubation compared to weaning outcome. For example, Tahvanainen

Table 5 Studies Examining the Prediction of Extubation Outcome

Study (Ref.)	Prevalence of success	Parameter	PPV	NPV
Tahvanainen (77)	0.81	VC > 10 mL/kg	0.83	0.5
		MIP < −30	0.74	0
		VE < 10 L/min	0.89	0.25
		$V_D/V_T < 0.6$	0.81	0.25
		MVV/VE > 2	0.86	0.24
		Urine volume > 500 mL/6 h	0.89	0.5
		RQ < 0.9	0.89	0.5
Krieger (111)	0.90	MIP ≤20 cm H_2O	0.91	0.22
		MIP ≤ 30 cm H_2O	0.92	0.21
		MIP ≤ 20 & VE < 10 L/min	0.93	0.19
		MIP ≤ 30 & VE < 10 L/min	0.93	0.15
		$Pao_2/Fio_2 > 238$ torr	0.90	0.10
		pH > 7.35	0.90	0.19
Lee (28)	0.83	$f/V_T < 105$	0.79	0.08
Epstein (75)	0.83	$f/V_T < 100$	0.83	0.40
Capdevila (19)	0.82	MIP > 50 cm H_2O	0.86	0.31
		f/V_T (>60)	0.92	0.36
		$P_{0.1}$ (<5 cm H_2O)	0.96	0.65
		$P_{0.1}/MIP$ (<0.09)	1.00	0.92
Epstein (22)	0.84	$f/V_T < 100$	0.86	0.28

VC, Vital capacity; MIP, maximal inspiratory pressure; VE, minute ventilation; V_D/V_T, dead space fraction; MVV, maximal voluntary ventilation; RQ, respiratory quotient; f/V_T, frequency-tidal volume ratio; $P_{0.1}$, airway occlusion pressure.

et al. found that vital capacity > 10 mL/kg, maximal inspiratory pressure < -30 cm H_2O, minute ventilation < 10 L/min, dead space < 0.6, and maximal voluntary ventilation (MVV) greater than twice the minute ventilation did not accurately separate reintubated patients from those successfully extubated (77). In contrast, Krieger and colleagues found that MIP and pH were lower in elderly patients who needed reintubation within 48 hours of successful extubation (111). Unfortunately, the mean absolute differences were small and the diagnostic accuracy marginal. These authors also found that total minute ventilation, $Paco_2$, Pao_2, and Pao_2/Fio_2 were similar between successful and failed extubations. Other studies also failed to identify differences in Pao_2/Fio_2, minute ventilation, vital capacity, maximal inspiratory pressure/negative inspiratory force when comparing successfully extubated to reintubated patients (7,10). Khan et al. noted that pediatric patients with extubation failure had higher values for the oxygenation index, Fio_2, mean airway pressure, and fraction of minute ventilation delivered by the ventilator compared to those with extubation success. In contrast, no differences were found for maximal inspiratory pressure (MIP) or the ratio of inspiratory pressure to MIP (Pi/MIP) (112).

Measurement of traditional predictors during, rather than prior to, the weaning trial may enhance accuracy. For example, Capdevila and coinvestigators found differences in mean values of vital capacity (0.80 vs. 1.2 mL, $p < 0.05$) and maximal inspiratory pressure (53 vs. 70, $p < 0.05$) between failure and success patients when measured 20 minutes into a T-piece trial (19).

Breathing Pattern and Individual Components

Of the numerous parameters studied over the past two decades, the breathing pattern [frequency–tidal volume ratio (f/V_T) or rapid shallow breathing index] has proven the most accurate noninvasive predictor of weaning outcome (15,108,110). Weaning success is likely when the f/V_T is $<100–105$ breaths/min/L. The likelihood of weaning failure has been very high when the f/V_T is >105 breaths/min/L. The basis for rapid shallow breathing is both complex and controversial. Initially it was hypothesized that rapid shallow breathing occurred as an adaptive response to load/capacity imbalance, that is, the pathophysiological cause for weaning failure. But, two recent studies found no correlation between the tension-time index (a measure of the load capacity interaction) and the f/V_T (32,41). Another hypothesis is that rapid shallow breathing contributes to weaning failure in COPD by worsening hyperinflation and dead space ventilation. As with traditional predictors, relatively few studies have exclusively examined the role of f/V_T in predicting outcome for extubated patients.

Several studies of adult patients have found no difference in mean values for respiratory frequency, tidal volume, and f/V_T when extubation success and extubation failure patients were directly compared (7,10,111). Similarly, Khan et al. found that respiratory rate (standardized for age) and the f/V_T did not discriminate between pediatric patients with failure and success (112). Specifically, these investigators found similar reintubation rates at an f/V_T of <4 breaths/min/ mL/kg (normal for an infant) and when the f/V_T was >16 breaths/min/mL/kg. They did note the risk of extubation failure increased with decreasing tidal volume adjusted to body weight. In contrast to the above studies, Del Rosario and coinvestigators found a lower tidal volume, higher respiratory rate, and higher f/V_T among patients with extubation failure (20).

When thresholds have been examined, positive predictive values have been similar to those reported for studies looking at weaning outcome, likely reflecting the similar definition of success and the high prevalence of extubation success in the populations tested (75). Nevertheless, up to 20% of patients predicted to succeed still fail, perhaps reflecting the distinct causes of extubation failure. For example, it was noted that most false positive (f/V_T < 100 breaths/min/L, but extubation failure) occurred because of congestive heart failure, upper airway obstruction, secretions, encephalopathy, or the onset of a new process (75). Another explanation is the threshold value selected, which may be lower (e.g., f/V_T < 100) for certain patient groups. This appears true for studies looking primarily at weaning outcome. For example, Jaeschke and coworkers reanalyzed the data of Yang and Tobin and found that 50% of patients with f/V_T values between 80 and 100 failed weaning compared to 95% with f/V_T > 100 and just 9% with f/V_T < 80 breaths/min/L (113). Vassilakopoulos et al. noted a substantial reduction in f/V_T (measured at the end of a weaning trial) when comparing weaning failure to weaning success, though the mean initial value was below 100 (32).

Several studies also suggest that lower thresholds may also be applicable to extubation prediction. Murciano and colleagues, studying COPD patients 24 hours after intubation and prior to extubation, noted a decrease in respiratory rate and increase in tidal volume over time among successfully extubated patients, compared to no change among those who failed. Calculating from their data, the f/V_T decreased from 70 to 35 breaths/min/L in those successfully extubated and remained at 68 breaths/min/L for those requiring reintubation within 48 hours (80). Capdevila et al., taking measurements 20 minutes into a T-piece trial, found trends toward higher respiratory rate (28 vs. 24 breaths/min) and lower tidal volume (0.46 vs. 0.53 mL) when comparing extubation failure to success (19). When combined into the f/V_T, values were significantly higher for those who failed (70 vs. 53 breaths/min/L, p < 0.05). Using a threshold value of 60 breaths/ min/L, the authors found a sensitivity of 0.73, specificity of 0.75, PPV of 0.92, and NPV of 0.36. Using a threshold of 100 breaths/min/L, the sensitivity was 97% with a specificity of 30%. Lastly, in a recently completed study, 60% of patients failing extubation with a f/V_T < 100 but >60 breaths/min/L demonstrated a significant fall ($>20\%$) in f/V_T at the time of eventual successful extubation (Epstein, personal communication). This effect was principally confined to patients failing from congestive heart failure or respiratory failure. Conversely, for patients failing from other etiologies, such as aspiration, increased respiratory secretions, encephalopathy, and upper airway obstruction, the breathing pattern did not become less rapid and shallow at the time of successful extubation. The implication of these studies is that using f/V_T thresholds below 100, for some patient groups, may substantially increase the capacity to predict extubation failure by reducing the number of false positives (e.g., improved PPV). In fact, recent work suggests that breathing pattern may increase the accuracy of predicting extubation outcome for certain patient populations. For example, a lower tidal volume (339 vs. 449 mL) and a trend toward a higher f/V_T (81 vs. 62 breaths/min/L) were noted among extubated COPD patients who required reintubation (26).

A risk of using lower thresholds is that the number of false negatives (e.g., patients predicted to fail who actually can be successfully extubated) will increase. In fact, studies indicate the NPV for the f/V_T is substantially lower for prediction of extubation compared to weaning outcome. One reason for this observation is the higher pretest probability of success. Another explanation, noted earlier, is that some patients who appear to fail weaning trials actually no longer require mechanical ventilation. This may occur if the imposed work of breathing is high or if nonventilatory factors manifest as the criteria used to categorize a patient as a weaning failure. For example, DeHaven et al. noted that $>90\%$ of patients with a respiratory rate of >30 breaths/min during a room air CPAP trial (89% with respiratory rate $\geq$ 38 breaths/min) were successfully extubated when the measured physiological work of breathing was not elevated (51). Many such patients were previously noted to have an f/V_T of >105 breaths/min/L (52). One explanation for the high false negative rate is the growing list of factors identified that increase the f/V_T including anxiety (114–118), female gender (22,23), narrow endotracheal tube size (22,52,119), sepsis/pneumonia (120), older age (23,121), supine positioning (122) increased temperature (23), and preceding lung disease (123). Therefore, a patient with a $f/V_T > 100$ breaths/min/L and failing a weaning trial because of a high imposed work of breathing (or a subjective criterion that may not truly indicate ventilator dependence) will be classified as a true negative. If the patient were to be successfully extubated, he would be reclassified as a false negative and the NPV of the test would decrease.

To summarize, breathing pattern and its components may have some limited utility in predicting extubation outcome but are far more accurate in predicting apparent weaning outcome. For patients at risk for a poor outcome after extubation failure, it is reasonable to decrease the f/V_T threshold to minimize the number of false positives. Conversely, when the risk associated with prolonged mechanical ventilation exceeds that of extubation failure or factors are present that increase the f/V_T, it is reasonable to increase the threshold to reduce the number of false negatives.

Respiratory Motion

Studies of chest wall and abdomen motion have been used to identify patients likely to fail weaning trials (124). Similarly, Krieger and Ershowsky used inductive plethysmography to compare successful to failed extubation (125). Respiratory rate (34 vs. 25 breaths/min) and the ratio of total compartmental displacement to tidal volume (TCD/V_T, a measure of ribcage-abdominal asynchrony) were higher in the 10 minutes immediately prior to reintubation compared to the last 10-minute epoch during the hour immediately following extubation in those who were successful. Either an increase in respiratory rate of >11 breaths/min, increase in TCD/V_T of >0.22 (compared to values for one hour prior), or respiratory alternans was present in all seven patients with extubation failure. Unfortunately, no differences were seen when these parameters were measured one hour prior to reintubation and compared to control measurements. Capdevila et al. found that "coordinated thoracoabdominal motion" had a PPV 0.85 and NPV 0.44 and "absence of sternocleidomastoid contraction" a PPV 0.87 and NPV 0.42 for extubation success (19). Use of these physical signs as predictors is limited by the lack of precise definitions. In addition, predictive accuracy is not significantly superior to the f/V_T.

Assessing Expiratory Function

The capacity to protect the airway and expel secretions with an effective cough is crucial for extubation success, but few studies have systematically examined the issue. Assessing this capacity has consisted principally of ensuring an adequate gag reflex, demonstrating a cough reflex when stimulated with a suction catheter and by the absence of excess secretions. Unfortunately no studies adequately address the issue of what constitutes excess secretions and how they should be quantified. Some use the frequency of necessary suctioning as a surrogate (e.g., no more than every 2 hours). Investigators have started to assess "effective cough" as a predictor of extubation outcome. Though their criteria were not specifically delineated, Capdevila et al. found that "effective cough" had a PPV of 0.86 and NPV of 0.40 in predicting extubation success (19). Recently, others have attempted to quantify expiratory capacity. In a study of 49 patients with primarily neuromuscular disease, Bach and Saporto found the peak cough flows (PCF) could predict extubation/decannulation outcome (68). Unassisted or assisted (after abdominal thrust at the instant of glottic opening) peak cough flows were measured using a peak flow meter. All patients with PCF > 160 L/min were successfully extubated/decannulated, defined as no respiratory symptoms or blood gas deterioration for 2 weeks. All patients with PCF $<$ 160 L/min failed, defined as the development of respiratory distress, decreased vital capacity and oxygen desaturation despite the use of noninvasive positive pressure ventilation and assisted coughing. Of the four patients with PCF $=$ 160 L/min, two succeeded and two failed. Vallverdu et al. measured maximal expiratory pressure (MEP) prior to the first weaning trial in 217 patients (9). Using a unidirectional valve to occlude the expiratory port (allowing patients to inspire but not expire) for 25–30 seconds, the most positive expiratory pressure generated was recorded. In acute respiratory failure patients and neurological patients, but not those with COPD, the MEP was lower among weaning failure patients. Using discriminant analysis, a lower MEP was shown to be an independent predictor of failure among neurological patients, most of whom were extubation rather than weaning failures. The MEP is useful because it may correlate with the efficacy of cough and the capacity to clear secretions (126). Threshold values of MEP to separate patients likely to fail from those likely to succeed have not yet been published.

Assessing for Upper Airway Obstruction (Cuff Leak Test)

The presence of the endotracheal tube prevents adequate direct evaluation of upper airway caliber and, when the airway is abnormally narrowed, serves to stent the airway open. Detection of an air leak when the balloon of the endotracheal tube is deflated has been used to assess upper airway patency (cuff leak test) (127,128). The absence of an audible air-leak suggests the presence of upper airway obstruction and increased risk for postextubation stridor. Fisher and Raper noted that 3 of 10 patients without a cuff leak (e.g., negative cuff leak test) required reintubation for postextubation stridor (127). In contrast, stridor did not develop in the 62 patients with a positive cuff leak test. More recently, Miller and Cole studied a quantitative cuff leak test in medical intensive care unit patients (57). While the patient breathed on assist control, the balloon was deflated and the expiratory tidal volume recorded for the next six breaths (Fig. 5). Using an average of the lowest three values they defined the cuff leak volume as the difference between inspiratory and average expiratory volume. The cuff leak volume measured within 24 hours of extubation was lower in those who developed postextubation stridor (180 vs. 360 mL, $p <$ 0.05). Using receiver operation curve analysis, a threshold value of 110 mL was identified. When the cuff leak volume was greater than 110 mL, 98% did not have stridor (PPV 0.98), whereas 80% developed stridor when the volume was less than 110 mL (NPV 0.80). Although the accuracy of this test seems good, the impact on care may be limited because less than 50% of patients with stridor actually need reintubation and the mortality for patients reintubated with stridor is not significantly different from successfully extubated patients (7,60,62,76). In addition, upper airway obstruction (in nontrauma populations) causes 20% or fewer of all cases of extubation failure.

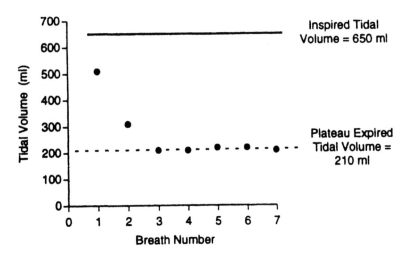

Figure 5 Sequential expired tidal volume after endotracheal tube balloon cuff deflation. (From Ref. 57.)

Work of Breathing

Numerous studies have examined work of breathing, as represented by the oxygen cost of breathing, pressure time product, or Campbell diagram, as a predictor of weaning outcome (129–132). Recently, investigators used esophageal manometry to determine work of breathing in patients failing weaning trials (51,52,133–136). Relatively few studies have examined the value of work of breathing (WOB) measurements in predicting extubation outcome. Levy et al. recently studied 24 patients on PSV 5–8 cm H_2O. Work of breathing, measured with esophageal manometry, was elevated (>0.75 J/L) in 10 patients, but 9 were still successfully extubated (136). Using esophageal manometry, Kirton and coworkers studied trauma patients, with tachypnea during a room air CPAP trial. Six were successfully extubated after total WOB was found to be low (<0.8 J/L) (Fig. 6) (52). Twenty of 21 others were successfully extubated after an elevated total WOB was found to be attributable to an increase in the imposed WOB. In a larger follow-up study of similar design, these authors studied extubation outcome in patients who had a respiratory rate of >30 and either a WOB ≤ 1.1 J/L or total WOB minus imposed WOB of ≤ 0.8 J/L (51). Among 105 patients, only 8 (7.8%) required reintubation within 72 hours. These studies nicely demonstrate that tachypnea may result from factors other than increased physiological work of breathing and by itself is insufficient as an extubation criterion.

Unfortunately, these studies do not fully examine the accuracy of an elevated physiological work of breathing in predicting extubation outcome. Because

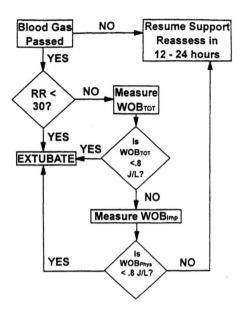

Figure 6 Extubation algorithm using work of breathing (WOB) measured with an esophageal balloon. Physiological WOB (WOB$_{phys}$) is equal to total WOB (WOB$_{tot}$) minus imposed WOB (WOB$_{imp}$). For blood gases to be "passed" the following criteria had to be satisfied: Pao$_2$ ≥ 55 mmHg, Paco$_2$ ≤ 45 mmHg, and pH ≥ 7.35. (From Ref. 52.)

they require special equipment, it is doubtful that these techniques will find widespread use. It is unclear whether work of breathing measurements will identify patients destined to fail extubation despite passing a weaning trial. The greatest utility may be application in patients who inexplicably fail weaning trials.

Occlusion Pressure

Airway occlusion pressure measured at 100 msec (P$_{100}$ or P$_{0.1}$) has been used to assess respiratory drive and as an indirect measurement of the demand on the respiratory system (137–140). When corrected for maximal inspiratory pressure (P$_{0.1}$/MIP), it may provide a numerical expression of the balance between load and capacity. Murciano et al. measured P$_{0.1}$ 24 hours after onset of mechanical ventilation and again prior to extubation in 16 patients with COPD. Among the 11 successfully extubated patients, the P$_{0.1}$ fell significantly from 7.4 cm H$_2$O to 3.9 cm H$_2$O. In contrast, the 5 patients with extubation failure had no improvement in P$_{0.1}$ over time (6.6 vs. 6.5 cm H$_2$O) (80). Del Rosario and colleagues also noted a higher P$_{0.1}$ and P$_{0.1}$/Pimax among patients with extubation failure (20). Capdevila and coworkers found that patients destined to fail extubation had higher $P_{0.1}$ (7.4 vs. 3.6 cm H_2O, $p = 0.001$) and $P_{0.1}/MIP$ values measured after 20 minutes of spontaneous breathing (19). For $P_{0.1}$, a cut-off of 5 cm H_2O led to a PPV of 0.96 and a NPV 0.65. For $P_{0.1}/MIP$, a cut-off of 0.09 led to a PPV of 1.0 and NPV 0.92. The ROC curves for either measurement had significantly greater areas under the curve than for f/V_T or MIP. Although these measurements require special equipment, the technological principles can be potentially adapted to modern ventilators. It should be noted that both $P_{0.1}$ and WOB are unlikely to detect patients at risk for extubation failure from upper airway obstruction, ineffective cough, excess secretions, or encephalopathy. These modalities are more likely to detect those at risk of load/capacity imbalance or possibly congestive heart failure. Given the very high mortality associated with these latter etiologies, the potential importance of adequate prediction and prevention is great.

Multivariate Predictors

Capdevila et al. studied the utility of 10 "classic weaning criteria" measured after 20 minutes of T-piece breathing including effective cough, coordinated thoracoabdominal movement, absence of sternocleidomastoid muscle participation, respiratory rate < 35 breaths/min, tidal volume > 5 mL/kg, vital capacity > 10 mL/kg, minute ventilation < 10 L/min; $Pao_2 > 60$ mmHg or $Sao_2 > 90\%$, $Paco_2 < 50$ mmHg or pH > 7.30, and chest radiograph showing no new pulmonary infiltrate or pleural effusion. Of the 67 patients satisfying at least 8 or 10 criteria, 12 (18%) required reintubation within 48 hours (19). Unfortunately, this rate of extubation failure is no different from studies that used fewer and simpler criteria.

Other Predictors

Tahvanainen and colleagues found that reintubated patients had lower urine volume and lower respiratory quotient values (77). In addition, 3 days prior to extubation 15% of successfully extubated compared to 44% of reintubated patients had positive blood cultures. Capdevila et al. found that half of patients with a new infiltrate or pleural effusion on chest radiograph failed extubation (19). In their large retrospective study, Rady and Ryan found that admission source, arterial vascular disease, pulmonary hypertension, presence of COPD or asthma, severe left ventricular dysfunction, cardiac shock, reduced hematocrit and albumin, elevated BUN, reduced oxygen delivery, and numerous operative factors were all predictors of extubation failure after cardiac surgery (14).

Monitoring Performance During a Weaning Trial

In two large prospective studies, Esteban and colleagues measured respiratory frequency, heart rate, systolic arterial pressure, and oxygen saturation every 15

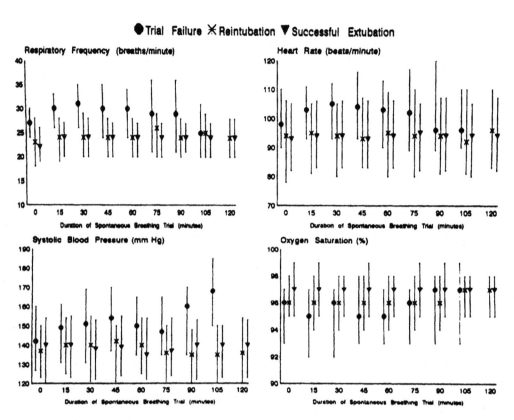

Figure 7 Median (25th–75th percentiles) respiratory frequency, heart rate, systolic blood pressure, and oxygen saturation for patients successfully extubated, reintubated patients (extubation failure) and patients failing a 2-hour spontaneous breathing trial. Using a comparison of the incremental area under the curve, there was no difference between extubation success and extubation failure. (From Ref. 7.)

minutes during a 2-hour trial of T-piece (30 or 120 min duration) or PSV (120 min, 7 cm H_2O) (7,11). Using the incremental area under the curve as a summary statistic, changes in these four variables during the successful weaning trial were not able to distinguish between patients who eventually required reintubation and those successfully extubated (Fig. 7).

VI. Treatment and Prevention of Extubation Failure

Clearly, some etiologies of extubation failure are reversible without the reinstitution of mechanical ventilation. For example, only a minority of patients failing from upper airway obstruction require reintubation (60,62). When postextubation stridor occurs, medical management usually consists of topical epinephrine and/ or corticosteroids. Routine use of dexamethasone prior to extubation does not appear to be more effective than placebo in reversing postextubation laryngeal edema in adults (60). Excessive postextubation secretions are typically treated with inhaled or nebulized bronchodilators, chest physiotherapy, and suctioning of the airway. Postextubation congestive heart failure is treated with diuretics, afterload reduction, and nitroglycerin. This strategy does appear to be effective in treating congestive heart failure occurring during weaning trials (43). When encephalopathy resulting from inadequate recovery from sedative agents leads to extubation failure, antidotes such as flumazenil and naloxone can be effective therapy.

The understanding that extubation failure is associated with increased mortality emphasizes the importance of preventing this outcome. On the other hand, if extubation failure cannot be prevented, then an alternative approach is to prevent the adverse consequences. The observation that patients with delayed reintubation experience higher mortality suggests that early reinstitution of ventilatory support may improve outcome. Physicians may delay reintubation in patients with initial signs of extubation failure, waiting to see if "medical" treatment proves effective. Because extubation failure often implies that "premature extubation" has occurred, its presence can be perceived as an error in decision making. Therefore, physicians may delay reintubation because it would confirm that an error in judgment had occurred. In contrast, "turning the patient around" with medical therapy alone would indicate that the decision to extubate had been the correct one.

Because physicians may be hesitant to resort to invasive ventilation at the earliest signs of distress, noninvasive ventilation has been employed in patients with respiratory failure after extubation (141–143). In a large observational study, Meduri et al. used noninvasive positive pressure ventilation for postextubation respiratory failure in 39 patients (17 with COPD) (142). Six failed to improve gas exchange, five developed complications and 13 (35%) required invasive ventilation. Three patients with upper airway obstruction were supported with NPPV for 18 hours while therapy with corticosteroids and racemic epinephrine was administered. Hilbert and colleagues recently conducted a case control study of noninvasive pressure support (NIPSV) in 30 COPD patients with hypercapneic respiratory failure within 72 hours of extubation (144). These were compared to 30 historical matched controls managed by traditional means. NIPSV was established at 20 ± 13 hours after extubation when respiratory distress was noted (f > 25 breaths/min, 20% increase in $Paco_2$, and pH < 7.35). Among the NIPSV groups fewer patients required invasive ventilation (20% vs. 67%, $p < 0.001$) and the length of ICU stay decreased (8 vs. 14 days, $p < 0.01$). In the control group, the period between extubation and reintubation was approximately 33 hours. Randomized controlled prospective studies examining the role of noninvasive ventilation in preventing extubation failure are needed. Development of accurate predictors are imperative because they would allow identification of a group that might benefit from "routine" use of noninvasive ventilation after extubation. Alternatively, there may be factors detectable in the early postextubation phase (e.g., subtle changes in vital signs, expiratory or inspiratory muscle function) that would signal impending extubation failure and the need for early ventilatory support.

VII. Unplanned Extubation Failure

Unplanned extubation is a major complication of translaryngeal intubation, occurring in 3–16% of mechanically ventilated patients (Table 6). Unplanned extubation can lead to sudden loss of airway control in a critically ill patient with unresolved respiratory failure who may be heavily sedated or paralyzed. Although infrequently reported, death can occur because of immediate complications of failed unplanned extubation (145–149). Unplanned extubation has been

Table 6 Studies of Unplanned Extubation

Study (Ref.)	ICU type	Frequency of unplanned extubation (%)	% Reintubated
Zwillich (97)	Multidisciplinary	8	47
Stauffer (61)	Multidisciplinary	13	
Coppolo (155)	Multidisciplinary	11	31
Little (163)	Pediatric, neonatal	8.9	
Vassal (145)	Medical	12	74
Maguire (164)	Multidisciplinary	5.8	71
Listello (153)	Multidisciplinary		48
Whelan (157)	Medical	7	78
Tindol (156)	Multidisciplinary	3	46
Tominaga (146)	Surgical	5	23
Christie (151)	Trauma, surgical		56
Atkins (150)	Multidisciplinary		74
Chevron (148)	Medical	16	37
Betbese (154)	Multidisciplinary	7	46
Mort (147)	Multidisciplinary	3[a]	30[a]
Boulain (149)	Medical, surgical	11	61
Epstein (152)	Medical	11	56

[a] Percentages from surgical ICUs only.

categorized as either deliberate or accidental, with the vast majority being the former. Deliberate unplanned extubation occurs when the patients pulls the endotracheal tube out by hand or ''tongues'' the tube out. Accidental unplanned extubation occurs when the tube becomes dislodged during nursing care, airway care, or transport or procedures.

After unplanned extubation, 23–78% of patients require reintubation. The overwhelming majority of patients with failed unplanned extubation (62–95%) are reintubated within the first 30–120 minutes (145,147,149–153). Respiratory distress or ventilatory failure (hypoxemia, hypercapnia, tachypnea, increased work of breathing) are the indications for reintubation in 79–91% of unplanned extubation failures (147,151,153). Problems with airway protection or an abnormal mental status have been noted in 8–19% of unplanned extubation failures.

Several studies have examined the rate of complications associated with reintubation for failure of unplanned extubation. Listello and Sessler noted only 5 complications in 81 reintubations (153). In contrast, Atkins observed that a complication rate of 22% including laryngeal edema, prolonged respiratory distress, aspiration, hypotension, and arrhythmias (150). Mort found that 41/57 (72%) patients suffered a total of 102 complications related to reintubation including hemodynamic complications (hypo- or hypertension, tachy- or bradycardia, other arrhythmia, cardiac arrest) and tracheal airway complications (multiple intubation attempts, hypoxemia, esophageal intubation, bronchospasm, right mainstem intubation, accidental extubation, inability to intubate, and cricothyrotomy) (147).

A number of investigators have defined factors that identify patients likely to fail unplanned extubation. The most important of these is the degree of ventilatory support at the time of unplanned extubation. Among patients on full support, 63–82% will require reintubation (152–154). In contrast, when unplanned extubation occurs during weaning trials, the reintubation rate is lower, ranging from 16 to 42%. The extubation failure rate is higher for cases of accidental (range 75–83%) than for deliberate unplanned extubation (range 11–66%) (145,148,151,154,155). Other risk factors associated with unplanned extubation failure include older age, APACHE II > 28, medical rather surgical patients chronic respiratory failure or pulmonary disease, duration of mechanical ventilation, insufficient recovery from the process that led to mechanical ventilation, presence of multiple organ failure, more than two coexisting medical problems, abnormal mental status with GCS < 11, sedation with Ramsay score of 4–6, $Fio_2 > 0.4$ or $Pao_2/Fio_2 < 200$–250, machine-delivered minute ventilation of >7–10 L/min, or ventilator rate > 6 breaths/min (145,148,153,154,156,157).

The majority of studies have detected no increase in mortality when comparing all patients with unplanned extubation to those without unplanned extubation (97,149,150,152,154). In contrast, the mortality is uniformally higher for unplanned extubation failure (range 28–51%) compared to those who do not need reintubation (range 0–21%) (148,150,152,153). Unlike the case with planned extubation, patients with unplanned extubation failure or success may differ significantly in severity of illness, presence of comorbid conditions, or other important factors. To better define the effect of unplanned extubation on outcome, a case-control study of 75 unplanned extubations was undertaken. For each case, two controls were matched for age, APACHE II score, indication for mechanical ventilation, presence of significant comorbid conditions, and gender. Overall mortality was similar between unplanned extubations and controls (32% vs. 30% controls). Mortality for failed unplanned extubation was not significantly elevated when compared to their controls (40% vs. 31%, $p = 0.28$), although increases in duration of mechanical ventilation, ICU stay, hospital stay, and need for transfer to a skilled nursing facility were reported (152). Therefore, in contrast to the experience with planned extubation failure, it appears that unplanned extubation failure does not lead to excess mortality. One explanation for this is the fact that 75% of unplanned failures have ventilatory support reestablished in less than one hour (86% in less than 12 hours). The rapid reinstitution of adequate ventilatory support may prevent deterioration and the subsequent development of organ dysfunction.

VIII. Summary

Numerous factors appear to influence the prevalence of extubation failure, including the patient population studied, patient age, duration of mechanical ventilation prior to extubation, and the use of sedation. Although the pathophysiological causes of weaning failure may also lead to extubation failure, the latter frequently results from entities such as upper airway obstruction, aspiration or an inability to manage pulmonary secretions, cardiac failure, and encephalopathy. Several investigators have now established that extubation failure is independently associated with an increase in the duration of mechanical ventilation, ICU and hospital stay, and, most importantly, an increase in hospital mortality. The etiology of extubation failure is known to be an important determinant of outcome, with patients failing because of airway problems having a lower mortality than those failing for other reasons.

Given the high associated mortality, prevention and treatment of extubation failure are of paramount importance. Unfortunately, traditional parameters, such as the f/V_T or the negative inspiratory force, used to predict weaning outcome have proved much less precise in predicting extubation outcome. Efforts aimed at the period just before (during weaning) or immediately after extubation may help accurately identify patients likely to experience extubation failure. Mortality rises with increasing time between extubation and reintubation, suggesting that clinical deterioration during the period without ventilatory support contributes to excess mortality. The implication of these observations is that early identification of those at risk followed by rapid reinstitution of ventilatory support has the potential to improve the outcome for patients with extubation failure.

References

1. Sahn SA, Lakshminarayan S. Bedside criteria for discontinuation of mechanical ventilation. Chest 1973; 63:1002–1005.
2. Mancebo J. Weaning from mechanical ventilation. Eur Respir J 1996; 9:1923–1931.
3. Ely EW, Baker AM, Dunagan DP, Burke HL, Smith AC, Kelly PT, Johnson MM, Browder RW, Bowton DL, Haponik EF. Effect on the duration of mechanical ventilation of identifying patients capable of breathing spontaneously. N Engl J Med 1996; 335:1864–1869.
4. Kollef MH, Shapiro SD, Silver P, St. John RE, Prentice D, Sauer S, Ahrens TS, Shannon W, Baker-Clinkscale D. A randomized, controlled trial of protocol-directed versus physician-directed weaning from mechanical ventilation. Crit Care Med 1997; 25:567–574.
5. Brochard L, Rauss A, Benito S, Conti G, Mancebo J, Rekik N, Gasparetto A, Lemaire F. Comparison of three methods of gradual withdrawal from ventilatory support during weaning from mechanical ventilation. Am J Respir Crit Care Med 1994; 150:896–903.
6. Esteban A, Frutos F, Tobin MJ, Alia I, Solsona JF, Valverdu I, Fernandez R, de la Cal MA, Benito S, Tomas R, Carriedo D, Macias S, Blanco J. A comparison of four methods of weaning patients from mechanical ventilation. N Engl J Med 1995; 332:345–350.
7. Esteban A, Alia I, Gordo F, Fernandex R, Solsona J, Vallverdu I, Macias S, Allegue J, Blanco J, Carriedo D, Leon M, de la Cal M, Taboada F, Velasco J, Palazon E, Carrizosa F, Tomas R, Suarez J, Goldwasser R. Extubation outcome after spontaneous breathing trials with t-tube or pressure support ventilation. Am J Respir Crit Care Med 1997; 156:459–465.
8. Tomlinson JR, Miller KS, Lorch DG, Smith L, Reines HD, Sahn SA. A prospective comparison of IMV and T-piece weaning from mechanical ventilation. Chest 1989; 96:348–352.
9. Vallverdu I, Calaf N, Subirana M, Net A, Benito S, Mancebo J. Clinical characteristics, respiratory functional parameters, and outcome of two-hour t-piece trial in patients weaning from mechanical ventilation. Am J Respir Crit Care Med 1998; 158:1855–1862.
10. Epstein SK, Ciubotaru RL, Wong JB. Effect of failed extubation on the outcome of mechanical ventilation. Chest 1997; 112:186–192.
11. Esteban A, Alia I, Tobin M, et al. Effect of spontaneous breathing trial duration on outcome of attempts to discontinue mechanical ventilation. Am J Respir Crit Care Med 1999; 159:512–518.

12. Reyes A, Vega G, Blancas R, Morato B, Moreno JL, Torrecilla C, Cereijo E. Early vs conventional extubation after cardiac surgery with cardiopulmonary bypass. Chest 1997; 112:193–201.

13. London M, Shroyer A, Jernigan V, Fullerton D, Wilcox D, Baltz J, Brown J, MaWhinney S, Hammermeister K, Grover F. Fast-track cardiac surgery in a department of veteran affairs patient population. Ann Thorac Surg 1997; 64:134–141.

14. Rady MY, Ryan T. Perioperative predictors of extubation failure and the effect on clinical outcome after cardiac surgery. Crit Care Med 1999; 27:340–347.

15. Jacob B, Chatila W, Manthous C. The unassisted respiratory rate/tidal volume ratio accurately predicts weaning outcome in postoperative patients. Crit Care Med 1997; 25:253–257.

16. Stone WM, Larson JS, Young M, Weaver AL, Lunn JJ. Early extubation after abdominal aortic reconstruction. J Cardiothorac Vasc Anest 1998; 12:174–176.

17. Demling RH, Read T, Lind LJ, Flanagan HL. Incidence and morbidity of extubation failure in surgical intensive care patients. Crit Care Med 1988; 16:573–577.

18. Daley B, Garcia-Perez F, Ross S. Reintubation as an outcome predictor in trauma patients. Chest 1996; 110:1577–1580.

19. Capdevila XJ, Perrigault PF, Perey PJ, Roustan JPA, d'Athis F. Occlusion pressure and its ratio to maximum inspiratory pressure are useful predictors for successful extubation following t-piece weaning trial. Chest 1995; 108:482–489.

20. Del Rosario N, Sasson CS, Chetty KG, Gruer SE, Mahutte CK. Breathing pattern during acute respiratory failure and recovery. Eur Respir J 1997; 10:2560–2565.

21. White DP, Douglas NJ, Pickett CK, Weil JV, Zwillich CW. Sexual influence on the control of breathing. J Appl Physiol 1983; 54:874–879.

22. Epstein SK, Ciubotaru RL. Influence of gender and endotracheal tube size on preextubation breathing pattern. Am J Respir Crit Care Med 1996; 154:1647–1652.

23. Gaebe G, Curley F, Sammon M. Physiologic correlates of rapid shallow breathing (F/VT) during weaning from mechanical ventilation (MV). Am J Respir Crit Care Med 1997; 155:A525.

24. Epstein S, Vuong V. Lack of influence of gender on outcome of mechanically ventilated medical intensive care unit patients. Chest 1999; 116:732–739.

25. Kollef MH, O'Brien JD, Silver P. The impact of gender on outcome from mechanical ventilation. Chest 1997; 111:434–441.

26. Nevins M, Epstein S. Effect of extubation failure on outcome of mechanical ventilation in patients with COPD. Am J Respir Crit Care Med 1999; 159:A373.

27. DeHaven CB, Hurst JM, Branson RD. Evaluation of two different extubation criteria: attributes contributing to success. Crit Care Med 1986; 14:92–94.

28. Lee KH, Hui KP, Chan TB, Tan WC, Lim TK. Rapid shallow breathing (frequency-tidal volume ratio) did not predict extubation outcome. Chest 1994; 105:540–543.

29. Scheinhorn DJ, Artinian BM, Catlin JL. Weaning from prolonged mechanical ventilation. The experience at a regional weaning center. Chest 1994; 105:534–539.

30. Esteban A, Anzueto A, Alia I, Tobin M, Benito S, Brochard L, Stewart T. Clinical characteristics of patients receiving mechanical ventilation. Am J Respir Crit Care Med 1999; 159:A47.

31. Civetta JM. Nosocomial respiratory failure or iatrogenic ventilator dependency. Crit Care Med 1993; 21:171–173.

32. Vassilakopoulos T, Zakynthinos S, Roussos C. The tension-time index and the frequency/tidal volume ratio are the major pathophysiologic determinants of weaning failure and success. Am J Respir Crit Care Med 1998; 158:378–385.

33. Gandia F, Blanco J. Evaluation of indexes predicting the outcome of ventilator weaning and value of adding supplemental inspiratory load. Intensive Care Med 1992; 18:327–333.

34. Nathan SD, Ishaaya AM, Koerner SK, Belman MJ. Prediction of minimal pressure support during weaning from mechanical ventilation. Chest 1993; 103:1215–1219.

35. Ishaaya AM, Nathan SD, Belman MJ. Work of breathing after extubation. Chest 1995; 107:204–209.

36. Jones D, Byrne P, Morgan C, Fraser I, Hyland R. Positive end-expiratory pressure vs T-piece extubation after mechanical ventilation. Chest 1991; 100:1655–1659.

37. Saura P, Blanch L, Mestre J, Valles J, Artigas A, Fernandez R. Clinical consequences of the implementation of a weaning protocol. Intensive Care Med 1996; 22:1052–1056.

38. Cohen IL, Bari N, Strosberg MA, Weinberg PF, Wacksman RM, Millstein BH, Fein IA. Reduction of duration and cost of mechanical ventilation in an intensive care unit by use of a ventilatory management team. Crit Care Med 1991; 19:1278–1284.

39. Ely E, Bennett P, Bowton D, Murphy S, Florance A, Haponik E. Large scale implementation of a respiratory therapist-driven protocol for ventilator weaning. Am J Respir Crit Care Med 1999; 159:439–446.

40. Kollef MH, Levy NT, Ahrens TS, Schaiff R, Prentice D, Sherman G. The use of continuous i.v. sedation is associated with prolongation of mechanical ventilation. Chest 1998; 114:541–548.

41. Jubran A, Tobin MJ. Pathophysiologic basis of acute respiratory distress in patients who fail a trial of weaning from mechanical ventilation. Am J Respir Crit Care Med 1997; 155:906–915.

42. Capdevila X, Perrigault PF, Ramonatxo M, Roustan JP, Peray P, d'Athis F, Prefaut C. Changes in breathing pattern and respiratory muscle performance parameters during difficult weaning. Crit Care Med 1998; 26:79–87.

43. Lemaire F, Teboul J-L, Cinotti L, Giotto G, Abrouk F, Macquin-Mavier I, Zapol WM. Acute left ventricular dysfunction during unsuccessful weaning from mechanical ventilation. Anesthesiology 1988; 69:171–179.

44. Hurford WE, Lynch KE, Strauss HW, Lowenstein E, Zapol WM. Myocardial perfusion as assessed by thallium 201 scintigraphy during the discontinuation of mechanical ventilation in ventilator-dependent patients. Anesthesiology 1991; 74:1007–1016.

45. Hurford WE, Favorito F. Association of myocardial ischemia with failure to wean from mechanical ventilation. Crit Care Med 1995; 23:1475–1480.

46. Holliday JE, Hyers TM. The reduction of weaning time from mechanical ventilation using tidal volume and relaxation biofeedback. Am Rev Respir Dis 1990; 141:1214–1220.

47. Weissman C. Flow-volume relationships during spontaneous breathing through endotracheal tubes. Crit Care Med 1992; 20:615–620.

48. Shapiro M, Wilson RK, Casar G, Bloom K, Teague RB. Work of breathing through different sized endotracheal tubes. Crit Care Med 1986; 14:1028–1031.

49. Bolder PM, Healy TE, Bolder AR, Beatty PC, Kay B. The extra work of breathing through adult endotracheal tubes. Anesth Analg 1986; 65:853–859.

50. Bersten AD, Rutten AJ, Vedig AE, Skowronski GA. Additional work of breathing imposed by endotracheal tubes, breathing circuits, and intensive care ventilators. Crit Care Med 1989; 17:671–677.

51. DeHaven CB, Kirton OC, Morgan JP, Hart AML, Shatz DV, Civetta JM. Breathing measurement reduces fals-negative classification of tachypneic preextubation trial failures. Crit Care Med 1996; 24:976–980.

52. Kirton OC, DeHaven CB, Morgan JP, Windsor J, Civetta JM. Elevated imposed work of breathing masquerading as ventilator weaning intolerance. Chest 1995; 108:1021–1025.

53. Wright PE, Marini JJ, Bernard GR. In vitro versus in vivo comparison of endotracheal tube airflow resistance. Am Rev Respir Dis 1989; 140:10–16.

54. Straus C, Louis B, Isabey D, Lemaire F, Harf A, Brochard L. Contribution of the endotracheal tube and the upper airway to breathing workload. Am J Respir Crit Care Med 1998; 157:23–30.

55. Colice G, Stukel T, Dain B. Laryngeal complications of prolonged intubation. Chest 1989; 96:877–884.

56. Whited R. A prospective study of laryngotracheal sequelae in long-term intubation. Laryngoscope 1984; 94:367–377.

57. Miller R, Cole R. Association between reduced cuff leak volume and postextubation stridor. Chest 1996; 110:1035–1040.

58. Kastanos N, Estopa Miro R, Marin Perez A, et al. Laryngotracheal injury due to endotracheal intubation: incidence, evolution and predisposing factors: a prospective long term study. Crit Care Med 1983; 11:362–367.

59. Rashkin M, Davis T. Acute complications of endotracheal intubation: relationship to reintubation, route, urgency and duration. Chest 1986; 89:165–167.

60. Darmon J-Y, Rauss A, Dreyfuss D, Bleichner G, Elkharrat D, Schlemmer B, Tenaillon A, Brun-Boisson C, Huet Y. Evaluation of risk factors for laryngeal edema after tracheal extubation in adults and its prevention by dexamethasone. Anesthesiology 1992; 77:245–251.

61. Stauffer JL, Olson DE, Petty TL. Complications and consequences of endotracheal intubation and tracheotomy. A prospective study of 150 critically ill adult patients. Am J Med 1981; 70:65–76.

62. Ho LI, Harn HJ, Lien TC, Hu PY, Wang JH. Postextubation laryngeal edema in adults. Risk factor evaluation and prevention by hydrocortisone. Intensive Care Med 1996; 22:933–936.

63. Pavlin EG, Holle RH, Schoene RB. Recovery of airway protection compared with ventilation in humans after paralysis with curare. Anesthesiology 1989; 70:381–385.

64. Burgess GE, Cooper JR, Marino RJ, et al. Laryngeal competence after tracheal extubation. Anesthesiology 1979; 51:73–77.

65. de Larminat V, Montravers P, Dureuil B, Desmonts J-M. Alteration in swallowing reflex after extubation in intensive care unit patients. Crit Care Med 1995; 23:486–490.

66. Leder S, Cohn S, Moller B. Fiberoptic endoscopic documentation of the high inci-

dence of aspiration following extubation in critically ill trauma patients. Dysphagia 1998; 13:208–212.

67. Tolep KA, Getch CL, Criner GJ. Swallowing dysfunction in patients receiving prolonged mechanical ventilation. Chest 1996; 109:167–173.

68. Bach J, Saporto L. Criteria for extubation and tracheostomy tube removal for patients with ventilatory failure. Chest 1996; 110:1566–1571.

69. Mier A, Laroche C, Agnew JE, Vora H, Clarke SW, Green M, Pavia D. Tracheobronchial clearance in patients with bilateral diaphragmatic weakness. Am Rev Respir Dis 1990; 142:545–548.

70. Aubier M, Trippenbach T, Roussos C. Respiratory muscle fatigue during cardiogenic shock. J Appl Physiol 1981; 51:499–508.

71. Mancini DM, Henson D, LaManca J, Levine S. Respiratory muscle function and dyspnea in patients with chronic congestive heart failure. Circulation 1992; 86: 909–918.

72. Nishimura Y, Maeda H, Tanaka K, Nakamura H, Hashimoto Y, Yokoyama M. Respiratory muscle strength and hemodynamics in chronic heart failure. Chest 1994; 105:355–359.

73. Chatila W, Ani S, Guaglianone D, Jacob B, Amoateng-Adjepong Y, Manthous C. Cardiac ischemia during weaning from mechanical ventilation. Chest 1996; 109: 1577–1583.

74. Esteban A, Alia I, Ibanez J, Benito S, Tobin MJ. Modes of mechanical ventilation and weaning. A national survey of Spanish hospitals. The Spanish Lung Failure Collaborative Group. Chest 1994; 106:1188–1193.

75. Epstein SK. Etiology of extubation failure and the predictive value of the rapid shallow breathing index. Am J Respir Crit Care Med 1995; 152:545–549.

76. Epstein SK, Ciubotaru RL. Independent effects of etiology of failure and time to reintubation on outcome for patients failing extubation. Am J Respir Crit Care Med 1998; 158:489–493.

77. Tahvanainen J, Salmenpera M, Nikki P. Extubation criteria after weaning from intermittent mandatory ventilation and continuous positive airway pressure. Crit Care Med 1983; 11:702–707.

78. Harel Y, Vardi A, Quigley R, Brink LW, Manning SC, Carmody TJ, Levin DL. Extubation failure due to post-extubation stridor is better correlated with neurologic impairment than with upper airway lesions in critically ill pediatric patients. Int J Pediatr Otorhinolaryngol 1997; 39:147–158.

79. Brochard L, Rua F, Lorino H, et al. Inspiratory pressure support compensates for the additional work of breathing caused by the endotracheal tube. Anesthesiology 1991; 75:739–745.

80. Murciano D, Boczkowski J, Lecocguic Y, Milic-Emili J, Patiente R, Aubier M. Tracheal occlusion pressure: a simple index to monitor respiratory muscle fatigue during acute respiratory failure in patients with chronic obstructive pulmonary disease. Ann Intern Med 1988; 108:800–805.

81. Menzies R, Gibbons W, Goldberg P. Determinants of weaning and survival among patients with COPD who require mechanical ventilation for acute respiratory failure. Chest 1989; 95:398–405.

82. Rieves RD, Bass D, Carter RR, Griffith JE, Norman JR. Severe COPD and acute

respiratory failure: correlates for survival at the time of tracheal intubation. Chest 1993; 104:854–860.

83. Connors AF, Dawson NV, Thomas C, Harrell FE, Desbiens N, Fulkerson WJ, Kussin P, Bellamy P, Goldman L, Knaus WA. Outcomes following acute exacerbations of severe chronic obstructive lung disease. Am J Respir Crit Care Med 1996; 154: 959–967.

84. Kaelin RM, Assimacopoulos A, Chevrolet JC. Failure to predict six-month survival of patients with COPD requiring mechanical ventilation by analysis of simple indices; a prospective study. Chest 1987; 92:971–978.

85. Doyle RL, Szaflarski N, Modin GW, Wiener-Kronish JP, Matthay MA. Identification of patients with acute lung injury: predictors of mortality. Am J Respir Crit Care Med 1995; 152:1818–1824.

86. Zilberberg MD, Epstein SK. Acute lung injury in the medical ICU: comorbid conditions, age, etiology, and hospital outcome. Am J Respir Crit Care Med 1998; 157: 1159–1164.

87. Suchyta MR, Clemmer TP, Elliott CG, Orme JF, Weaver LK. The adult respiratory distress syndrome: a report on survival and modifying factors. Chest 1992; 101: 1074–1079.

88. Crawford SW, Schwartz DA, Petersen FB, Clark JG. Mechanical ventilation after marrow transplantation: risk factors and clinical outcome. Am Rev Respir Dis 1988; 137:682–687.

89. Crawford SW, Petersen FB. Long-term survival from respiratory failure after marrow transplantation for malignancy. Am Rev Respir Dis 1992; 145:510–514.

90. Staikowsky F, Lafon B, Guidet B, Denis M, Mayaud C, Offenstadt G. Mechanical ventilation for *Pneumocystis carinii* pneumonia in patients with the acquired immunodeficiency syndrome. Is the prognosis really improved? Chest 1993; 104:756–762.

91. Rosen MJ, Clayton K, Schneider RF, Fulkerson W, Rao AV, Stansell J, Kvale PA, Glassroth J, Reichman LB, Wallace JM, Hopewell PC. Intensive care of patients with HIV infection: utilization, critical illnesses, and outcomes. Pulmonary Complications of HIV Infection Study Group. Am J Respir Crit Care Med 1997; 155:67–71.

92. Matuschak GM, Shaw BW, Jr. Adult respiratory distress syndrome associated with acute liver allograft rejection: resolution following hepatic retransplantation. Crit Care Med 1987; 15:878–881.

93. Zimmerman JE, Wagner DP, Seneff MG, Becker RB, Sun X, Knaus WA. Intensive care unit admissions with cirrhosis: risk-stratifying patient groups and predicting individual survival. Hepatology 1996; 23:1393–1401.

94. Schuster DP, Marion JM. Precedents for meaningful recovery during treatment in a medical intensive care unit: outcome in patients with hematologic malignancy. Am J Med 1983; 75:402–408.

95. Schapira DV, Studnicki J, Bradham DD, Wolff P, Jarrett A. Intensive care, survival, and expense of treating critically ill cancer patients. JAMA 1993; 269:783–786.

96. Fedullo A, Swinburned A, Wahl G, Bixby K. Acute cardiogenic pulmonary edema treated with mechanical ventilation: factors determining in-hospital mortality. Chest 1991; 99:1220–1226.

97. Zwillich CW, Pierson DJ, Creagh CE, Sutton FD, Schatz E, Petty TL. Complications of assisted ventilation. A prospective study of 354 consecutive episodes. Am J Med 1974; 57:161–170.

98. Schwartz D, Matthay M, Cohen N. Death and other complications of emergency airway management in critically ill adults. Anesthesiology 1995; 82:367–376.

99. Rashkin MC, Davis T. Acute complications of endotracheal intubation: relationship to reintubation, route, urgency, and duration. Chest 1986; 89:165–167.

100. Torres A, Aznar R, Gatell JM, Jimenez P, Gonzalez J, Ferrer A, Celis R, Rodriguez-Roisin R. Incidence, risk, and prognosis factors of nosocomial pneumonia in mechanically ventilated patients. Am Rev Respir Dis 1990; 142:523–528.

101. Torres A, Gatell JM, Aznar E, el-Ebiary M, Puig de la Bellacasa J, Gonzalez J, Ferrer M, Rodriguez-Roisin R. Re-intubation increases the risk of nosocomial pneumonia in patients needing mechanical ventilation. Am J Respir Crit Care Med 1995; 152:137–141.

102. Wood KA, Lewis L, Von Harz B, Kollef MH. The use of noninvasive positive pressure ventilation in the emergency department: results of a randomized clinical trial. Chest 1998; 113:1339–1346.

103. Esteban A, Anzueto A, Alia I, Tobin M, Benito S, Brochard L, Stewart T. Mortality of patients receiving mechanical ventilation. Am J Respir Crit Care Med 1999; 159:A47.

104. Pingleton SK. Complications of acute respiratory failure. Am Rev Respir Dis 1988; 137:1463–1493.

105. Fagon JY, Chastre J, Hance AJ, Montravers P, Novara A, Gibert C. Nosocomial pneumonia in ventilated patients: a cohort study evaluating attributable mortality and hospital stay. Am J Med 1993; 94:281–288.

106. Harris SK, Bone RC, Ruth WT. Gastrointestinal hemorrhage in patients in a respiratory intensive care unit. Chest 1977; 72:301–304.

107. Epstein S, Picken H. Application of decision analysis principles to predicting weaning and extubation outcome. Clin Pulm Med 1997; 4:283–291.

108. Chatila W, Jacob B, Guaglionone D, Manthous CA. The unassisted respiratory rate-tidal volume ratio accurately predicts weaning outcome. Am J Med 1996; 101:61–67.

109. Dojat M, Harf A, Touchard D, Laforest M, Lemaire F, Brochard L. Evaluation of a knowledge-based system providing ventilatory management and decision for extubation. Am J Respir Crit Care Med 1996; 153:997–1004.

110. Yang KL, Tobin MJ. A prospective study of indexes predicting the outcome of trials of weaning from mechanical ventilation. N Engl J Med 1991; 324:1445–1450.

111. Krieger BP, Ershowsky PF, Becker DA, Gazeroglu HB. Evaluation of conventional criteria for predicting successful weaning from mechanical ventilatory support in elderly patients. Crit Care Med 1989; 17:858–861.

112. Khan N, Brown A, Venkataraman ST. Predictors of extubation success and failure in mechanically ventilated infants and children. Crit Care Med 1996; 24:1568–1579.

113. Jaeschke R, Meade M, Guyatt G, Keenan S, Cook D. How to use diagnostic test

articles in the intensive care unit: diagnosing weanability using the f/Vt. Crit Care Med 1997; 25:1514–1521.

114. Corson JA, Grant JL, Moulton DP, Green RL, Dunkel PT. Use of biofeedback in weaning paralyzed patients from respirators. Chest 1979; 76:543–545.

115. Blumenstein B, Beslav I, Bar-Eli M, Tenenbaum G, Weinstein Y. Regulation of mental states and biofeedback techniques: effects on breathing pattern. Biofeed Self-Reg 1995; 20:169–183.

116. LaRicchia PJ, Katz RH, Peters JW, Atkinson GW, Weiss T. Biofeedback and hypnosis in weaning from mechanical ventilators. Chest 1985; 87:267–269.

117. Mador MJ, Tobin MJ. Effect of alterations in mental activity on the breathing pattern in healthy subjects. Am Rev Respir Dis 1991; 144:481–487.

118. Tobin MJ, Chadha TS, Jenouri G, Birch SJ, Gazeroglu HB, Sackner MA. Breathing patterns: normal subjects. Chest 1983; 84:202–205.

119. Mehta S, Nelson G, Buczko G, Levy M. The effect of endotracheal tube size on respiratory frequency. Am J Respir Crit Care Med 1998; 147:A224.

120. Amoateng-Adjepong Y, Jacob BK, Ahmad M, Manthous CA. The effect of sepsis on breathing pattern and weaning outcomes in patients recovering from respiratory failure. Chest 1997; 112:472–477.

121. Krieger BP, Isber J, Breitenbucher A, Throop G, Ershowsky P. Serial measurements of the rapid-shallow-breathing index as a predictor of weaning outcome in elderly medical patients. Chest 1997; 112:1029–1034.

122. Vitacca M, Clini E, Spassini W, Scaglia L, Negrini P, Quadri A. Does the supine position worsen respiratory function in elderly subjects? Gerontology 1996; 42: 46–53.

123. Tobin MJ, Chadha TS, Jenouri G, et al. Breathing patterns 2. Disease subjects. Chest 1983; 84:286–294.

124. Tobin MJ, Perez W, Guenther SM, Semmes BJ, Mador MJ, Allen SJ, Lodato RF, Dantzker DR. The pattern of breathing during successful and unsuccessful trials of weaning from mechanical ventilation. Am Rev Respir Dis 1986; 134:1111–1118.

125. Krieger BP, Ershowsky P. Noninvasive detection of respiratory failure in the intensive care unit. Chest 1988; 94:254–261.

126. Truwit J, Marini J. Evaluation of thoracic mechanics in the ventilated patient: primary measurements. J Crit Care 1988; 3:133–140.

127. Fisher MM, Raper RF. The "cuff lead" test for extubation. Anaesthesia 1992; 47: 10–12.

128. Kemper K, Benson M, Bishop M. Predictors of post-extubation stridor in pediatric trauma patients. Crit Care Med 1991; 19:352–355.

129. Shikora SA, Benotti PN, Johannigman JA. The oxygen cost of breathing may predict weaning from mechanical ventilation better than the respiratory rate to tidal volume ratio. Arch Surg 1994; 129:269–274.

130. Hubmayr RD, Loosbrock LM, Gillespie DJ, Rodarte JR. Oxygen uptake during weaning from mechanical ventilation. Chest 1988; 94:1148–1155.

131. Fiastro JF, Habib MP, Shon BY, Campbell SC. Comparison of standard weaning parameters and the mechanical work of breathing in mechanically ventilated patients. Chest 1988; 94:232–238.

132. Annat GJ, Viale JP, Dereymez CP, Bouffard YM, Delafosse BX, Motin JP. Oxygen cost of breathing and diaphragmatic pressure time index: measurement in patients with COPD during weaning with pressure support ventilation. Chest 1990; 98:411–414.

133. Banner MJ, Kirby RR, Blanch PB, Layon AJ. Decreasing imposed work of the breathing apparatus to zero using pressure-support ventilation. Crit Care Med 1993; 21:1333–1338.

134. Banner MJ, Kirby RR, Kirton OC, DeHaven CB, Blanch PB. Breathing frequency and pattern are poor predictors of work of breathing in patients receiving pressure support ventilation. Chest 1995; 108:1338–1344.

135. Gluck EH, Barkoviak MJ, Balk RA, Casey LC, Silver MR, Bone RC. Medical effectiveness of esophageal balloon pressure manometry in weaning patients from mechanical ventilation. Crit Care Med 1995; 23:504–509.

136. Levy MM, Miyasaki A, Langston D. Work of breathing as a weaning parameter in mechanically ventilated patients. Chest 1995; 108:1018–1020.

137. Whitelaw WA, Derenne JP, Milic-Emili J. Occlusion pressure as a measure of respiratory center output in conscious man. Respir Physiol 1975; 23:181–199.

138. Sassoon CSH, Te TT, Mahutte CK, Light RW. Airway occlusion pressure; an important indicator for successful weaning in patients with chronic obstructive pulmonary disease. Am Rev Respir Dis 1987; 135:107–113.

139. Sassoon CSH, Mahutte CK. Airway occlusion pressure and breathing pattern as predictors of weaning outcome. Am Rev Respir Dis 1993; 148:860–866.

140. Montgomery AB, Holle RHO, Neagley SR, Pierson DJ, Schoene RB. Prediction of successful ventilator weaning using airway occlusion pressure and hypercapnic challenge. Chest 1987; 91:496–499.

141. Magel JR, McArdle WD, Toner M, Delio DJ. Metabolic and cardiovascular adjustment to arm training. J Appl Physiol 1978; 45:75–79.

142. Meduri GU, Turner RE, Abou-Shala N, Wunderink RG, Tolley E. Noninvasive positive pressure ventilation via face mask: first-line intervention in patients with acute hypercapnic and hypoxemic respiratory failure. Chest 1996; 109:179–193.

143. Wysocki M, Tric L, Wolff M, Millet H, Herman B. Noninvasive pressure support ventilationin patients with acute respiratory failure. A randomized comparison with conventional therapy. Chest 1995; 107:761–768.

144. Hilbert G, Gruson D, Portel L, Gbikpi-Benissan G, Cardinaud J. Noninvasive pressure support ventilation in COPD patients with postextubation hypercapnic respiratory insufficiency. Eur Respir J 1998; 11:1349–1353.

145. Vassal T, Anh NG, Gabillet JM, Guidet B, Staikowsky F, Offenstadt G. Prospective evaluation of self-extubations in a medical intensive care unit. Intensive Care Med 1993; 19:340–342.

146. Tominaga G, Rudzwick H, Scannell G, Waxman K. Decreasing unplanned extubations in the surgical intensive care unit. Am J Surg 1995; 170:586–590.

147. Mort T. Unplanned tracheal extubation outside the operating room: a quality improvement audit of hemodynamic and tracheal airway complications associated with emergent tracheal intubation. Anesth Analg 1998; 86:1171–1176.

148. Chevron V, Menard JF, Richard JC, Girault C, Leroy J, Bonmarchand G. Un-

planned extubation: risk factors of development and predictive criteria for reintubation. Crit Care Med 1998; 26:1049–1053.

149. Boulain T. Unplanned extubations in the adult intensive care unit: a prospective multicenter study. Association des Reanimateurs du Centre-Ouest. Am J Respir Crit Care Med 1998; 157:1131–1137.

150. Atkins PM, Mion LC, Mendelson W, Palmer RM, Slomka J, Franko T. Characteristics and outcomes of patients who self-extubate from ventilatory support: a case-control study. Chest 1997; 112:1317–1323.

151. Christie JM, Dethlefsen M, Cane RD. Unplanned endotracheal extubation in the intensive care unit. J Clin Anesth 1996; 8:289–293.

152. Epstein S. Effect of unplanned extubation on outcome of mechanically venilated medical intensive care unit patients: a case control study. Am J Respir Crit Care Med 1999; 159:A372.

153. Listello D, Sessler CN. Unplanned extubation. Clinical predictors for reintubation. Chest 1994; 105:1496–1503.

154. Betbese AJ, Perez M, Bak E, Rialp G, Mancebo J. A prospective study of unplanned endotracheal extubation in intensive care unit patients. Crit Care Med 1998; 26: 1180–1186.

155. Coppolo DP, May JJ. Self-extubations. A 12-month experience. Chest 1990; 98: 165–169.

156. Tindol GA, Jr., DiBenedetto RJ, Kosciuk L. Unplanned extubations. Chest 1994; 105:1804–1807.

157. Whelan J, Simpson SQ, Levy H. Unplanned extubation. Predictors of successful termination of mechanical ventilatory support. Chest 1994; 105:1808–1812.

158. Schachter EN, Tucker D, Beck GJ. Does intermittent mandatory ventilation accelerate weaning? JAMA 1981; 246:1210–1214.

159. Stauffer JL, Fayter NA, Graves B, Cromb M, Lynch JC, Goebel P. Survival following mechanical ventilation for acute respiratory failure in adult men. Chest 1993; 104:1222–1229.

160. Mohsenifar Z, Hay A, Hay J, Lewis MI, Koerner SK. Gastric intramuralpH as a predictor of success or failure in weaning patients from mechanical ventilation. Ann Intern Med 1993; 119:794–798.

161. Leitch EA, Moran JL, Grealy B. Weaning and extubation in the intensive care unit. Clinical or index-driven approach? Intensive Care Med 1996; 22:752–759.

162. Davis K, Jr., Campbell RS, Johannigman JA, Valente JF, Branson RD. Changes in respiratory mechanics after tracheostomy. Arch Surg 1999; 134:59–62.

163. Little LA, Koenig JC, Jr., Newth CJ. Factors affecting accidental extubations in neonatal and pediatric intensive care patients. Crit Care Med 1990; 18:163–165.

164. Maguire GP, DeLorenzo LJ, Moggio RA. Unplanned extubation in the intensive care unit: a quality-of-care concern. Crit Care Nurs Q 1994; 17:40–47.

22

"Pulling the Plug"
Ethical Considerations in the Withholding and Withdrawal of Mechanical Ventilation

JOHN M. LUCE

University of California
San Francisco, California

I. Introduction

Mechanical ventilation is a medical intervention that supports patients who otherwise would die from acute or chronic respiratory failure or other conditions. Although several forms of mechanical ventilation have been used for this purpose, including negative-pressure ventilation achieved with an "iron lung" or chest cuirass, positive-pressure ventilation is the form most commonly employed today. Furthermore, although positive-pressure ventilation can be delivered through a tightly fitting face mask, a technique called noninvasive ventilation, it is most commonly administered via an endotracheal or tracheotomy tube. Thus, endotracheal intubation remains an essential component of mechanical ventilation for most patients in critical care units.

Mechanical ventilation can be used in a variety of settings; for example, patients with chronic respiratory failure can receive either negative- or positive-pressure ventilation at home or in long-term care facilities. Nevertheless, most patients with acute respiratory failure are ventilated in intensive care units (ICUs), where more nursing attention and oversight are available. Indeed, ICUs were originally developed to house and treat patients with neuromuscular weakness due to poliomyelitis and patients who were recovering from general anesthesia and surgery. Today, mechanical ventilation is synonymous with critical care medicine in the minds of many people, and it is not unusual to find that most patients in a given medical-surgical ICU are receiving positive-pressure ventilation.

Because mechanical ventilation can save and sustain life, it is rightly regarded as "one of the most important high-technology advances in contemporary medicine," in the words of Schneiderman and Spragg (1). At the same time, however, mechanical ventilation is seen as a source of ethical dilemmas because some patients supported by it may never recover from their underlying illnesses. Examples include chronic obstructive pulmonary disease causing chronic respiratory failure or multiple organ system failure requiring ongoing ventilatory support. Patients with these illnesses and conditions may themselves question the desirability of continuing treatment indefinitely, as may their families and other surrogates. Similarly, physicians may wonder whether initiating or continuing mechanical ventilation is appropriate for patients with advanced cancer or a persistent vegetative state.

In some underdeveloped countries, the ethical dilemmas created by mechanical ventilation relate to the relative unavailability of ventilators (and ICUs, for that matter) and the large number of acutely or chronically ill patients who might benefit from them. Such dilemmas usually involve the issue of distributive justice and the allocation of scarce medical resources. In the United States, Canada, and other developed nations, however, mechanical ventilators, like ICUs, are ubiquitous, at least in urban areas. As a result, at issue is not what patients should have access to mechanical ventilation but, rather, in which patients this treatment is more likely to cause harm than to confer benefit.

In part because it is so well known to the public and to health professionals, mechanical ventilation have become a symbol of both the therapeutic potential and the ethical complexity of modern medicine. As one manifestation of this symbolism, the term "pulling the plug," which might apply to disconnecting any piece of electrically powered equipment, is not only widely used to describe limiting life-sustaining treatment in general, but is also specifically identified with termination of mechanical ventilation. In this regard, "pulling the plug" refers not only to the act of removing the ventilator from the patient or never starting ventilation in the first place, but also to the state of mind of the persons who sanction or perform the act. Thus, "pulling the plug" is tantamount to "calling it quits," giving up hope," "letting nature take its course," and "ending dependence on a machine."

II. Case Law

Another reason for the symbolic importance of mechanical ventilation is that most case law regarding the withholding and withdrawal of life support in the

United States has come from situations in which mechanical ventilation was not started or was removed. The first such case was that of Karen Ann Quinlan in 1976 (2), in which the father of a girl who was in a persistent vegetative state petitioned the court to be appointed guardian with the power to discontinue ventilation. The lower court denied the petition, but the New Jersey Supreme Court reversed the decision. In doing so, the court argued that patients such as Ms. Quinlan had a right to privacy that allowed them to refuse unwanted medical interventions.

The New Jersey Supreme Court reasoned that patients generally would accept or refuse treatment based on its ability to support sentient life over mere biological existence. Having concluded that had Ms. Quinlan been capable of making decisions herself, she would have forgone therapy that could only prolong biological life but not sentient life, the court decided that her right to privacy would be abrogated if it prevented the exercise of that right on her behalf. The court, therefore, granted the father's petition, allowing him to exercise "substituted judgment" for his daughter and stated that life support could be withdrawn if her physicians and a hospital ethics committee agreed that such support did not alter Ms. Quinlan's underlying condition. After such agreement was reached, the ventilator was removed from Ms. Quinlan, who breathed without the ventilator for many years.

The 1983 case of *Barber v. Los Angeles County Superior Court* (3) involved two California physicians whose patient, Mr. Herbert, suffered cardiopulmonary arrest after revision of an ileostomy. Five days later, after determining that his coma was irreversible and with the consent of his family, the physicians withdrew mechanical ventilation along with intravenous fluids and nutrition. The physicians then were accused of murder by a district attorney. After the case was heard by several courts, the California Court of Appeals ruled that because the physicians considered it medically futile to continue treatment and obtained the agreement of Mr. Herbert's family, they had performed their duty to the patient and were not guilty of murder.

In reaching its decision, the Court of Appeals rejected the idea that removing mechanical ventilation once it had been initiated was ethically different from not starting mechanical ventilation to begin with. Instead, it argued, any and all therapies can be withheld or withdrawn if they are not beneficial or are disproportionately burdensome. In the court's words, "Even though these life support devices are, to a degree, 'self-propelled,' each pulse of the respirator or each drop of fluid introduced into the patient's body by intravenous feeding devices is comparable to a manually administered injection or item of medications. Hence, 'disconnecting' of the mechanical devices is comparable to withholding the manually administered injection or medication."

In *Quinlan* and *Barber*, the courts made it abundantly clear that patients and their surrogates can refuse mechanical ventilation. Nevertheless, the court's position on whether patients and surrogates can successfully demand mechanical ventilation is less certain. The 1991 case of Helen Wanglie (4) involved an elderly woman who had a cardiopulmonary arrest during an attempt at weaning from mechanical ventilation at a long-term care facility. She was returned to Hennepin County Medical Center in Minneapolis in a vegetative state. Ms. Wanglie's physician recommended to her husband and children that life-sustaining therapy be withdrawn. However, the family insisted that it be continued because they and Mrs. Wanglie valued life at all costs.

Eventually a new physician told the family that he did not wish to continue mechanical ventilation because it would not heal Mrs. Wanglie's lungs nor end her unconsciousness and was not beneficial. After the family tried and failed to find another facility willing to care for the patient, the medical center asked a district court first to appoint a conservator other than Mr. Wanglie to decide if ventilation was beneficial and, second, for a hearing to determine whether ventilation was required if its benefit could not be confirmed. The court refused to replace Mr. Wanglie on the grounds that he could best represent his wife's interests. Because Mrs. Wanglie died before a hearing could be held, the issues of whether ventilation was beneficial and whether physicians could override family wishes were not resolved.

The most recent case to explore whether physicians can override family wishes involved another elderly woman named Catherine Gilgunn, who was being cared for at Massachusetts General Hospital (5). Mrs. Gilgunn was comatose with multiple medical problems. Although her husband and two of her daughters agreed to physician recommendations for a do-not-resuscitate (DNR) order, another daughter disagreed, and the DNR order was rescinded. At a subsequent meeting to discuss the DNR order, this daughter stormed out after physicians recommended limiting further treatment.

After this event, the other two daughters agreed to reinstate the DNR order, and the ventilator was removed from Mrs. Gilgunn. The daughter who had refused the DNR order then brought action against her mother's physicians and the hospital on the basis of her own suffering. Subsequently, a Suffolk County Superior Court jury absolved the physicians and the hospital of liability, apparently because they believed that Mrs. Gilgunn could not benefit from mechanical ventilation even if she might have wanted to be kept alive. Thus, for the first time, a U.S. jury determined that life-sustaining treatment may be discontinued despite the objections of patients or their surrogates.

III. Limiting Treatment

Although cases such as *Gilgunn* suggest that life support can be withheld or withdrawn unilaterally on the part of physicians, it must be stressed that almost all decisions to limit treatment are reached through a consensus involving caregivers, patients, and their families. Furthermore, such decisions are increasingly commonplace, at least in ICUs. In this regard, observational studies from ICUs at the University of Minnesota (6) and the University of Rochester (7) and at several academic and community hospitals in Canada (8,9) have demonstrated that the majority of patients who die do so after the withholding or withdrawal of life support. In addition, sequential studies (10,11) conducted in the medical-surgical ICUs of two hospitals affiliated with the University of California, San Francisco (UCSF), indicate that the incidence of withholding and withdrawal of life support increased from 51% of patients in 1987–1988 to 90% of patients in 1992–1993.

Perhaps the best illustration of how common treatment is limited in America comes from an observational study (12) of end-of-life care involved over a 6-month period in 1994 and 1995 in 131 ICUs at 110 hospitals with critical care training programs in 38 states. A total of 24,502 patients were admitted to these ICUs during the study period, 6303 of whom died (9% ICU mortality rate). Of the 6303 patients who died, 393 were brain dead. Of the 5910 remaining patients who faced end-of-life decisions, 74% received less than full ICU support; the median proportions of ICU deaths after full support, including cardiopulmonary resuscitation (CPR), full support without CPR, withholding of life support, and withdrawal of life support, were 23, 22, 10, and 38%, respectively.

Although limiting treatment was common in the study ICUs, there was wide variation in practice among them, with ranges of 4–79%, 0–83%, 0–67%, and 0–79% in the four categories listed in the previous paragraph (12). Variation was not related to ICU type (medical, surgical, medical-surgical, or other), hospital type (academic, community, public, veterans, other), region of the country, number of admissions, or mortality. However, a pattern was noted in the two regions of the United States that included states with strict legal standards for withdrawal of support by surrogate decision makers. Thus, ICUs in New York and Missouri had lower proportions of deaths preceded by withdrawal of life support than did the Middle Atlantic and Midwest regions.

In addition to reflecting the influence of state statutes, the wide variation in end-of-life care observed in American ICUs presumably results in differences among the types of patients admitted to the units, their attitudes and those of their surrogates, and the attitudes of the physicians caring for them. Regarding physician attitudes, one survey (13) of critical care practitioners who were members of the American Thoracic Society revealed that most such practitioners consider limiting treatment appropriate in many circumstances and that they incorporate some concept of futility into decision making at the bedside. Another survey (14) using clinical vignettes demonstrated that internists at the University of Pennsylvania preferred to withdraw therapy if it supported organs that failed for natural rather than iatrogenic reasons. Treatment that was recently instituted rather than long-standing resulted in immediate death rather than prolonged death or in delayed death in the face of with diagnostic uncertainty. In keeping with these attitudes, the internists chose to withdraw, in order, blood products, hemodialysis, vasopressors, total parenteral nutrition, antibiotics, mechanical ventilation, tube feedings, and finally intravenous fluids. Many of the respondents to this survey probably had limited contact with critically ill patients. Furthermore, their choices of therapies to withdraw were expressed in response to hypothetical situations, not real events. Finally, the responses were restricted to the withdrawal of a single form of life support, whereas in reality more than a single form may be withdrawn sequentially or at the same time. Nevertheless, the study suggests that removing mechanical ventilation is difficult for many physicians, including some who work in ICUs.

Despite this difficulty, and despite the symbolic importance of mechanical ventilation, most studies of withholding and withdrawal of life support from critically ill patients suggest that mechanical ventilation sometimes is not administered and frequently is removed. For example, in the studies (10,11) from medical-surgical ICUs associated with UCSF, mechanical ventilation was the second most commonly withheld intervention after vasopressors and was the intervention most commonly withdrawn after reductions in the inspired oxygen fraction (FIO_2), ventilation rate, and level of positive end-expiratory pressure (PEEP). In the study (7) from the University of Rochester, 27 of 28 patients from whom life support was withdrawn were receiving mechanical ventilation, and 23 had it discontinued; 4 continued to be ventilated but died after other treatments were removed. And in the study (6) from the University of Minnesota, which included non-ICU and ICU patients, 26 of 52 patients in whom treatment was limited were being mechanically ventilated; of these 26 patients, 11 died while receiving ventilatory support, 8 died during incremental decreases or support (including reduction in the FIO_2, ventilator rate, or PEEP level), and 6 died within hours of extubation.

IV. Terminal Weaning

The process of reducing the FIO_2, ventilator rate, and PEEP level before removing the ventilator or extubating the patient is called terminal weaning. As first described by Grenvik (15) in 1983, terminal weaning was developed to avoid abruptly discontinuing treatment in such a way that "might be interpreted with intent to kill." In terminal weaning from mechanical ventilation, Grenvik and his associates "continue to analyze arterial blood gases in order to know how close the patient may be to a final cardiac arrest or whether the patient surprisingly may be able to maintain his or her spontaneous breathing sufficiently for a temporary time period (compare the situation of Karen Ann Quinlan, who continued to breathe spontaneously for more than 7 years after discontinuation of mechanical ventilation, although in a permanently unconscious condition). According to Grenvik,

> Terminal weaning proceeds quickly, over several hours rather than several days. Many patients die in this phase. A few survive to the point of spontaneous breathing and, occasionally, we are able to extubate these patients. Some need to remain intubated to avoid sudden airway obstruction which causes a relatively abrupt, rather than the intended peaceful, death taking place over a few hours. In the past, a tracheostomy was performed to avoid the airway obstruction/suffocation type of death; this procedure is avoided today, as it does not benefit the patient. For those patients with gasping or other distressful signs, we provide increments of morphine IV, 1–2 mg at a time, to decrease reflex response to hypoxia and also to reduce metabolism and, thus, oxygen demand. This therapy provides comfort to the relatives who want their loved one to die quietly without "signs of suffering." Further, it has a comforting effect on the ICU personnel.

Terminal weaning has taken many forms since Grenvik first described it, and debate (16,17) has occurred about how quickly the process should be performed. The most expeditious approach, which is referred to as rapid extubation, is to simply extubate patients and give them supplemental oxygen or, more commonly, room air to breathe. This approach is certainly direct, and it offers the potential advantage of allowing the parents of infants and pediatric patients to hold them without being encumbered by the ventilator and its tubing. Whether rapid extubation decreases the chance that patients of all ages can survive without artificial support is unclear.

In 1994, Faber-Langendoen (18) published the results of a survey of 273 members of the Society of Critical Care Medicine who were involved in ventilator management. Fifteen percent of the respondents almost never withdrew mechanical ventilation from patients forgoing life-sustaining treatment; 37% did so less than half of the time. Of physicians who withdrew ventilators, 33% preferred terminal weaning, 13% preferred rapid extubation, and the remainder preferred both methods. Reasons for preferring extubation included the directness of the action, family perceptions, and patient comfort; reasons for preferring weaning included patient comfort, family perceptions, and the belief that weaning was less active. Narcotic analgesics and benzodiazepine sedatives were used by the majority of physicians when withdrawing ventilators, and 6% used neuromuscular blocking agents at least occasionally.

V. Pain Control

The first observational study (19) of the ordering and administration of sedatives and analgesics during the withholding and withdrawal of life support was conducted in the two medical-surgical ICUs in hospitals affiliated with UCSF and published in 1992. These drugs were given to 75% of the patients in this study; the only patients who did not receive them were considered incapable of benefiting because they were so comatose. The median time until death following the forgoing of life-sustaining treatment was 3.5 hours in the patients who received drugs and 1.3 hours in the patients who did not. Physicians ordered drugs to decrease pain, anxiety, and air hunger; to comfort families; and to hasten death—in no instance was hastening death the only reason cited. The amounts of benzodiazepines and opiates averaged 2.2 mg/h of diazepam and 3.3 mg/h of morphine sulfate in the 24 hours before withholding and withdrawal of life support and 9.8 mg/h and 11.2 mg/h in the 24 hours thereafter. Neuromuscular blocking agents were not permitted for any patients from whom mechanical ventilation was removed.

Although drug administration did not appear to hasten death in the study from two UCSF-affiliated hospitals, that hastening death was cited as a reason for ordering sedatives and analgesics seems inconsistent with the ethical principle of the double effect. This principle holds that drugs may be given to relieve suffering (the ethically permissible effect) even if death is hastened (the ethically objectionable effect). This is the case only as long as the ethically permissible and not the ethically objectionable effect is intended and the ethically objectionable effect is not the means to the ethically permissible one. If sedatives and analgesics are administered only in doses sufficient to prevent or treat pain, agitation, and air hunger, the intention to relieve suffering seems primary and the action may be considered ethical. However, if doses in excess of that amount are given, the intention to hasten death seems primary and the action may be considered unethical.

Consistent with this view, it appears unlikely that sedatives and analgesics were administered primarily to hasten death in the UCSF study (19). Indeed, when asked about their attitudes, physicians participating in the study said that because they could not quantify suffering, they preferred to err on the side of giving larger rather than smaller doses of drugs. They also stated that they saw no reason to prolong pain, agitation, and air hunger once the decision to withhold and withdraw life support was made. Although the physicians were aware that sedatives and analgesics could hasten death due to their hemodynamic and respiratory depressant quality, they were far from certain that such depression actually occurred.

Although the optimal way to administer the sedatives and analgesics during the withholding and withdrawal of life support is a matter of debate, there is no question that neuromuscular blocking agents are contraindicated in this situation. This results from the fact that neuromuscular blocking agents cannot relieve suffering, although they can hasten death. More important, blocking agents may make it impossible for health care professionals to gauge pain, agitation, and air hunger and to give appropriate agents to treat these conditions. Another drug that has no place during the forgoing of life-sustaining treatment is potassium chloride, whose only potential therapeutic purpose is to reverse hypokalemia, an abnormality that rarely requires correction during the withholding and withdrawal of life support.

Despite general agreement among physicians regarding the advisability of administering sedatives and analgesics during the removal of mechanical ventilation from dying patients, little is known about how satisfactorily terminal weaning actually occurs. Following an earlier publication (20), Campbell and colleagues (21) recently described rapid terminal weaning in 31 patients at Detroit Receiving Hospital. Most of the patients in this observational study were neurologically depressed due to anoxic or metabolic encephalopathy. The average length of time until weaning from the ventilator, but not the extubation, was 15 minutes, with some patients living considerably longer. One third of the patients were extubated after being removed from the ventilator; their average duration of survival was 45 hours. In fact, two of the extubated patients survived and were discharged to hospices within the community. Fully one third of the patients required no sedatives or analgesia, presumably because of their already depressed level of consciousness. Among the patients given narcotic analgesics and benzodiazepines, no correlation was detected between the amounts of drugs used, the duration of weaning, and survival thereafter. Assessment of the patients' relative wakefulness with a portable cerebral function monitor and evaluation of their degree of agitation and discomfort with bedside ranking scales demonstrated that the patients were comfortable at baseline and at the end of the weaning process. The study investigators concluded that "withdrawal of mechanical ventilation using a rapid terminal weaning procedure is a humane method in unconscious patients."

The realities of critical care practice are such that patients frequently are comatose before terminal weaning or rapid extubation are initiated, a factor that accounts for the finding that not all patients required drugs to achieve adequate sedation in the studies from Detroit Receiving Hospital. Indeed, the observational studies (10,11) from UCSF cited earlier in this chapter demonstrated that, in the ICU, decisions to withhold and withdraw life support are more often made by surrogates than by patients. Only occasionally are critically ill patients conscious at the start of terminal weaning, whether or not it is followed by extubation. Most of these patients have long-standing medical conditions such as chronic obstructive pulmonary disease or neuromuscular disease.

Unfortunately, no investigators have specifically focused on groups of patients with chronic illness who undergo terminal weaning. Nevertheless, in 1992 two physicians (22) from the Oregon Health Sciences University described the anguish they experienced in disconnecting the ventilator from a man who had spent 6 weeks in an iron lung as a young adult and remained ventilator-free until the age of 67, when he developed postpolio syndrome. The patient then went on a positive-pressure ventilator, on which he became dependent. At his request and with the consent of his family, the physicians administered intravenous morphine sulfate and midazolam to the patient until he was relaxed and comfortable but still conscious; they then discontinued the ventilator. The patient subsequently slipped into a coma, and 45 minutes after discontinuation his breathing became irregular and stopped. Although the physicians' consciences were clear after the event, they acknowledged how difficult it was to remove support from a conscious patient who knew he would then die.

Although the patient described above died in an ICU, he was similar in many ways to other patients with chronic illnesses who undergo terminal weaning in long-term care centers or in their homes. Discontinuing support in such patients is complicated by the fact that they often remain awake and aware until shortly before their death. Yet terminal weaning also may be easier because the patients have come to terms with their underlying conditions over months or years. Furthermore, the ethical principles that justify withholding and withdrawal of life support in general and removing mechanical ventilation in particular are the same in all settings. These principles are (1) that patients or their surrogates may refuse any and all medical interventions, (2) that physicians and other health professionals are not obligated to provide futile care, (3) that life-sustaining treatments should be limited if they are more burdensome than beneficial, and (4) that, whenever possible, patients should not die in pain.

VI. Summary and Conclusions

The field of medical ethics, particularly in the ICU, has evolved remarkably in the quarter century since the Karen Quinlan case established the role of surrogates in end-of-life decisions. Subsequently, the concepts of limiting therapy, medical futility, and terminal weaning have taken hold, and the belief that withdrawing life support is tantamount to withholding it in the first place has gained wide acceptance. As a consequence, most ICU patients who die today do so after limitation or withdrawal of support, whereas 25 years ago full support was often administered to the end, and "codes" were commonplace. However, end-of-life decision making remains an often agonizing process for clinicians and families alike, and controversy persists relating to how to define medical futility, how to terminally wean patients, and how best to medicate them. Nonetheless, if clinicians keep basic principles of medical ethics in mind—that the patient's interest must be served first, that in terminal situations, the decision is not between life and death, but rather how death will proceed, and that medications should be used with the primary goal of optimizing comfort, not hastening death—then the "plug" can be pulled in the most humane fashion.

References

1. Schneiderman LJ, Spragg RG. Ethical decisions in discontinuing mechanical ventilation. N Engl J Med 1988; 318:984–988.

2. In re: Quinlan, 70 N.J. 10, 355A. 2d 647, *cert. denied*, 429 U.S. 922 (1976).
3. Barber and Los Angeles County Superior Court, 195 Cal. Rptr. 484, 147 Cal. App. 3d 1006 (1983).
4. In re: Helen Wanglie, 450 (Dist. Ct. Probates Ct Div) PX-91-280. Minn. Hennepin Co.
5. Luce JM. Withholding and withdrawal of life support from critically ill patients. West J Med 1997; 167:411–416.
6. Faber-Langendoen K, Bartels DM. Process of forgoing life-sustaining treatment in a university hospital: an empirical study. Crit Care Med 1992; 20:570–577.
7. Lee DKP, Swinburne AJ, Fedullo AJ, Wahl GW. Withdrawing care: experience in a medical intensive care unit. JAMA 1994; 271:1358–1361.
8. Keenan SP, Busche KD, Chen LM, McCarthy L, Inman KJ, Sibbald WJ. A retrospective review of a large cohort of patients undergoing the process of withholding or withdrawal of life support. Crit Care Med 1997; 25:1324–1331.
9. Keenan SP, Busche KD, Chen LM, Esmail R, Inman KJ, Sibbald WJ. Withdrawal and withholding of life support in the intensive care unit: a comparison of teaching and community hospitals. Crit Care Med 1998; 26:245–251.
10. Smedira NG, Evans BH, Grais LS, Cohen NH, Lo B, Cooke M, Schecter WP, Fink C, Epstein-Jaffe E, May C, Luce JM. Withholding and withdrawal of life support from the critically ill. N Engl J Med 1990; 322:309–315.
11. Prendergast TJ, Luce JM. Increasing incidence of withholding and withdrawal of life support from the critically ill. Am J Respir Crit Care Med 1997; 155:15–20.
12. Prendergast TJ, Claessens MT, Luce JM. A national survey of end-of-life care for critically ill patients. Am J Respir Crit Care Med 1998; 158:1163–1167.
13. Asch DA, Hansen-Flaschen J, Lanken PN. Decisions to limit or continue life-sustaining treatment by critical care physicians in the United States: conflicts between physicians' practices and patients' wishes. Am J Respir Crit Care Med 1995; 151:288–292.
14. Christakis, NA, Asch DA. Biases in how physicians choose to withdraw life support. Lancet 1993; 342:642–646.
15. Grenvik A. "Terminal weaning": discontinuance of life-support therapy in the terminally ill patient. Crit Care Med 1983; 11:394–395.
16. Gianakos D. Terminal weaning. Chest 1995; 108:1405–1406.
17. Gilligan T, Raffin TA. Rapid withdrawal of support. Chest 1995; 108:1407–1408.
18. Faber-Langendoen K. The clinical management of dying patients receiving mechanical ventilation: a survey of physician practice. Chest 1994; 106:880–888.
19. Wilson WC, Smedira NG, Fink C, McDowell JA, Luce JM. Ordering and administration of sedatives and analgesics during the withholding and withdrawal of life support from critically ill patients. JAMA 1992; 267:949–953.
20. Campbell ML, Carlson RW. Terminal weaning from mechanical ventilation. Am J Crit Care Med 1993; 2:354–358.
21. Campbell ML, Bizek KS, Thill M. Patient responses during rapid terminal weaning from mechanical ventilation: a prospective study. Crit Care Med 1999; 27:73–77.
22. Edwards MJ, Tolle SW. Disconnecting a ventilator at the request of a patient who knows he will then die: the doctor's anguish. Ann Intern Med 1992; 117:254–256.

AUTHOR INDEX

Italic numbers give the page on which the complete reference is listed.

SUBJECT INDEX

A

Abdominal aortic surgery, 105
Abdominal wall muscles, 656
AC, asthma, 335
Acetylcysteine, asthma, 345
Acidemia, asthma, 336–337
Acinetobacter, 641
Acquired immunodeficiency syndrome
    (AIDS), 474–475
  cost, 474
  costs, 90
  mask CPAP, 474–475
  NPPV, 475
Acute hypercapnic respiratory failure, hos-
    pitalization, 600
Acute hypoxemic respiratory failure, non-
    invasive ventilation, 583–584
Acute lung injury (ALI), 14
  heart–lung interactions, 679–680
Acute pulmonary edema, NPPV, 141–142
Acute respiratory distress syndrome
    (ARDS), 14–21, 393–433, 469–
    470
  alveolar recruitment, 398–405, 626–627
  APRV, 416–417
  ASPIDS, 431–432
  decelerating flow, 405–406
  demographics, 17
  HFO, 628
  HFV, 417–422
  incidence, 16–17

[Acute respiratory distress syndrome
    (ARDS)]
  INO, 422–425
  IRV, 412–414
  ITPV, 430–431
  liquid ventilation, 425–429
  long-term morbidity, 19–20
  long-term survival, 19
  lung volume protection, 408–410
  mask CPAP, 469–470
  NPPV, 142, 470
  partial liquid ventilation, 628
  $PEEP_i$, 232
  permissive hypercapnia, 410–412
  pressure-controlled decelerating flow,
    406–407
  prone positioning, 414–416
  PV curve, 397–398
  quality of life, 20–21
  risk factors, 17–18
  short-term mortality, 18–19
  surfactant therapy, 627–628
  TGI, 429–430
  tidal volume reduction, 625–626
  ventilator settings, 69–71
  VILI, 394–398
  volume-cycled decelerating flow, 407–
    408
  weaning protocol, 126–127
Acute respiratory failure (ARF),
  causes, 4, 7–13
  defined, 2–3

813

Bronchodilators, excessive postextubation
    secessions, 728

C

CABG, continuous intravenous midazo-
    lam, 265–266
    vs. propofol, 265
Cardiac failure, extubation failure, 706–
    707
Cardiac ischemia, 520–521
Cardiogenic pulmonary edema (CPE),
    465–469
    mask CPAP, 467–468
    mask ventilation, 465–466
    NPPV, 468–469
    positive pressure ventilation, develop-
      ment, 41
    weaning, 679
Cardiovascular instability, 594
Case law, 744–746
CBF, continuous intravenous midazolam,
    268
Central respiratory monitoring unit, 93
Cerebral blood flow (CBF), continuous in-
    travenous midazolam, 268
Cerebral cortex, pain, 250
CESAR ventilator, 198–199
Chest physiotherapy, excessive postextuba-
    tion secessions, 728
Chest radiography,
    endobronchial intubation, 294
    endotracheal tube position, 303
CHF,
    extubation failure, 699
    heart-lung interactions, 680–681
    postextubation, treatment, 728
    weaning, 555–556
Chile, ventilator settings, 70
Chlorpromazines, delirium, ICU, 254
Chronic obstructive pulmonary disease
    (COPD), 7, 21–28, 353–385
    acute respiratory failure, invasive me-
      chanical ventilation, 374–384
    autoPEEP, 357–367
    CPAP, 365–366
    critical illness, 362
    extubation failure, 699
      mortality, 709
    flow volume loops, 357
    heart-lung interactions, 679
    hospitalization, 600
    hypoxemia, 361

[Chronic obstructive pulmonary disease
    (COPD)]
    increased airway resistance, 354–355
    in-hospital mortality, 15
    in-hospital survival time, Kaplan-Meier
      analysis, 554
    invasive mechanical ventilation,
      autoPEEP, 377–378
      end-of-life decision making, 383–
        384
      hyperinflation, 374–377
      patient-ventilator synchrony, 379–380
      permissive hypercapnia, 378–379
      prognosis, 383
      weaning, 380–383
    invasive *vs.* noninvasive support ventila-
      tion, 591–592
    long-term survival, 24–27
    NIVM failure, cause, 593–594
    noninvasive ventilation,
      initiation, 371–373
      patient selection, 368–371
      strategy, 373–374
    NPPV, algorithm, 373
    prolonged mechanical ventilation, sur-
      vival, 582
    quality of life, 27–28
    respiratory muscles,
      blood supply, 361–362
      dysfunction, 355–357
    short-term mortality, 22–24
    therapy, complications, 362–363
    weaning, 553–555, 580–581
      noninvasive ventilation, 556
      survival, 581–582
Classic weaning criteria, 726
Clinical decision making, 113
Clinical practice, standardization, 115
Clinical quality improvement, 116
Clonidine, pain, ICU, 258–259
Closed loop ventilation (CLV), 223–239
    computer decision support systems, 224
    future, 238–239
    gas exchange, 225–226
    goal, 224
    I:E ratio, 237
    inputs, 225, 234
    mechanics, 226–233
    outputs, 234
    $P_{0.1}$, 233
    respiratory rate, 234–237
    tidal volume, 234–237
    weaning, 237–238

[Noninvasive positive pressure ventilation
(NPPV)]
postoperative respiratory failure, 471–
472
restrictive lung diseases, 143
trauma, 144, 473
weaning facilitation, 144–145
Noninvasive positive pressure ventilation
(NPPV)-assisted bronchoscopy,
477
Noninvasive pressure support ventilation,
vs. invasive pressure support ventilation, 587
Noninvasive respiratory care unit, 597
Noninvasive ventilation,
early extubation, 590
vs. endotracheal intubation, 584
exclusion, causes, 584
vs. invasive ventilation, 594–595
rationale, 138
sequential use, 598
weaning, 586–597
clinical trials, 586–593
future, 597–599
limitations, 596–597
rationale, 593–595
Nosocomial events, health care providers,
111
Nosocomial pneumonia, 582–583
epidemiology, 636–637
ICU, mortality, 637
pathogens, 637
ventilator equipment, 44
NPPV (*see* Noninvasive positive pressure
ventilation)
acute setting, ventilator settings, 148
NPPV-assisted bronchoscopy, 477
Nurse staffing rations, ICU protocols,
113
Nutrition, VAP prevention, 644

O

OAD, 453–456
Obstructive airway disease (OAD), 453–
456
Obstructive diseases, NPPV, 141
Obstructive sleep apnea (OSA), 459–
460
mask CPAP, 460
NPPV, 460
Occlusion pressure, extubation outcome
prediction, 725–726

Open intensive care unit (ICU), 119–
120
Opiates, dyspnea, 277
Opioids,
asthma, 343
intubation, 291
Oregon Health Sciences University, 751
Organ system failure,
agitation,
ICU, 270–272
Oronasal masks, 145–146
COPD, 371
Orotracheal tubes, 304–305
OSA, 459–460
mask CPAP, 460
NPPV, 460
Outcome prediction, mechanical ventila-
tion, ICU, 95
Oxygen, described, 38
Oxygen analyzers, VAP prevention, 644
Oxygenation,
CLV, 226
NPPV, ICU, 149
Oxygen cost of breathing, 518–519
Oxygen demand, 656
Oxygen toxicity, 44

P

$P_{0.1}$, 233
P450, 271
Pain,
avoidance, 250–251
control, 749–752
ICU, 248–251
treatment, 250, 255–259
mediators, 249
physiology, 255–256
stress factors, 249
Pancuronium, asthma, 343
P_{aO2}/P_{AO2} ratio, accuracy, 510
PAP, INO, 424
Paralysis, asthma, 342–344
Paralytics, asthma, 343
Partial liquid ventilation,
ARDS, 628
VILI, 622–625
Partial lung ventilation (PLV), 426–428
Patient compliance, lack, 593
Patient populations, extubation failure,
694
Patient respiratory drive ($P_{0.1}$), 233
Patient-ventilator dyssynchrony, 593